# CURRENT CLINICAL PATHOLOGY

ANTONIO GIORDANO, MD, PhD

Director, Sbarro Institute for Cancer Research and Molecular
Medicine and Center for Biotechnology
Temple University
Philadelphia, PA, USA

*SERIES EDITOR*

More information about this series at http://www.springer.com/series/7632

This series includes monographs dealing with important topics in surgical pathology, cytopathology hematology, and diagnostic laboratory medicine. It is aimed at practicing hospital based pathologists and their residents providing them with concise up-to- date reviews and state of the art summaries of current problems that these physicians may encounter in their daily practice of clinical pathology.

Luigi Pirtoli
Giovanni Luca Gravina
Antonio Giordano

Editors

# Radiobiology of Glioblastoma

## Recent Advances and Related Pathobiology

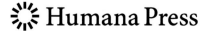 Humana Press

*Editors*
Luigi Pirtoli
Section of Radiation Oncology
Department of Medicine
Surgery and Neurosciences
University of Siena
Siena, Italy

Antonio Giordano
Sbarro Institute for Cancer Research
  and Molecular Medicine
Center for Biotechnology
Temple University
Philadelphia, PA, USA

Giovanni Luca Gravina
Department of Applied Clinical and
  Biotechnological Sciences
University of L'Aquila
L'Aquila, Italy

ISSN 2197-781X            ISSN 2197-7828   (electronic)
Current Clinical Pathology
ISBN 978-3-319-28303-6    ISBN 978-3-319-28305-0   (eBook)
DOI 10.1007/978-3-319-28305-0

Library of Congress Control Number: 2016938820

Printed on acid-free paper

This Humana Press imprint is published by Springer Nature
The registered company is Springer International Publishing AG Switzerland

*This book is dedicated to our patients, in particular to those affected by tumors with a very poor prognosis, as glioblastoma currently is, as research has unfortunately not provided favorable survival outcomes as of yet; to our mentors, who have oriented our lives toward professional and scientific commitments; and to our families, who have sustained our efforts in implementing this volume.*

# Foreword

*Le vent se lève! ... il faut tenter de vivre!*

(Paul Valéry, Cimetière Marin, 1920)

Toward the end of 2013, Antonio Giordano suggested I should prepare for publication a book on radiobiology of glioblastoma, my main field of scientific interest. Initially, I had some qualms about the difficulty in implementing such an issue and on its possible usefulness, given the tremendous accumulation of knowledge on this subject in recent years and the present, modest impact of most of these disclosures on therapy outcome. Nevertheless, the idea appealed to me because many of the striking radiobiology experimental results presently achieved are not satisfactorily addressed by suitable clinical trials. A comprehensive coverage of the modern, mechanistic, pathobiology-grounded radiobiology topics of possible clinical relevance through selected contributions seemed to be appropriate, considering the possible translational perspectives. Therefore, I decided to take up the challenge after ensuring the cooperation for this task with Antonio Giordano himself, as a prominent pathobiology scientist in oncology, and with Giovanni Luca Gravina, a radiation oncologist and biologist of established reputation, both of whom have honored me with their friendship.

Glioblastoma patients may achieve, at most, median survivals of 12–15 months and 25 % and 5 % 2- and 5-year overall survival rates, respectively, after current therapy. From a radiobiological point of view, the most relevant problem is the radiation resistance of glioblastoma, which in the vast majority of cases recurs in the primary site after radiotherapy. The empirically developed principles of radiation dose fractionation and modulation over time, for improved tumor control/normal tissue damage ratios, do not enable improved tumor control with radiation doses higher than 60 Gy, differently from most other cancers. Technology alone does not seem able to overcome this situation. The impressive progress in medical imaging and in radiotherapy facilities, in fact, now safely provide a very precise tumor localization and radiation high-dose delivery in a few sessions, activating also cell-death pathways different from those involved in killing cancer cells with conventional schedules, but the results of specially designed clinical trials have been disappointing. However, hallmarks in the framework of molecular classification, genome-wide characterization, membrane receptors, epigenetic features, signal pathways, and immune domain are shown to be inherently related to the prognosis of glioblastoma and, in some cases, are predictive of a response to current postoperative therapy methods, including radiotherapy. Targeting or modulating these determinants by "biological" agents is a promising approach for improving radiation effectiveness, as documented in numerous preclinical disclosures. However, glioblastoma is a complex and elusive disease, and these attempts have been unsuccessful in the clinical setting so far, probably due to molecular signaling redundancy, clonal selection (or emergence) of resistant phenotypes under treatment, or difficulty in penetrating blood–brain barrier by the drugs. In conclusion, further research is warranted, for a more fitting, "individually featured" radiotherapy of glioblastoma with radiation optimization and enhancement grounded on pathobiology knowledge, an approach which is more and more frequently implemented in other tumors. Translational aspects are relevant to this regard. Identification of suitable markers should continue through the use of large database collections including pathological, biological, and clinical data to establish reliable correlations with advanced statistical methods, so that preclinical research may select the most plausible working hypotheses for clinical trial design.

I hope this book will contribute to this purpose or at least in facilitating communication among the involved professionals and researchers.

Siena, Italy                                                                                                    Luigi Pirtoli
23 October 2015                                                                                  luigipirtoli@gmail.com

# Preface

There has been a clear-cut change in the mentality of oncologists in the last decades. Up to the end of the past century, in fact, any therapeutic approach to cancer could be assigned to one of the following two categories: treatment for definitive cure or otherwise palliation. In the former setting, the real possibility of achieving definitive healing of the disease sometimes justified treatment-related side effects or damages of not negligible severity, whereas in the latter orientation—whose intent was a only a reasonable improvement in life expectancy and/or symptoms relief—a milder therapeutic conduct was more advisable. This scenario has been radically modified by the rise of more effective and safer surgical, radiation, and drug therapies, with the consequence that also in patients whose cancer could not be eradicated, it could be changed into a chronic disease in many cases with an approach more active than in the past, allowing survival times often exceeding the fateful 5-year threshold and a satisfactory quality of life.

Unfortunately, this is not the case of glioblastoma: with current therapies, one half of the affected patients decease within 1 year from the diagnosis and long-term survivors are extremely rare, amounting to no more than 5 % at 5 years. But resigning to a palliation outcome is generally seen as inappropriate by the medical community and by the patients and their relatives. However, due to the frailty of the brain, surgical ablation is necessarily incomplete in most cases, and radiation therapy can be delivered only within precise dose and volume constraints. Even the most advanced radiotherapy technology scarcely impacts on tumor control, and associated chemotherapy may improve outcome only to a limited extent. Furthermore, relevant treatment-related damages may occur. So, much effort is presently made to enhance the effectiveness and safety of the available therapeutic tools.

One major determinant of therapy failure in glioblastoma, in fact, is its inherent resistance to radiation that, in light of the most recent radiobiology disclosures, can be appropriately considered as an "adaptive strategy" of the tumor against the radiation threat, which is more effective than in other cancers. The enormously improved knowledge of the natural history of glioblastoma in the fields of gene and mechanistic molecular biology, achieved in the last decades, seems to point the way to effectively cope with radiation resistance, by specifically targeting its underlying molecular determinants. However, much research is still needed, as the first clinical trials on molecular targeting agents have produced modest results. This may be due sometimes to working hypotheses not thoroughly verified in the preclinical setting but, in general, to the great complexity of the disease and the redundancy of its biological machinery. Another cause may be the insufficient communication between preclinical and clinical researchers. There is also the need of new translational tools, besides clinical trials, such as large database collection and advanced statistical methodology.

We collected in this book authoritative information by some authors of the highest repute, giving a context to, and focusing on, clinical, laboratory, and translational radiation biology research on glioblastoma and its related pathobiology field. Also subjects such as particle therapy, radiation tolerance of normal brain, immunology, and nanomaterial technology are dealt with, with special reference to their respective correlated radiobiology topics. Our intent was mainly to promote the reciprocal understanding and insight among researchers and professionals in radiation and medical oncology, pathology, biology, and medical physics, in order to improve cooperation among them. Glioblastoma, although relatively rare, is in the spotlight due to the extreme complexity of its biological machinery, which represents a challenge for research, due to the necessity to disclose multiple new targets suitable for innovative therapies and unconventional approaches. These investigations might elucidate aspects of relevant interest also in other neoplasms. We hope that the efforts and the time devoted to the accomplishment of this book have obtained a useful and stimulating state-of-the-art assessment for the readers.

Siena, Italy                                                               Luigi Pirtoli
L'Aquila, Italy                                                  Giovanni Luca Gravina
Philadelphia, PA, USA                                                Antonio Giordano

# Acknowledgments

We are sincerely grateful to all contributors for their outstanding work and continuous engagement. Their expertise, readiness, and clear exposition have allowed us to exceed all our expectations.

Our special thanks go to Richard Hruska and Susan Westendorf of Springer, for their invaluable suggestions and precious help to make the book a reality.

L.P., G.L.G., and A.G.

# Contents

# Contributors

**Anna Rita Alitto** Radiation Oncology Department, Gemelli-ART, Università Cattolica S. Cuore, Rome, Italy

**A. Antonosante** Department of Life, Health and Environmental Sciences, University of L'Aquila, L'Aquila, Italy

**Mario Balducci** Radiation Oncology Department, Gemelli-ART, Università Cattolica S. Cuore, Rome, Italy

**G. Belmonte** Tuscany Tumor Institute, Unit of Radiation Oncology, Department of Medicine, Surgery and Neurosciences, University of Siena, Siena, Italy

**E. Benedetti** Sbarro Institute for Cancer Research and Molecular Medicine and Center for Biotechnology, Temple University, Philadelphia, PA, USA

Department of Medicine, Surgery and Neurosciences, University of Siena, Siena, Italy

**Paolo Borghetti** Radiation Oncology Department, University and Spedali Civili, Brescia, Italy

**Michela Buglione** Radiation Oncology Department, University and Spedali Civili, Brescia, Italy

**Kevin Camphausen** Radiation Oncology Branch, National Cancer Institute, National Institutes of Health, Bethesda, MD, USA

**Silvia Chiesa** Radiation Oncology Department, Gemelli-ART, Università Cattolica S. Cuore, Rome, Italy

**A. Cimini** Department of Life, Health and Environmental Sciences, University of L'Aquila, L'Aquila, Italy

Sbarro Institute for Cancer Research and Molecular Medicine and Center for Biotechnology, Temple University, Philadelphia, PA, USA

**Sergio Comincini** Department of Technology and Biotechnology, University of Pavia, Italy

**Benjamin Cooper** Radiation Oncology, NYU Langone Medical Center, New York, NY, USA

**L. Cristiano** Sbarro Institute for Cancer Research and Molecular Medicine and Center for Biotechnology, Temple University, Philadelphia, PA, USA

Department of Medicine, Surgery and Neurosciences, University of Siena, Siena, Italy

**M. D'Angelo** Department of Life, Health and Environmental Sciences, University of L'Aquila, L'Aquila, Italy

**Andrea Damiani** Radiation Oncology Department, Gemelli-ART, Università Cattolica S. Cuore, Rome, Italy

**Isacco Desideri** Radiotherapy Unit, Department of Experimental and Clinical Biomedical Sciences, University of Florence, Firenze, Italy

**Beatrice Detti** Radiation Oncology Unit, Azienda Ospedaliero–Universitaria Careggi, Florence, Italy

**Nicola Dinapoli** Radiation Oncology Department, Gemelli-ART, Università Cattolica S. Cuore, Rome, Italy

**Luciana Dini** Department of Biological and Environmental Science and Technology (Di.S.Te.B.A.), University of Salento, Lecce, Italy

**Marco Durante** Helmholtzzentrum für Schwerionenforschung GmbH (GSI), Darmstadt, Germany

**Francesca De Felice** Department of Radiological, Oncological and Anatomo-Pathological Sciences, University "Sapienza" of Rome, Rome, Italy

**Milena Ferro** Radiation Oncology Department, Gemelli-ART, Università Cattolica S. Cuore, Rome, Italy

**A. Fidoamore** Department of Life, Health and Environmental Sciences, University of L'Aquila, L'Aquila, Italy

**Alba Fiorentino** Radiation Oncology Department, Sacro Cuore-Don Calabria Hospital, Negrar, Italy

**Silvia Formenti** Radiation Oncology, NYU Langone Medical Center, New York, NY, USA

**Giulio Francolini** Radiation Oncology Unit, Azienda Ospedaliero–Universitaria Careggi, Florence, Italy

**Roberto Gatta** Radiation Oncology Department, Gemelli-ART, Università Cattolica S. Cuore, Rome, Italy

**Chiara Gerini** Radiotherapy Unit, Department of Experimental and Clinical Biomedical Sciences, University of Florence, Firenze, Italy

**Antonio Giordano** Sbarro Institute for Cancer Research and Molecular Medicine and Center for Biotechnology, Temple University, Philadelphia, PA, USA

Department of Medicine, Surgery and Neurosciences, University of Siena, Siena, Italy

**Encouse Golden** Radiation Oncology, NYU Langone Medical Center, New York, NY, USA

**Giovanni Luca Gravina** Department of Applied Clinical and Biotechnological Sciences, University of L'Aquila, Rome, Italy

**Daniela Greto** Radiation Oncology Unit, Azienda Ospedaliero— Universitaria Careggi, Florence, Italy

**Alexander Helm** Helmholtzzentrum für Schwerionenforschung GmbH (GSI), Darmstadt, Germany

Trento Institute for Fundamental Physics and Applications (TIFPA), Italy

**Gianluca Ingrosso** Radiation Oncology Unit, University of Rome "Tor Vergata", Rome, Italy

**Andra Krauze** Radiation Oncology Branch, National Cancer Institute, National Institutes of Health, Bethesda, MD, USA

**Lorenzo Livi** Radiotherapy Unit, Department of Experimental and Clinical Biomedical Sciences, University of Florence, Firenze, Italy

**Mauro Loi** Radiotherapy Unit, Department of Experimental and Clinical Biomedical Sciences, University of Florence, Firenze, Italy

**Stefano Maria Magrini** Radiation Oncology Department, University and Spedali Civili - Brescia, Brescia, Italy

**Monica Mangoni** Radiotherapy Unit, Department of Experimental and Clinical Biomedical Sciences, University of Florence, Firenze, Italy

**Elisa Meldolesi** Radiation Oncology Department, Gemelli-ART, Università Cattolica S. Cuore, Rome, Italy

**Clelia Miracco** Tuscany Tumor Institute, Florence, Italy

Unit of Pathological Anatomy, Department of Medicine, Surgery and Neurosciences, University of Siena, Siena, Italy

**Daniela Musio** Department of Radiological, Oncological and Anatomo-Pathological Sciences, University "Sapienza" of Rome, Rome, Italy

**Silvia Palumbo** Unit of Radiation Oncology, Department of Medicine, Surgery and Neurosciences, University of Siena, Siena, Italy

**Elisa Panzarini** Department of Biological and Environmental Science and Technology (Di.S.Te.B.A.), University of Salento, Lecce, Italy

**Nadia Pasinetti** Radiation Oncology Department, Spedali Civili, University of Brescia, Brescia, Italy

**Piernicola Pedicini** I.R.C.C.S. Regional Cancer Hospital C.R.O.B., Rionero-in-Vulture, PZ, Italy

**Sara Pedretti** Radiation Oncology Department, Spedali Civili, University of Brescia, Brescia, Italy

**Luigi Pirtoli** Tuscany Tumor Institute, Florence, Italy

Unit of Radiation Oncology, Department of Medicine, Surgery and Neurosciences, University of Siena, Siena, Italy

**Riccardo Santoni** Radiation Oncology Unit, University of Rome "Tor Vergata", Rome, Italy

**Cody Schlaff** Radiation Oncology Branch, National Cancer Institute, National Institutes of Health, Bethesda, MD, USA

**Silvia Scoccianti** Radiation Oncology Unit, Azienda Ospedaliero—Universitaria Careggi, Florence, Italy

**Uma Shankavaram** Radiation Oncology Branch, National Cancer Institute, National Institutes of Health, Bethesda, MD, USA

**Joshua Silverman** Radiation Oncology, NYU Langone Medical Center, New York, NY, USA

**Mariangela Sottili** Radiotherapy Unit, Department of Experimental and Clinical Biomedical Sciences, University of Florence, Firenze, Italy

**Luigi Spiazzi** Physics Department, Spedali Civili Hospital, Brescia, Italy

**Lidia Strigari** Laboratory of Medical Physics and Expert Systems, Regina Elena National Cancer Institute, Rome, Italy

**Anita Tandle** Radiation Oncology Branch, National Cancer Institute, National Institutes of Health, Bethesda, MD, USA

**Walter Tinganelli** Helmholtzzentrum für Schwerionenforschung GmbH (GSI), Darmstadt, Germany

Trento Institute for Fundamental Physics and Applications (TIFPA), Italy

**Paolo Tini** Tuscany Tumor Institute, Florence, Italy

Unit of Radiation Oncology, University Hospital of Siena (Azienda Ospedaliera Universitaria Senese), Istituto Toscano Tumori, Siena, Italy

**Vincenzo Tombolini** Department of Radiological, Oncological and Anatomo-Pathological Sciences, University "Sapienza" of Rome, Rome, Italy

Fondazione Eleonora Lorillard Spencer Cenci, Rome, Italy

**Marzia Toscano** Tuscany Tumor Institute, Florence, Italy

Unit of Radiation Oncology, Department of Medicine, Surgery and Neurosciences, University of Siena, Siena, Italy

**Luca Triggiani** Radiation Oncology Department, University and Spedali Civili - Brescia, Brescia, Italy

**Vincenzo Valentini** Radiation Oncology Department, Gemelli-ART, Università Cattolica S. Cuore, Rome, Italy

**Ralph Vatner** Radiation Oncology, NYU Langone Medical Center, New York, NY, USA

# Introduction and Background

Luigi Pirtoli, Giovanni Luca Gravina,
and Antonio Giordano

Glioblastoma (GB) accounts for 54 % of primary brain tumors, with an incidence of about five new cases for every 100,000 per year, and after aggressive multimodal treatments, prognosis remains poor, with a 5-year Overall Survival (OS) rate barely reaching 5 %, as extensively documented in the section of this book dedicated to prognostic parameters of GB. Maximum achievable safe surgical resection, and limited-volume radiotherapy (RT) with concurrent and sequential chemotherapy (CHT) based on the alkylating agent Temozolomide (TMZ) [1], achieve 40, 15, and 7–8 % OS rates, respectively at 1-, 2-, and 3-years. These present standards of treatment mostly stem from studies dating back to the seventies of the last century [2, 3], and progressively evolving through subsequent clinical trials.

A great deal of medical literature is dedicated to GB, with increasing frequency over time. Most recent articles on GB, in fact, begin with the statement that prognosis has not improved, despite the numerous research findings on its underlying genomic and molecular mechanisms. This is due at least in part to the difficulty in improving patient outcomes, given the elusive nature of this disease with respect to therapeutic innovations, including those in the RT domain. Radiation is one of the most used and useful tool against cancer, including GB, and knowledge of its mechanisms of action on biological substrates is of the utmost importance in oncology. Radioresistance of GB is one challenge for Radiation Biology (RB) that has emerged from the clinical setting, and important questions raised by clinical experiences are addressed by basic RB laboratory research. However, RB is a scarcely known discipline outside of the inner circle of the radiological science scholars, and we are convinced that a comprehensive and updated coverage of this subject is warranted, that is, the aim of this book. The researchers and the practitioners studying GB in the domains of radiation and medical oncology, pathology, biology, and physics may profit from reciprocal scientific contributions collected in a lineup fitting the present state-of-the-art.

L. Pirtoli (✉)
Tuscany Tumor Institute, Florence, Italy

Unit of Radiation Oncology, Department of Medicine, Surgery and Neurosciences, University of Siena, Siena, Italy
e-mail: luigipirtoli@gmail.com

G.L. Gravina
Department of Radiological, Oncological, and Anatomo-Pathological Sciences, University of Rome "La Sapienza", Rome, Italy

A. Giordano
Sbarro Institute for Cancer Research and Molecular Medicine and Center for Biotechnology, Temple University, Philadelphia, PA, USA

Department of Medicine, Surgery and Neurosciences, University of Siena, Siena, Italy

© Springer International Publishing Switzerland 2016
L. Pirtoli et al. (eds.), *Radiobiology of Glioblastoma*, Current Clinical Pathology,
DOI 10.1007/978-3-319-28305-0_1

We dedicated the first section of the book to RB topics emerging from clinical studies on GB. These include research regarding RT dose, volume and fractionation, CHT associated with RT, RT modalities alternative to the current photon irradiation, mathematical modeling of treatment parameters, prognostic parameters and markers, and radiation tolerance of normal brain. The second part addresses preclinical research domains of particular relevance for GB. These include related basic experimental RB; immune system and GB microenvironment; genetic and epigenetic determinants in tumor initiation and progression; GB microenvironment in its relationship with hypoxia and glioma stem cell-related radiation resistance; cell-death pathways and radiation; miRNA manipulation in modifying radiation resistance of GB; and nanoparticle research. The third and last section of the book deals with translational issues, specifically preclinical models for GB RB, present attempts to correlate molecular RB with clinical RB, and the perspectives of large databases and ontologic models for the correlation of results derived from preclinical and clinical data. Many of these contributions are unavoidably overlapping, reflecting contiguous fields of research and the scientific interests of the authors, who are often watchful for collateral disclosures influencing their work. In our opinion, this is an added value and not redundancy.

## Prognostic Markers and Treatment Strategies

The largely incomplete information on tumor initiation and progression of GB and its almost universally fatal course have driven research for many years towards an analytic approach of both patient- and treatment-related prognostic factors conditioning life expectancy. Respectively, these include age, performance, and neurological status, as well as extent of surgical resection, RT and CHT [4], which have been analyzed in the past in an attempt to identify parameters for the best benefit/risk ratio of therapy. The traditional approach to biological and clinical radiation

oncology investigation in this field for a long time consisted mainly of mathematical modeling of in vitro and in vivo experimental results, or of data from clinical series. The vast majority of available reports show that RT acts as a prognostic factor just as a dichotomic parameter: the related survival advantage exists, as compared to surgery alone, but this is not dose-dependent according to a continuous dose-effectiveness function above 60 Gy, as normally happens in solid tumors. A recent mathematical analysis of GB patients undergoing RT-CHT seems to theoretically indicate that increments of outcome might occur up to a tumor control probability of 85 % with a RT total dose of 74 Gy in 30 daily fractions of 2.2 Gy each over 6 weeks [5]. This hypothesis needs to be confirmed in a clinical setting, but it is unlikely to deliver such an RT treatment without increasing the probability of normal tissue complication beyond acceptable levels, even using the most advanced irradiation techniques.

Only recently, pathobiology research has unveiled information that is conceivably suitable for identifying prognostic parameters. We are aware, in fact, that GB is a biologically complex disease, and that patient- and treatment-related prognostic parameters may reflect inherent tumor initiation and progression features, and different response to treatment. GB regrowth in the primary site, that is, in the full-dose RT region, is the most common failure of RT, even if it improves survival over surgery alone, as previously mentioned.

The recent assessment of the "genomic landscape" of GB [6], and the improved knowledge of signaling pathways, have led to great expectations from biologically targeted therapies, specifically monoclonal antibodies (mAb) and tyrosine-kinase inhibitors (TKI), as well as active and passive immune therapy [7, 8]. However, the numerous clinical trials undertaken on these grounds have generally yielded unsatisfactory results. Possible hypotheses for explaining these failures include molecular signaling redundancy and cross-talk; clonal selection (or emergence) of resistant phenotypes under treatment; preclinical studies mainly addressing tumor-initiating or early growth factors and not late tumor progression mechanisms; difficulty of the drugs in penetrating the blood–brain barrier (BBB), etc. [9]. In addition, integrating the above-mentioned agents with radiation, as well as modern refinements of imaging and radiation-dose delivery techniques, have not produced substantially improved outcomes. However, molecular radiobiology, in general, has rapidly evolved over the last two decades, paralleling the improved knowledge of DNA damage and repair mechanisms, intra- and intercellular signaling pathways and microenvironmental factors, as well as tumor profiling biomarkers and molecular targeting [10]. GB, in particular, is presently the subject of much scientific discussion regarding ionizing radiation under this new perspective. The recent molecular classification of GB TCGA (The Genome Cancer Atlas) addressed recurrent genomic abnormalities in GB, which resulted in a gene-expression/molecular classification of GB into proneural, neural, classical, and mesenchymal subtypes [11]. An aggressive postsurgical therapy (that is, RT with > 3 cycles of chemotherapy, vs. a less intensive management), yielded a significantly reduced mortality in the classical and mesenchymal subtype, a borderline impact on survival in the neural subtype, and no effect on the proneural subtype.

## Inherent GB Radiation Resistance and Failure in Radiosensitizing GB by Targeting Key Signal Molecules

Radioresistance of GB is attributable to both intracellular and microenvironmental factors [12]. Radiation-induced cell death in solid tumors is mostly due to DNA double-strand break (DSB), and enhanced DNA DSB repair may occur and improve radiation resistance: the PI3K-Akt pathway, downstream of several membrane receptors (particularly the erbB family members) may be activated and potentiate DSB repair after radiation, besides constitutively stimulating tumor growth and invasion [13]. *EGFR* amplification (present in about 40 % of GBs) promotes resistance to RT in preclinical studies through the activation of DNA PKcs (DNA-

dependent protein kinase catalytic subunit) leading mainly to nonhomologous end joining (NHEJ) DNA DSB repair. Furthermore, experimental evidence indicates that the link between EGFR signaling and DSB repair occurs by the PI3K-Akt or MAPK (mitogen-activated PK) pathways [14]. A frequent (30–50 %) mutant form of EGFR is expressed in GB, specifically the EGFR variant III (EGFRvIII or ΔEGFR). Its deletion of the extracellular domain (exons 2–7) constitutively activates a high stimulation of the PI3K/Akt/mTOR pathway, and confers radiation resistance [15]. Some authors [16–18] have considered the relationship between increased cell-survival signaling by EGFR and *TP53* mutations and apoptosis. For a long time, in fact, apoptosis has been supposed to be the main type of programmed cell death (PCD) after anticancer treatments, including RT [19–22]. However, evidence exists that other types of PCD are induced by CHT and RT, such as autophagy-related or type-II PCD, and regulated necrosis (including necroptosis, type III PCD) [21–23] These pathways are not necessarily mutually exclusive, as previously believed. Even if autophagy is important in many cancers as a protective mechanism against radiation [10], it can act both as a pro-survival mechanism and as a pro-death mechanism, the latter observed in GB [24]. Autophagy-related cell death is one of the metabolic pathways inhibited by EGFR, which can act via mTOR or by direct inhibition of Beclin1, a cytoplasmic protein that induces autophagy by binding to the Vps34-Vps15 core [25, 26]. We could experimentally demonstrate, for instance, that combined EGFR and autophagy modulation impact on radiation and TMZ sensitivity (that is, clonal inhibition) in human GB cell lines [27]. Similarly, in patients undergoing RT and TMZ, low-EGFR- and high Beclin1-expressing GBs have a significantly better median survival, as compared to other ones showing high-EGFR and both high- and low-Beclin1 expression, after standard RT-TMZ [28].

Some failures of mAb or of TKI against EGFR in achieving favorable results in clinical trials might be due, at least in part, to the lack of a concurrent inhibition of the downstream cell-death pathway's activity. PI3K-mTOR and EGFR inhibitors, as well as PDGFR, VEGF, and p53 inhibitors, are the subject of very recent, extensive, and thorough reviews (e.g., [9]). Some authors considered, in particular, the relationships of these pathways with the related genomic significant mutations [8], as identified in TGCA of GB [6].

However, these studies do not primarily address RT enhancement, but in general the effectiveness of biological targeting drugs, both as single- or dual-agents, or in combination with current RT-CHT schedules. From a radiobiological point of view, further study is necessary: in fact, many trials associate "targeting" drugs with RT without previous preclinical in vitro and in vivo investigations exhaustively grounding their effectiveness as radiation enhancers on sound proofs-of-principle [12].

## Glioma Stem Cells

Another main factor causing GB resistance to radiation therapy is its intrinsic composition including heterogeneous cell populations—that is, a cellular hierarchy deriving from glioma stem cells (GSCs) through multiple genetic and epigenetic events [29–31]: inducing quiescence, altered cell-cycle control, activation of the DNA-repair pathways and complex interactions with the tumor microenvironment. Irradiated GBs contain more GSCs than unexposed ones, thus suggesting that GSCs have a role in radiation resistance [32]. GSCs may also have a fundamental role in promoting tumor neo-angiogenesis [33, 34], as suggested by high VEGF expression, and by their possibility to differentiate into endothelial tumor cells [35, 36] or pericytes [37]. Neo-angiogenesis may also depend on hypoxia-inducible factor (HIF)-mediated recruitment of bone marrow-derived cells restoring GB vascularity damaged by radiation [38].

Hypoxia, due to its general and well-known property of reducing the effect of radiation-induced reactive oxygen species (ROS) damage on DNA by restraining their combination with oxygen [39], has a relevant role in radiation resistance of GB, which is a highly hypoxic tumor. Furthermore, specialized hypoxic sites (the so-

called "niches") composed of GB-associated stromal cells, immune cells, and non-cellular components provide signals promoting the GSC phenotype [40–43]. GSCs located in these niches usually express the CD133/prominin-1 marker, used for their identification, enrichment, and as a prognostic marker. However, it is questioned whether glioma and normal brain stem cells can be univocally discriminated by CD133 positivity. Genome-wide-based analyses have demonstrated that GSCs express a multiple-gene signature, existing in GSCs but not in normal brain SCs, correlating with survival [44]. This report also shows that characteristic Hedgehog- and Wnt-pathway alterations, such as active β-catenin, were present only in GB GSCs. Interestingly β-catenin, as well as Gli-1 enhanced immunohistochemistry expression level, negatively conditioned GB patients' survival after standard RT-TMZ in our experience [45].

The clinical implications of the radiobiological research on cancer SC are currently the subject of ongoing studies, both for predictive bioassays and for combination of novel systemic treatments with RT [46].

## Epigenetic Events

Radiation and CHT resistance, as well as other features of the aggressiveness of GB, may result from epigenetic events, such as alterations in the gene methylation status, conditioning the radiation or CHT effect in DNA gene sequence disruption and repair. Different DNA methylation alterations exist between radiation-sensitive and -resistant cells [47]. Furthermore, radiation may induce modifications, such as phosphorylation or changes in the methylation status of histones [48]. About half of GBs harbor somatic mutations determining DNA methylation, histone modification, and nucleosome positioning [49].

Methylation of the O6-methylguanine-DNA methyl-transferase (MGMT) gene showed a significant median survival benefit for GB patients undergoing RT-TMZ, as compared to those with the same feature undergoing RT only (21.7 vs. 15.3 months, respectively; $p = 0.007$). On the contrary, the difference between the same treatment groups, out of nonmethylated-MGMT GB patients, did not attain statistical significance, in 206 patients included in an EORTC-NCIC trial [50]. A meta-analysis study on 2018 high-grade glioma patients included in 20 reports showed that MGMT gene silencing was significantly associated with improved survival in patients undergoing RT-TMZ; this advantage was less significant in those receiving only RT, and null in those receiving neither TMZ nor RT [51]. However, causal interpretation of these results requires caution: a sample classification only according to the methylated and nonmethylated status for a gene may be dependent on the relationship between the overall CpG island methylation, the CpG methylation at individual sites, and the effectiveness of gene silencing, that is dependent in turn on the location within the gene [52]. DNA methylation may also involve other epigenetic modifications of chromatin, and the methyl-CpG-binding domain (MBD) proteins connected with histone deacetylases (HDACs) and histone methyl-transferase (HMTs), functionally affecting the regulation of transcription. Furthermore, these events may regulate HIF effects at the DNA and histone levels, as extensively reported by Cimini et al. in a dedicated section of this book.

Antiepileptic drugs may affect therapeutic outcome of GB patients undergoing current RT-TMZ schedules, by MGMT-independent mechanisms, and due to HDAC inhibition and the consequent histone acetylation that loosens up the chromatin structure, making DNA more accessible to anticancer drugs and enhancing the cytotoxic effect of radiation. This is the case of Valproic acid (VPA) [53], which also induces apoptosis independently of the p53 status [54], induces autophagy as a cell-death pathway in GB, and may increase the bioavailability of TMZ by reducing the clearance of the metabolite that methylates DNA. GB patients submitted to RT-TMZ and treated with VPA, in fact, have enjoyed a better survival benefit, as compared to those not undergoing VPA medication or receiving other antiepileptic drugs in an EORTC/NCIC trial [55]. Further studies are warranted, in order to assess whether the activity of VPA in enhanc-

ing RT-TMZ in GB is mainly due to HDAC inhibition, or to an increased TMZ bioavailability or to other bioeffects, as indicated above. Other antiepileptic drugs are presently under evaluation in this area of research, but the main interest at the moment is focused on TMZ- and not on radiation-enhancement, which, however, deserves consideration.

MicroRNAs (or miRs, small noncoding RNA sequences of an average of 23 nucleotides) may exert an epigenetic downregulation of target genes. Overexpression of miR-181a sensitizes U87-MG (malignant glioma) cells to radiation and downregulates mRNA and protein expression of BCL-2, a protein that regulates apoptotic cell death. MiRNA expression profiles after IR exposure in the U87-MG cells showed downregulation of miR-181a. Transient overexpression of miR-181a sensitized these cells to IR and led to downregulation of mRNA and protein level of BCL-2. BCL-2 is associated with radioresistance but also it plays a protective role against apoptotic cell death and is frequently overexpressed in human tumor cells [56, 57]. Growth arrest and apoptosis, due to radiation, can be enhanced by inhibition of miR-21 in U251GBM cells through overriding G2-M arrest [58]. GB cell line radiation resistance can be mediated through regulation of cell-cycle genes, such as PDCD4 and hMSH2 by miR-21 [59]. There is sound preclinical evidence showing that also many other miRNAs may modulate the radiation resistance of GB, conditioning downstream both the PI3K/Akt and the ATM/Chk2/p53 pathways, as reported by Comincini et al. in this book. These authors speculate that, given the short time in which a large number of radiobiological studies on miRNAs in GB have been published (that is, over the past 10 years or so) it is reasonable to expect rapid and significant clinical developments.

## Immunity and Radiation Response of Glioblastoma

Differently from a former concept, brain is not immune-privileged, particularly if a breakdown of the BBB takes place, like in the case of GB, which develops abnormal vasculature and tumor-associated inflammation. Immunotherapy of GB has been developed, through passive (mAb, cytokine-mediated therapies and adoptive cell transfer) and active immunity agents (peptide- and cell-based approaches). Immunology subjects and immunotherapy are dealt with in most recent updates on emerging strategies against GB [60–63] and many prospective phase-I to -III clinical trials are presently ongoing on this subject. However, the topic of an immunity-based approach to overcome GB refractoriness to radiation is specifically addressed more rarely, both in laboratory and clinical experimental contexts. In this book, Cooper et al. deal specifically with radiation-induced immune response against GB, as well as with the interference of the brain/tumor microenvironment with effective antitumor immunity. Radiation may have several adverse effects on immunity, such as those systemically occurring during limited-volume, fractionated RT for GB, due to exposure to circulating lymphocytes. Over a complete RT course (60 Gy in 6 weeks, 5 fractions of 2 Gy per week) lymphocytes may drop by 50 % of the baseline count [64] due to radiation-induced apoptosis. Immunosuppressive effects may also be due to TMZ- and steroid-induced leukopenia. Furthermore, the GB microenvironment itself may exert an immunosuppressive influence, and immune checkpoints may inhibit immune cell proliferation and activity.

These effects make it difficult to detect a possible antitumor immunity in the clinical setting and the role of radiation in its modulation. Preclinical experimental radiobiology approaches are therefore necessary, such as those undertaken in mice submitted to a focally collimated, stereotactic single-fraction 10 Gy irradiation of an orthotopic tumor deriving from GL261 glioma cells, followed by activation of 4-1BB (or CD137, a member of TNF superfamily, a co-stimulatory molecule), and blockade of CTLA-4 (or CD 152, Cytotoxic T-lymphocyte Antigen 4, an immune checkpoint downregulating the immune system) [65]. This triple-therapy schedule achieved a median survival of 66.5 days, vs. 22.5 days ($p < 0.05$) in mice undergoing only the 4-1BB/CTLA-4 manipulation, and 24 days

($p < 0.01$) in those submitted to irradiation alone. The primary tumor site showed increased CD4+ and CD8+ infiltrating lymphocytes after triple-therapy; depletion by monoclonal Abs of CD4+ inhibited the antitumor efficacy of triple-therapy, whereas depletion of CD8+ did not interfere with triple-therapy efficacy and allowed a longer survival compared with controls. Long-term-surviving animals achieved also memory response and rejected a subsequent growth of GL261 glioma cells, implanted in the flank. Some clinical trials are presently ongoing, taking into account also similar co-signal balances in other animal-model experiments [66, 67], and adopting programmed cell death (PD-1) immune checkpoint-inhibiting monoclonal Abs, such as Pidilizumab and Nivolumab. However, RT exerts multiple favorable and sometimes unfavorable effects on GB, based on different domains of cell-mediated and humoral immunity, which need in-depth evaluation and are the subject of intensive research [7].

Vaccination with DCs loaded with an *EGFRvIII* (a mutant form of *EGFR* present in about 30–40 % of GBs) specific peptide, induced immune response and a relevant improvement in prognosis out of a small series of patients [68]. This led to the development of a prospective trial in the adjuvant setting after chemoradiation [69], showing good results in a comparison with matched controls. The preliminary results of the ACT-III trial, addressing Rindopepimut (a vaccine consisting of the unique EGFRvIII peptide sequence conjugated with keyhole limpet hemocyanin), delivered in conjunction with TMZ and after chemoradiation in GB, were published very recently [70]. This study raises remarkable interest, due to a median overall survival of 21.8 months and 3-year survival of 26 %, out of 65 EGFRvIII+ GB patients, to a fourfold anti-EGFR antibody increase in 85 % of patients, and to the EGFRvIII+/EGFRvIII-conversion in 4/6 recurring patients. These outcomes are under evaluation in a random phase-III trial (ACT-IV). However, the above results derive primarily from investigating the subject of vaccine therapy against *EGFRvIII* in GB, with no particular radiobiological meaning. The subject of immunotherapy against *EGFRvIII* in conjunction with radiation is stimulating, and not yet sufficiently addressed in preclinical experiments that are suitable for specific therapeutic developments.

## Evolving Radiation Techniques, Particle Therapy, and Immunity

The recent evolution of image tools (CT, MRI, radionuclide methods) and radiation therapy planning and dose delivering has generally provided high conformality in RT of GB. Ionizing particle beams, as compared to photons, have the peculiarity of more selective dose deposition at a definite depth (Bragg's peak). Proton beam irradiation of GB has a better conformity index (CI, which is the ratio between the planned target volume of a tumor and the healthy tissue volume that receives a significant dose as regards radiation tolerance) compared to the most sophisticated photon RT techniques presently available [71]. This may spare critical structures of the healthy brain from severe damage, thus allowing very high-dose irradiation of GB and possibly improving local tumor control. Heavy ion beams (e.g., carbon ions) add to this selective dose deposition, also producing the advantage of a high ionization density (expressed as Linear Energy Transfer, or LET). This achieves a high relative biological effectiveness (RBE), due to inactivating events very close to each other along particles' paths, spaced out ranges comparable to the size of biological molecules like DNA. Therefore, more effects of charged particle irradiation are direct and irreparable, with a lesser dependence on parameters like dose fractionation, oxygenation, stem cell resistance, etc., than X- or γ-ray photon irradiation. However, it is difficult to demonstrate the clinical benefits of ion-beam methods, mainly due to the very limited availability of dedicated facilities. Nevertheless, the present trend towards hypofractionated photon RT, which derives from the selective, high-gradient linear-accelerator-based RT techniques and image-guided irradiation, might further develop in the near future with charged particles.

From a radiobiological standpoint, the focal RT high-dose deposition with stereotactic RT or particle therapy is attractive for many reasons. At very high doses, vascular radiation damage may become dominant, impairing tumor nutrient supply and oxygenation. Endothelial cell apoptosis steeply increases above fractions of 10 Gy [72], and a devascularizing effect becomes evident at image studies after doses of 18–24 Gy [73]. Further, radiation may induce cell necrosis in tumors [74] besides apoptosis and autophagy-related cell death, especially after high-dose delivery, and inflammation response is always present in this case. Immunity is a main pathophysiological domain involved in this context, as inflammatory status may promote the antigen-specific immunity through DC maturation, internalization of apoptosis- and necrosis-derived tumor cell molecules, and presentation of antigens to T cells, thus countering the poor immunogenicity of clinically developed tumors [75]. The presence in the microenvironment, after irradiation, of the so-called DAMPs (damage-associated molecular patterns) [76], like ATP and the high-mobility group protein 1 (HMGB1), activates TLR4 (toll-like receptor 4) in CD8+ T-lymphocytes (shown to be correlated with radiation success). Calreticulin translocation to the cell surface (CRT) may in turn induce the capture of tumor antigens by dendritic cells (DC), which also mature due to HMGB1, thus initiating an immune response against the tumor [77]. In tumors characterized by systemic metastases, these processes are involved in the so-called "abscopal effect", which is a regression effect beyond direct cytotoxicity of radiation on tumor cells, occurring on primary or metastatic sites after focal irradiation of a single tumor site (revised in [78]). However, many mechanisms are involved in radiation-induced immunity against cancer, which are the subject of intensive preclinical research for its enhancement also in the clinical setting, e.g., through vaccination, immunomodulation, and adoptive cell transfer for a synergic approach with RT. These studies are ongoing also for GB [77] and are the subject of a dedicated section of this book.

## The State-of-the-Art in GB Radiobiology, Related Pathobiology, and Their Clinical Relevance

It is becoming a truism to state that the progress made in clinical and molecular oncology and radiobiology has made it possible to switch from a population-based approach to a personalized treatment. The main advantage of combining information derived from both preclinical and clinical settings lies in the real opportunity of selecting specific molecular-oriented subjects, who will most likely benefit from a particular treatment in accordance with their "molecular profile", or to select patients at risk of adverse events. For instance, the close integration between molecular biology and imaging may favor a reliable functional clinical evaluation of a number of biological events, previously identified only by pathology or laboratory assays, allowing a proper patient selection for the most effective therapeutic approach.

We now have a better understanding of the mechanisms sustaining the processes responsible, at the biological and clinical levels, for the aggressive radioresistant phenotypes of GB. At the same time, the important advances being made in our knowledge of biological processes might ground strategies for enhanced radiation response, as well as reduced toxicity of organs at risk. With particular regard to GB, progress in characterization, quantification, and timing of biological processes might improve the growing body of current evidence in the diagnostic and therapeutic fields, such as imaging and RT. This hopefully will allow for both the identification of subjects with specific molecular profiles and for this reason more responsive to ionizing radiation and strategies suitable for enhancing GB radiation sensitivity in radioresistant phenotypes.

However, advances in molecular-based approaches presently have the most striking consequences in an overwhelming amount of new drugs, able to modify cellular systems at the genetic, epigenetic, and signaling pathway levels in the preclinical setting, and in the introduction of a multitude of diagnostic tools able to monitor individual molecular and biological processes with improving sensitivity and specificity. These achievements have dramatically augmented our understanding of the molecular bases of GB, and putatively should improve clinical outcomes, but this is not yet the rule. The presently available, enormous body of biological knowledge likely requires reliable processes for translation into the clinical setting. This might be a major challenge for the near future. In this regards, as previously stated, the aim of this book is to provide some selected contributions that might facilitate reciprocal understanding and communication among the main players in radiation research and clinical management of GB.

## References

1. Stupp R, Tonn JC, Brada M, et al. On behalf of the ESMO Guidelines Working Group: high-grade malignant glioma: ESMO clinical practice guidelines for diagnosis, treatment and follow-up. Ann Oncol. 2010;21:190–3.
2. Salazar OM, Rubin P, Donald JF, Feldstein ML. High-dose radiation therapy in the treatment of glioblastoma multiforme. Int J Radiat Oncol Biol Phys. 1976;1:717–27.
3. Walker MD, Strike TA, Sheline GE. Analysis of dose-effect relationship in the radiotherapy of malignant gliomas. Int J Radiat Oncol Biol Phys. 1979;5:1715–31.
4. Curran Jr WJ, Scott CB, Horton J, et al. Recursive partitioning analysis of prognostic factors in three Radiation Therapy Oncology Group malignant glioma trials. J Natl Cancer Inst. 1993;85:704–10.
5. Pedicini P, Fiorentino A, Simeon V, et al. Clinical radiobiology of glioblastoma multiforme: estimation of tumor control probability from various radiotherapy fractionation schemes. Strahlenther Onkol. 2014;190:925–32.
6. Brennan C, Verhaak RGW, McKenna A, et al. The somatic genomic landscape of glioblastoma. Cell. 2013;155:462–77.
7. Patel MA, Kim JE, Ruzevick J, et al. The future of glioblastoma therapy: synergism of standard of care and immunotherapy. Cancers. 2014;6:1953–85.
8. Prados MD, Byron SA, Tran NL, et al. Towards precision medicine in glioblastoma: the promise and the challenges. Neuro Oncol. 2015;17:1051–63. doi:10.1093/neuronc/nov031:1-10.
9. Bastien JL, McNeill KA, Fine HA. Molecular characterization of glioblastoma, target therapy, and clinical results to date. Cancer. 2014;121:502–10.
10. Baumann M, Bodis S, Dikomey E, et al. Molecular radiation biology/oncology at its best: cutting edge research presented at the 13th international Wofsberg

meeting on molecular radiation biology/oncology. Radiother Oncol. 2013;108:357–61.

11. Verhaak RGW, Hoadley KA, Purdom E, et al. An integrated genomic analysis identifies clinically relevant subtypes of glioblastoma characterized by abnormalities in PDGFRA, IDH1, EGFR and NF1. Cancer Cell. 2010;17(1):98. doi:10.1016/J.ccr2009.12.020.

12. Cohen-Jonathan Moyal E. Du laboratoire vers la clinique: expérience du glioblastoma pur moduler la radiosensibilité tumorale. Cancer Radiother. 2012;16:25–8.

13. Toulany M, Rodemann HP. Potential of Akt mediated repair in radioresistance of solid tumors overexpressing erbB-PI3K-Akt pathway. Transl Cancer Res. 2013;2:190–202.

14. Hatampaa KJ, Burma S, Zhao D, Habib AA. Epidermal growth factor receptor in glioma: signal transduction, neuropathology, imaging, and radioresistance. Neoplasia. 2010;12:675–84.

15. Mukheriee B, McEllin B, Camacho CV, et al. EGFRvIII and DNA double strand break repair: a molecular mechanism for radioresistance in glioblastoma. Cancer Res. 2009;69:4252–9.

16. Mellinghoff IK, Wang MY, Vivanco I, et al. Molecular determinants of the response of glioblastoma to EGFR kinase inhibitors. N Engl J Med. 2005;353:2012–24.

17. Krakstad C, Chekenya M. Survival signaling and apoptosis resistance in glioblastomas: opportunities for target therapies. Mol Cancer. 2010;9:135. http://www.molecular-cancer.com/content/9/1/135

18. Taylor TE, Furnari FB, Cavanee WK. Targeting EGFR for treatment of glioblastoma: molecular basis to overcome resistance. Curr Cancer Drug Targets. 2012;12:197–209.

19. Wong R. Apoptosis in cancer: from pathogenesis to treatment. J Exp Clin Cancer Res. 2011;30:87. doi:10.1186/1756-9966-30-87.

20. Balcer-Kubiczek EK. Apoptosis in radiation therapy: a double edged sword. Exp Oncol. 2012;34:277–85.

21. Ma H, Rao L, Wang HL, Mao ZW, et al. Transcriptome analysis of glioma cells for the dynamic response to irradiation and dual regulation of apoptosis genes: a new insight into radiotherapy for glioblastoma. Cell Death Dis. 2013;4, e895. doi:10.1038/cddis.2013.412.

22. Mirzayans R, Andrais B, Scott A, et al. Ionizing radiation-induced responses in human cells with differing TP53 status. Int J Mol Sci. 2013;14:22409–35.

23. Galluzzi L, Vitale I, Abrams JM, et al. Molecular definitions of cell death subroutines: recommendations of the Nomenclature Committee on Cell Death 2012. Cell Death Differ. 2012;19:107–20.

24. Miracco C, Palumbo S, Pirtoli L, Comincini S. Autophagy in human brain cancer: therapeutic implications. In: Hayat MA, editor. Autophagy: cancer, other pathologies, inflammation, immunity, infection, and aging, vol. 5. San Diego: Elsevier/Academic Press; 2015. p. 105–20.

25. Kang R, Zeh HJ, Lotze MT, Tang D. The beclin1 network regulates autophagy and apoptosis. Cell Death Differ. 2011;18:571–80.

26. Wei Y, Zou Z, Becker N, et al. XEGFR-mediated beclin1 phosphorylation in autophagy suppression, tumor progression, and tumor chemoresistance. Cell. 2013;154:1269–84.

27. Palumbo S, Tini P, Toscano M, et al. Combined EGFR and autophagy modulation impairs cell migration and enhances radiosensitivity in human glioblastoma cells. J Cell Physiol. 2014;229:1863–73.

28. Tini P, Belmonte G, Toscano M et al. Combined epidermal growth factor receptor and beclin1 autophagic protein expression analysis identifies different clinical presentations, responses to chemo- and radiotherapy, and prognosis in glioblastoma. BioMed Res Int. 2015; ID 208076. http://dx.doi.org/10.1159/2015/208076

29. Schonberg DL, Lubelski D, Miller TE, Rich JN. Brain tumor stem cells: molecular characteristics and their impact on therapy. Mol Aspects Med. 2014;39:82–101.

30. Carrasco-Garcia E, Sampron N, Aldaz P, et al. Therapeutic strategies targeting glioblastoma stem cells. Recent Pat Anticancer Drug Discov. 2013;8:216–27.

31. Altaner C. Glioblastoma and stem cells. Neoplasma. 2008;55:369–74.

32. Bao S, Wu Q, McLendon RE, Hao Y, et al. Glioma stem cells promote radioresistance by preferential activation of the DNA damage response. Nature. 2006;444:756–60.

33. Bao S, Wu Q, Sathornsumetee S, Hao Y, et al. Stem cell-like glioma cells promote tumor angiogenesis through vascular endothelial growth factor. Cancer Res. 2006;66:7843–8.

34. Wang J, Ma Y, Cooper MK. Cancer stem cells in glioma: challenges and opportunities. Transl Cancer Res. 2013;2:429–41.

35. Wang R, Chadalavada K, Wilshire J, et al. Glioblastoma stem-like cells give rise to tumour endothelium. Nature. 2010;468:829–33.

36. Ricci-Vitiani L, Pallini R, Biffoni M, et al. Tumour vascularization via endothelial differentiation of glioblastoma stem-like cells. Nature. 2010;468:824–8.

37. Cheng L, Huang Z, Zhou W, et al. Glioblastoma stem cells generate vascular pericytes to support vessel function and tumor growth. Cell. 2013;153:139–52.

38. Kioi M, Vogel H, Schultz G, et al. Inhibition of vasculogenesis, but not angiogenesis, prevents the recurrence of glioblastoma after irradiation in mice. J Clin Invest. 2010;120:694–705.

39. Horsman MR, Overgaard J. The oxygen effect and tumor microenvironment. In: Steel G, editor. Basic clinical radiobiology. London: Arnold; 2002. p. 158–68.

40. Persano L, Rampazzo E, Della Puppa A, Pistollato F, et al. The three-layer concentric model of glioblastoma: cancer stem cells, microenvironmental regulation, and therapeutic implications. Scientific World Journal. 2011;11:1829–41.

41. Shiao SL, Ganesan AP, Rugo HS, Coussens LM. Immune microenvironments in solid tumors: new targets for therapy. Genes Dev. 2011;25:2559–72.

42. Hanahan D, Coussens LM. Accessories to the crime: functions of cells recruited to the tumor microenvironment. Cancer Cell. 2012;21:309–402.

43. Yang L, Lin C, Wang L, Guo H, et al. Hypoxia and hypoxia-inducible factors in glioblastoma multiforme progression and therapeutic implications. Exp Cell Res. 2012;318:2417–26.

44. Sandberg CJ, Altschuler G, Jeong J, et al. Comparison of glioma stem cells to neural stem cells from the adult human brain identifies dysregulated Wnt-signaling and a fingerprint associated with clinical outcome. Exp Cell Res. 2013;319:2230–43.

45. Rossi M, Magnoni L, Miracco C, et al. β-catenin and Gli1 are prognostic markers in glioblastoma. Cancer Biol Ther. 2011;11:1–9.

46. Bütof R, Dubrowska A, Baumann N. Clinical perspectives of cancer stem cell research in radiation oncology. Radiother Oncol. 2013;108:388–96.

47. Chaudry MA, Omaruddin RA. Different DNA methylation alterations in radiation-sensitive and -resistant cells. DNA Cell Biol. 2012;31:657–63.

48. Kim J-G, Park M-T, Heo K, et al. Epigenetics meets radiation biology as a new approach in cancer treatment. Int J Mol Sci. 2013;14:45059–73.

49. Dawson MA, Kouzarides T. Cancer epigenetics: from mechanism to therapy. Cell. 2012;150:12–27.

50. Hegi ME, Diserens AC, Gorlia T, et al. MGMT gene silencing and benefit from temozolomide in glioblastoma. N Engl J Med. 2005;352:997–1003.

51. Olson R, Brastianos PK, Palma DA. Prognostic and predictive value of epigenetic silencing of MGMT in patients with high grade gliomas: a systematic review and meta-analysis. J Neuroncolol. 2011;105:325–35.

52. Van Vlodrop IJ, Niessen HE, Derks S, et al. Analysis of promoter CpG island hypermethylation in cancer: location, location, location! Clin Cancer Res. 2011;17:4225–31.

53. Van Nifterik KA, Van den Berg J, Slotman BJ, et al. Valproic acid sensitizes human glioma cells for temozolomide and γ-radiation. J NeuroOncol. 2012;107:61–7.

54. Chen CH, Chang YJ, Ku MS, et al. Enhancement of temozolomide-induced apoptosis by valproic acid in human glioma cell lines through redox regulation. J Mol Med (Berl). 2011;89:303–15.

55. Weller M, Gorlia T, Cairncross JG, et al. Prolonged survival with valproic acid use in the EORTC/NCIC temozolomide trial for glioblastoma. Neurology. 2011;77:1156–64.

56. Hara T, Omura-Minamisawa M, Kang Y, et al. Flavopiridol potentiates the cytotoxic effects of radiation in radioresistant tumor cells in which p53 is mutated or Bcl-2 is overexpressed. Int J Radiat Oncol Biol Phys. 2008;71:1485–95.

57. Chen G, Zhu W, Shi D, et al. MicroRNA-181a sensitizes human malignant glioma U87MG cells to radiation by targeting Bcl-2. Oncol Rep. 2010;23:997–1003.

58. Li Y, Zhao S, Zhen Y, Li Q, et al. A miR-21 inhibitor enhances apoptosis and reduces G(2)-M accumulation induced by ionizing radiation in human glioblastoma U251 cells. Brain Tumor Pathol. 2011;28:209–14.

59. Chao TF, Xiong HH, Liu W, et al. MiR-21 mediates the radiation resistance of glioblastoma cells by regulating PDCD4 and hMSH2. J Huazhong Univ SciTechnol Med Sci. 2013;33:525–9.

60. Carlsson SK, Brothers SP, Wahlestedt C. Emerging treatment strategies for glioblastoma multiforme. EMBO Mol Med. 2014;6:1359–70.

61. Thomas AA, Ernstoff MS, Fadul CE. Immunotherapy for the treatment of glioblastoma. Cancer J. 2012;18:59–68.

62. Wilson TA, Karajannis MA, Harter DH. Glioblastoma multiforme: state of the art and future therapeutics. Surg Neurol Int. 2014;5:64. doi:10.4103/2152-7806.132138.

63. Veliz I, Loo Y, Castillo O, et al. Advances and challenges in the molecular biology and treatment of glioblastoma—is there any hope for the future. Ann Transl Med. 2015;3(1):7. doi:10.3978/j.issn.2305-5839-2014.10.06.

64. Weeke E. The development of lymphopenia in uremic patients undergoing extracorporeal irradiation of the blood with portable beta units. Radiat Res. 1973;56:554–9.

65. Belcaid Z, Phallen JA, Zeng J, et al. Focal radiation therapy combined with 4-1BB activation and CTLa-4 blockade yields long-term survival and a protective antigen-specific memory response in a murine glioma model. PLos One. 2014;9:e101764. doi:10.1371/journal.pone.0101764.

66. Zitvogel L, Kroemer G. Targeting PD-1/PD-L1 interactions for cancer immunotherapy. Oncoimmunology. 2012;1:1223–5.

67. Shindo Y, Yoshimura K, Kuramasu A, et al. Combination immunotherapy with 4-1BB activation and PD-1 blockade enhances antitumor efficacy in a mouse model of subcutaneous tumor. Anticancer Res. 2015;35:129–36.

68. Sampson JH, Archer GE, Mitchell DA, et al. An epidermal growth factor receptor variant III-targeted vaccine is safe and immunogenic in patients with glioblastoma multiforme. Mol Cancer Ther. 2009;8:2773–9.

69. Sampson JH, Heimberger AB, Archer GE, Aldape KD, Friedman AH, Friedman HS, et al. Immunologic escape after prolonged progression-free survival with epidermal growth factor receptor variant III peptide vaccination in patients with newly diagnosed glioblastoma. J Clin Oncol. 2010;28:4722–9.

70. Schuster J, Lai RK, Recht LD, et al. A phase II, multicenter trial of rindopepimut (CDX-110) in newly diagnosed glioblastoma: the ACT III study. Neuro Oncol. 2015;17:854–61.

71. Rosenschöld PMA, Engelholm S, Ohlhues L, et al. Photon and proton therapy planning comparison for malignant glioma based on CT, FDG-PET, DTI-MRI and fiber tracking. Acta Oncol. 2011;50:777–83.

72. Garcia-Barros M, Paris F, Cordon-Cardo C, et al. Tumor response to radiotherapy regulated by endothelial cell apoptosis. Science. 2003;300:1155–9.

73. Yamada Y, Bilsky MH, Lovelock DM, et al. High-dose, single-fraction image-guided intensity-modulated radiotherapy for metastatic spinal lesions. Int J Radiat Oncol Biol Phys. 2008;71:484–90.

74. Kondo T. Radiation-induced cell-death and its mechanisms. Rad Emergency Med. 2013;2:1–14.

75. Finkelstein SE, Timmermann R, McBride WH, et al. The confluence of stereotactic ablative radiotherapy and tumor immunology. Clin Dev Immunol. 2011;2011:439752. doi:10.1155/2011/439752.

76. Srikrishna G, Freeze HH. Endogenous damage-associated molecular pattern molecules at the cross-roads of inflammation and cancer. Neoplasia. 2009;11:615–28.

77. Durante M, Reppingen N, Held KD. Immunologically augmented cancer treatment using modern radiotherapy. Trends Mol Med. 2013;19:565–82.

78. Park B, Yee C, Lee K-M. The effect of radiation on the immune response to cancers. Int J Mol Sci. 2014;15:927–43.

**Part I**

**From Bedside to Bench: Radiobiological
Topics Arising from Clinical Studies**

# The "Radioresistance" of Glioblastoma in the Clinical Setting, and the Present Therapeutic Options

**2**

Michela Buglione, Luca Triggiani, Paolo Borghetti,
Sara Pedretti, Nadia Pasinetti,
and Stefano Maria Magrini

## Radiotherapy: Clinical Historical Landmarks

External Beam Radiotherapy (EBRT) has been the cornerstone of the therapeutic approach to glioblastoma (GBM) for the last 50 years. In the 1970s and early 1980s, data on level-I evidence data became available, thanks to several studies [6, 7], including the prospective phase-III trial conducted by the Brain Tumor Study Group (BTSG 6901) [8]. This study demonstrated the efficacy of radiotherapy (RT) as postoperative treatment. Overall survival (OS) was better in the two arms including RT, compared with surgery alone or chemotherapy alone (BCNU) [8]. In addition, Walker et al. demonstrated a radiation dose–effect relationship in a series of 420 patients treated on Brain Tumor Cooperative Group protocols (BTCG), and the dose of 60 Gy was established as the standard of care [9].

The treatment of GBM dramatically changed after the encouraging findings from a Phase-III joint EORTC-NCIC trial [5]. This trial, first published by Stupp and colleagues in 2005 and then updated in 2010 with 5-year data, demonstrated a remarkable improvement in median survival (MST) (14.6 months vs. 12.1 months) and 5-year OS (9.8 % vs. 1.9 %; HR, 0.63; $p < .0001$) with the use of concomitant Temozolomide (TMZ) and radiation with adjuvant TMZ [5, 10]. In this study, an acceptable additional toxicity was observed in the combined modality group; concomitant treatment resulted in grade 3 or 4 hematologic toxic effects in 7 % of patients. The benefit of TMZ was particularly striking in patients having the MGMT (O-6-methyl-guanine DNA methyltransferase) DNA-repair gene silenced by promoter methylation [11].

In recent years, literature on the treatment of GBM has been characterized by different promising Phase-II trials unconfirmed in subsequent Phase-III trials.

High-grade gliomas are a very interesting topic for radiation oncologists, but they still represent a frontier to be conquered.

## Dose Escalation and Hypofractionation

GBM is considered one of the most radioresistant solid tumors in humans and has inherent radiation resistance pathways [12, 13]. They are characterized by an extremely high local failure rate

M. Buglione (✉) • L. Triggiani • S.M. Magrini
P. Borghetti • N. Pasinetti
Radiation Oncology Department, University and
Spedali Civili - Brescia, Brescia, Italy
e-mail: michela.buglione@unibs.it

S. Pedretti
Radiation Oncology Department, Spedali Civili,
University of Brescia, Brescia, Italy

© Springer International Publishing Switzerland 2016
L. Pirtoli et al. (eds.), *Radiobiology of Glioblastoma*, Current Clinical Pathology,
DOI 10.1007/978-3-319-28305-0_2

despite dose escalation, with local recurrence rates approaching 90 % [14, 15]. Resistance may also be induced by some biologic factors within the tumor and some tumor microenvironment features [16, 17]. Moreover, in few cases, the proper doses of radiation can hardly be delivered because of the limited dose tolerance of the surrounding organs at risk. Further dose intensification using higher radiation doses and altered fractionation were pursued, but failed to provide a clear clinical benefit.

In the pre-TMZ era, Nelson et al. reported on the joint study of the Radiation Therapy Oncology Group (RTOG) and the Eastern Cooperative Oncology Group (ECOG). It randomized 253 patients into two treatment groups: whole-brain irradiation (60 Gy) and 60 Gy plus a 10 Gy boost to limited volume. The median survival times were 9.3 months and 8.2 months respectively, with no additional benefit for the group receiving the higher radiation doses [18]. Given these results, 60 Gy has been considered as the standard dose in postoperative radiotherapy and has been adopted in most clinical trials.

However, the poor outcome associated with standard therapy was conditioned by recurrences occurring within the irradiated field. In their renowned paper of 1980, Hochberg and Pruitt reported the use of CT scans to determine that about 90 % of GBM recurrences occurred no farther than 2 cm from the boundary of the primary tumor [19]. Those data were also confirmed by Wallner and associates [20].

For this reason, the role of radiation dose escalation in the management of GBM has been the object of a larger clinical effort. In a multicenter phase-I trial (RTOG 98-03), dose escalation was conducted using 3D-conformal irradiation. Here, a four-step dose escalation strategy from 66 to 84 Gy was studied, but no benefit was detected in progression-free survival (PFS). In fact, even when a dose at 80 Gy was reached, 90 % of patients failed within the high-dose-region [21]. These data have been confirmed in 2002 by a retrospective study by Chan JL et al., where an infield recurrence rate of 80 % also in patients treated to 90 Gy was demonstrated. Chan et al. published the results of 34 patients with GBM

treated using 3D conformal IMRT to a dose of 90 Gy. At a median follow-up of 11.7 months, median survival was 11.7 months, and 1- and 2-year survivals were 47.1 % and 12.9 %, respectively, comparable to historical controls [22].

In the post-TMZ era, dose escalation remains a crucial investigational option, as a pattern of failure, characterized by local progression or recurrence, still exists. Recently, an increase in survival in patients with GBM with no increment in the incidence of severe toxicity has been reported by some dose escalation studies using IMRT [23, 24]. Direct dosimetric comparison of IMRT and 3D-CRT has clearly shown that IMRT improves target dose conformity, reduces doses to organs at risk, and achieves comparable or slightly better target coverage [25, 26]. In a recent study, Tsien et al. demonstrated that doses of 66–81 Gy delivered by IMRT over 6 weeks, with concomitant and adjuvant TMZ, resulted in a lower infield recurrence rate in groups that received higher doses. PFS was 9.0 months (95 % CI, 6.0–11.7) and median OS was 20.1 months [23]. In a recent review by Badiyan et al. all the clinical studies carried out—between 2000 and 2012—using high-dose radiotherapy HDRT (>60 Gy) and TMZ and standard dose radiotherapy (SDRT) (60 Gy at 2 Gy per fraction) with TMZ were considered. OS and PFS rates for patients who received HDRT versus SDRT were 12.4 % versus 13.2 % ($P = 0.71$), and 5.6 % versus 4.1 % ($P = .54$), respectively. The result of Badiyan's review was that clinical outcomes for patients with GBM do not seem to be improved by moderate radiation therapy dose escalation above 60 Gy with concurrent TMZ [27]. These data were confirmed by large retrospective series [28].

An advantage in cell-killing of intrinsically radioresistant cancer cells, like the ones in GBM, has been demonstrated in in vitro models of [24, 29, 30]. More heavily hypofractionated treatments have therefore been tested for dose escalation to translate to the clinic this advantage in cell-killing. In the Iuchi study, few favorably selected patients were treated with a total dose of 48–68 Gy (260 BEDGy3) and fractional doses of 6–8.5 Gy. Patients treated with tumor BED ranging from 80 to 140 Gy8, obtained the best results and showed improved local control; local recurrence occurred in only 6/25 patients (25 %). These data and those reported by other groups testing the same strategy are however flawed by the nature of the patient population treated (highly selected) [24].

## Hyperfractionation

Hyperfractionated schedules were also used by some clinical trials. GBM cells are known to be relatively rapid proliferating cells and a greater number of daily fractions would increase the chance of radiating them during a more sensitive cell-cycle phase. Furthermore, GBM is a very hypoxic tumor: at smaller radiation doses per fraction, cell-killing is less dependent on oxygen, which could be an advantage, especially if the site of the most hypoxic areas is known in advance. Under these circumstances, in several groups hyperfractionated or accelerated regimens have been utilized as a means to escalate dose, using twice, three-times, and even four-times-daily fractionation [31–34]. Unfortunately, in most clinical trials, a statistical benefit in terms of OS was not achieved even by the "low dose per fraction" strategy [31, 33]. Only in the study of Shin et al. was an improvement in survival using three fractions a day shown. In this study, 69 patients were randomized to 61.4 Gy in 69 fractions of 0.89 Gy over 4.5 weeks or to conventional fractionation to 58 Gy in 30 fractions given once daily over 6 weeks. Median survival in the two groups was 39 and 27 weeks, respectively, and the 1-year survival rates were 41 % and 20 %, respectively ($p < .001$) [34]. The prospective, randomized, phase-I/II RTOG 83-02 trial, examined dose escalation using twice-daily fractionation. Patients were randomized to one or four different dose arms (64.8, 72, 76.8, or 81.6 Gy) using twice-daily fractions of 1.2 Gy. Initial results suggested the superiority of the 72 Gy hyperfractionated schedule but, in a subsequent Phase-III trial, no OS improvement was demonstrated [35]. Patients also received chemotherapy with BCNU. In the final report on all 747 patients, there were no significant differences in MST between the treatment arms. Late toxicities were slightly increased with higher doses. [35]. In a phase-III trial (RTOG 9006), conventional radiotherapy (60 Gy in 30 daily fractions) with hyperfractionated RT to 72 Gy in sixty 1.2 Gy fractions given twice daily were compared. No difference in OS was found [36]. Several other accelerated hyperfractionation regimens to doses over 70 Gy have been investigated, also without significant improvements in survival [37]. Prados and colleagues used a hyperfractionation schedule of 1.6 Gy twice daily to a total dose of 70.4 Gy, also to determine the activity of difluoromethylornithine (DFMO), a compound that inhibits sublethal and potentially lethal damage repair. Unfortunately, survival was not improved by either intervention [38] (Table 2.1).

## Stereotactic Radiosurgery and Stereotactic Radiation Therapy

Stereotactic Radiosurgery (SRS) and Stereotactic Radiation Therapy (SRT) are types of highly hypofractionated radiotherapy delivery. While achievability and efficacy of the combination of conformal radiotherapy and SRS or SRT have, to date, been confirmed in many retrospective studies, they have only been supported in some prospective studies. Mehta and colleagues reported a 2-year survival rate of 28 % in 31 patients treated with EBRT (54 Gy in 1.8 Gy/fraction) plus SRS boost (15–35 Gy, $m = 18.75$ Gy), which was significantly superior to the 9.7 % in the previous RTOG study [39]. Loeffler et al reported on 37 patients with GBM treated with fractionated radiotherapy to 59.4 Gy followed by a STR boost to a median dose of 12 Gy. After a median follow-up period of 19 months, a 76 % survival rate was reported [40]. A group of 115 GBM patients who received conformal radiation therapy and a stereotactic boost was described by Sarkaria and colleagues. The median survival time was 96 weeks. It was questioned whether these results represented a real benefit from SRS or simply the effect of a selection bias, since only smaller lesions, in patients with a good performance status, showing a dimensional response after the

**Table 2.1** Hyperfractionation

| Authors | Dose fraction | Treatments/day | Total dose | Results |
|---------|---------------|----------------|------------|---------|
| Shin et al. [34] | 0.89 | 3 | 61.4 Gy | 1-and 2-year actuarial survival rate is 54 % and 21 %. |
| Curran et al. [35] | 1.2 | 2 | 64.8, 72, 76.8 or 81.6 Gy | Survival rates at 2 and 5 years were: 21 % and 11 %, and 4 %, respectively |
| Nelson [36] | 1.2 | 2 | 72 Gy | – |
| Prados et al. [38] | 1.6 | 2 | 70.4 | OS: 5.7 months |
| | | | | PFS 2.7 months |

first EBRT phase were usually selected for the SRS boost [41]. Subsequently, in an effort to delineate the role of SRS, a prospective multicenter randomized phase-III trial (RTOG 93-05) was conducted by the RTOG to assess the efficacy of SRS followed by standard adjuvant radiochemotherapy for newly diagnosed GBM. In this trial, 203 patients were randomly assigned to receive either 60 Gy of EBRT at 2 Gy/fraction with BCNU or SRS prior to EBRT and BCNU. The tumor dose was volume-dependent, ranging from 15 to 24 Gy in compliance with the established maximum safely tolerated doses. The median overall survival (OS) was 13.5 months for the SRS group and 13.6 months for the standard treatment group at a median follow-up of 61 months. An improvement of patient survival failed to be demonstrated by the study. Moreover, SRS was not related to a better quality of life, or neurologic function [42].

GBMs are most commonly large, diffusively infiltrative tumors with substantial surrounding edema, known to possibly harbor microscopic disease, reducing the likelihood of success of SRS. Currently the role of SRS in the adjuvant setting for GBM is not well defined. Although adjuvant treatment did not prove to be beneficial, attention still remains focused on SRS for the treatment of recurrent GBM [43–45] (Table 2.2).

## Brachytherapy

Brachytherapy refers to the use of implanted radioactive material at the site of the tumor and is usually used for focal dose escalation. In this field, it is well known that higher radiation doses

**Table 2.2** SRS STR

| Authors | EBRT (Gy) | Boost | Results |
|---------|-----------|-------|---------|
| Mehta et al. [39] | 54 | SRS boost (15–35 Gy, $m=18.75$ Gy) | 1- and 2-years survival were 38 % and 28 % |
| Loeffler et al. [40] | 59.4 | STR boost to a median dose of 12 Gy | – |
| RTOG 93-05 [42] | 60 | SRS boost (15 to 24 Gy) | the median survival was 13.5 months |

may otherwise significantly increase the risk of brain necrosis [46]. Both permanent and temporary radioactive implants have been placed in the brain of GBM patients. In most studies, including two prospective randomized trials [47, 48], high-dose rate implants (40–70 cGy/h) were used to treat GBM. This approach, however, was associated with a high incidence of radiation-induced changes, requiring treatment with steroids for almost all patients, and repeated surgery rates up to 50 %. Furthermore, no significant survival benefits were achieved by this approach, compared with standard treatment regimens [47, 48]. Another technique is the application of low-dose-rate implants (3–8 cGy/h). It has been demonstrated that this approach was associated with only minimal permanent deficits; radiation-induced changes were almost absent [49, 50].

The results obtained in 56 patients with GBM treated with temporary 125I interstitial implants were reported by Prados and colleagues. Patients received EBRT (median, 59.4 Gy), in most cases with concomitant chemotherapy (hydroxyurea), followed by interstitial implant. Eight patients (14 %) survived 3 years or longer, and 16 (29 %) survived 2 years or longer. A second operation was necessary in 50 % of the patients to remove symptomatic localized necrosis produced by the implant. Prolonged steroid use was necessary in many patients [51]. Brachytherapy was used by Laperriere et al. as a boost to conventional radiotherapy in patients with GBM. Patients were randomized to EBRT (50 Gy in 25 fractions) alone ($n=69$) or EBRT plus a temporary stereotactic 125 I implant delivering a minimum peripheral tumor dose of 60 Gy ($n=71$). Median survival was not significantly different in the two arms (13.8 vs. 13.2 months; $p=.49$) [47]. The results of the BTCG—NIH Trial 8701 reported by Selker et al. support these findings. In this randomized, prospective trial, 299 patients with newly diagnosed GBM received surgery, EBRT, and chemotherapy (BCNU) with or without an interstitial radiotherapy boost with 125 I. Survival was not prolonged by treatment with an interstitial boost, compared with conventional treatment [48] (Table 2.3).

## Radiation Volume and the Changing Delineation Concepts

Over the years, the approach of radiotherapy to GBM has evolved. At first, the entire brain volume was covered by means of large opposed lateral fields. In 1989, Shapiro et al. published data from BTCG trial 8001, where the randomization

**Table 2.3** Brachytherapy

| Authors | EBRT (Gy) | Boost | Results |
|---|---|---|---|
| Prados et al. [51] | median 59.4 | temporary 125I interstitial implants | 2-years survival rate 29 % |
| Laperriere et al. [47] | 50 | implant delivering a minimum peripheral tumor dose of 60 Gy | Median survival was 13.8 months |
| Selker et al. [48] | 50 | temporary stereotactic 125I | The median survival was 9.7 months |

was altered during the trial to compare partial brain irradiation (PBI) with whole-brain radiotherapy (WBI). No differences in OS or changes in the patterns of failure were observed [52]. Accordingly, WBI is generally not needed to treat GBM. Nowadays, two main practice guidelines for the definition of the volumes and for the dose prescription are enforced: the EORTC and the RTOG.

In EORTC, a single-phase technique is favored, consisting of 30 daily fractions of 2 Gy. The gross tumor volume (GTV) is defined as the region of enhancement in preoperative T1 magnetic resonance imaging (MRI) in patients who underwent biopsy, while in the patients who underwent resection (total/subtotal) GTV corresponds to tumor bed plus any residual enhancing tumor . This is expanded by 2–3 cm to create the clinical target volume (CTV). The planning target volume (PTV) encloses the CTV with a margin of 0.5–0.7 cm, depending on the technique used (3D, IMRT, or others). In RTOG, on the other hand, a cone-down technique is favored, using two different volumes. The GTV in RTOG protocols is similarly defined as in EORTC advice, while the CTV is created including the edema shown on the CT/MRI scan (T2/FLAIR hyperintensity). This is then expanded 2.0 cm to create the PTV1 and it is treated using a total dose of 46 Gy in 23 fractions. The PTV2 is smaller, including GTV with a margin of 2.5 cm (without edema) plus margins related to set up error. PTV2 should be treated with an additional 14 Gy in 7 fractions (total cumulative dose 60 Gy). The mentioned guidelines to PTV margins definition are controversial. The extent of the treated brain volume is associated with the potential development of neurotoxicity; the incidence of these side effects might be reduced by a decrease of the treated volume [53]. RT margin reduction is especially important in treatment regimens that incorporate hypofractionation schedules. Nevertheless, margin reductions could be associated with an increased risk of marginal misses. The pattern of failure in 62 consecutive patients treated with 60 Gy and concurrent TMZ (97 %) was analyzed by McDonald et al. A mean PTV1 margin ranging between 1.05 and 1.3 cm off the GTV was selected, and patients were treated with a total PTV boost margin of 1 cm or less. Radiographic tumor progression developed in 43 of 62 patients at 12 months, with a median time to progression (TTP) of 7 months. It was observed that through the use of limited margins, only 5 % and 2 % of patients had respectively a marginal failure and distant failure, with a median follow-up between 12 and 15 months. These data support the notion that limited GTV–CTV margins for GBM do not lead to an increase in local failures [54].

Minniti et al compared relapse patterns in 105 patients planned using the EORTC technique of GTV delineation, encompassing the resection cavity and any residual tumor detected in postoperative T1-weighted MRI with a 2-cm margin to create the CTV. CTV–PTV margin was 3 mm. All the patients were treated with conformal radiotherapy (60 Gy in 30 fractions) plus concomitant and adjuvant chemotherapy (TMZ). The patients were retrospectively rescheduled, when the disease relapsed, using the RTOG guideline and the target radiation coverage (EORTC vs. RTOG) of the site of recurrence was directly compared. No significant difference between the two techniques, in the fraction of "in field" relapses, was documented; however, a significantly greater volume of healthy brain tissue demonstrated to be treated using the RTOG two-phase technique [15].

It was demonstrated by Brandes et al. that patients with MGMT methylation developed fewer recurrences in or close to the radiotherapy treatment field, suggesting a clinically evident radiosensitizing effect of TMZ [55]. Further studies are needed to highlight the relationship between individual molecular variations and patterns of relapse, in order to develop future individualized radiotherapy plans.

## Radiation Volume and the Use of Advanced Imaging Techniques

Treatment failure for GBM is mainly caused by the invasion of GBM cells into the normal tissue brain. Nowadays, conventional imaging is not able to detect the actual extent of the tumor. Even

the higher spatial resolution of MRI failed to allow direct visualization of the tumor margins. It has been shown, by some postmortem studies, that approximately between 20 and 27 % of GBMs have limited invasion (less than 1 cm from the edge of the gross tumor), 20 % have more extensive invasion (more than 3 cm from the gross tumor), and 8 % show disseminated spread [56, 57]. These groups should be treated differently; however, at present, GBM cannot be treated according to the extent of microscope invasion. The potential of biomarkers for tumor invasion imaging is an active field of research. Biological images are needed in Radiotherapy both to spare normal brain tissue and to better target GBM microscopic extension into the brain parenchyma. Biologic imaging could be referred to as a way to depict physiologic, metabolic, and functional processes, also to noninvasively measure the biologic features of tumors or normal tissues. Significant information on cellular proliferation, angiogenesis, hypoxia, and metabolic activity could be supplied to radiation oncology by functional and molecular imaging techniques (diffusion and perfusion MRI, magnetic resonance spectroscopy (MRS), and positron emission tomography (PET)).

MRS can provide biochemical changes in the brain tissue, particularly when tumors are present. On MRS, the chemical composition (metabolites) of normal brain tissue can be differentiated from the tumor tissue. The metabolites detectable with proton MRS include, among others, N-acetylaspartate (NAA) and choline-containing compounds (Cho), and could act as potential biomarkers for tumor activity. Cho is a membrane component that reflects the metabolism of cellular membrane turnover; NAA is a marker for neuronal density that is decreased in tumors due to neuronal loss. GBM shows an increase in the Cho/NAA ratio due to a marked high resonance in the spectral region of Cho and a low NAA resonance [58]. These data could be significant for radiation oncology to define the CTV in GBM. Ken et al. published a phase-II trial that integrates in 16 patient 3D MRS images in the treatment planning process for GBM, to guide the treatment delivery. A simultaneous boost technique (SIB) with intensity-modulated radio-therapy (IMRT) was chosen to simultaneously deliver higher doses (72 Gy) to "high-risk" sub-volumes; the GTV2 was defined as the MRS abnormality (Cho/NAA ≥ 2.00). No difference in the pattern of recurrences was described [59]. In another prospective Phase-II trial, Einstein et al. reported the results of 35 GBM patients treated with defining high-risk tumor volumes using postoperative MRS (elevated Cho/NAA ratio in excess of 2:1) to deliver a SRS boost (single fraction of 15–24 Gy). All patients received in addition EBRT to a total dose of 60 Gy in 2 Gy daily fractions. Mean Survival Time was 20.8 months, and it equalled the historical control. In this study the local control was not specifically analyzed [60]. MRS is nowadays performed to differentiate brain tumor recurrence from radionecrosis [61].

PET is an imaging modality widely used in oncology for clinical staging, monitoring of treatment efficacy, and follow-up to detect disease recurrence. Conventional (18)F-FDG-PET is of limited relevance for GBM imaging, due to high levels of glucose uptake by normal brain and the resulting unfavourable signal-to-noise ratio. In contrast, 11C-methionine (MET) and 18F-fluoroethyl-L-tyrosine (FET) are more helpful in brain tumor imaging than 18F-FDG [62]. In 2012, Piroth et al. published a prospective phase-II study in which they used postoperative FET-PET to define the CTV receiving a boost dose up to 72 Gy at 2.4 Gy per fraction with IMRT technique. OS and PFS were 14.8 months and 7.8 months, respectively. In this study the authors demonstrated that postoperative tumor volume in FET-PET has an independent significant influence on DFS and OS of patients with GBM [63].

Although some interesting results have been achieved by using sophisticated imaging modalities applied to radiation treatment planning, it has not been possible to develop dose escalation programs that are able to overcome GBM radioresistance. However, better ways to define the target volume could be identified by past research programs and others now in progress, thanks to a more accurate "anatomic" localization of the tumor biological features. This is particularly relevant to the association of radiation and target therapies to treat a very heterogeneous neoplasm like GBM.

## Molecularly Targeted Therapies and Radiotherapy

Combinations of different "biologically active" drugs with radiotherapy provide alternative strategies to improve the OS in GBM patients. The main research strategies addressed the possible role of EGFR and VEGF inhibitors.

The *epidermal growth factor receptor (EGFR)* is considered one of the most attractive therapeutic targets for GBM. The gene encoding EGFR is amplified in approximately 40 % of GBMs, especially in the classical subtype (80 %) [64]. EGFR tyrosine kinase inhibitors (TKIs), gefitinib and erlotinib have been used in patients with recurrent GBMs, but only minimal activity and no OS benefit have occurred [65, 66]. A Radiation Therapy Oncology Group (RTOG) phase-I/II trial (RTOG 0211), including 147 patients with newly diagnosed GBM, investigated the combination of gefitinib and radiotherapy followed by gefitinib maintenance until the time of relapse. PFS was 5.1 months and OS was 11 months, which is comparable to historical controls receiving radiotherapy alone [67]. A Phase-II trial by Qaddoumi studied the role of Erlotinib during and after RT in children with newly diagnosed high-grade gliomas. 41 patients were enrolled, 21 with GBM; the 2-year PFS was 19 months. The outcome was not improved by the use of erlotinib during and after RT [68].

Most of the drugs evaluated in clinical trials interfere with the *vascular epidermal grown factor (VEGF)* pathway, blocking directly the receptor or using monoclonal antibody directed against VGEF (bevacizumab). GBM blood vessels are structurally abnormal, contributing to an adverse microenvironment characterized by a low oxygen tension; VEGF inhibitors "normalize" structurally and functionally abnormal tumor vasculature. Radioresistance is promoted by this microenvironment and the delivery of chemotherapy is impaired [69]. Two major phase-III trials were performed, one by the RTOG (RTOG-0825) in the USA [70] and one, AVAGlio, mostly run in Centres in Europe [71]. In both studies, in newly diagnosed GBM, a standard "Stupp" regimen was compared to the association of bevacizumab and TMZ plus RT. The results from both trials were presented at the 2013 Meeting of the American Society of Clinical Oncology and subsequently published. PFS was significantly prolonged in both trials and the quality of life was preserved in the AVAGlio trial, but not in RTOG-0825. Unfortunately, OS was not improved. Upon subgroup analysis, it was not possible to identify specific subgroups of patients who particularly benefitted from bevacizumab. Therefore, at present, the use of bevacizumab is approved by the Federal Drug Administration (FDA) as a monotherapy only in recurrent GBM. The approval was based on demonstration of durable objective response rates observed in two single-arm Phase-II trials, AVF3708g and NCI 06-C-0064E [72, 73]. Furthermore, bevacizumab could play an important role in the therapy for CNS radiation necrosis. As a matter of fact, radiation necrosis can be considered an ongoing process from endothelial cell dysfunction to tissue hypoxia and necrosis, accompanied by the release of a vasoactive protein, like the vascular endothelial growth factor (VEGF) that can lead to progressive blood–brain barrier dysfunction and brain edema [74].

Vatalanib is an oral TKI that specifically targets TK signalling of VEGFR. In a Phase I/II trial performed by EORTC, 19 patients with newly diagnosed GBM were treated with vatalanib in combination with standard treatment. The planned randomized phase-II trial was discontinued right at the start due to industry decision not to further develop this agent [75].

Sorafenib is a small molecular inhibitor of several tyrosine protein kinases (VEGFR and PDGFR) (tyrosine kinase inhibitor or TKI) and Raf kinases. A Phase-I dose escalation trial was conducted to evaluate the safety and efficacy of sorafenib in combination with standard treatment (RT + TMZ) in patients with newly diagnosed GMB, or in combination with hypofractionated stereotactic RT alone in patients with recurrent GMB [76].

Apart from EGFR and VEGF blockade, other biological pathways aroused the interest of clinical researchers as possible targets for the association of radiotherapy and targeted therapy.

Farnesyltransferase inhibitors (FTIs) have been shown to have radiosensitizing properties in preclinical models [77]. The combination of RT and FTI (tipifarnib) was studied in a phase-II clinical trial; the association of tipifarnib with radiotherapy showed promising OS results, but no increase in TTP compared to historical data [78].

Cilengitide is a novel small molecule that selectively blocks the activation of the $\alpha\nu\beta3$ and $\alpha\nu\beta5$ integrins and has been studied in GBM. Integrins are a family of cell surface receptors that play different important roles in most biological cells' activity. The $\alpha\nu\beta3$ and $\alpha\nu\beta5$ integrins are overexpressed in GBM cells and in tumor vasculature. Integrins, in addition to VEGF, are key mediators of angiogenesis and tumor growth. Unfortunately, the results of two large phase-III trials showed that the addition of cilengitide to RT and TMZ for the treatment of newly diagnosed GBM does not improve PFS and OS compared to RT and TMZ alone [79, 80]. The considerable radiochemoresistance of GBM cells is underlined by these clinical data, and the possible presence of a particular subpopulation of cells responsible for local recurrence is also suggested.

The use of immunotherapy with radiotherapy is one of the modern challenges. No clinical data for GBM have been produced yet by this approach, but it is certainly an exciting future research field. For example, researches and ongoing clinical studies are being conducted to evaluate the role of the programmed death-1 (PD-1)/PD-ligand1 (PD-L1) pathway in cancers. It has been demonstrated by recent preclinical data that a combination of radiosurgery with immunotherapy with anti-PD1 blockade produces long-term survivors in GBM-challenged mice [82]. Ionizing radiation is a potent immune-modulator through several mechanisms: the increased availability and reliability of new drugs that modulate the immune response

**Table 2.4** Targeted therapy

| Anti EGFR | | | |
|---|---|---|---|
| Authors | Drug | Patients | Results |
| Chakravarti et al. [67] | Gefitinib | 147 | *PFS: 4.9 months* |
| | | | *OS: 11.1 months* |
| Qaddoumi et el [68] | Erlotinib | 21 | *PFS: 19 months* |
| *Anti-VEFG/Anti-VEGFR* | | | |
| RTOG-0825 [70] | Bevacizumab | 637 | *PFS 10.7 months* |
| | | | *OS: 15.7 months* |
| Avaglio [71] | Bevacizumab | 921 | *PFS: 10.6 months* |
| | | | *OS: 16.8 months* |
| Brandes et al. [75] | Vatalanib | 19 | *PFS: 6.8 months* |
| | | | *OS: 17.3 months* |
| Den et al. [76] | Sorafenib | 11 | *OS: 18 months* |
| *Anti αvβ3 and αvβ5 integrins* | | | |
| Stupp et al. [80] | Cilengitide | 52 | *PFS: 6 months* |
| | | | *OS: 16.1 months* |
| *Other* | | | |
| Ducassou et al. [79] | Tipifarnib | 27 | *OS 20 months* |

could represent, in the next future, a powerful synergistic approach. Table 2.4.

# References

1. Central Brain Tumor Registry of the United States (CBTRUS). CBTRUS statistical report: primary brain and central nervous system tumors diagnosed in the United States in 2004–2007. 2011. www.cbtrus.org/2011-npcr-seer/web-0407-report-3-3-2011.pdf. Accessed 16 Aug 2011.
2. Louis DN, Ohgaki H, Wiestler OD, Cavenee WK, Burger PC, Jouvet A, Scheithauer BW, Kleihues P. The 2007 WHO classification of tumours of the central nervous system. Acta Neuropathol. 2007;114(2):97–109. doi:10.1007/s00401-007-0243-4.
3. Dunn GP, Rinne ML, Wykosky J, Genovese G, Quayle SN, Dunn IF, Agarwalla PK, Chheda MG, Campos B, Wang A, Brennan C, Ligon KL, Furnari F, Cavenee WK, Depinho RA, Chin L, Hahn WC. Emerging insights into the molecular and cellular basis of glioblastoma. Genes Dev. 2012;26(8):756–84.
4. Huse JT, Phillips HS, Brennan CW. Molecular subclassification of diffuse gliomas: seeing order in the chaos. Glia. 2011;59:1190–9.
5. Stupp R, Mason WP, van den Bent MJ, Weller M, Fisher B, Taphoorn MJ, Belanger K, Brandes AA, Marosi C, Bogdahn U, Curschmann J, Janzer RC, Ludwin SK, Gorlia T, Allgeier A, Lacombe D, Cairncross JG, Eisenhauer E, Mirimanoff RO. Radiotherapy plus concomitant and adjuvant temozolomide for glioblastoma. N Engl J Med. 2005;352(10):987–96.
6. Shapiro WR, Young DF. Treatment of malignant glioma. A controlled study of chemotherapy and irradiation. Arch Neurol. 1979;33:494–500.
7. Walker MD, Green SB, Byar DP, Alexander Jr E, Batzdorf U, Brooks WH, Hunt WE, MacCarty CS, Mahaley Jr MS, Mealey Jr J, Owens G, Ransohoff 2nd J, Robertson JT, Shapiro WR, Smith Jr KR, Wilson CB, Strike TA. Randomized comparisons of radiotherapy and nitrosoureas for the treatment of malignant glioma after surgery. N Engl J Med. 1980;303:1323–9.
8. Walker MD, Alexander Jr E, Hunt WE, MacCarty CS, Mahaley Jr MS, Mealey Jr J, Norrell HA, Owens G, Ransohoff J, Wilson CB, Gehan EA, Strike TA. Evaluation of BCNU and/or radiotherapy in the treatment of anaplastic gliomas. A cooperative clinical trial. J Neurosurg. 1978;49:333–43.
9. Walker MD, Strike TA, Sheline GE. An analysis of dose-effect relationship in the radiotherapy of malignant gliomas. Int J Radiat Oncol Biol Phys. 1979;5(10):1725–31.
10. Stupp R, Hegi ME, Mason WP, van den Bent MJ, Taphoorn MJ, Janzer RC, Ludwin SK, Allgeier A, Fisher B, Belanger K, Hau P, Brandes AA, Gijtenbeek J, Marosi C, Vecht CJ, Mokhtari K, Wesseling P, Villa S, Eisenhauer E, Gorlia T, Weller M, Lacombe D, Cairncross JG, Mirimanoff RO. Effects of radiotherapy with concomitant and adjuvant temozolomide versus radiotherapy alone on survival in glioblastoma in a randomised phase III study. 5-year analysis of the

EORTC-NCIC trial. Lancet Oncol. 2009;10(5):459–66. doi:10.1016/S1470-2045(09)70025-7.

11. Hegi ME, Diserens AC, Gorlia T, Hamou MF, de Tribolet N, Weller M, Kros JM, Hainfellner JA, Mason W, Mariani L, Bromberg JE, Hau P, Mirimanoff RO, Cairncross JG, Janzer RC, Stupp R. MGMT gene silencing and benefit from temozolomide in glioblastoma. N Engl J Med. 2005;352(10):997–1003.

12. Bao S, Wu Q, McLendon RE, Hao Y, Shi Q, Hjelmeland AB, Dewhirst MW, Bigner DD, Rich JN. Glioma stem cells promote radioresistance by preferential activation of the DNA damage response. Nature. 2006;444:756–60.

13. Wang J, Wakeman TP, Lathia JD, Hjelmeland AB, Wang XF, White RR, Rich JN, Sullenger BA. Notch promotes radioresistance of glioma stem cells. Stem Cells. 2010;28:17–28.

14. Lee SW, Fraass BA, Marsh LH, Herbort K, Gebarski SS, Martel MK, Radany EH, Lichter AS, Sandler HM. Patterns of failure following high-dose 3-D conformal radiotherapy for high-grade astrocytomas: a quantitative dosimetric study. Int J Radiat Oncol Biol Phys. 1999;43(199):79–88.

15. Minniti G, Amelio D, Amichetti M, Salvati M, Muni R, Bozzao A, Lanzetta G, Scarpino S, Arcella A, Enrici RM. Patterns of failure and comparison of different target volume delineations in patients with glioblastoma treated with conformal radiotherapy plus concomitant and adjuvant temozolomide. Radiother Oncol. 2010;97(3):377–81.

16. Calabrese C, Poppleton H, Kocak M, Hogg TL, Fuller C, Hamner B, Oh EY, Gaber MW, Finklestein D, Allen M, Frank A, Bayazitov IT, Zakharenko SS, Gajjar A, Davidoff A, Gilbertson RJ. A perivascular niche for brain tumor stem cells. Cancer Cell. 2007;11(1):69–82.

17. Jamal M, Rath BH, Williams ES, Camphausen K, Tofilon PJ. Microenvironmental regulation of glioblastoma radioresponse. Clin Cancer Res. 2010;16(24):6049–59.

18. Nelson DF, Diener-West M, Horton J, Chang CH, Schoenfeld D, Nelson JS. Combined modality approach to treatment of malignant gliomas–re-evaluation of RTOG 7401/ECOG 1374 with long-term follow-up: a joint study of the Radiation Therapy Oncology Group and the Eastern Cooperative Oncology Group. NCI Monogr. 1988;6:279–84.

19. Hochberg FH, Pruitt A. Assumptions in the radiotherapy of glioblastoma. Neurology. 1980;30:907–11.

20. Wallner KE, Galicich JH, Krol G, Malkin MG, Arbit E. Patterns of failure following treatment for glioblastoma multiforme and anaplastic astrocytoma. Int J Radiat Oncol Biol Phys. 1989;16:1405–9.

21. Tsien C, Moughan J, Michalski JM, Gilbert MR, Purdy J, Simpson J, Kresel JJ, Curran WJ, Diaz A, Mehta MP, Radiation Therapy Oncology Group Trial 98-03. Phase I three-dimensional conformal radiation dose escalation study in newly diagnosed glioblastoma: Radiation Therapy Oncology Group Trial 98-03. Int J Radiat Oncol Biol Phys. 2009;73:699–708.

22. Chan JL, Lee SW, Fraass BA, Normolle DP, Greenberg HS, Junck LR, Gebarski SS, Sandler HM. Survival and failure patterns of high-grade gliomas after three-dimensional conformal radiotherapy. J Clin Oncol. 2002;20(6):1635–42.

23. Tsien CI, Brown D, Normolle D, Schipper M, Piert M, Junck L, Heth J, Gomez-Hassan D, Ten Haken RK, Chenevert T, Cao Y, Lawrence T. Concurrent temozolomide and dose-escalated intensity-modulated radiation therapy in newly diagnosed glioblastoma. Clin Cancer Res. 2012;18:273–9.

24. Iuchi T, Hatano K, Narita Y, Kodama T, Yamaki T, Osato K. Hypofractionated high-dose irradiation for the treatment of malignant astrocytomas using simultaneous integrated boost technique by IMRT. Int J Radiat Oncol Biol Phys. 2006;64:1317–24.

25. Chan MF, Schupak K, Burman C, Chui CS, Ling CC. Comparison of intensity-modulated radiotherapy with three-dimensional conformal radiation therapy planning for glioblastoma multiforme. Med Dosim. 2003;28:261–5.

26. Buglione M, Spiazzi L, Saiani F, Costa L, Shehi B, Lazzari B, Uccelli C, Pasinetti N, Borghetti P, Triggiani L, Donadoni L, Pedretti S, Magrini SM. Neuro-Oncology Group, Spedali Civili, Brescia University, Brescia, Italy. Three-dimensional conformal radiotherapy, static intensity-modulated and helical intensity-modulated radiotherapy in glioblastoma. Dosimetric comparison in patients with overlap between target volumes and organs at risk. Tumori. 2014;100(3): 272–7.

27. Badiyan SN, Markovina S, Simpson JR, Robinson CG, DeWees T, Tran DD, Linette G, Jalalizadeh R, Dacey R, Rich KM, Chicoine MR, Dowling JL, Leuthardt EC, Zipfel GJ, Kim AH, Huang J. Radiation Therapy Dose Escalation for Glioblastoma Multiforme in the Era of Temozolomide. Int J Radiat Oncol Biol Phys. 2014;90(4): 877–85. pii: S0360-3016(14)03493-2. doi: 10.1016/j.ijrobp.2014.07.014.

28. Scoccianti S, Magrini SM, Ricardi U, Detti B, Buglione M, Sotti G, Krengli M, Maluta S, Parisi S, Bertoni F, Mantovani C, Tombolini V, De Renzis C, Lioce M, Fatigante L, Fusco V, Muto P, Berti F, Rubino G, Cipressi S, Fariselli L, Lupattelli M, Santoni R, Pirtoli L, Biti G. Patterns of care and survival in a retrospective analysis of 1059 patients with glioblastoma multiforme treated between 2002 and 2007: a multicenter study by the Central Nervous System Study Group of Airo (Italian Association of Radiation Oncology). Neurosurgery. 2010;67(2):446–58.

29. Narayana A, Yamada J, Berry S, Shah P, Hunt M, Gutin PH, Leibel SA. Intensity-modulated radiotherapy in high-grade gliomas: clinical and dosimetric results. Int J Radiat Oncol Biol Phys. 2006;64:892–7.

30. Floyd NS, Woo SY, Teh BS, Prado C, Mai WY, Trask T, Gildenberg PL, Holoye P, Augspurger ME, Carpenter LS, Lu HH, Chiu JK, Grant 3rd WH, Butler

EB. Hypofractionated intensity-modulated radiotherapy for primary glioblastoma multiforme. Int J Radiat Oncol Biol Phys. 2004;58:721–6.

31. Payne DG, Simpson WJ, Keen C, Platts ME. Malignant astrocytoma: hyperfractionated and standard radiotherapy with chemotherapy in a randomized prospective clinical trial. Cancer. 1982;50(11):2301–6.

32. Douglas BG, Worth AJ. Superfractionation in glioblastoma multiforme-results of a phase II study. Int J Radiat Oncol Biol Phys. 1982;8(10):1787–94.

33. Fulton DS, Urtasun RC, Shin KH, Geggie PH, Thomas H, Muller PJ, Moody J, Tanasichuk H, Mielke B, Johnson E. Misonidazole combined with hyperfractionation in the management of malignant glioma. Int J Radiat Oncol Biol Phys. 1984;10(9):1709–12.

34. Shin KH, Muller PJ, Geggie PH. Superfractionation radiation therapy in the treatment of malignant astrocytoma. Cancer. 1983;52(11):2040–3.

35. Werner-Wasik M, Scott CB, Nelson DF, Gaspar LE, Murray KJ, Fischbach JA, Nelson JS, Weinstein AS, Curran Jr WJ. Final report of a phase I/II trial of hyperfractionated and accelerated hyperfractionated radiation therapy with carmustine for adults with supratentorial malignant gliomas. Radiation Therapy Oncology Group Study 83-02. Cancer. 1996;77(8):1535–43.

36. Scott C, Curran JW, Yung W, Scarantino C, Urtasun R, Movsas B, Jones C, Simpson J, Fischbach A, Petito C, Nelson J. Long term results of RTOG 9006: a randomized trial of hyperfractionated radiotherapy (RT) to 72.0 Gy & carmustine vs standard RT & carmustine for malignant glioma patients with emphasis on anaplastic astrocytoma (AA) patients [abstract]. Proc Ann Meet Am Soc Clin Oncol. 1998;17: 401a.

37. Curran Jr WJ, Scott CB, Nelson JS, Weinstein AS, Phillips TL, Murray K, Fischbach AJ, Yakar D, Schwade JG, Powlis WD. A randomized trial of accelerated hyperfractionated radiation therapy and bis-chloroethyl nitrosourea for malignant glioma. A preliminary report of Radiation Therapy Oncology Group 83-02. Cancer. 1992;70(12):2909–17.

38. Prados MD, Wara WM, Sneed PK, McDermott M, Chang SM, Rabbitt J, Page M, Malec M, Davis RL, Gutin PH, Lamborn K, Wilson CB, Phillips TL, Larson DA. Phase III trial of accelerated hyperfractionation with or without difluromethylornithine (DFMO) versus standard fractionated radiotherapy with or without DFMO for newly diagnosed patients with glioblastoma multiforme. Int J Radiat Oncol Biol Phys. 2001;49(1):71–7.

39. Mehta MP, Masciopinto J, Rozental J, Levin A, Chappell R, Bastin K, Miles J, Turski P, Kubsad S, Mackie T. Stereotactic radiosurgery for glioblastoma multiforme: report of a prospective study evaluating prognostic factors and analyzing long-term survival advantage. Int J Radiat Oncol Biol Phys. 1994;30(3):541–9.

40. Loeffler JS, Alexander E, Shea WM, Wen PY, Fine HA, Kooy HM, Black PM. Radiosurgery as part of the initial management of patients with malignant gliomas. J Clin Oncol. 1992;10(9):1379–85.

41. Sarkaria JN, Mehta MP, Loeffler JS, Buatti JM, Chappell RJ, Levin AB, et al. Radiosurgery in the initial management of malignant gliomas: survival comparison with the RTOG recursive partitioning analysis. Radiation Therapy Oncology Group. Int J Radiat Oncol Biol Phys. 1995;32(4):931–41.

42. Souhami L, Seiferheld W, Brachman D, et al. Randomized comparison of stereotactic radiosurgery followed by conventional radiotherapy with carmustine to conventional radiotherapy with carmustine for patients with glioblastoma multiforme: report of Radiation Therapy Oncology Group 93-05 protocol. Int J Radiat Oncol Biol Phys. 2004;60:853–60.

43. Van Kampen M, Engenhart-Cabillic R, Debus J, Fuss M, Rhein B, Wannenmacher M. The radiosurgery of glioblastoma multiforme in cases of recurrence. The Heidelberg experiences compared to the literature [in German]. Strahlenther Onkol. 1998;174:19–24.

44. Combs SE, Widmer V, Thilmann C, Hof H, Debus J, Schulz-Ertner D. Stereotactic radiosurgery (SRS): treatment option for recurrent glioblastoma multiforme (GBM). Cancer. 2005;104(10):2168–73.

45. Chamberlain MC, Barba D, Kormanik P, Shea WM. Stereotactic radiosurgery for recurrent gliomas. Cancer. 1994;74:1342–7.

46. Lawrence YR, Li XA, el Naqa I, Hahn CA, Marks LB, Merchant TE, Dicker AP. Radiation dose-volume effects in the brain. Int J Radiat Oncol Biol Phys. 2010;1:76.

47. Laperriere NJ, Leung PM, McKenzie S, Milosevic M, Wong S, Glen J, Pintilie M, Bernstein M. Randomized study of brachytherapy in the initial management of patients with malignant astrocytoma. Int J Radiat Oncol Biol Phys. 1998;41(5):1005–11.

48. Selker RG, Shapiro WR, Burger P, Blackwood MS, Arena VC, Gilder JC, Malkin MG, Mealey Jr JJ, Neal JH, Olson J, Robertson JT, Barnett GH, Bloomfield S, Albright R, Hochberg FH, Hiesiger E, Green S. The Brain Tumor Cooperative Group NIH Trial 87–01: a randomized comparison of surgery, external radiotherapy, and carmustine versus surgery, interstitial radiotherapy boost, external radiation therapy and carmustine. Neurosurgery. 2002;51(2):343 55; discussion 355–347.

49. Voges J, Treuer H, Schlegel W, Pastyr O, Sturm V. Interstitial irradiation of cerebral gliomas with stereotactically implanted iodine-125 seeds. Acta Neurochir Suppl (Wien). 1993;58:108–11.

50. Voges J, Sturm VV. Interstitial irradiation with stereotactically implanted I-125 seeds for the treatment of cerebral glioma. Crit Rev Neurosurg. 1999;9(4):223–33.

51. Gutin PH, Prados MD, Phillips TL, Wara WM, Larson DA, Leibel SA, Sneed PK, Levin VA, Weaver KA, Silver P, et al. External irradiation followed by an interstitial high activity iodine-125 implant "boost" in the initial treatment of malignant gliomas: NCOG

study 6G-82-2. Int J Radiat Oncol Biol Phys. 1991;21(3):601–6.

52. Shapiro WR, Green SB, Burger PC, Mahaley Jr MS, Selker RG, VanGilder JC, Robertson JT, Ransohoff J, Mealey Jr J, Strike TA, et al. Randomized trial of three chemotherapy regimens and two radiotherapy regimens and two radiotherapy regimens in postoperative treatment of malignant glioma. Brain Tumor Cooperative Group Trial 8001. J Neurosurg. 1989;71(1):1–9.

53. Soussain C, Ricard D, Fike JR, Mazeron JJ, Psimaras D, Delattre JY. CNS complications of radiotherapy and chemotherapy. Lancet. 2009;374(9701):1639–51.

54. McDonald MW, Shu HK, Curran Jr WJ, Crocker IR. Pattern of failure after limited margin radiotherapy and temozolomide for glioblastoma. Int J Radiat Oncol Biol Phys. 2011;1:79(1).

55. Brandes AA, Tosoni A, Franceschi E, Sotti G, Frezza G, Amistà P, Morandi L, Spagnolli F, Ermani M. Recurrence pattern after temozolomide concomitant with and adjuvant to radiotherapy in newly diagnosed patients with glioblastoma: correlation with MGMT promoter methylation status. J Clin Oncol. 2009;27(8):1275–9.

56. Halperin EC, Bentel G, Heinz ER, Burger PC. Radiation therapy treatment planning in supratentorial glioblastoma multiforme: an analysis based on post mortem topographic anatomy with CT correlations. Int J Radiat Oncol Biol Phys. 1989;17:1347–50.

57. Burger PC, Dubois PJ, Schold Jr SC, Smith Jr KR, Odom GL, Crafts DC, Giangaspero F. Computerized tomographic and pathologic studies of the untreated, quiescent, and recurrent glioblastoma multiforme. J Neurosurg. 1983;58:159–69.

58. McKnight TR, dem Bussche MH, Vigneron DB, Lu Y, Berger MS, McDermott MW, Dillon WP, Graves EE, Pirzkall A, Nelson SJ. Histopathological validation of a three-dimensional magnetic resonance spectroscopy index as a predictor of tumor presence. J Neurosurg. 2002;97(4):794–802.

59. Ken S, Vieillevigne L, Franceries X, Simon L, Supper C, Lotterie JA, Filleron T, Lubrano V, Berry I, Cassol E, Delannes M, Celsis P, Cohen-Jonathan EM, Laprie A. Integration method of 3D MR spectroscopy into treatment planning system for glioblastoma IMRT dose painting with integrated simultaneous boost. Radiat Oncol. 2013;8:1. doi:10.1186/1748-717X-8-1.

60. Einstein DB, Wessels B, Bangert B, Fu P, Nelson AD, Cohen M, Sagar S, Lewin J, Sloan A, Zheng Y, Williams J, Colussi V, Vinkler R, Maciunas R. Phase II trial of radiosurgery to magnetic resonance spectroscopy-defined high-risk tumor volumes in patients with glioblastoma multiforme. Int J Radiat Oncol Biol Phys. 2012;84(3):668–74. doi:10.1016/j.ijrobp.2012.01.020.

61. Philipp K, Franziska D, Tobias B, Matthias S, Martin K, Norbert G, Maximilian R. Differentiation of local tumor recurrence from radiation-induced changes after stereotactic radiosurgery for treatment of brain metastasis:

case report and review of the literature. Radiat Oncol. 2013;8:52. doi:10.1186/1748-717X-8-52.

62. Jacobs AH, Thomas A, Kracht LW, Li H, Dittmar C, Garlip G, Galldiks N, Klein JC, Sobesky J, Hilker R, Vollmar S, Herholz K, Wienhard K, Heiss WD. 18F-fluoro-l-thymidine and 11C-methylmethionine as markers of increased transport and proliferation in brain tumors. J Nucl Med. 2005;46(12):1948–58.

63. Piroth MD, Pinkawa M, Holy R, Klotz J, Schaar S, Stoffels G, Galldiks N, Coenen HH, Kaiser HJ, Langen KJ, Eble MJ. Integrated boost IMRT with FET-PET-adapted local dose escalation in glioblastomas. Results of a prospective phase II study. Strahlenther Onkol. 2012;188(4):334–9.

64. Verhaak RG, Hoadley KA, Purdom E, Wang V, Qi Y, Wilkerson MD, Miller CR, Ding L, Golub T, Mesirov JP, Alexe G, Lawrence M, O'Kelly M, Tamayo P, Weir BA, Gabriel S, Winckler W, Gupta S, Jakkula L, Feiler HS, Hodgson JG, James CD, Sarkaria JN, Brennan C, Kahn A, Spellman PT, Wilson RK, Speed TP, Gray JW, Meyerson M, Getz G, Perou CM, Hayes DN, Cancer Genome Atlas Research Network. Integrated genomic analysis identifies clinically relevant subtypes of glioblastoma characterized by abnormalities in PDGFRA, IDH1, EGFR, and NF1. Cancer Cell. 2010;17(1):98–110. doi:10.1016/j.ccr.2009.12.020.

65. Rich JN, Reardon DA, Peery T, Dowell JM, Quinn JA, Penne KL, Wikstrand CJ, Van Duyn LB, Dancey JE, McLendon RE, Kao JC, Stenzel TT, Ahmed Rasheed BK, Tourt-Uhlig SE, Herndon 2nd JE, Vredenburgh JJ, Sampson JH, Friedman AH, Bigner DD, Friedman HS. Phase II trial of gefitinib in recurrent glioblastoma. J Clin Oncol. 2004;22(1):133–42.

66. Prados MD, Lamborn KR, Chang S, Burton E, Butowski N, Malec M, Kapadia A, Rabbitt J, Page MS, Fedoroff A, Xie D, Kelley SK. Phase 1 study of erlotinib HCl alone and combined with temozolomide in patients with stable or recurrent malignant glioma. Neuro Oncol. 2006;8(1):67–78.

67. Chakravarti A, Wang M, Robins HI, Lautenschlaeger T, Curran WJ, Brachman DG, Schultz CJ, Choucair A, Dolled-Filhart M, Christiansen J, Gustavson M, Molinaro A, Mischel P, Dicker AP, Bredel M, Mehta M. RTOG 0211: a phase 1/2 study of radiation therapy with concurrent gefitinib for newly diagnosed glioblastoma patients. Int J Radiat Oncol Biol Phys. 2013;85(5):1206–11. doi:10.1016/j.ijrobp.2012.10.008.

68. Qaddoumi I, Kocak M, Pai Panandiker AS, Armstrong GT, Wetmore C, Crawford JR, Lin T, Boyett JM, Kun LE, Boop FA, Merchant TE, Ellison DW, Gajjar A, Broniscer A. Phase II trial of Erlotinib during and after radiotherapy in children with newly diagnosed high-grade gliomas. Front Oncol. 2014;4:67. doi:10.3389/fonc.2014.00067.

69. Jain RK, di Tomaso E, Duda DG, Loeffler JS, Sorensen AG, Batchelor TT. Angiogenesis in brain tumours. Nat Rev Neurosci. 2007;8(8):610–22.

70. Mark R. Gilbert, James Dignam, Minhee Won, Deborah T. Blumenthal, Michael A. Vogelbaum, Kenneth D. Aldape, Howard Colman, Arnab Chakravarti, Robert Jeraj, Terri S. Armstrong, Jeffrey Scott Wefel, Paul D. Brown, Kurt A. Jaeckle, David Schiff, James Norman Atkins, David Brachman, Maria Werner-Wasik, Ritsuko Komaki, Erik P. Sulman and Minesh P. Mehta. RTOG 0825: Phase III double-blind placebo-controlled trial evaluating bevacizumab (Bev) in patients (Pts) with newly diagnosed glioblastoma (GBM). 2013 ASCO Annual Meeting. Abstract 1. Presented June 2, 2013.

71. Chinot OL, de La Motte RT, Moore N, Zeaiter A, Das A, Phillips H, Modrusan Z, Cloughesy T. AVAglio: Phase 3 trial of bevacizumab plus temozolomide and radiotherapy in newly diagnosed glioblastoma multiforme. Adv Ther. 2011;28(4):334–40. doi:10.1007/s12325-011-0007-3.

72. Friedman HS, Prados MD, Wen PY, Mikkelsen T, Schiff D, Abrey LE, Yung WK, Paleologos N, Nicholas MK, Jensen R, Vredenburgh J, Huang J, Zheng M. Cloughesy T.J Bevacizumab alone and in combination with irinotecan in recurrent glioblastoma. Clin Oncol. 2009;27(28):4733–40. doi:10.1200/JCO.2008.19.8721.

73. Kreisl TN, Kim L, Moore K, Duic P, Royce C, Stroud I, Garren N, Mackey M, Butman JA, Camphausen K, Park J, Albert PS, Fine HA. Phase II trial of single-agent bevacizumab followed by bevacizumab plus irinotecan at tumor progression in recurrent glioblastoma. J Clin Oncol. 2009;27(5):740–5. doi:10.1200/JCO.2008.16.3055.

74. Levin VA, Bidaut L, Hou P, Kumar AJ, Wefel JS, Bekele BN, Prabhu S, Loghin M, Gilbert MR, Jackson EF. Randomized double-blind placebo-controlled trial of bevacizumab therapy for radiation necrosis of the CNS. Int J Radiat Oncol Biol Phys. 2011;79(5):1487–95.

75. Brandes AA, Stupp R, Hau P, Lacombe D, Gorlia T, Tosoni A, Mirimanoff RO, Kros JM, van den Bent MJ. EORTC study 26041-22041: phase I/II study on concomitant and adjuvant temozolomide (TMZ) and radiotherapy (RT) with PTK787/ZK222584 (PTK/ZK) in newly diagnosed glioblastoma. Eur J Cancer. 2010;46(2):348–54. doi:10.1016/j.ejca.2009.10.029.

76. Den RB, Kamrava M, Sheng Z. A phase I study of the combination of sorafenib with temozolomide and radiation therapy for the treatment of primary and recurrent high-grade gliomas. Int J Radiat Oncol Biol Phys. 2013;85(2):321–8.

77. Delmas C, Heliez C, Cohen-Jonathan E, End D, Bonnet J, Favre G, Toulas C. Farnesyltransferase inhibitor, R115777, reverses the resistance of human glioma cell lines to ionizing radiation. Int J Cancer. 2002;100(1):43–8.

78. Ducassou A, Uro-Coste E, Verrelle P, Filleron T, Benouaich-Amiel A, Lubrano V, Sol JC, Delisle MB, Favre G, Ken S, Laprie A, De Porre P, Toulas C, Poublanc M, Cohen-Jonathan ME. αvβ3 Integrin and fibroblast growth factor receptor 1 (FGFR1): prognostic factors in a phase I-II clinical trial associating continuous administration of tipifarnib with radiotherapy for patients with newly diagnosed glioblastoma. Eur J Cancer. 2013; 49(9):2161–9. doi:10.1016/j.ejca.2013.02.033.

79. Stupp R, Hegi ME, Gorlia T, Erridge SC, Perry J, Hong YK, Aldape KD, Lhermitte B, Pietsch T, Grujicic D, Steinbach JP, Wick W, Tarnawski R, Nam DH, Hau P, Weyerbrock A, Taphoorn MJ, Shen CC, Rao N, Thurzo L, Herrlinger U, Gupta T, Kortmann RD, Adamska K, McBain C, Brandes AA, Tonn JC, Schnell O, Wiegel T, Kim CY, Nabors LB, Reardon DA, van den Bent MJ, Hicking C, Markivskyy A, Picard M, Weller M. Cilengitide combined with standard treatment for patients with newly diagnosed glioblastoma with methylated MGMT promoter (CENTRIC EORTC 26071-22072 study): a multicentre, randomised, open-label, phase 3 trial. Lancet Oncol. 2014;15(10):1100–8. doi:10.1016/S1470-2045(14)70379-1.

80. Deng L, Liang H, Burnette B, Beckett M, Darga T, Weichselbaum RR, Fu YX. Irradiation and anti-PD-L1 treatment synergistically promote antitumor immunity in mice. J Clin Invest. 2014;124(2):687–95. doi:10.1172/JCI67313.

# Radiobiological Hints from Clinical Studies

3

Silvia Scoccianti, Riccardo Santoni, Beatrice Detti,
Gianluca Ingrosso, Daniela Greto,
and Giulio Francolini

## Introduction

Glioblastoma (GBM) is the most common primary brain tumor in adults. The standard treatment is surgery followed by radiotherapy plus concomitant and sequential temozolomide. Despite multimodality treatment, the prognosis is still poor and the median overall survival (mOS) among patients with newly diagnosed glioblastoma is in the range of 12–15 months. Outcome for recurrent GBM (rGBM) is even worse with a mOS of 6 months with conventional salvage therapies.

Several microenvironmental factors influence the residual tumor cells after surgery, making them acquire the traits of cancer stem cells (high self-renewal capacity and DNA-breakage repair capacity). These cells are able to resist to radiochemotherapy, to proliferate and, lastly, to result in the recurrent disease. A growing body of data indicate a crucial role for intercellular communication in the tumor stroma interface in GBM development and therapy refractoriness [1]. Cross-talks between microglia or endothelium and glioma contribute to tumor growth and invasion. Recently, several targeted agents have been developed as potential inhibitors of molecular genetic and signal transduction pathways involved in the resistance to radiation therapy-induced damage, including those of VEGF (Vascular Endothelial Growth Factor), EGFR (Epidermal Growth Factor Receptor), integrin signaling, and mTOR (mammalian target of rapamycin) signaling. Some of these agents have been tested in clinical studies in association with radiotherapy. In this chapter, we provide a brief overview of the clinical series with the most important targeted agents against glioblastoma, focusing on the experiences in which they are used together with radiotherapy. Moreover, hypothetical causes for failures of targeted therapies for glioblastoma are listed.

## VEGF Antagonists

Blocking of proangiogenic mechanisms may improve the radiotherapy efficacy. GBM angiogenesis is driven mainly by VEGF signaling through its tyrosine kinase receptor VEGFR2/KDR. Blockade of VEGF with bevacizumab (a humanized monoclonal antibody against VEGF) was associated with good response rates in clinical trials in patients with rGBM.

Positive outcomes have been obtained with the addition of bevacizumab (BEV) to radiotherapy

S. Scoccianti (✉) • B. Detti • D. Greto • G. Francolini
Radiation Oncology Unit, Azienda Ospedaliero—
Universitaria Careggi, Florence, Italy
e-mail: silvia.scoccianti@unifi.it

R. Santoni • G. Ingrosso
Radiation Oncology Unit, University of Rome
"Tor Vergata", Rome, Italy

© Springer International Publishing Switzerland 2016
L. Pirtoli et al. (eds.), *Radiobiology of Glioblastoma*, Current Clinical Pathology,
DOI 10.1007/978-3-319-28305-0_3

in the recurrent setting (see Table 3.1). Radiotherapy technique varied from single session radiosurgery to conventionally fractionated radiotherapy. Median survival ranged between 8.4 and 34.2 months. The majority of these trials are retrospective; all of them included patients with other high-grade gliomas (HGG) and some of them included also patients with relapsing low-grade gliomas (LGG). Rate of severe toxicity was inferior to 15 % of the cases. The ongoing RTOG 1205 trial aims to confirm the advantages of the addition of BEV to re-irradiation in the relapsing GBM in a prospective setting.

Based on these clinical experiences, two phase-III trials for assessing the role of bevacizumab in addition to standard radiotherapy and temozolomide in newly diagnosed patients were opened (RTOG 0825 trial [9] and AVAGLIO trial [10]). Both these trials found significant improvement in terms of progression-free survival (PFS) (RTOG 0825 trial: bevacizumab + standard therapy arm: median PFS 10.7 months; standard therapy: median PFS 7.3 months; AVAGLIO trial: bevacizumab + standard therapy arm: median PFS 10.6 months; standard therapy: median PFS 6.2 months) but both of them failed in demonstrating advantages in terms of overall survival (RTOG 0825 trial: bevacizumab + standard therapy arm: mOS 15.7 months; standard therapy: mOS 16.1 months; AVAGLIO trial: bevacizumab + standard therapy arm: mOS 16.8 months; standard therapy: mOS 16.7 months).

The reasons why anti-VEGF therapy failed in improving overall survival are still under investigation. A study on autoptic specimens of patients treated with cediranib, a pan-VEGFR tyrosine kinase inhibitor, showed a change in growth pattern of rGBM after antiangiogenic treatment [11]. The recurrence after anti-VEGF treatment is not characterized by a second wave of angiogenesis because tumor endothelial cells expressed molecular markers specific to the blood–brain barrier, indicative of a lack of revascularization despite the discontinuation of therapy. In addition, lower tumor cellularity,

decreased pseudopalisading necrosis, and blood vessels with normal molecular expression and morphology were found. So, this study demonstrated that, rGBM after antiangiogenic therapy, instead of switching to alternative angiogenesis pathways, exhibit a more infiltrative phenotype. A reasonable hypothesis is that anti-VEGF therapy could be efficient in blocking tumor growth due to neoangiogenesis but it is not efficient in blocking tumor growth due to the co-opting of preexisting vessels or due to the generation of new vessels through the colonization of circulating endothelial cells, in a process called "vasculogenesis". Preclinical evidence pointed toward a key role for treatment-induced recruitment of protumor bone marrow–derived cells (BMDCs) [12]. These cells may differentiate in endothelial progenitors and produce new vessels. The recruitment of BMDCs into the tumor is mainly mediated by the interaction between a chemokine called SDF-1 and its receptor, CXCR4 [13]. The pharmacological inhibition of this interaction is possible through a drug called AMD3100. The ongoing trial NCT01339039 is currently testing this agent in addition to BEV in recurrent HGG. Among myeloid BMDCs, tumor-associated macrophages (TAMs) have been shown to mediate escape from antiangiogenic therapy in preclinical models. TAMs may promote tumor progression and spread despite vascular targeting. Lu-Emerson et al. examined the role of macrophages in patients with recurrent glioblastoma, comparing autopsy brain specimens from patients with recurrent glioblastoma who received antiangiogenic treatment with brain specimens from patients who did not receive antiangiogenic therapy [14]. Among the antiangiogenic-treated patients, an increase of macrophages both in the tumor bulk and infiltrative areas was shown. Of note, an increased number of macrophages correlated with poor overall survival. These data suggest that among bone marrow-derived cells, TAMs may represent a potential biomarker of resistance and a potential therapeutic target in recurrent glioblastoma.

**Table 3.1** Clinical studies of bevacizumab (BEV) plus radiotherapy in relapsing high-grade gliomas (HGG)

| | Radiotherapy technique | Pt number | Histology | Median dose (Gy) | Median fraction dose (Gy) | Overall survival, OS (months) | Progression-free survival, PFS (months) | Rate of severe toxicity (%) |
|---|---|---|---|---|---|---|---|---|
| Gutin et al. [2] | Hypofractionated stereotactic radiotherapy | 25 (20 GBM) | HGG | 30 | 6 | Median OS 12.5 months Actuarial 12-months OS 54 % | Actuarial 6-months-PFS 65 % | 12 |
| Cuneo et al. [3] | Radiosurgery | 63 (49 GBM) | HGG | 15 | 15 | Median OS 10 months Actuarial 12-months OS 50 % | Median PFS 6 months | 10–14 |
| Shapiro et al. [4] | Hypofractionated stereotactic radiotherapy | 24 (20 GBM) | HGG | 30 | 6 | Median 12.2 months | Median PFS 6.8 months | 11 |
| Niyazi et al. [5] | 3D conformal radiotherapy | 30 (21 GBM) | HGG LGG | 36 | 2 | Median 10.3 months | Median PFS 6.3 months | 6 |
| Fliegerr et al. [6] | 3D conformal radiotherapy or IMRT | 71 (52 GBM) | HGG | 36 | 2 | Median 34.2 months | Median PFS 5.6 months | 7 |
| Hundsberger et al. [7] | 3D conformal radiotherapy or IMRT | 14 (8 GBM) | HGG LGG | 41.6 | 2.66 | Median 8.4 months | Median PFS 5.7 months | 14 |
| Cabrera et al. [8] | Hypofractionated stereotactic radiotherapy | 15 (8 GBM) | HGG | 21.5 | 24/18/5 | Median 14.4 months | Median PFS 3.9 months | 6.7 |
| Shapiro et al. [4] | Hypofractionated stereotactic radiotherapy | 24 (20 GBM) | HGG | 30 | 5 | Median 32.1 months | Median PFS 7.5 months | 12.5 |

## EGFR Antagonists

EGFR represents an attractive molecular target in patient with HGG because overexpression of this receptor is present in 40–50 % of patients with GBM. EGFR signaling results in an increase in GBM cell invasion, infiltration, and proliferation and lead to inhibition of apoptosis and induction of angiogenesis [15]. Furthermore, the presence of EGFRvIII mutant (a pathological variation of EGFR with a constitutively activated extracellular domain) has been demonstrated in glioma stem cells and it defines HGG with a worse prognosis [16], whereas high EGFR expression is an independent prognostic factor in GBM treated with standard therapy [16, 17]. Moreover, EGFR overexpression in GBM correlates with radioresistance [17–19].

EGFR signaling can be inhibited with small-molecule tyrosine kinase inhibitors such as erlotinib (Tarceva) and gefitinib (Iressa) or with targeted monoclonal antibodies (mAb) such as cetuximab and nimotuzumab.

Erlotinib is a inhibitor of EGFR tyrosine kinase with antitumor activity in lung and pancreatic cancer. In preclinical studies in GBM cell lines, this agent had activity against cell lines that harbor the EGFRvIII mutant receptor [20], whereas in phase-I or -II studies erlotinib was shown to have some antitumor activity in rGBM [21, 22].

In the recent years, two phase-II studies tested erlotinib together with TMZ and radiotherapy in newly diagnosed GBM, obtaining conflicting results.

Prados et al. [23] reported about the addition of erlotinib to RT+TMZ in a phase-II trial that enrolled 65 patients: the median survival of 19.3 months was better than that reported for historical controls. On the contrary, Peereboom et al. [24] did not confirm the efficacy of erlotinib in combination with the standard regimen of concurrent RT and TMZ in 27 patients with newly diagnosed GBM enrolled in a phase-II trial. Authors concluded that erlotinib was not an efficient agent (median PFS 2.8 months, median OS 8.6 months) and had an unacceptable toxicity

(four treatment-related deaths) that caused early closure of the trial.

The RTOG 0211 [25] trial tried to determine the efficacy of gefitinib in combination with radiotherapy for newly diagnosed GBM. Treatment consisted of daily oral gefitinib during the radiotherapy and after radiation treatment for 18 months or until progression. Gefitinib did not add any advantage in terms of survival: median survival of these patients was similar to that in a historical control cohort treated with RT alone.

The use of cetuximab, a chimeric IgG monoclonal antibody that targets the extracellular domain of the EGFR, is supported by preclinical models. This agent seems to be more efficient in inhibiting the EGFRvIII mutant as compared with small EGFR inhibitors. The capability of crossing the blood–brain barrier is demonstrated by some phase-I trials that showed the presence of these mAb within resected glioma tissues. Belda-Iniesta et al. [26] showed long-term responses for cetuximab in three cases of recurrent glioblastoma. Neyns et al. [27] conducted a phase-II trial in which patients were stratified according to the amplification status of the EGFR gene. This trial showed not only the absence of a significant correlation between outcome and EGFR amplification status but also that cetuximab has a low activity in patients with relapsing HGG [only 5 out of 55 patients (9 %) had a durable disease control (longer than 9 months) and improved overall survival].

Given the synergistic effect of EGFR inhibition with cetuximab and RT, further investigations of the use of cetuximab in association with radiotherapy in the treatment of newly diagnosed GBM are needed. Interim results of a phase I/II study of chemoradiation therapy with temozolomide and cetuximab in patients with newly diagnosed GBM [28] showed promising outcome in terms of PFS (PFS at 6 months=81 %, PFS at 12 months=37 %), as well as overall survival (OS at 12 months=87 %).

Some recent studies reported conflicting results obtained with nimotuzumab, a humanized monoclonal antibody against EGFR, used in combination with RT±TMZ. Wang et al. [29]

did not find any advantage in terms of survival in 26 patients with newly diagnosed GBM treated with nimotuzumab, RT, and TMZ, whereas Solomon et al. [30] found a survival gain after combining nimotuzumab and radiotherapy in a series of 35 HGG. Nimotuzumab showed a trend towards efficacy in the subgroup of MGMT non-methylated GBM patients when tested in 142 patients enrolled in a phase-III trial for newly diagnosed glioblastoma, in addition to standard radiotherapy and temozolomide [31].

Some predictive factors for response to tyrosine kinase inhibitors have been identified for other types of cancer (mutations in the tyrosine kinase pocket [32], EGFR copy-number [33], Akt activation [34]). Unfortunately, prospective trials did not show such a relationship in glioblastoma. In a phase-II trial of gefitinib in patients with relapsing GBM [35], EGFR protein expression and gene status and EGFRvIII protein expression were not associated with response or survival. Similarly, EGFR copy-number, Akt activation, and protein expression did not have a predictive role in another prospective trial that tested the use of gefitinib in recurrent HGG [36]. No association has been found between the expression of EGFRvIII and PTEN in GBM patients by Gallego et al. [37] who performed a prospective trial and showed that erlotinib had minimal efficacy also in patients with high protein expression for EGFRvIII and PTEN. EGFR amplification and EGFRvIII expression did not have any impact on the response rate to erlotinib in the 26034 trial by EORTC [38].

In conclusion, EGFR inhibitors have shown only moderate clinical activity when used as single agents in patients with GBM. Definition of molecular biomarkers as determinants to EGFR inhibitors response in GBM is crucial in order to select patients who might benefit from therapy: further prospective trials with standardized methods for assessment of molecular markers are strongly required.

The poor efficacy of EGFR inhibitors can also be explained with the fact that glioblastoma has a very complex signaling network that is not only driven by EGFR. Since alternative kinase signaling pathways may be activated in GBM cells, the

inhibition of a single tyrosine kinase inhibitor may not be sufficient to significantly block downstream oncogenic signaling.

## Inhibition of Integrins Signaling

Integrins are a family of cell–cell and cell–extracellular matrix adhesion molecules mediating the interaction of tumor cells with their microenvironment. Hereby, integrins transmit molecular signals influencing processes involved in tumor angiogenesis and invasion such as cell shape, survival, proliferation, and migration. Moreover, integrins have a role in the regulation of apoptosis because integrin-mediated adhesion promotes cell survival [39].

In particular, $\alpha v\beta 3$ and $\alpha v\beta 5$ integrins, involved both in angiogenesis and cell migration and proliferation, are expressed at low levels in normal cells and overexpressed in some malignancies such as melanoma, breast, prostate, and pancreatic cancer cells [40, 41]; therefore, integrins have been considered as a promising therapeutic target [42] because their patterns in cancer cells differ from those of their parent tissues, potentially allowing selective targeting.

In glioblastoma, overexpression of $\alpha v\beta 3$ and $\alpha v\beta 5$ integrin is well documented as well [43–45].

Integrin inhibitors are expected to normalize the tumor vasculature through an antiangiogenic mechanism, and they are also expected to enhance the effects of radiation therapy and chemotherapy [46].

In the preclinical glioma models and in vivo studies, integrin antagonists were shown to induce apoptosis of glioma cells and efficiently enhance the effect of radiotherapy [47, 48].

Abdollahi et al. [49] tested the interaction of radiotherapy and integrin antagonist, showing that the radiosensitivity of endothelial cells was enhanced by the concurrent administration of the integrin antagonist.

For those reasons the combination of integrin antagonists and radiotherapy was thought to represent a rational approach in glioma treatment. Cilengitide is an inhibitor of both integrin receptors αvβ3 and αvβ5 [50–52] competitively blocking binding of integrin ligands and it was tested for the treatment of newly diagnosed and recurrent glioblastoma. Objective and durable responses in patients with glioblastoma were shown in phase-I [53, 54] and -II trials. Reardon et al. [55] conducted a phase-II trial to assess the efficacy of cilengitide in 81 patients with relapsing glioblastoma, obtaining a PFS at 6 months of 10–15 % and a median OS ranging between 6.5 and 9 months. Two years later, the authors reported updated results on survival, showing a 4-year survival rate of 2.4 in patients treated with the lower dose, and 10.0 % in patients treated with higher dose of cilengitide [56]. More recently, similar outcomes in terms of PFS were obtained by Gilbert et al. [57].

In 2009 Nabors et al. reported a phase-II randomized trial evaluating lower (500 mg) and higher (2000 mg) doses cilengitide plus standard temozolomide and radiotherapy in newly diagnosed glioblastoma patients; they showed a median survival of 18.9 months [58].

The addition of cilengitide to radiotherapy and temozolomide in patients with newly diagnosed glioblastoma was shown to improve the outcome in patients with methylated MGMT gene promoter in a phase-I/II trial [59], suggesting a synergy between cilengitide and temozolomide chemotherapy in chemosensitive tumors.

Unfortunately, the promising activity of cilengitide was not confirmed in a recently published randomised phase-III trial: the addition of cilengitide (dose of 2000 mg intravenously twice weekly on days 1 and four concomitantly to radiotherapy and standard temozolomide, followed by maintenance cilengitide, for non-progressive patients, up to 18 months) did not significantly improve outcome in the enrolled 545 patients with newly diagnosed glioblastoma with methylated MGMT gene promoter [60]. This trial was limited to patients with methylated MGMT promoter, based mainly on a slightly increased cilengitide activity in this subgroup compared with patients with unmethylated MGMT promoter [61]. Neither progression-free survival nor overall survival was significantly prolonged, and the authors stated that an HR of

1.02 for overall survival suggests absence of any activity.

The reasons why the phase-III trial failed in confirming the antitumor activity of cilengitide that was shown in phase-I and -II trials may be various.

First of all, unfavorable pharmacokinetics of the drug may partly explain these negative results. A different schedule of administration of the drug may be more efficient: for example a continuous administration may be more appropriate to fulfill a proper antiangiogenic pressure considering the short serum half-life of cilengitide (about 2–4 h) [60, 61]. Indeed, low doses of cilengitide have been even reported to have proangiogenic activity in experimental tumor models, by contrast with inhibition at higher doses [62].

Second, some errors in the assessment of the imaging with overestimation of the results could be done in the previous trials because cilengitide might induce some normalization of the blood–brain barrier, suggesting a false response [60].

Third, it is noteworthy that the phase-II trials conducted in glioblastoma did not have a control group without cilengitide and this could be an important point to explain why the positive results noted in phase-II trials did not translate into the findings of the phase-III trial.

Finally, the restriction to patients with methylated MGMT promoter is not based on robust data and it may worsen the results, since a phase-II trial showed that cilengitide activity was irrespective of MGMT status. [63].

## Mammalian Target of Rapamycin Inhibitors

Changes in genomic, transcriptional, and post-transcriptional levels of proteins and protein kinases and their transcriptional factor effectors contribute to the inherent resistance of cancer to radiotherapy and chemotherapy [64]. The phosphatase and tensin homologue deleted in chromosome ten (PTEN)/phosphatidylinositol 3′ kinase (PI3K)/Akt/mammalian targets of rapamycin (mTOR)/nuclear factor kappa B

(NF-kB) and other signaling cascades play a critical role in the transmission of signals from growth factor receptors to regulate gene expression and prevent cell death [65]. In particular, PI3K/Akt and mTOR could be considered as a single pathway interacting with many other pathways. The activity of the PI3K/Akt and the mTOR pathway is often constitutively upregulated in tumors as a result of excessive stimulation by growth factor receptors, as well as mutation in the PTEN tumor suppressor gene regulating the PI3K-dependent activation of Akt signaling [66].

Mammalian target of rapamycin is a serine/threonine kinase ubiquitously expressed in mammalian cells and is a key protein evolutionarily conserved, indeed embryonic mutations in mTOR proved to be lethal. In normal cells, mTOR is controlled by positive and negative upstream regulators. Positive regulators include growth factors and their receptors, such as the members of the human epidermal growth factor receptor (HER) family and associated ligands, and vascular endothelial growth factor receptors (VEGFRs) and their ligands, which transmit signals to mTOR through the PI3K/Akt. Negative regulators of mTOR activity include PTEN that inhibits signaling through the PI3K/Akt pathway and the tuberous sclerosis complex (TSC) 1 (hamartin) and TSC2 (tuberin). Another negative regulator, LKB1, is in an energy-sensing pathway upstream to TSC. Mammalian target of rapamycin activity is carried out by two distinct complexes: mTORC1 and mTORC2. The mTORC1 complex is made up of mTOR, Raptor, mLST8, and PRAS40. It is extremely sensitive to rapamycin and thus represents the target of first generation mTOR inhibitors. It also activates S6K and inactivates 4EBP1, leading to protein translation and cell growth. The mTORC2 complex is composed of mTOR, Rictor, Sin1, and mLST8. It is less sensitive to rapamycin and its role in normal cell function and oncogenesis has not been well clarified. However, it is known to activate Akt, thereby promoting cell proliferation and survival. The canonical pathway of mTOR activation depends on mitogen-driven signaling through PI3K/Akt, although alternative non-Akt-dependent activation through the RAS/MEK/ERK pathway is now recognized [66]. Altogether mTOR activation leads to increased synthesis of multiple proteins. These include several that have been implicated in the pathogenesis of multiple tumors, e.g., cyclin D1, which allows progression of cells through the cell cycle and HIF, which drive the expression of proangiogenic growth factors such as VEGF.

The genomic characterization of glioblastoma defined several molecular aberrations and copy-number changes [67] opening the possibility of using novel agents that target specific pathways regulating glioblastoma growth and resistance, in combination with the standard therapeutic platform (i.e., radiotherapy and temozolomide).

In vitro and in vivo data suggested that mTOR inhibitors may modify the activation of PI3K/Akt pathway influencing the expression of cell-cycle regulatory or anti-apoptotic proteins. In particular when used in combination with radiation, preclinical studies have demonstrated that mTOR inhibitors can enhance glioblastoma response to radiation by affecting both tumor vasculature and tumor cell viability through different mechanisms: activation of apoptosis, induction of cell cycle arrest and upregulation of autophagy [68–70]. In addition, combined radiation and mTOR inhibitor treatment decreases tumor vessels density and blood flow in vivo [71].

Rapamycin (sirolimus) is an antifungal agent with immunosuppressive properties, that showed a broad anticancer activity [72]; sirolimus analogs, with a more favorable pharmacokinetic (i.e., temsirolimus, everolimus, and ridaforolimus), are mTOR inhibitors used as anticancer agents. All these drugs are small-molecule inhibitors that function intracellularly, forming a complex with the FK506-binding protein-12 (FKBP-12) that is then recognized by mTOR. The resulting complex prevents mTOR activity, leading to inhibition of cell-cycle progression, survival, and angiogenesis. All mTOR inhibitors affect only mTORC1 and not mTORC2 [73].

Several phase-II clinical trials evaluating the use of mTOR inhibitors for the treatment of recurrent glioblastoma were published, whereas only some phase-I trials to assess the feasibility of association of mTOR inhibitors with radio-therapy and temozolomide in newly diagnosed glioblastoma were conducted.

The NCCTG dose-escalation phase-I trial (N027D) analyzed the integration of Temsirolimus (CCI-779) with radiotherapy and temozolomide, in patients with newly diagnosed GBM [74]. The first patients were treated with Temsirolimus combined with radiotherapy/ TMZ followed by adjuvant Temsirolimus and TMZ. After excessive infectious toxicities, and based on preclinical studies with mTOR inhibi-tors that show significant radiosensitizing effects in animal models, the trial design was modi-fied and Temsirolimus was delivered only dur-ing concurrent RT/TMZ, followed by adjuvant TMZ monotherapy. The recommended phase-II dose and schedule of i.v. temsirolimus in newly diagnosed GBM patients is 50 mg/week com-bined only during concomitant radiotherapy and temozolomide.

The NCCTG phase-I trial N057K enrolled 18 patients with newly diagnosed GBM [75]. All patients received weekly everolimus (EVEROLIMUS) in combination with standard chemoradiotherapy, followed by Everolimus in combination with adjuvant temozolomide. Everolimus at 70 mg/week is the recommended phase-II dosage for use in combination with stan-dard chemoradiotherapy in GBM. With a median follow-up of 8.4 months (range 1.8–15.9), 10 of 18 patients had a progression of disease.

In the recurrent setting, temsirolimus [76, 77], sirolimus [78], and everolimus [79] were tested in single arm phase-II trials. In two of these stud-ies mTOr inhibitors were associated with EGFR antagonists. Poor outcome in terms of PFS were reached (6-months-PFS ranging from 2 to 8 %) while median OS ranged from 4.4 to 8.5 months.

Recently a new generation of compounds, the so-called "dual PI3k/mTOR inhibitors", seems to inhibit not only PI3K class-I isoforms, but also mTORC1 and mTORC2; in theory this combined activity would lead to the strongest inhibition of the whole PI3K/mTOR pathway [80]. In particular NVP-BEZ235, a dual PI3K/ mTOR inhibitor seems to inhibit the DNA dam-age response (DDR). Ionizing radiation induces DNA double-strand breaks (DSBs) [81] that can be either repaired through the error-prone non-homologous end joining (NHEJ) pathway or the error-free homologous recombination pathway, in which the phosphoinositide 3-kinase (PI3K)-like kinases, DNA-PKcs (DNA-dependent protein kinase catalytic subunit) and ATM (ataxia-telangiectasia mutated), respectively, are centrally involved [82, 83]. NVP-BEZ235 seems to potently inhibit both ATM and DNA-PKcs, thereby attenuating both homologous recombi-nation and NHEJ and resulting in unprecedented radiosensitization in a panel of glioblastoma cell lines [84]. NVP-BEZ235 can cross the blood–brain barrier (BBB) and in vivo studies have shown its efficacy in controlling tumor growth in both subcutaneous and orthotopic tumor models, when administered in combination with ionizing radiation [85]. Thus, these novel agents target-ing PI3K/Akt/mTOR seem to be promising for improving clinical results in glioblastoma.

In the case of mTOR inhibitors, the poor per-meability of the BBB for most mTOR inhibitors may justify the failure in the few clinical experi-ences in patients with glioblastoma. Molecular screening for potentially high-yield subsets of tumors, such as those with PTEN mutations, may be needed to identify optimal tumors to treat.

## Conclusions

Unfortunately, to date, most promising agents have failed to significantly improve the clinical outcome in patients with glioblastoma. These repeatedly failed efforts underscore the complex-ity of this tumor type, and warrant improved pre-clinical models and further clinical trials. Since in the GBM cells, multiple pathways are coacti-vated and, in addition, several tumor suppres-sor genes are lost, probably only combinations of targeted agents may work. As an example, a phase-II trial of radiation therapy, temozolomide, erlotinib, and bevacizumab for initial treatment of glioblastoma was recently published [86]. This combination was well tolerated and significantly improved PFS (mPFS 13.5 months) but, again, the overall survival did not improve. In conclusion, much remains to be learned regarding the optimal combination of multi-pathways-targeted therapies with standard chemoradiotherapy, but maybe investigation of combined target inhibition will lead to the improvement of the poor results observed with a single-target approach.

## References

1. Debus J, Abdollahi A. For the next trick: new discoveries in radiobiology applied to glioblastoma. Am Soc Clin Oncol Educ Book. 2014:e95–9. doi: 10.14694/EdBook_AM.2014.34.e95.
2. Gutin PH, Iwamoto FM, Beal K, Mohile NA, Karimi S, Hou BL, et al. Safety and efficacy of bevacizumab with hypofractionated stereotactic irradiation for recurrent malignant gliomas. Int J Radiat Oncol Biol Phys. 2009;75(1):156–63.
3. Cuneo KC, Vredenburgh JJ, Sampson JH, Reardon DA, Desjardins A, Peters KB, et al. Safety and efficacy of stereotactic radiosurgery and adjuvant bevacizumab in patients with recurrent malignant gliomas. Int J Radiat Oncol Biol Phys. 2012;82(5):2018–24.
4. Shapiro LQ, Beal K, Goenka A, Karimi S, Iwamoto FM, Yamada Y, et al. Patterns of failure after concurrent bevacizumab and hypofractionated stereotactic radiation therapy for recurrent high-grade glioma. Int J Radiat Oncol Biol Phys. 2013;85(3):636–42.
5. Niyazi M, Ganswindt U, Schwarz SB, Kreth FW, Tonn JC, Geisler J, et al. Irradiation and bevacizumab in high-grade glioma retreatment settings. Int J Radiat Oncol Biol Phys. 2012;82(1):67–76.
6. Flieger M, Ganswindt U, Schwarz SB, Kreth FW, Tonn JC, la Fougère C, et al. Re-irradiation and bevacizumab in recurrent high-grade glioma: an effective treatment option. J Neurooncol. 2014;117(2):337–45.
7. Hundsberger T, Brügge D, Putora PM, Weder P, Weber J, Plasswilm L. Re-irradiation with and without bevacizumab as salvage therapy for recurrent or progressive high-grade gliomas. J Neurooncol. 2013;112(1):133–9.
8. Cabrera AR, Cuneo KC, Desjardins A, Sampson JH, McSherry F, Herndon 2nd JE, et al. Concurrent stereotactic radiosurgery and bevacizumab in recurrent malignant gliomas: a prospective trial. Int J Radiat Oncol Biol Phys. 2013;86(5):873–9.
9. Gilbert MR, Dignam JJ, Armstrong TS, Wefel JS, Blumenthal DT, Vogelbaum MA. A randomized trial of bevacizumab for newly diagnosed glioblastoma. N Engl J Med. 2014;370(8):699–708.
10. Chinot OL, Wick W, Mason W, Henriksson R, Saran F, Nishikawa R. Bevacizumab plus radiotherapy-temozolomide for newly diagnosed glioblastoma. N Engl J Med. 2014;370(8):709–22.
11. di Tomaso E, Snuderl M, Kamoun WS, Duda DG, Auluck PK. Fazlollahi glioblastoma recurrence after cediranib therapy in patients: lack of "rebound" revascularization as mode of escape. Cancer Res. 2011;71(1):19–28.
12. Kioi M, Vogel H, Schultz G, Hoffman RM, Harsh GR, Brown JM. Inhibition of vasculogenesis, but not angiogenesis, prevents the recurrence of glioblastoma after irradiation in mice. J Clin Invest. 2010;120(3): 694–705.
13. Kozin SV, Kamoun WS, Huang Y, Dawson MR, Jain RK, Duda DG. Recruitment of myeloid but not endothelial precursor cells facilitates tumor regrowth after local irradiation. Cancer Res. 2010;70(14):5679–85.
14. Lu-Emerson C, Snuderl M, Kirkpatrick ND, Goveia J, Davidson C, Huang Y, et al. Increase in tumor-associated macrophages after antiangiogenic therapy is associated with poor survival among patients with recurrent glioblastoma. Neuro Oncol. 2013;15(8): 1079–87.
15. Lund-Johansen M, Bjerkvig R, Humphrey PA, Bigner SH, Bigner DD, Laerum OD. Effect of epidermal growth factor on glioma cell growth, migration, and invasion in vitro. Cancer Res. 1990;50(18):6039–44.
16. Shinojima N, Tada K, Shiraishi S, Kamiryo T, Kochi M, Nakamura H, et al. Prognostic value of epidermal growth factor receptor in patients with glioblastoma multiforme. Cancer Res. 2003;63(20):6962–70.
17. Watanabe K, Tachibana O, Sata K, Yonekawa Y, Kleihues P, Ohgaki H. Overexpression of the EGF receptor and p53 mutations are mutually exclusive in the evolution of primary and secondary glioblastomas. Brain Pathol. 1996;6(3):217–23.
18. Barker FG, Simmons ML, Chang SM, Prados MD, Larson DA, Sneed PK, et al. EGFR overexpression and radiation response in glioblastoma multiforme. Int J Radiat Oncol Biol Phys. 2001;51(2):410–8.
19. Chakravarti A, Chakladar A, Delaney MA, Latham DE, Loeffler JS. The epidermal growth factor receptor pathway mediates resistance to sequential administration of radiation and chemotherapy in primary human glioblastoma cells in a RAS-dependent manner. Cancer Res. 2002;62(15):4307–15.
20. Halatsch ME, Gehrke EE, Vougioukas VI, Bötefür IC, A-Borhani F, Efferth T. Inverse correlation of epidermal growth factor receptor messenger RNA induction and suppression of anchorage-independent growth by OSI-774, an epidermal growth factor receptor tyrosine kinase inhibitor, in glioblastoma multiforme cell lines. J Neurosurg. 2004;100(3):523–33.
21. Prados MD, Lamborn KR, Chang S, Burton E, Butowski N, Malec M. Phase 1 study of erlotinib HCl alone and combined with temozolomide in patients with stable or recurrent malignant glioma. Neuro Oncol. 2006;8(1):67–78.
22. Vogelbaum MA, Peereboom D, Stevens G, Barnett GH, Brewer C. Response rate to single agent therapy with the EGFR tyrosine kinase inhibitor erlotinib in recurrent glioblastoma multiforme: results of a phase

II study. Proceedings of the ninth meeting of the society for neuro-oncology 2004;384.

23. Prados MD, Chang SM, Butowski N, DeBoer R, Parvataneni R, Carliner H, et al. Phase II study of erlotinib plus temozolomide during and after radiation therapy in patients with newly diagnosed glioblastoma multiforme or gliosarcoma. J Clin Oncol. 2009;27(4):579–84.

24. Peereboom DM, Shepard DR, Ahluwalia MS, Brewer CJ, Agarwal N, Stevens GH, et al. Phase II trial of erlotinib with temozolomide and radiation in patients with newly diagnosed glioblastoma multiforme. J Neurooncol. 2010;98(1):93–9.

25. Chakravarti A, Wang M, Robins HI, Lautenschlaeger T, Curran WJ, Brachman DG, et al. RTOG 0211: a phase 1/2 study of radiation therapy with concurrent gefitinib for newly diagnosed glioblastoma patients. Int J Radiat Oncol Biol Phys. 2013;85(5):1206–11.

26. Belda-Iniesta C, Carpeño Jde C, Saenz EC, Gutiérrez M, Perona R, Barón MG. Long term responses with cetuximab therapy in glioblastoma multiforme. Cancer Biol Ther. 2006;5(8):912–4.

27. Neyns B, Sadones J, Joosens E, Bouttens F, Verbeke L, Baurain JF, et al. Stratified phase II trial of cetuximab in patients with recurrent high-grade glioma. Ann Oncol. 2009;20(9):1596–603.

28. Combs SE, Schulz-Ertner D, Hartmann C, Welzel T, Timke C, Herfarth KK, et al. Erbitux (Cetuximab) plus temozolomide as radiochemotherapy for primary glioblastoma (GERT): interim results of a phase I/II study. Int J Radiat Oncol Biol Phys. 2008;72(1S): S10–1.

29. Wang Y, Pan L, Sheng XF, Chen S, Dai JZ. Nimotuzumab, a humanized monoclonal antibody specific for the EGFR, in combination with temozolomide and radiation therapy for newly diagnosed glioblastoma multiforme: first results in Chinese patients. Asia Pac J Clin Oncol. 2014. doi: 10.1111/ajco.12166.

30. Solomon MT, Miranda N, Jorrín E, Chon I, Marinello JJ, Alert J, et al. Nimotuzumab in combination with radiotherapy in high grade glioma patients: a single institution experience. Cancer Biol Ther. 2014;15(5): 504–9.

31. Westphal M, Bach F. Final results of a randomized phase III trial of nimotuzumab for the treatment of newly diagnosed glioblastoma in addition to standard radiation and chemotherapy with temozolomide versus standard radiation and temoziolamide. J Clin Oncol 30, 2012, suppl abstr 2033,

32. Jänne PA, Gurubhagavatula S, Yeap BY, Lucca J, Ostler P, Skarin AT, et al. Outcomes of patients with advanced non-small cell lung cancer treated with gefitinib (ZD1839, "iressa") on an expanded access study. Lung Cancer. 2004;44(2):221–30.

33. Cappuzzo F, Hirsch FR, Rossi E, Bartolini S, Ceresoli GL, Bemis L, et al. Epidermal growth factor receptor gene and protein and gefitinib sensitivity in non-small-cell lung cancer. J Natl Cancer Inst. 2005;97(9):643–55.

34. Han SW, Kim TY, Jeon YK, Hwang PG, Im SA, Lee KH, et al. Optimization of patient selection for gefitinib in non-small cell lung cancer by combined analysis of epidermal growth factor receptor mutation, K-ras mutation, and Akt phosphorylation. Clin Cancer Res. 2006;12(8):2538–44.

35. Rich JN, Reardon DA, Peery T, Dowell JM, Quinn JA, Penne KL, et al. Phase II trial of gefitinib in recurrent glioblastoma. J Clin Oncol. 2004;22(1):133–42.

36. Franceschi E, Cavallo G, Lonardi S, Magrini E, Tosoni A, Grosso D, et al. Gefitinib in patients with progressive high-grade gliomas: a multicentre phase II study by Gruppo Italiano Cooperativo di Neuro-Oncologia (GICNO). Br J Cancer. 2007;96(7): 1047–51.

37. Gallego O, Cuatrecasas M, Benavides M, Segura PP, Berrocal A, Erill N, et al. Efficacy of erlotinib in patients with relapsed gliobastoma multiforme who expressed EGFRVIII and PTEN determined by immunohistochemistry. J Neurooncol. 2014;116(2): 413–9.

38. van den Bent MJ, Brandes AA, Rampling R, Kouwenhoven MC, Kros JM, Carpentier AF, et al. Randomized phase II trial of erlotinib versus temozolomide or carmustine in recurrent glioblastoma: EORTC brain tumor group study 26034. J Clin Oncol. 2009;27(8):1268–74.

39. Stupack DG, Puente XS, Boutsaboualoy S, Storgard CM, Cheresh DA. Apoptosis of adherent cells by recruitment of caspase-8 to unligated integrins. J Cell Biol. 2001;155(3):459–70.

40. Ruegg C, Mariotti A. Vascular integrins: pleiotropic adhesion and signaling molecules in vascular homeostasis and angiogenesis. Cell Mol Life Sci. 2003;60(6):1135–57.

41. Avraamides CJ, Garmy-Susini B, Varner JA. Integrins in angiogenesis and lymphangiogenesis. Nat Rev Cancer. 2008;8(8):604–17.

42. Alghisi GC, Ruegg C. Vascular integrins in tumor angiogenesis: mediators and therapeutic targets. Endothelium. 2006;13(2):113–35.

43. Schnell O, Krebs B, Wagner E, Romagna A, Beer AJ, Grau SJ, et al. Expression of integrin alphavbeta3 in gliomas correlates with tumor grade and is not restricted to tumor vasculature. Brain Pathol. 2008;18(3):378–86.

44. Taga T, Suzuki A, Gonzalez-Gomez I, Gilles FH, Stins M, Shimada H, et al. Alpha vintegrin antagonist emd 121974 induces apoptosis in brain tumor cells growing on vitronectin and tenascin. Int J Cancer. 2002;98(5):690–7.

45. Bello L, Francolini M, Marthyn P, Zhang J, Carroll RS, Nikas DC, et al. Alpha(v) beta3 and alpha(v) beta5 integrin expression in glioma periphery. Neurosurgery. 2001;49(2):380–9.

46. Ruegg C, Alghisi GC. Vascular integrins: therapeutic and imaging targets of tumor angiogenesis. Recent Results Cancer Res. 2010;180:83–101.

47. Wild-Bode C, Weller M, Rimner A, Dichgans J, Wick W. Sublethal irradiation promotes migration and invasiveness of glioma cells: implications for radiotherapy of human glioblastoma. Cancer Res. 2001;61(6): 2744–50.

48. Mikkelsen T, Brodie C, Finniss S, Berens ME, Rennert JL, Nelson K, et al. Radiation sensitization of glioblastoma by cilengitide has unanticipated schedule-dependency. Int J Cancer. 2009;124(11):2719–27.

49. Abdollahi A, Griggs DW, Zieher H, Roth A, Lipson KE, Saffrich R, et al. Inhibition of alpha(v) beta3 integrin survival signaling enhances antiangiogenic and antitumor effects of radiotherapy. Clin Cancer Res. 2005;11:6270–9.

50. Xiong JP, Stehle T, Zhang R, Joachimiak A, Frech M, Goodman SL, et al. Crystal structure of the extracellular segment of integrin alphaVbeta3 in complex with an arg-gly-asp ligand. Science. 2002;296(5565):151–5.

51. Goodman SL, Hölzemann G, Sulyok GA, Kessler H. Nanomolar small molecule inhibitors for alphaV (beta)6, alphaV (beta)5, and alphaV(beta)3 integrins. J Med Chem. 2002;45(5):1045–51.

52. Nisato RE, Tille JC, Jonczyk A, Goodman SL, Pepper MS. AlphaV beta 3 and alphav beta 5 integrin antagonists inhibit angiogenesis in vitro. Angiogenesis. 2003;6(2):105–19.

53. Nabors B, Mikkelsen T, Rosenfeld S, Hochberg F, Shastry Akella N, Fisher J, et al. A phase I and correlative biology study of cilengitide in patients with recurrent malignant glioma. J Clin Oncol. 2007;25(13):1651–7.

54. MacDonald TJ, Stewart CF, Kocak M, Goldman S, Ellenbogen RG, Phillips P, et al. Phase I clinical trial of cilengitide in children with refractory brain tumors: pediatric brain tumor consortium study pbtc-012. J Clin Oncol. 2008;26(6):919–24.

55. Reardon DA, Fink KL, Mikkelsen T, Cloughesy TF, O'Neill A, Plotkin S, et al. Randomized phase II study of cilengitide, an integrin-targeting arginine-glycine-aspartic acid peptide, in recurrent glioblastoma multiforme. J Clin Oncol. 2008;26(34):5610–7.

56. Fink N, Mikkelsen T, Nabors LB, Ravin P, Plotkin SR, Schiff D, et al. Long-term effects of cilengitide, a novel integrin inhibitor, in recurrent glioblastoma: a randomized phase II study. J Clin Oncol 2010;28(suppl; abstr, 2010).

57. Gilbert MR, Kuhn J, Lamborn KR, Lieberman F, Wen PY, Mehta M, et al. Cilengitide in patients with recurrent glioblastoma: the results of NABTC 03-02, a phase II trial with measures of treatment delivery. J Neurooncol. 2012;106(1):147–53.

58. Nabors L, NABTT 0306: A randomized phase II trial of EMD 121974 in conjunction with concomitant and adjuvant temozolomide with radiation therapy in patients with newly diagnosed glioblastoma multiforme (GBM). Proc Am Soc Clin Oncol, J Clin Oncol 2009.

59. Stupp R, Hegi ME, Neyns B, Goldbrunner R, Schlegel U, Clement PM, et al. Phase I/IIa study of cilengitide and temozolomide with concomitant radiotherapy followed by cilengitide and temozolomide maintenance therapy in patients with newly diagnosed glioblastoma. J Clin Oncol. 2010;28(16):2712–8.

60. Stupp R, Hegi ME, Gorlia T, Erridge SC, Perry J, Hong YK, et al. Cilengitide combined with standard treatment for patients with newly diagnosed glioblastoma with methylated MGMT promoter (CENTRIC EORTC 26071-22072 study): a multicentre, randomised, open-label, phase 3 trial. Lancet Oncol. 2014;15(10):1100–8.

61. Chinot O. Cilengitide in glioblastoma: when did it fail? Lancet Oncol. 2014;15(10):1044–5.

62. Reynolds AR, Hart IR, Watson AR, Welti JC, Silva RG, Robinson SD, et al. Stimulation of tumour growth and angiogenesis by low concentrations of RGD-mimetic integrin inhibitors. Nat Med. 2009;15:392–400.

63. Nabors LB, Mikkelsen T, Hegi ME, Batchelor T, Lesser G, Peereboom D, et al. A safety run-in and randomized phase 2 study of cilengitide combined with chemoradiation for newly diagnosed glioblastoma (NABTT 0306). Cancer. 2012;118:5601–7.

64. Okada H, Mak TW. Pathways of apoptotic and non-apoptotic death in tumour cells. Nat Rev Cancer. 2004;4:592–603.

65. McCubrey JA, Steelman LS, Abrams SL, Lee JT, Chang F, Bertrand FE, et al. Roles of the RAF/MEK/ERK and PI3K/PTEN/AKT pathways in malignant transformation and drug resistance. Adv Enzyme Regul. 2006;46:249–79.

66. Hay N, Sonenberg N. Upstream and downstream of mTOR. Genes Dev. 2004;18:1926–45.

67. Cancer Genome Atlas Research Network. Comprehensive genomic characterization defines human glioblastoma genes and core pathways. Nature. 2008;455:1061–8.

68. Eshleman JS, Carlson BL, Mladek AC, Kastner BD, Shide KL, Sarkaria JN. Inhibition of the mammalian target of rapamycin sensitizes U87 xenografts to fractionated radiation therapy. Cancer Res. 2002;62(24):7291–7.

69. Anandharaj A, Cinghu S, Park WY. Rapamycin-mediated mTOR inhibition attenuates surviving and sensitizes glioblastoma cells to radiation therapy. Acta Biochim Biophys Sin (Shangai). 2011;43(4):292–300.

70. Kim KW, Mutter RW, Cao C, Albert JM, Freeman M, Hallahan DE, et al. Autophagy for cancer therapy through inhibition of pro-apoptotic proteins and mammalian target of rapamycin signaling. J Biol Chem. 2006;281(48):36883–90.

71. Shinohara ET, Cao C, Niermann K, Mu Y, Zeng F, Hallahan DE, et al. Enhanced radiation damage of tumor vasculature by mTOR inhibitors. Oncogene. 2005;24(35):5414–22.

72. Seghal SN, Baker H, Vézina C. Rapamycin (AY-22,989), a new antifungal antibiotic. II. Fermentation, isolation and characterization. J Antibiot. 1975;28:727–32.

73. Faivre S, Kroemer G, Raymond E. Current development of mTOR inhibitors as anticancer agents. Nat Rev Drug Discov. 2006;5:671–88.

74. Sarkaria JN, Galanis E, Wu W, Dietz AB, Kaufmann TJ, Gustafson MP, et al. Combination of temsirolimus

(CCI-779) with chemoradiation in newly diagnosed glioblastoma multiforme (NCCTG trial N027D) is associated with increased infectious risk. Clin Cancer Res. 2010;16(22):5573–80.

75. Sarkaria JN, Galanis E, Wu W, Peller PJ, Giannini C, Brown PD, et al. North Central Treatment Group phase I trial N057K of everolimus (RAD001) and temozolomide in combination with radiation therapy in patients with newly diagnosed glioblastoma multiforme. Int J Radiat Oncol Biol Phys. 2011;81(2): 468–75.

76. Chang SM, Wen P, Cloughesy T, Greenberg H, Schiff D, Conrad C, et al. Phase II study of CCI-779 in patients with recurrent glioblastoma multiforme. Invest New Drugs. 2005;23:357–61.

77. Galanis E, Buckner JC, Maurer MJ, Kreisberg JI, Ballman K, Boni J, et al. Phase II trial of temsirolimus (CCI-779) in recurrent glioblastoma multiforme: a North Central Cancer Treatment Group Study. J Clin Oncol. 2005;23(23):5294–304.

78. Reardon DA, Vredenburgh JJ, Desjardins A, Peters K, Gururangan S, Sampson JH, et al. Effect of CYP3A-inducing antiepileptics on sorafenib exposure: results of a phase II study of sorafenib plus daily temozolomide in adults with recurrent glioblastoma. J Neurooncol. 2011;101:57–66.

79. Kreisl TN, Lassman AB, Mischel PS, Rosen N, Scher HI, Teruya-Feldstein J, et al. A pilot study of everolimus and gefitinib in the treatment of recurrent glioblastoma (GBM). J Neurooncol. 2009;92:99–105.

80. Martelli AM, Chiarini E, Evangelisti C, Cappellini A, Buontempo F, Bressanin D, et al. Two hits are better than one: targeting both phosphatidylinositol 3-kinase and mammalian target of rapamycin as a therapeutic strategy for acute leukemia treatment. Oncotarget. 2012;3:371–94.

81. Jackson SP, Bartek J. The DNA-damage response in human biology and disease. Nature. 2009;462:1071–8.

82. Shiloh Y, Ziv Y. The ATM protein kinase: regulating the cellular response to genotoxic stress, and more. Nat Rev Mol Cell Biol. 2013;14:197–210.

83. Wang C, Lees-Miller SP. Detection and repair of ionizing radiation-induced DNA double strand breaks: new developments in nonhomologous end joining. Int J Radiat Oncol Biol Phys. 2013;86:440–9.

84. Mukherjee B, Tomimatsu N, Amancherla K, Camacho CV, Pichamoorthy N, Burma S. The dual PI3K/mTOR inhibitor NVP-BEZ235 is a potent inhibitor of ATM- and DNA-PKcs-mediated DNA damage responses. Neoplasia. 2012;14:34–43.

85. Rodrigo C, del Alcazar G, Hardebeck MC, Mukherjee B, Tomimatsu N, Gao X, et al. Inhibition of DNA double-strand break repair by the dual PI3K/mTOR inhibitor NVP-BEZ235 as a strategy for radiosensitization of glioblastoma. Clin Cancer Res. 2013;20(5):1235–48.

86. Clarke JL, Molinaro AM, Phillips JJ, Butowski NA, Chang SM, Perry A, et al. A single-institution phase II trial of radiation, temozolomide, erlotinib, and bevacizumab for initial treatment of glioblastoma. Neuro Oncol. 2014;16(7):984–90.

# Chemoradiotherapy: Radiation Total Dose and Fractionation

**4**

Silvia Chiesa, Mario Balducci, Milena Ferro,
Anna Rita Alitto, and Vincenzo Valentini

## Introduction

Glioblastoma Multiforme (GBM) accounts for more than 50 % of all primary malignant brain tumors in adults [1, 2]. More than 30 years of clinical trials have been conducted but only recently the standard treatment has been defined for primary GBM. The introduction of temozolomide (TMZ) allowed a survival improvement in newly diagnosed GBM. Nowadays the standard treatment for naive GBM includes the surgical resection followed by radiotherapy and concurrent plus adjuvant chemotherapy (CT) with temozolomide [3]. The prognosis remains dismal with a long-term survival of 2–5 % at 5 years and a median overall survival of around 14 months [3]. Local failure continues to be the main cause of mortality and research trends are focusing on genomic and/or molecular analysis to improve outcomes.

## Chemoradiation Therapy: Primary Treatment

Chemoradiation therapy, following surgery when indicated, is the main modality in the treatment of newly diagnosed GBM. A multidisciplinary approach is encouraged to define an individualized therapeutic plan. This section describes the evolution of the standard care and investigation trends in radiotherapy, chemotherapy, and in combined approaches.

## External Beam Radiation Therapy

More than six decades of clinical trials investigated the use of RT in the treatment of malignant gliomas. Between the 1970s and the 1990s, the first randomized trials demonstrated the survival benefit of a postoperative radiation therapy [4]. A conventionally fractionated total dose of 60 Gy to a limited field of the brain is currently considered as the standard of care.

### Conventional Postoperative Radiation Versus No Radiation

Since the mid-1970s, patients with malignant gliomas have been randomized to receive postoperative RT; five out of six trials [5–10] reported a statistically significant survival benefit favoring postoperative RT compared with best supportive care (BSC) only or single- or multi-agent CT

S. Chiesa (✉) • M. Balducci • M. Ferro • A.R. Alitto
V. Valentini
Radiation Oncology Department, Gemelli-ART,
Università Cattolica S. Cuore,
L.go Agostino Gemelli, 8, Rome 00168, Italy
e-mail: silvia.chiesa.md@gmail.com

© Springer International Publishing Switzerland 2016
L. Pirtoli et al. (eds.), *Radiobiology of Glioblastoma*, Current Clinical Pathology,
DOI 10.1007/978-3-319-28305-0_4

without radiation (RR 0.81; 95 % confidence interval 0.74–0.88, $p<0.10$). (Table 4.1)

In a randomized study (90 % GBM), the Brain tumor Study Group (BTSG 6901 [7], BTSG 7201 [8]) demonstrated a significant median survival benefit in postoperative RT compared with BSC ($p=0.001$), with BCNU alone ($p=0.013$) or with others nitrosoureas ($p=0.0003$) without benefit with concomitant chemotherapy.

On the contrary, the Scandinavian Glioblastoma Study Group [9] observed the superiority of postoperative irradiation using bleomycin agent. The median overall survival reported in these randomized trials ranged from 5.75 to 11.2 weeks. This finding suggested that further studies were required.

## Radiation Volume

*Whole brain* irradiation was the main modality employed in early clinical trials. Since the beginning of 1990s, with better tumor localization due to the computed tomography and magnetic resonance imaging (MRI), the advent of conformal radiotherapy and the knowledge that high doses of whole brain irradiation induced neurocognitive impairment with slowly progressive dementia, studies were carried out to explore the impact of *partial brain* radiation on survival [11, 12] and on patterns of failure [13–15]. The Brain Tumor Cooperative Trial 8001 [12] and the study published by Kita et al. [11] did not observe any statistically significant differences between whole brain and focal volume irradiation. One additional small randomized trial observed not only equivalent outcomes but also a significant lower toxicity in long-term survivors who received focal irradiation [16].

Several studies have been conducted to evaluate the pattern of treatment failure in high-grade gliomas. Some authors [14, 17, 18] studied the *patterns of recurrence* after WBRT and observed that 95 % were within the resected area or within 3 cm of the presurgical tumor margin. These data were the same in case of a partial brain irradiation [15, 19, 20]. For clinical target volume (CTV), some investigators correlated peritumoral edema with the infiltrating tumors cells [3, 11, 12, 17] and recommended edema plus 2 cm margins, as reported in several RTOG studies [21–24]. Others, upon observing that recurrences were mainly central, in field or marginal (80–90 %) and only 10–20 % outside the irradiated field [25, 26], recommended the use of a margin of 2–3 cm around the enhancement area. Table 4.2 shows the two CTV's strategies in partial brain irradiation. The MDACC experience

**Table 4.1** Post-operative radiotherapy versus no radiotherapy in randomized studies- modified by Laperrière [4]

| Study [ref] | Treatment | Dose (Gy)/no. Fractions | No pts randomized | Target volume | Median survival (weeks) | P value overall survival | RR for 1 year mortality |
|---|---|---|---|---|---|---|---|
| Shapiro et al. [5] | CT | - | 16 | WB | 30 | NR | 1.13 |
| | RT+CT | 60 | 17 | | 44.5 | | |
| Andersen et al. [6] | Surgery | – | 57 | NR | 15 | <0.005 | 0.86 |
| | RT | 45/25 | 51 | | 23 | | |
| Walker et al. [7] | Surgery | – | 42 | WB | 14 | 0.001 | 0.79 |
| | RT | 50–60/25–35 | 93 | | 36 | | |
| Walker et al. [8] | CT | – | 111 | NR | 31 | 0.003 | 0.85 |
| | RT | 60/30–35 | 118 | | 37 | | |
| Kristiansen et al. [9] | Surgery | – | 38 | Supratentorial | 23 | NR | 0.69 |
| | RT+/–CT | 45/25 | 80 | | 47 | Significant | |
| Sandberg-Wollheim et al. [10] | CT | – | 87 | WB | 42 | 0.028 | 0.70 |
| | RT+CT | 58/27 | 84 | | 62 | | |

*RT* radiotherapy, *CT* chemotherapy, *NR* not reported

[27] showed that CTV delineation based on a 2-cm margin did not seem to alter the central pattern of failure for patients with GBM. Mc Donald et al. [28] found that use of total planning target volume (PTV) margins of less than 1 cm resulted in 93 % in field failures, further indicating that there was likely to be no recurrence detriment of a reduced margin. In most cases, the target volumes are defined according to RTOG or EORTC guidelines (Table 4.2).

## Radiation Total Dose and Fractionation

In GBM, the recommended radiation dose to the CTV is 60 Gy in *conventional fractionation* (30–33 fractions). In poorly performing patients or in elderly patients with particularly poor prognosis, a hypo-fractionated accelerated course is effective and allows the completion of the treatment in 2–4 weeks. Fractionation schedules include 34 Gy/10 fr, 40.05/15 fr, or 50 Gy/20 fr [29, 30]. The standard of care over time is the result of first studies demonstrating a survival benefit for doses beyond 60 Gy and further experiences failed to demonstrate a real advantage of dose escalation regimens. The results of three randomized trials performed by BTSG (BTSG 6601 [31], BTSG 6901 [7], BTSG 7201 [8]) were pooled in a large study on 621 patients demonstrating a survival improvement with higher doses (45vs 50vs 55vs 60 Gy with a median survival of 3.4-7-8-10.5 months, respectively). A Medical Research Council (UK) large randomized trial further confirmed the standard dose of 60 Gy in 30 fractions, compared to 45 Gy in 20 fractions. The conventional fractionation to 60 Gy correlated with a statistically significant benefit of median survival from 9 to 12 months ($p=0.007$). The joint study

of the RTOG/ECOG randomized 626 patients and failed to show any advantage of 70 Gy over 60 Gy [32].

Some authors investigated other approaches to *altered fractionation* considering some radiobiological aspects such as shorter overall treatment time, reduced neoplastic cell repopulation or more favorable cell cycle phase redistribution with better radiobiological effects. *Hyperfractionated* schedules, increasing the chance of irradiating neoplastic cells in the more radiosensitivity phase of cell cycle and obtaining a less oxygen dependent cell killing, were evaluated in six randomized studies (Table 4.3). None of the studies, except Shin et al. [35], observed any significant survival benefit for the experimental arm.

A valid alternative could be a *hypofractionation* scheme based on low $\alpha/\beta$ ratio of GBM suggested by experimental [52, 53] and clinical trials [43, 54]. This shortened regimen is considered an appropriate treatment option for most malignant glioma patients with poor prognosis, such as the elderly, or those with poor performance status. Kleinbeg et al. [43] reported a study of 219 patients treated with 51 Gy in 17 fractions in 5.5 weeks with similar survival results to standard regimens in poor prognostic groups with less patient effort and cost. Other hypo-fractionated regimes are 30 Gy in 6 fractions, 30 Gy in 10 fractions, 36 in 12 fractions, 37.5 in 15 fractions, and 42 in 14 fractions. On the contrary in analyzing 108 randomized patients, Glinski et al. [44] demonstrated a survival advantage of a hypo-fractionated regimen consisting of three courses of treatment separated by a 1-month interval in 44 patients with GBM (23 vs. 10 % at 2 years, $p<0.05$).

**Table 4.2** Guidelines for treatment volume delineation

| Guidelines | Phase | Treatment volume | Total dose/fractionation |
|---|---|---|---|
| RTOG | Phase I/II | Contrast enhancing lesion + peri-tumoral edema + 2 cm margin to PTV | 46 Gy/2 Gy |
| | Phase II/II | Contrast enhancing lesion in preoperative MRI + 2.5 cm margin to PTV | 14 Gy/2 Gy |
| EORTC | Phase I/I | Contrast enhancing lesion + 2 or 3 cm margins to CTV | 50–60 Gy/1.8–2 Gy |

*PTV* planning target volume, *CTV* clinical target volume

**Table 4.3** Overview of altered fractionation studies

| Study | Radiotherapy dose/no fractions | no patients | Median survival altered fractionated RT ± vs. conventional RT (weeks) | Significance |
|---|---|---|---|---|
| Hyper-fractionation | | | | |
| Payne et al. [33] | 36–40Gy/60 | NR[a] | 48[b] | NS |
| Shin et al. [34] | 50 Gy/50 | 35 | 56 vs. 39 | NS |
| Shin et al. [35] | 61.4 Gy/69 | 43 | 39 vs. 27 | 0.007 |
| Ludgate et al. [36] | 47.6 Gy/63 + 10 Gy/5 | 42 | 46 vs. 32 | NS |
| Deutsch et al. [37] | 66 Gy/60 | 154 | 45[c] vs. 43[c] | NS |
| Scott et al. [38] | 72 Gy/60 | NR[d] | 44 vs. 49 | 0.44 |
| Accelerated | | | | |
| Horiot et al. [39] | 30 Gy/15/1 week +30 Gy/15/1 week | NA | NA | NR |
| Brada et al. [40] | 55 Gy/34 twice/daily | 211 | 40 | NS |
| RTOG 8302 [41] | 48–54.4 Gy/30 or 34 twice daily | 305 | 42 | NS |
| Chen et al. [42] | 60 Gy/10 | 16 | 66 | NR |
| Hypo-fractionated | | | | |
| Kleinberg et al. [43] | 30 Gy/10 + 21 Gy/7 | 219 | 20–32 | NR |
| Glinski [44] | 20 Gy/5 × 2 courses + 10Gy/5[e] | 108 | 68 | NS $P<0.05$[f] |
| Bauman 1994 [45] | 30 Gy/10 | 29 | 24 | NR |
| Ford et al. [46] | 36 Gy/12 | 32 | 16 | NS |
| Hoegler and Davey [47] | 37.5 Gy/15 | 25 | 32 | NR |
| Slotman et al. [48] | 42 Gy/14 | 30 | 36 | NR |
| Accelerated hypo-fractionated | | | | |
| Prados, et al. [49] | 70 Gy/44 | 231 | 41 vs. 42 | NS |
| Massaccesi et al. [50] | 70 Gy/25 | 40 | 68 | NR |
| Iuchi et al. [51] | 68 Gy/8 to PTV1 | 46 | 20 | NR |

[a]The number of patients randomized per treatment group is not reported; the total no of randomized patients is 168
[b]Median overall survival for the whole sample
[c]Median survival is reported considering the evaluable patients (282: 142 for hyper-fractionated RT and 140 for conventional RT)
[d]A total of 172 patients were randomized but the number for treatment group was not reported
[e]The three courses were separated by 1-month intervals

*NR* not reported, *NS* not significant, *NA* not available, *PTV* planning target volume

The *accelerated* RT aim, limiting the overall treatment time, reduces the chance of cell repopulation during the treatment. The EORTC's study [39] randomized 340 patients to receive conventional radiotherapy or 30 Gy in 1 week administered by 3 fractions of 2 Gy per day with an interval of 4 h. The results demonstrated only the feasibility without an increased toxicity or a survival benefit. The same results were reported by RTOG 8302 trial [41] where 305 patients were randomized to receive 48 or 54.4 Gy in 30 or 34

fractions with a low toxicity rate in accelerated radiation.

Alternative fractionation schemes were also used to design *dose escalation* approaches. The total radiation dose that may be delivered to brain tumors is limited by normal tissue toxicity but technical advances in radiotherapy have become prevalent over the last years: intensity-modulated radiotherapy (IMRT) and volumetric modulated arc therapy (VMAT) allow the delivery of steep dose gradients at the target volume, reducing exposure to adjacent normal tissues and allowing highly conformal radiotherapy [55, 56]. Dose escalation protocols to test the feasibility and the benefit are increasingly becoming a field of interest, although randomized studies did not demonstrate any advantage over conventionally fractionated doses. Using hyper-fractionated regimen, Scott et al. [38] administered 72Gy, while Deutsch et al. [37] delivered 66 Gy without any significant advantage. In a phase III trial, Prados and colleagues [49] delivered an accelerated hyper-fractionated schedule of 70.4 Gy at 1.6 twice daily observing the same survival as the conventional dose patients. The RTOG investigated dose escalation strategy testing four different hyper-fractionated arms to total dose of 64.8, 72, 76.8, and 81.6 [21]. The late toxicity increase for higher doses and the most efficient dose level of 72 Gy was employed in further studies (RTOG 90-06 [38]), but no superiority was demonstrated compared to conventional schedule of 60 Gy.

Since the advance of IMRT in the 1990s, various studies have evaluated the possibility of escalating the biological effective dose (BED) investigating the clinical feasibility of IMRT with altered fractionation schedules. An improvement in the BED is feasible using a *simultaneous integrated boost* administered with *IMRT technique* or using fractionated stereotactic radiosurgery to escalate the dose to the target volume, to minimize adjacent tissue dose and maximize radiobiological parameters of total dose and dose per fraction. The feasibility of this strategy concomitant to chemotherapy has been demonstrated. Chen et al. [42] reported an acceptable toxicity when 60 Gy are delivered in IMRT 6 Gy fraction within 2 weeks (BED for GBM of 119.4 Gy, equivalent dose in 2 Gy per fraction-EQD2 for normal brain 108.9 Gy). Iuchi and colleagues [57] delivering a BED higher than 90 Gy achieved an excellent local control rate. Morganti et al. in an Italian phase I dose escalation study demonstrated the feasibility of an accelerated IMRT plus temozolomide. The dose to tumor bed plus margins was escalated from 60 Gy to 62.5, 65, 67.5, and 70 Gy (BED of 92.8 Gy) with no grade >2 of late neurotoxicity after a median follow-up of 25 months [50, 58].

Chan et al. [59] and Lee et al. [20] collected results of dose escalation protocols and reported a feasibility of the intensification of local radiotherapy without any change in the pattern of failure, primarily central or "in field."

*Radiosurgery* has been used for local irradiation in both new and recurrent GBM, with several modalities to escalate the dose to the primary or recurrent disease. Because at least 80 % of gliomas fall within 2 cm of the primary high dose level local radiation and because radiosurgery allows a highly local conformal irradiation, several authors investigated the use of radiosurgery as a boost after external beam radiotherapy in retrospective studies [60, 61]. Sarkaria et al. [60] retrospectively pooled the data from the Joint Center for Radiation Therapy, from the University of Wisconsin, and from the University of Florida, of 115 patients treated with a combination of surgery, external beam radiation therapy (54 or 59 Gy), and linac-based radiosurgery (12 or 13.8 Gy). An improvement of 2-year median survival ($p = 0.01$) was observed mainly in worse prognostic classes.

The promising results of a better survival than for the historical controls heavily influenced the following prospective studies, focused primarily on brain metastases and recurrent malignant brain tumors [62]. In the pre-temozolomide era, the first prospective trials exploring radiosurgery or fractionated stereotactic (FSRT) boost were performed by RTOG Group. In the RTOG 9305 [63], 203 patients were randomized to receive or not receive postoperative radiosurgery and EBRT (60 Gy) plus BCNU; the lesion size was within 4 cm and the radiosurgical dose ranged from 15 to 24 according to RTOG 9005 [62]. The phase II prospective trial RTOG 0023 [64], exploring a concomitant schedule of FSRT of 5 or 7 Gy per fraction to obtain a total dose of 70 or 78 Gy followed by standard BCNU schedule. Both of the two prospective trials failed to demonstrate a survival advantage of SRS or FSRT and the debate still remains open. From the advent of IMRT, the interest in radiosurgery has slowly decreased even if some prospective experiences with promising results in temozolomide era were reported [65].

*Brachytherapy* has been also investigated to escalate the dose because of its rapid dose decrease outside the high dose volume and of its relative sparing of normal tissues. Two randomized trials have been completed for newly GBM. Laperrière et al. (1998) [66] randomized 140 patients to EBRT delivering 50 Gy in 25 fractions over 5 weeks or EBRT plus high activity $^{125}$I implanted to an additional peripheral dose of 60 Gy. The BTCG performed a second randomized trial [67] (BTDG8701) involving 270 patients receiving EBRT plus BCNU followed by 60 Gy with $^{125}$I brachytherapy or without. Both studies failed to demonstrate a significant survival advantage of brachytherapy in newly malignant gliomas.

Nowadays the standard treatment is conventional RT with a total dose of 60 Gy. Hypofractionated protocols using high precision techniques such as IMRT or volumetric arc therapy should be confirmed by prospective randomized studies.

## Chemotherapy

Optimal chemotherapy for GBM is still unclear despite the standard regimen with Temozolomide (TMZ). Temozolomide has emerged as a major advance to improved patients survival. The Phase III 26981 trial, performed by EORTC/NCIC, demonstrated that concurrent (75 mg/m$^2$/day for <7 week) and adjuvant (150–200 mg/m$^2$/day on 5 days every 28 days for at least 6 maintenance cycles) chemoradiotherapy with TMZ conferred a 2.5-months survival benefit if compared to radiotherapy alone [3].

Before this study, the addition of chemotherapy to primary radiotherapy was investigated in several studies. Two meta-analysis [68, 69], including a large Medical Research Council trial [70], suggested only modest improvement in survival. Lipophilic alkylators have been the first successful drug able to cross the blood–brain barrier (BBB) and to damage DNA in order to kill the cycling of malignant cell population.

*Nitrosourea* has been used since the 1960s in several clinical trials. The BTSG 6901 [7] employed BCNU (80 mg/m$^2$/day for 3 days every 6–8 weeks) alone or in combination with RT compared with BSC or radiotherapy alone. The BCNU allowed for a better overall survival than the BSC but no significant advantage compared to radiotherapy alone. Another large intergroup cooperative study [32] compared two chemoradiation regimens and the use of BCNU resulted as being better tolerated and conferred a higher overall survival.

The PCV schedule of procarbazine, lomustine and vincristine, established in the 1970s, remains a major component of clinical practice and was investigated in several clinical trials, demonstrating a survival of adjuvant administration. A randomized trial [71] reported a doubling of median survival with PCV regimen compared to BCNU in malignant gliomas which previously received 60 Gy of RT plus hydroxyurea.

*Temozolomide* is a lipophilic alkylating drug that methylates of O-6 position of guanine preventing tumor cell proliferation, leading to the double strand breaks. It is able to penetrate the BBB, and it undergoes a spontaneous degradation at physiological pH to 3-methyl (triazen-1-yl) imidazole-4-carboxamide (MTIC). The DNA-repair enzyme O-6-methylguanine DNA methyl-transferase (MGMT) confers resistance to alkylated agents, therefore the methylation of the MGMT promoter, which inactivates transcription of the gene, predicts drug sensitivity [72–76]. Temozolomide was not initially developed for glioblastoma, but has attracted the interest of researchers after the observation of generic phase I trials. The promising results of preclinical studies [76, 77], conducted on glioma cells which used Temozolomide as radiosensitizer, and the employment of TMZ in recurrent patients, were followed by the landmark demonstration of improved outcome when used in combination with RT, suggesting an additive or synergistic interaction, as reported previously in the phase II study [3] and successively in the phase III randomized trial performed by EORTC and NCI-Canada (NCI-C) [3, 78]. Median and 2-years overall survival were better if compared with RT alone (12.1 vs. 14.6 months and 26 % vs. 10, $p < 0.001$ respectively).

Several questions remain regarding the optimal dosing schedule in combination with radiotherapy, the optimal number of adjuvant cycle and the role of concomitant or adjuvant TMZ, although there is some indication that adjuvant TMZ is more important than the low-dose concomitant treatment [79].

In order to optimize the deployment of this clear leader, *alternative dosing schedules* have been explored. A phase III trial tested *dose-dense* (dd) and metronomic dosing in the post-chemoradiation adjuvant phase. Another phase III trial RTOG 0525 [80] was designed to compare two adjuvant TMZ schedules, dd vs. standard dose (sd) in order to prolong MGMT depletion with a major dose intensity. However, intensified TMZ schedules are not superior to standard dose in clinical trials.

In the post-TMZ era, other phase III trials tested the use of nitrosourea and cisplatin or nimustine (ACNU) and CDDP. The promising therapeutic role of a combination of hydrophilic agents such as platinum and lipophilic drugs as nitrosourea in GBM patients [81, 82] and platinum's recognized role as a known radiosensitizer were investigated in a phase III trial using BCNU and CDDP with a significant 1.5-month improvement in overall survival with the intention to treat analysis, not confirmed considering only eligible patients. The rather small benefit and the increased toxicity as ototoxicity prevents further application of the combined regimen [83].

The use of a neo-adjuvant ACNU-CDDP followed by RT and TMZ in a Korean study was terminated prematurely due to hematologic toxicities [84], while the association with procarbazine was terminated in a Japanese study due to its failure in efficacy and safety when compared with ACNU alone.

The use of an aggressive combination of multiple conventional cytotoxic drugs does not correlate with superiority in survival outcomes, while presenting a high risk of serious side effects.

The standard chemotherapy remains TMZ, concomitant to conventional RT to 60 Gy and adjuvant for 6–12 cycles.

## Target Therapies

Advances in genomics have significantly improved our knowledge of the molecular features of glioblastoma, and allowed for its classification into molecular subtypes [85–87]. This has translated into the development of prognostic and predictive biomarkers, and the identification of specific targets for potential treatments.

Targeted cancer therapies are drugs or other substances that block the growth and spread of cancer by interfering with specific molecules involved in tumor growth and progression pathways.

Angiogenesis is a significant, complex and critical process in GBM [88]. Pathologically, malignant gliomas are characterized by endothelial proliferation and neovascularization. The *anti-angiogenic agents* are perhaps the most developed and studied, and the assessment of their use alone or in combination with a cytotoxic agent in the setting of progressive glioblastoma is a field of investigation and the use in GBM is supported by evidence: GBM is a highly vascularized tumor [89]; the vascular normalization theory assumes that there are normal vessels among the aberrant ones that leads drug administration [90]; the steroid like effect of VEGF (vascular endothelial growth factor) inhibition, because VEGF normally increases the vascular permeability; the activation of malignant cells by VEGF activity.

The VEGF is the best described and the most influential growth factor. *Bevacizumab* is a humanized monoclonal antibody to VEGF-A. Its development has been convoluted. It has been investigated in naive glioblastoma, concomitantly with TMZ and RT. AVAglio [91] and RTOG 0825 [23] trials failed to demonstrate a significant survival benefit. The progression-free survival (PFS) seems to have increased, while the results in terms of quality of life are controversial, showing worse condition and decline in neurocognitive function in RTOG trial and a good stable performance status in AVAglio study. Overall, the current data cannot justify the use of Bevacizumab in the first-line setting of GBM treatment [92].

Even if prospective and randomized studies have been performed, the advantage of target therapies still remains open to discussion and debate.

## Chemoradiation Therapy: Treatment at Progression or Recurrence

GBM is an aggressive disease and, despite standard of care therapy, it relapses in 90 % of patients. The optimum management for recurrent glioma has not been established. A variety of treatment such as repeated surgery, high precision radiotherapy techniques, chemotherapy, and supportive care should all be considered in multidisciplinary setting in order to carry out an appropriate and personalized treatment. Given the biological complexity of GBM predictive response in recurrence remains difficult to define. Median overall survival and PFS at 6 months remain the best end point available for assessing therapeutic outcome.

## Repeated Surgery

Surgery should be considered in selected patients with progressive or recurrent GBM. Studies on repeated surgery do not show a consistent benefit when compared with no reoperation [93–96] but a more favorable prognosis is associated with a younger age (<70 years), a smaller tumor volume (<50 cm$^3$), and a preoperative KPS greater than 80 % [97, 98], especially when surgery is followed by systemic adjuvant therapy [99–101].

The repeated surgery could be considered in selected cases.

## Radiation Therapy

Radiotherapy offers a local, non-systemic treatment alternative that should be considered at the time point of recurrence.

A *conventional regimen* is indicated in the case of secondary malignant gliomas not previously irradiated. In the setting of re-irradiation, there is a lack of prospective trials. Based on retrospective series, repeated radiotherapy remains a palliative option for selected patients.

A KPS >60 %, a tumor size of up to 40 mm, and a time to progression >6 months from surgery are the eligibility criteria for a repeated radiation treatment [102]. It is well established that local failure is the most common pattern of recurrence and that the risk of treatment-related side effects increases with target size as well as a RT escalation dose.

In the setting of previous partial brain irradiation and recurrence within the volume irradiated with a high dose, it is not advisable to administer another conventional course of irradiation to the recurrence site plus margins.

Over recent years conventional RT has improved and the advent of modern high precision techniques, such as stereotactic radiosurgery (SRS) or fractionated *stereotactic radiotherapy* (FSRT) or hypo-fractionated stereotactic radiotherapy (HFSRT), as well as the improvement in imaging modalities, has enabled the radiation oncologist to accurately describe the target volume and to individually define the optimal treatment.

*SRS* is a highly conformal, noninvasive technique, in which the total dose is delivered in a single fraction. Radiation therapy oncology Group (RTOG) 90-05 [62] demonstrated in recurrent brain tumors or in brain metastasis that SRS is safe and feasible and established the maximum tolerated dose for single fraction as following: 24 Gy, 18 Gy, and 15 Gy for tumors <20 mm, 21–30 mm, and 31–40 mm in maximum diameter. Unacceptable CNS toxicity was more likely in patients with larger tumors, whereas local tumor control was most dependent on the type of recurrent tumor and the treatment unit. Several studies confirmed its feasibility but that it should be reserved for smaller lesions.

In an experiment carried out in Minnesota [103] for 26 GBM treated with 20 Gy, 31 % of patients presented severe toxicity and 14 % a necrosis with an 8 months as median survival rate. At Harvard University [104] 13 Gy were delivered in 86 GBM with a 22 % of side effects.

Combs et al. [105] do not report any toxicity in 32 GBM treated with 17 Gy. The higher rate of severe effect reported in the first study might be due to the largest treatment volume (28 cm$^3$ vs. 10.1 and 10 cm$^3$).

In *FSRT*, the therapeutic dose is divided into a number of conventional fractions, exploiting the radiobiological advantage of fractionation and reducing the treatment side effects. It should be used for small lesions and therefore could be used as alternative to SRS, but it is also safe in the case of larger volumes.

Cho et al. [106] confirmed the major feasibility of FSRT compared with SRS; delivering 2.5 Gy in 15 fractions to 15 GBM and registering 8 % of toxicity instead of 30 % as delivering 17 Gy in single fraction. A large patient series of 172 patients was evaluated in the University of Heidelberg by Combs et al. [107] observing a median overall survival of 21 months.

The *HFSRT* technique can exploit the radiobiological advantage of fractionation and of accelerated treatment, reducing the overall treatment time which is a relevant issue in this setting of patients. Shepherd et al. [108] observed a higher risk of brain impairment for doses >40 Gy, testing a total dose range of 20–50 Gy at 5 Gy for fraction with 36 % of steroid-dependent toxicity and 6 % of reoperation. Hudes et al. [109] published the result of a dose escalation study from 24 to 35 Gy in median fraction of 3 Gy to 20 patients with no toxicity, no repeated surgery, and median survival of 10.5 months.

It is noteworthy that the choice between SRS, FSRT, and HFSRT appears to provide a reasonable median overall survival of approximately 6–12 months as reported in Table 4.4. The choice should be personalized, depending on the size and location of the lesion, its link with effected area of the brain, as well as the risk of side effects according to the previous radiation dose.

*IMRT* is another modern technique that allows a better dose conformity and sparing of the organ at risk, but requires a longer preparation time and increasing of the dose inhomogeneity into the target and the distribution of low doses around the target volume.

Therefore, IMRT has been investigated in small series of patients [131], and no dose limiting toxicity was observed at 35 Gy in 10 fractions after previous 60 Gy [109] and a good tolerance has been reported with 6×5 Gy [131].

Another technique that has been used in recurrent lesion smaller than 6 cm is the interstitial *brachytherapy* using high activity iodine 125 ($^{125}$I) or iridium-192 ($^{192}$I). Seed implants can produce inhomogeneous radiation dose distribution with 64 % of repeated surgery for radionecrosis. The $^{125}$I seeds can be used for permanent or temporary implants: permanent implants with a low-dose rate reduce the complication rate and allow for the same results as temporary high activity implants [132, 133]. Permanent brachytherapy produces a total dose rate of between 100 and 400 Gy and 50–65 Gy are applied over 4–12 days with median overall survival of 10.5–12 months [132–134]. With the use of temporary brachytherapy, a median overall survival from 9.1 to 12.3 was observed.

A novel alternative and temporary brachytherapy technique is the intracavitary low dose rate called Glia-site brachytherapy. Here a balloon catheter is placed in the resection cavity and used as a spherical source of low dose rate radiation. However, no conclusion can be reached regarding this device, and studies combining temozolomide and fractionated RT have been planned within the New Approaches to Brain Tumor Therapy (NABTT) CNS consortium.

*Hyperthermia* is an additional potential modality of treatment, which consists in increasing the antitumor action of chemotherapy and radiotherapy when the temperature is between 44 and 46 °C. The best evidence is reported in a randomized trial performed by Sneed et al. [135] in which 79 patients with focal tumor were randomized to brachytherapy with or without hyperthermia; a better survival was observed in the group receiving hyperthermia (31 % vs. 15 % at 2 years).

The use of *proton therapy* is reported in a few limited studies and selected cases, which are not considered sufficient to establish definitive evidence.

**Table 4.4** Studies of patients with recurrent gliomas treated with stereotactic radiotherapy

| Study | Median dose | No patients | Median OS (mo) | Toxicity |
|---|---|---|---|---|
| SRS | | | | |
| Chamberlain et al. [110] | 13.4×1 | 20 | 8 | – |
| Cho et al. [106] | 17×1 | 46 (27 GBM) | 11 | 22 % |
| Combs et al. [111] | 15×1 | 32 | 10 | – |
| Hall et al. [103] | 20×1 | 35 | 8 | 31 % with reoperation |
| Shrieve et al. [104] | 13×1 | 86 | 10.2 | 22 % reoperation rate; 48 %risk of reoperation |
| Biswas et al. [112] | 15×1 | 18 | 5.3 | RN in 1 pt |
| Kong et al. [113] | 16×1 | 65 | 13 | RN in 22 % |
| Patel et al. [114] | 18×1 | 26 | 8.4 | RN in 1 pt |
| Sirin et al. [115] | 16×1 | 19 | 9.3 | No gr>3 |
| Elliot et al. [116] | 15×1 | 16 | 12.9 | RN in 2 pt |
| Skeie et al. [117] | 12.2×1 | 51 | 12 | 908 % |
| Lederman et al. [118] | 6×x1 | 88 | 7 | 12 % reoperation |
| Larson et al. [119] | 15×1 | 14 | 8.8 | NR |
| Cuneo et al. [120] | 18×1 | 16 | 4 | RN in 19 % |
| Park et al. [121] | 16×1 | 11 | 12 | 9 % |
| FSRT | | | | |
| Cho et al. [106] | 2.5×15 | 15 | 7.1 | 8 % |
| Combs et al. [107] | 2×18 | 59 | 8 | RN in 1 pt |
| Niyazi et al. [122] | 2×18 | 22 | 5.8 (all pts) | G3 in 1 pt |
| Hundsberger et al. [123] | 2.67×15 | 8 | 9 (all pts) | RN in 1 pt |
| HFSRT | | | | |
| Hudes et al. [109] | 30/3 Gy/fr | 19 | 10.5 | 0 % |
| Shepherd et al. [108] | 20–50/5 Gy/fr | 29 | 11 | 36 % |
| Patel et al. [114] | 36/6 Gy/fr | 10 | 7.5 | – |
| Kim et al. [124] | 25/5 Gy/fr | 4 | 7.6 (all pts) | RN in 1 pt |
| Minniti et al. [125] | 30/6 Gy7fr | 38 | 12.4 (all) | G3 in 7 % |
| Combined with BVZ | | | | |
| Fogh et al. [126] | 35 /3.5 Gy/fr | 105 | 10 | G3 in 1 pt |
| Gutin et al. [127] | 30/6 Gy/fr | 20 | 13 | G3 in 3 pts |
| Cuneo et al. [120] | 18×1 or 25/5 Gy/fr | 33 | 11 | RN in 5 % |
| Torcuator et al. [128] | 18×1 or 36/6 Gy/fr | 18 | 7 | – |
| Park et al. [121] | 16×1 | 11 | 18 | – |
| Mckenzie et al. [129] | 30/6 Gy/fr | 30 | 8.6 (all pts) | RN in 3 pts |
| Cabrera et al. [130] | 18×1 | 8 | 14.4 | G3 in 1 pt |

*SRS* stereotactic radiosurgery, *FSRT* conventionally fractionated stereotactic radiotherapy, *HFSRT* hypofractionated stereotactic radiotherapy, *RN* radionecrosis, *NR* not reported

Nowadays re-irradiation is a valid palliative option in recurrent gliomas. The advance of techniques and technology allows for personalized treatment in selected cases but its use needs to be investigated in further studies.

## Chemotherapy

A broad range of chemotherapy agents have been and are being evaluated in the setting of recurrent GBM in monotherapy or combined trials.

Several studies have evaluated the efficacy and safety of *TMZ*, albeit few of the trials were conducted as prospective randomized controlled design. A randomized prospective phase II study demonstrating the significant superiority of TMZ over procarbazina with a PFS at 6 months of 21 % compared to 8 % ($p=0.008$) [136]. Other prospective single arm studies [137, 138] were carried out to test the standard dosing of TMZ but, given the incomplete success and occasional observation, alternative dose regimens were explored. After Stupp et al. [3], a protracted *dose-dense* (dd) temozolomide was investigated in the randomized study BR12 carried out by Brada et al. [139] without a survival or PFS benefit compared with a standard dose. Abacioglu et al. [140] tested TMZ 100 mg/m$^2$ for 21 consecutive days in a 28 day cycle, observing modest activity and a manageable toxicity. The DIRECTOR trial [141] evaluated 2 dose-intense regimens of TMZ (120 mg/m$^2$/day 1 week on/1 week off vs. 80 mg/m$^2$/day 3 week on/1 week off) in patients experiencing a first relapse after at least 2 cycles of TMZ, no earlier than 180 days after first surgery and no earlier than 90 days after completion of radiotherapy. The data is currently being processed.

The three-arm trial by Brada et al. compared different schedules of TMZ, sd or dd, to PCV schedule in chemotherapy-naive patients [139]. The sdTMZ is superior to PCV in terms of quality of life and more effective than ddTMZ in terms of survival.

TMZ *rechallenge* with a variety of metronomic schedules was employed in several studies [142–147], including 40–100 mg/m$^2$/day given for 21–365 consecutive days, as well as alternating 1 week on/1 week off. It resulted in a PFS-6 rate of 23–58.3 % with a median OS rate of 5.1–13 months. The RESCUE study [145] examined the benefit of TMZ rechallenge based on the TMZ free interval and it observed that those who experienced early progression obtained the most benefit from this schedule with a PFS6 of 27.3 % and a median OS of 3.6 months when progression is made while receiving TMZ and before 6 cycle adjuvant TMZ.

A *one week on–one week off* regimen was investigated by Wick et al. obtaining a response rate of 10 % and a PFS-6 rate of 44–48 % without substantial hematopoietic adverse events. The problem with these studies is that no patient had received prior chemotherapy.

Considering the small number of patients in most studies and the wide range of TMZ regimens tested, there was no evidence that one metronomic schedule was better than another in terms of safety; however, compared with the standard 5 of 28 day regimen, the dose-dense schedule is associated with an increased incidence of lymphocytopenia [148].

Over the last years phase I and II studies have investigated the advantages of using TMZ in *combination* with cisplatin, fotemustine, interferon, irinotecan, or procarbazine/lomustine/vincristine or target therapies but no single combination has clearly emerged as more effective than just TMZ alone.

Since the approval of TMZ in 1999, *nitrosoureas* (carmustine, lomustine, nimustine, procarbazine), which were previously employed in the first-line treatment of GBM, were moved into the second line therapy, and used alone or in combination regimens for recurrent disease. The efficacy and the feasibility of nitrosoureas are similar, although carmustina is related with a higher non-hematological toxicity. The PFS at 6 months ranged from 13 to 24.5 % and median OS ranged from 5.1 to 11.1 months considering the use of carmustine alone [149–151], lomustine [152–154], or fotemustine [155–158].

Other chemotherapeutic agents have been examined and others are currently being investigated but the data available is not conclusive for a standard treatment of recurrent GBM.

A standard chemotherapy in recurrence has not been established yet. Similar results could be obtained by using both old and new drugs.

## Target Therapies

The *anti-angiogenetic agents* are the most developed and studied target therapies in recurrent GBM.

*Bevacizumab (BCZ)* has been approved by FDA in recurrence setting after the promising results of two studies. The first prospective randomized phase II study by Friedmann et al. [159] provides a well-documented superiority in terms of PFS at 6 months and median OS (42.6 % and 9.2 months) of BCZ alone or in combination with irinotecan when compared with standard cytotoxic agents ($p < 0.0001$) [160, 161]. The adding of irinotecan did not increase the outcome rates. The second report by Kreisl et al. (2009) [162] described the experience of BVZ alone in 48 patients with a PFS-6 rate of 29 % and an overall response rate of 35 %.

Further prospective analysis of combined regimes with cytotoxic agent did not show any clear benefit over BVZ alone, while the timing and the dosage still remain to be established.

Unfortunately, toxicities of this regimen require discontinuation and seem to be associated with substantial and rapid tumor progression [163–165].

The anti-angiogenetic agents remain the most investigated therapies, but the efficacy needs to be confirmed by further prospective trials.

## Combined Modality Therapies with Radiotherapy

To optimize the treatment results obtained by re-irradiation, the addition of chemotherapy may offer some specific benefit. However, the combined approach might be less tolerated and it should be considered with caution.

Some investigators explored the association of conventional or hypo-fractionated radiotherapy with lomustine (CCNU) [166] concurrent to 34.5 Gy at 1.5 Gy for fraction, with CDDP [167] concurrent to hypo-fractionated RT (35–42 Gy at 3.5–6 Gy for fraction), or with paclitaxel receiving 18–36 Gy at 4–9 Gy/fr [118], or with topotecan treated with 30 Gy in 6 fractions [168]. The median overall survival ranged from 7 in the case of paclitaxel to 13.7 months when radiotherapy was concurrent to lomustine and CDDP.

Another combined modality is the association with target therapies, especially anti-angiogenetic drugs. The paradoxical angiogenetic effect of radiotherapy by the up-regulation of hypoxia factor might be modulated by the use of anti-angiogenetic agents. The combination of Bevacizumab (BVZ)

and SRS or HFSRT seems to provide a survival benefit and to reduce adverse radiation effects if it is compared with other exclusive modalities, although no prospective trials directly compare RT with BVZ versus BVZ alone.

A prospective trial of HFSRT and BVZ at Memorial Sloan Kettering Cancer Center [127] reported the feasibility of the combined treatment with a median overall survival of 12 months. The feasibility was also reported also by Cabrera et al. [130] in a group of 15 patients with recurrent GBM, showing maximal grade 3 toxicity in only 1 patient. A retrospective study [120] comparing the SRS alone and the combination with BVZ showed a significantly higher survival benefit, although these patients received several drugs after SRS, and a lower rate of radionecrosis.

The RTOG 1205 is currently randomized in patients with recurrent GBM to receive BVZ alone or in combination with HFSRT and the overall survival is the primary end point.

Alternatively, several authors have proposed a novel combined palliative regimen with low doses of fractionated radiotherapy (LD-FRT) as chemo-potentiator. In vitro studies demonstrated a low dose hypersensitivity (<1 Gy) in some glioma cell lines that was not predicted by the linear quadratic model, with an increased cell kill per unit dose [169, 170]; preclinical studies [171, 172] demonstrated a synergistic effect between LD-FRT and multiple chemotherapeutic alkylating agents. Recurrence during TMZ received CDDP (30 mg/mq on days 1,8,15), fotemustine (40 mg/mq on days 2,9,16) and concurrent LD-FRT 0.3 twice daily concurrent, while recurrence after 4 months from the end of adjuvant TMZ was treated by TMZ (150–200 mg/m² on days 1–5) concomitant with LD-FRT 0.4 twice daily. The combined regimen resulted feasible and median PFS and overall survival were 5 and 8 months, respectively [173, 174].

## Elderly

The elderly are a heterogeneous population and the optimal treatment depends on performance status, functional, cognitive, and physiological conditions. Elderly patients who have a good performance status favored a maximal safe resection [175–178]. The survival benefit of adjuvant treatment compared with BSC alone has been demonstrated by a series of prospective and retrospective trials, without any significant compromise of quality of life or neurocognitive function.

The phase II ANOEF trial (Association des Neuro-Oncologue D'Expression Française trial) showed the feasibility of TMZ as alternative to BSC, while a randomized and a prospective single arm trial demonstrated the significant advantage of RT (50 Gy in 28 fractions [179] or 30 Gy in 10 fractions [45]).

The choice between RT and TMZ should be based on the assessment of the MGMT promoter methylation status: patients with MGMT methylated tumors obtain the major advantage from treatment with TMZ [30, 180]. The optimal dose and fractionation remain to be defined.

Some randomized trials [29, 30] agreed that hypo-fractionated RT is not inferior to standard RT in respect to survival and quality of life with a better safety profile and a significant survival advantage in patients older than 70 years (7 vs. 5.2 months $p = 0.02$) [30].

Some studies have demonstrated a survival benefit in the elderly treated with combined treatments of RT and concurrent and adjuvant TMZ, that might be considered in selected patients with good performance status [181]. Its use might be limited by the high incidence of radiation induced neurological toxicity [182].

The hypo-fractionated RT in combination with TMZ might be an alternative. The study reported a median OS of 12.4 months administering 40 Gy in 15 fractions over 3 weeks [179]. Data from the recently closed multicenter, randomized EORTC26062/22061-NCIC-CTG C.6 trial [183], that explored the advantage of hypo-fractionated RT with or without concomitant and adjuvant TMZ.

Therefore, elderly patients with good performance status might be candidates for maximal resection followed by combined radiation and chemotherapy. A monotherapy strategy with temozolomide or hypo-fractionated RT should be considered in fragile, elderly patients with poor performance status and limited life expectancy depending on MGMT promoter methylation.

## Research Trends

Numerous therapeutic strategies for both newly and recurrent GBM are still undergoing. Several research trends can be identified to highlight the future trends. New microsurgical assistant systems such as intraoperative MRI and fluorescence-guided resection need to be validated. Unpublished and ongoing phase III trials are investigating new delivery technique in RT such as IMRT plus TMZ (NCT01507506), or the combination of standard RT with other chemotherapeutic agents such as lomustine (NCT01149109), or BCNU and O6-benzylguanine (NCT00017147) and are testing altered fractionations in short course RT in elderly patients (NCT01450449). Optimal usage of modified TMZ schedules, target agents against growth factors or small module kinases or immunotherapy in association with standard radio-chemotherapy are being studied to balance feasibility and efficacy as well as individualized treatment depending on biomarkers stratification.

Gene therapy, photodynamic therapy, and novel therapeutic modalities are all modern and interesting fields of investigation. Low voltage, intermediate-frequency alternating electric fields (AEFs) are a novel anti-cancer modality for the treatment of GBM approved in April 2011 by the FDA. Pilot studies [184] have demonstrated that electric fields of 100–300 kHz can influence tumor cell division and promising but as yet unconfirmed results have been reported in a phase III trial by Stupp et al. [185] carried out using the NovoTTF device.

In the last 10 years clinical practice is leading to a personalized medicine. Some authors propose a patient-specific accelerated failure time (AFT) survival model, resulting from 721 newly diagnosed patients with glioblastoma, in order to calculate the incremental survival advantages associated with incremental changes in extent of surgical resection (EOR), while also taking into account age, Karnofsky performance status, and adjuvant therapy with radiotherapy and/or TMZ [186]. The predictive accuracy improves by 21.5–25.9 % over current extent of surgical resection (EOR)-threshold-only models, determining the personalized relationship between survival and EOR during the management decision making process, before surgery or before adjuvant therapy. Studies based on different population-based datasets will be conducted in order to develop predictive models that allow physicians to share decisions with patients regarding a wider concept of personalized treatment.

# References

1. Crocetti E, Trama A, Stiller C, Caldarella A, Soffietti R, Jaal J, et al. Epidemiology of glial and non-glial brain tumours in Europe. Eur J Cancer. 2012;48(10):1532–42. doi:10.1016/j.ejca.2011.12.013.
2. Dolecek TA, Propp JM, Stroup NE, Kruchko C. CBTRUS statistical report: primary brain and central nervous system tumors diagnosed in the United States in 2005–2009. Neuro Oncol. 2012;14 Suppl 5:1–49. doi:10.1093/neuonc/nos218.
3. Stupp R, Mason WP, van den Bent MJ, Weller M, Fisher B, Taphoorn MJ, European Organisation for Research and Treatment of Cancer Brain Tumor and Radiotherapy Groups, National Cancer Institute of Canada Clinical Trials Group, et al. Radiotherapy plus concomitant and adjuvant temozolomide for glioblastoma. N Engl J Med. 2005;352(10):987–96.
4. Laperriere N, Zuraw L, Cairncross G, Cancer Care Ontario Practice Guidelines Initiative Neuro-Oncology Disease Site Group. Radiotherapy for newly diagnosed malignant glioma in adults: a systematic review. Radiother Oncol. 2002;64(3):259–73.
5. Shapiro WR, Young DF. Treatment of malignant glioma. A controlled study of chemotherapy and irradiation. Arch Neurol. 1976;33:494–500.
6. Andersen AP. Postoperative irradiation of glioblastomas. Results in a randomized series. Acta Radiol Oncol. 1978;17:475–84.
7. Walker MD, Alexander Jr E, Hunt WE, MacCarty CS, Mahaley Jr MS, Mealey Jr J, et al. Evaluation of BCNU and/or radiotherapy in the treatment of anaplastic gliomas. A cooperative clinical trial. J Neurosurg. 1978;49:333–43.
8. Walker MD, Green SB, Byar DP, Alexander Jr E, Batzdorf U, Brooks WH, et al. Randomized comparisons of radiotherapy and nitrosoureas for the treatment of malignant glioma after surgery. N Engl J Med. 1980;303:1323–9.
9. Kristiansen K, Hagen S, Kollevold T, Torvik A, Holme I, Nesbakken R, et al. Combined modality therapy of operated astrocytomas grade III and IV. Confirmation of the value of postoperative irradiation and lack of potentiation of bleomycin on survival time: a prospective multicenter trial of the Scandinavian Glioblastoma Study Group. Cancer. 1981;47:649–52.
10. Sandberg-Wollheim M, Malmstrom P, Stromblad LG, Anderson H, Borgström S, Brun A, et al. A randomized study of chemotherapy with procarbazine, vincristine, and lomustine with and without radiation therapy for astrocytoma grades 3 and/or 4. Cancer. 1991;68:22–9.
11. Kita M, Okawa T, Tanaka M, Ikeda M. Radiotherapy of malignant glioma-prospective randomized clinical study of whole brain vs. local irradiation [In Japanese]. Gan No Rinsho. 1989;35:1289–94.
12. Shapiro WR, Green SB, Burger PC, Mahaley Jr MS, Selker RG, VanGilder JC, et al. Randomized trial of three chemotherapy regimens and two radiotherapy regimens in postoperative treatment of malignant glioma. Brain Tumor Cooperative Group Trial 8001. J Neurosurg. 1989;71:1–9.
13. Hochberg FH, Pruitt A. Assumptions in the radiotherapy of glioblastoma. Neurology. 1980;30:907–11.
14. Wallner KE, Galicich JH, Krol G, Arbit E, Malkin MG, et al. Patterns of failure following treatment for glioblastoma multiforme and anaplastic astrocytoma. Int J Radiat Oncol Biol Phys. 1989;16:1405–9.
15. Liang BC, Thornton Jr AF, Sandler HM, Greenberg HS, et al. Malignant astrocytomas: focal tumor recurrence after focal external beam radiation therapy. J Neurosurg. 1991;75:559–63.
16. Sharma RR, Singh DP, Pathak A, Khandelwal N, Sehgal CM, Kapoor R, et al. Local control of high-grade gliomas with limited volume irradiation versus whole brain irradiation. Neurol India. 2003;51(4):512–7.
17. Gaspar LE, Fisher BJ, Macdonald DR, LeBer DV, Halperin EC, Schold Jr SC, et al. Supratentorial malignant glioma: patterns of recurrence and implications for external beam local treatment. Int J Radiat Oncol Biol Phys. 1992;24:55–7.
18. DeSchryver A, Greitz T, Forsby N, Brun A. Localized shaped field radiotherapy of malignant glioblastoma multiforme. Int J Radiat Oncol Biol Phys. 1976;1:713–6.
19. Garden AS, Max MH, Yung WKA, Bruner JM, Woo SY, Moser RP, et al. Outcome and pattern of failure following limited volume irradiation for malignant astrocytomas. Radiation Oncol. 1991;20:99–110.
20. Lee SW, Fraass BA, Marsh LH, Herbort K, Gebarski SS, Martel MK, Radany EH, et al. Patterns of failure following high-dose 3-D conformal radiotherapy for high grade astrocytomas: a quantitative dosimetric

study. Int J Radiat Oncol Biol Phys. 1999; 43(1):79–88.

21. Nelson DF, Curran Jr WJ, Scott C, et al. Hyperfractionated radiation therapy and bischlorethyl nitrosourea in the treatment of malignant glioma—possible advantage observed at 72.0 Gy in 1.2 Gy B.I.D. fractions: report of the Radiation Therapy Oncology Group Protocol 8302. Int J Radiat Oncol Biol Phys. 1993;25:193–207.

22. Urtasun RC, Kinsella TJ, Farnan N, DelRowe JD, Lester SG, Fulton DS, et al. Survival improvement in anaplastic astrocytoma, combining external radiation with halogenated pyrimidines: final report of RTOG 86-12, Phase I-II study. Int J Radiat Oncol Biol Phys. 1996;36:1163–7.

23. Gilbert MR, Dignam J, Won M, Blumenthal DB, Vogelbaum MA, Aldape KD et al. Radiation Therapy Oncology Group. RTOG 0825: Phase III double-blind placebo-controlled trial of conventional concurrent chemoradiation and adjuvant temozolomide plus bevacizumab versus conventional concurrent chemoradiation and adjuvant temozolomide in patients with newly diagnosed glioblastoma. J Clin Oncol. 2013;31. Suppl; abstr 1

24. Colman H, Berkey BA, Maor MH, Groves MD, Schultz CJ, Vermeulen S, Nelson DF, Mehta MP, Yung WK, Radiation Therapy Oncology Group. Phase II Radiation Therapy Oncology Group trial of conventional radiation therapy followed by treatment with recombinant interferon-beta for supratentorial glioblastoma: results of RTOG 9710. Int J Radiat Oncol Biol Phys. 2006;66(3):818–24.

25. Brandes AA, Tosoni A, Franceschi E, Sotti G, Frezza G, Amista P, et al. Recurrence pattern after temozolomide concomitant with and adjuvant to radiotherapy in newly diagnosed patients with glioblastoma: correlation with MGMT promoter methylation status. J Clin Oncol. 2009;27:1275–9. doi:10.1200/JCO.2008.19.4969.

26. Minniti G, Amelio D, Amichetti M, Salvati M, Muni R, Bozzao A, et al. Patterns of failure and comparison of different target volume delineations in patients with glioblastoma treated with conformal radiotherapy plus concomitant and adjuvant temozolomide. Radiother Oncol. 2010;97(3):377–81. doi:10.1016/j.radonc.2010.08.020.

27. Chang EL, Akyurek S, Avalos T, Rebueno N, Spicer C, Garcia J, et al. Evaluation of peritumoral edema in the delineation of radiotherapy clinical target volumes for glioblastoma. Int J Radiat Oncol Biol Phys. 2007;68(1):144–50.

28. McDonald MW, Shu HK, Curran Jr WJ, Crocker IR. Pattern of failure after limited margin radiotherapy and temozolomide for glioblastoma. Int J Radiat Oncol Biol Phys. 2011;79(1):130–6. doi:10.1016/j.ijrobp.2009.10.048.

29. Roa W, Brasher PM, Bauman G, Anthes M, Bruera E, Chan A, et al. Abbreviated course of radiation therapy in older patients with glioblastoma multiforme:

a prospective randomized clinical trial. J Clin Oncol. 2004;22(9):1583–8.

30. Malmström A, Grønberg BH, Marosi C, Stupp R, Frappaz D, Schultz H, et al. Temozolomide versus standard 6-week radiotherapy versus hypofractionated radiotherapy in patients older than 60 years with glioblastoma: the Nordic randomised, phase 3 trial. Lancet Oncol. 2012;13(9):916–26.

31. Walker MD, Strike TA, Sheline GE. An analysis of dose-effect relationship in the radiotherapy of malignant gliomas. Int J Radiat Oncol Biol Phys. 1979;5(10):1725–31.

32. Chang CH, Horton J, Schoenfeld D, Salazer O, Perez-Tamayo R, Kramer S, et al. Comparison of postoperative radiotherapy and combined postoperative radiotherapy and chemotherapy in the multidisciplinary management of malignant gliomas. A joint Radiation Therapy Oncology Group and Eastern Cooperative Oncology Group study. Cancer. 1983;52(6):997–1007.

33. Payne DG, Simpson WJ, Keen C, Platts ME. Malignant astrocytoma: hyperfractionated and standard radiotherapy with chemotherapy in a randomized prospective clinical trial. Cancer. 1982;50:2301–6.

34. Shin KH, Muller PJ, Geggie PH. Superfractionation radiation therapy in the treatment of malignant astrocytoma. Cancer. 1983;52:2040–3.

35. Shin KH, Urtasun RC, Fulton D, Geggie PH, Tanasichuk H, Thomas H, et al. Multiple daily fractionated radiation therapy and misonidazole in the management of malignant astrocytoma. A preliminary report. Cancer. 1985;56:758–60.

36. Ludgate CM, Douglas BG, Dixon PF, Steinbok P, Jackson SM, Goodman GB, et al. Superfractionated radiotherapy in grade III, IV intracranial gliomas. Int J Radiat Oncol Biol Phys. 1988;15:1091–5.

37. Deutsch M, Green SB, Strike TA, Burger PC, Robertson JT, Selker RG, et al. Results of a randomized trial comparing BCNU plus radiotherapy, streptozotocin plus radiotherapy, BCNU plus hyperfractionated radiotherapy, and BCNU following misonidazole plus radiotherapy in the postoperative treatment of malignant glioma. Int J Radiat Oncol Biol Phys. 1989;16:1389–96.

38. Scott CB, Curran WJ, Yung WKA, et al. Long-term results of RTOG-90-06. A randomized trial of hyperfractionated radiotherapy to 72 Gy and carmustina vs. standard RT and carmustina for malignant glioma patients with emphasis on anaplastic astrocytoma patients. J Clin Oncol. 1998;17:401.

39. Horiot JC, van den Bogaert W, Ang KK, Van der Schueren E, Bartelink H, Gonzalez D, et al. European Organization for Research on Treatment of Cancer Trials using radiotherapy with multiple fractions per day. Front Radiat Ther Oncol. 1988;22:149–61.

40. Brada M, Sharpe G, Rajan B, Britton J, Wilkins PR, Guerrero D, et al. Modifying radical radiotherapy in high grade gliomas; shortening the treatment time

through acceleration. Int J Radiat Oncol Biol Phys. 1999;43(2):287–92.

41. Werner-Wasik M, Scott CB, Nelson DF, Gaspar LE, Murray KJ, Fischbach JA, et al. Final report of a phase I/II trial of hyperfractionated and accelerated hyperfractionated radiation therapy with carmustine for adults with supratentorial malignant gliomas. Radiation Therapy Oncology Group Study 83-02. Cancer. 1996;77:1535–43.

42. Chen C, Damek D, Gaspar LE, Waziri A, Lillehei K, Kleinschmidt-DeMasters BK, et al. Phase I trial of hypofractionated intensity-modulated radiotherapy with temozolomide chemotherapy for patients with newly diagnosed glioblastoma multiforme. Int J Radiat Oncol Biol Phys. 2011;81:1066–74. doi:10.1016/j.ijrobp.2010.07.021.

43. Kleinberg LR, Slick T, Enger C, Grossman S, Brem H, Wharam Jr MD, et al. Short course radiotherapy is an appropriate option for most malignant glioma patients. Int J Radiat Oncol Biol Phys. 1997;38:31–6.

44. Glinski B. Postoperative hypofractionated radiotherapy versus conventionally fractionated radiotherapy in malignant gliomas. A preliminary report on a randomized trial. J Neurooncol. 1993;16:167–72.

45. Bauman GS, Gaspar LE, Fisher BJ, Halperin EC, Macdonald DR, Cairncross JG. A prospective study of short- course radiotherapy in poor prognosis glioblastoma multiforme. Int J Radiat Oncol Biol Phys. 1994;29(4):835–9. PMID: 8040031.

46. Ford JM, Stenning SP, Boote DJ, Counsell R, Falk SJ, Flavin A, et al. A short fractionation radiotherapy treatment for poor prognosis patients with high grade glioma. Clin Oncol (R Coll Radiol). 1997;9(1):20–4.

47. Hoegler DB, Davey P. A prospective study of short course radiotherapy in elderly patients with malignant glioma. J Neurooncol. 1997;33:201–4.

48. Slotman BJ, Kralendonk JH, van Alphen HA, Kamphorst W, Karim AB, et al. Hypofractionated radiation therapy in patients with glioblastoma multiforme: results of treatment and impact of prognostic factors. Int J Radiat Oncol Biol Phys. 1996;34:895–8.

49. Prados MD, Wara WM, Sneed PK, McDermott M, Chang SM, Rabbitt J. Phase III trial of accelerated hyperfractionation with or without difluoromethylornithine (DFMO) versus standard fractionated radiotherapy with or without DFMO for newly diagnosed patients with glioblastoma multiforme. Int J Radiat Oncol Biol Phys. 2001;49(1):71–7.

50. Massaccesi M, Ferro M, Cilla S, Balducci M, Deodato F, Macchia G, et al. Accelerated intensity-modulated radiotherapy plus Temozolomide in patients with glioblastoma: a phase I dose-escalation study (ISIDE-BT-1). Int J Clin Oncol. 2013;18(5):784–91. doi:10.1007/s10147-012-0462-0.

51. Iuchi T, Hatano K, Kodama T, Sakaida T, Yokoi S, Kawasaki K, et al. Phase 2 trial of hypofractionated high-dose intensity modulated radiation therapy with concurrent and adjuvant temozolomide for newly diagnosed glioblastoma. Int J Radiat Oncol

Biol Phys. 2014;88(4):793–800. doi:10.1016/j.ijrobp.2013.12.011.

52. Hasegawa M, Niibe H, Mitsuhashi N, Yamakawa M, Kato S, Furuta M, et al. Hyperfractionated and hypofractionated radiation therapy for human malignant glioma xenograft in nude mice. Jpn J Cancer Res. 1995;86:879–84.

53. Budach W, Gioioso D, Taghian A, Stuschke M, Suit HD. Repopulation capacity during fractionated irradiation of squamous cell carcinomas and glioblastomas in vitro. Int J Radiat Oncol Biol Phys. 1997;39:743–50.

54. Hulshof MCCM, Schimmel EC, Bosch DA, et al. Hypofractionation in glioblastoma multiforme. Radiother Oncol. 2000;54:143–8.

55. Fuller CD, Choi M, Forthuber B, Wang SJ, Rajagiriyil N, Salter BJ, et al. Standard fractionation intensity modulated radiation therapy (IMRT) of primary and recurrent glioblastoma multiforme. Radiat Oncol. 2007;2:26.

56. Narayana A, Yamada J, Berry S, Shah P, Hunt M, Gutin PH, et al. Intensity-modulated radiotherapy in high-grade gliomas: clinical and dosimetric results. Int J Radiat Oncol Biol Phys. 2006;64:892–7.

57. Iuchi T, Hatano K, Narita Y, Kodama T, Yamaki T, Osato K, et al. Hypofractionated high dose irradiation for the treatment of malignant astrocytomas using simultaneous integrated boost technique by IMRT. Int J Radiat Oncol Biol Phys. 2006;64:1317–24.

58. Morganti AG, Balducci M, Salvati M, Esposito V, Romanelli P, Ferro M, et al. A phase I dose escalation study (ISIDE-BT-1) of accelerated IMRT with temozolomide in patients with glioblastoma. Int J Radiat Oncol Biol Phys. 2010;77:92–7.

59. Chan JL, Lee SW, Fraass BA, Normolle DP, Greenberg HS, Junck LR, et al. Survival and failure patterns of high-grade gliomas after three-dimensional conformal radiotherapy. J Clin Oncol. 2002;20:1635–42.

60. Sarkaria JN, Mehta MP, Loeffler JS, Buatti JM, Chappell RJ, Levin AB, et al. Radiosurgery in the initial management of malignant gliomas: survival comparison with the RTOG recursive partitioning analysis. Radiation Therapy Oncology Group. Int J Radiat Oncol Biol Phys. 1995;32(4):931–41.

61. Loeffler JS, Alexander 3rd E, Shea WM, Wen PY, Fine HA, Kooy HM, et al. Radiosurgery as part of the initial management of patients with malignant gliomas. J Clin Oncol. 1992;10:1379–85.

62. Shaw E, Scott C, Souhami L, Dinapoli R, Bahary JP, Kline R, et al. Radiosurgery for the treatment of previously irradiated recurrent primary brain tumors and brain metastases: initial report of radiation therapy oncology group protocol (90-05). Int J Radiat Oncol Biol Phys. 1996;34(3):647–54.

63. Souhami L, Seiferheld W, Brachman D, Podgorsak EB, Werner-Wasik M, Lustig R, et al. Randomized comparison of stereotactic radiosurgery followed by conventional radiotherapy with carmustine to conventional radiotherapy with carmustine for patient

with glioblastoma multiforme: report of Radiation Therapy Oncology Group 93-05 protocol. Int J Radiat Oncol Biol Phys. 2004;60(3):853–60.

64. Cardinale R, Won M, Choucair A, Gillin M, Chakravarti A, Schultz C, et al. A phase II trial of accelerated radiotherapy using weekly stereotactic conformal boost for supratentorial glioblastoma multiforme: RTOG 0023. Int J Radiat Oncol Biol Phys. 2006;65(5):1422–8.

65. Balducci M, Apicella G, Manfrida S, Mangiola A, Fiorentino A, Azario L, et al. Single-arm phase II study of conformal radiation therapy and temozolomide plus fractionated stereotactic conformal boost in high-grade gliomas: final report. Strahlenther Onkol. 2010;186(10):558–64. doi:10.1007/s00066-010-2101-x.

66. Laperriere NJ, Leung PM, McKenzie S, Milosevic M, Wong S, Glen J, et al. Randomized study of brachytherapy in the initial management of patients with malignant astrocytoma. Int J Radiat Oncol Biol Phys. 1998;41(5):1005–11.

67. Selker RG, Shapiro WR, Burger P, Blackwood MS, Arena VC, Gilder JC, et al. The Brain Tumor Cooperative Group NIH Trial 87–01: randomized comparison of surgery, external radiotherapy, and carmustine versus surgery, interstitial radiotherapy boost, external radiation therapy, and carmustine. Neurosurgery. 2002;51(2):343–55. PMID: 12182772; discussion 355–7.

68. Fine HA, Dear KB, Loeffler JS, Black PM, Canellos GP. Meta-analysis of radiation therapy with and without adjuvant chemotherapy for malignant gliomas in adults. Cancer. 1993;71(8):2585–97. PMID: 8453582.

69. Stewart LA. Chemotherapy in adult high-grade glioma: a systematic review and meta-analysis of individual patient data from 12 randomised trials. Lancet. 2002;359:1011–8.

70. Party MRCBTW. Randomized trial of procarbazine, lomustine, and vincristine in the adjuvant treatment of high-grade astrocytoma: a Medical Research Council trial. J Clin Oncol. 2001;19:509e518.

71. Levin VA, Wara WM, Davis RL, Vestnys P, Resser KJ, Yatsko K, et al. Phase III comparison of BCNU and the combination of procarbazine, CCNU, and vincristine administered after radiotherapy with hydroxyurea for malignant gliomas. J Neurosurg. 1985;63(2):218–23.

72. Gerson SL. MGMT: its role in cancer aetiology and cancer therapeutics. Nat Rev Cancer. 2004;4(4):296–307.

73. Hegi ME, Diserens AC, Gorlia T, Hamou MF, de Tribolet N, Weller M, et al. MGMT gene silencing and benefit from temozolomide in glioblastoma. N Engl J Med. 2005;352:997e1003.

74. Brennan CW, Verhaak RG, McKenna A, Campos B, Noushmehr H, Salama SR, et al. The somatic genomic landscape of glioblastoma. Cell. 2013;155:462e477. doi:10.1016/j.cell.2013.09.034.

75. Weller M, Stupp R, Reifenberger G, Brandes AA, van den Bent MJ, Wick W, et al. MGMT promoter methylation in malignant gliomas: ready for personalized medicine? Nat Rev Neurol. 2010;6:39–51. doi:10.1038/nrneurol.2009.197.

76. Friedman HS, McLendon RE, Kerby T, Dugan M, Bigner SH, Henry AJ, et al. DNA mismatch repair and O6-alkylguanine-DNA alkyltransferase analysis and response to Temodal in newly diagnosed malignant glioma. J Clin Oncol. 1998;16(12):3851–7.

77. van Rijn J, Heimans JJ, van den Berg J, van der Valk P, Slotman BJ. Survival of human glioma cells treated with various combination of temozolomide and X-rays. Int J Radiat Oncol Biol Phys. 2000;47(3):779–84.

78. Stupp R, Hegi ME, Mason WP, van den Bent MJ, Taphoorn MJ, Janzer RC. Effects of radiotherapy with concomitant and adjuvant temozolomide versus radiotherapy alone on survival in glioblastoma in a randomised phase III study: 5-year analysis of the EORTC-NCIC trial. Lancet Oncol. 2009;10(5):459–66. doi:10.1016/S1470-2045(09)70025-7.

79. Balducci M, Fiorentino A, De Bonis P, Chiesa S, Mangiola A, Mattiucci GC, et al. Concurrent and adjuvant temozolomide-based chemoradiotherapy schedules for glioblastoma. Hypotheses based on two prospective phase II trials. Strahlenther Onkol. 2013;189:926e931. doi:10.1007/s00066-013-0410-6.

80. Gilbert MR, Wang M, Aldape KD, Stupp R, Hegi M, Jaeckle KA, et al. RTOG 0525: a randomized phase III trial comparing standard adjuvant temozolomide (TMZ) with a dose-dense (dd) schedule in newly diagnosed glioblastoma (GBM). J Clin Oncol. 2011;29:51.

81. Grossman SA, Wharam M, Sheidler V, Kleinberg L, Zeltzman M, Yue N, et al. Phase II study of continuous infusion carmustine and cisplatin followed by cranial irradiation in adults with newly diagnosed high-grade astrocytoma. J Clin Oncol. 1997;15:2596–603.

82. Grossman SA, O'Neill A, Grunnet M, Mehta M, Pearlman JL, Wagner H, et al. Phase III study comparing three cycles of infusional carmustine and cisplatin followed by radiation therapy with radiation therapy and concurrent carmustine in patients with newly diagnosed supratentorial glioblastoma multiforme: Eastern Cooperative Oncology Group Trial 2394. J Clin Oncol. 2003;21:1485–91.

83. Marshall NE, Ballman KV, Michalak JC, Schomberg PJ, Burton GV, Sandler HM, et al. Ototoxicity of cisplatin plus standard radiation therapy vs. accelerated radiation therapy in glioblastoma patients. J Neuro Oncology. 2006;77:315–20.

84. Kim IH, Park CK, Heo DS, Kim CY, Rhee CH, Nam DH, et al. Radiotherapy followed by adjuvant temozolomide with or without neoadjuvant ACNU-CDDP chemotherapy in newly diagnosed glioblastomas: a prospective randomized controlled

multicenter phase III trial. J Neurooncol. 2011;103:595–602. doi:10.1007/s11060-010-0427-y.

85. Cancer Genome Atlas Research Network. Comprehensive genomic characterization defines human glioblastoma genes and core pathways. Nature. 2008;455(7216):1061–8. doi:10.1038/nature07385.

86. Brennan C, Momota H, Hambardzumyan D, Ozawa T, Tandon A, Pedraza A, et al. Glioblastoma subclasses can be defined by activity among signal transduction pathways and associated genomic alterations. PLoS One. 2009;4(11), e7752. doi:10.1371/journal.pone.0007752.

87. Cheng YK, Beroukhim R, Levine RL, Mellinghoff IK, Holland EC, Michor F. A mathematical methodology for determining the temporal order of pathway alterations arising during gliomagenesis. PLoS Comput Biol. 2012;8(1), e1002337. doi:10.1371/journal.pcbi.1002337.

88. Bao S, Wu Q, Sathornsumetee S, Hao Y, Li Z, Hjelmeland AB, et al. Stem cell-like glioma cells promote tumor angiogenesis through vascular endothelial growth factor. Cancer Res. 2006;66(16): 7843–8.

89. Folkman J. Angiogenesis: an organizing principle for drug discovery? Nat Rev Drug Discov. 2007;6:273e286.

90. Jain RK. Normalizing tumor vasculature with anti-angiogenic therapy: a new paradigm for combination therapy. Nat Med. 2001;7:987e989.

91. Chinot OL, de La Motte RT, Moore N, Zeaiter A, Das A, Phillips H, et al. AVAglio: Phase 3 trial of bevacizumab plus temozolomide and radiotherapy in newly diagnosed glioblastoma multiforme. Adv Ther. 2011;28(4):334–40. doi:10.1007/s12325-011-0007-3. PMID: 21432029.

92. Batchelor TT, Reardon DA, de Groot JF, Wick W, Weller M. Antiangiogenic therapy for glioblastoma: current status and future prospects. Clin Cancer Res. 2014;20(22):5612–9. doi:10.1158/1078-0432.CCR-14-0834.

93. Chaichana KL, Zadnik P, Weingart JD, Olivi A, Gallia GL, Blakeley J, et al. Multiple resections for patients with glioblastoma: prolonging survival. J Neurosurg. 2013;118:812–20. doi:10.3171/2012.9.JNS1277.

94. Hoover JM, Nwojo M, Puffer R, Mandrekar J, Meyer FB, Parney IF, et al. Surgical outcomes in recurrent glioma: clinical article. J Neurosurg. 2013;118:1224–31. doi:10.3171/2013.2.JNS121731.

95. Ammirati M, Galicich JH, Arbit E, Liao Y. Reoperation in the treatment of recurrent intracranial malignant gliomas. Neurosurgery. 1987;21:607–14.

96. Pinsker M, Lumenta C. Experiences with reoperation on recurrent glioblastoma multiforme. Zentralbl Neurochir. 2001;62:43–7.

97. Barbagallo GM, Jenkinson MD, Brodbelt AR. 'Recurrent' glioblastoma multiforme, when should we reoperate? Br J Neurosurg. 2008;22(3):452–5. doi:10.1080/02688690802182256.

98. Park JK, Hodges T, Arko L, Shen M, Dello Iacono D, McNabb A, et al. Scale to predict survival after surgery for recurrent glioblastoma multiforme. J Clin Oncol. 2010;28(24):3838–43. doi:10.1200/JCO.2010.30.0582.

99. Brandes AA, Bartolotti M, Franceschi E. Second surgery for recurrent glioblastoma: advantages and pitfalls. Expert Rev Anticancer Ther. 2013;13:583–7. doi:10.1586/era.13.32.

100. De Bonis P, Fiorentino A, Anile C, Balducci M, Pompucci A, Chiesa S, et al. The impact of repeated surgery and adjuvant therapy on survival for patients with recurrent glioblastoma. Clin Neurol Neurosurg. 2013;115:883–6. doi:10.1016/j.clineuro.2012.08.030.

101. Mandl ES, Dirven CM, Buis DR, Postma TJ, Vandertop WP, et al. Repeated surgery for glioblastoma multiforme: only in combination with other salvage therapy. Surg Neurol. 2008;69:506–9. doi:10.1016/j.surneu.2007.03.043.

102. Dhermain F, de Crevoisier R, Parker F, Cioloca C, Kaliski A, Beaudre A, et al. Role of radiotherapy in recurrent gliomas. Bull Cancer. 2004;91(11):883–9.

103. Hall WA, Djalilian HR, Sperduto PW, Cho KH, Gerbi BJ, Gibbons JP, et al. Stereotactic radiosurgery for recurrent malignant gliomas. J Clin Oncol. 1995;13:1642–8.

104. Shrieve DC, Alexander III E, Wen PY, Fine HA, Kooy HM, Black PM, et al. Comparison of stereotactic radiosurgery and brachytherapy in the treatment of recurrent glioblastoma multiforme. Neurosurgery. 1995;36:275–82.

105. Combs SE, Schulz-Ertner D, Thilmann C, Edler L, Debus J. Treatment of cerebral metastases from breast cancer with stereotactic radiosurgery. Strahlenther Onkol. 2004;180:590–6.

106. Cho KH, Hall WA, Gerbi BJ, Higgins PD, McGuire WA, Clark HB. Single dose versus fractionated stereotactic radiotherapy for recurrent high-grade gliomas. Int J Radiat Oncol Biol Phys. 1999;45:1133–41.

107. Combs SE, Thilmann C, Edler L, Debus J, Schulz-Ertner D. Efficacy of fractionated stereotactic reirradiation in recurrent gliomas: long-term results in 172 patients treated in a single institution. J Clin Oncol. 2005;23:8863–9.

108. Shepherd SF, Laing RW, Cosgrove VP, Warrington AP, Hines F, Ashley SE, et al. Hypofractionated stereotactic radiotherapy in the management of recurrent glioma. Int J Radiat Oncol Biol Phys. 1997;37:393–8.

109. Hudes RS, Corn BW, Werner-Wasik M, Andrews D, Rosenstock J, Thoron L, et al. A phase I dose escalation study of hypofractionated stereotactic radiotherapy as salvage therapy for persistent or recurrent malignant glioma. Int J Radiat Oncol Biol Phys. 1999;43:293–8.

110. Chamberlain MC, Barba D, Kormanik P, Shea WM, et al. Stereotactic radiosurgery for recurrent gliomas. Cancer. 1994;74:1342–7.

111. Combs SE, Widmer V, Thilmann C, Hof H, Debus J, Schulz-Ertner D. Stereotactic radiosurgery (SRS): treatment option for recurrent glioblastoma multiforme (GBM). Cancer. 2005;104:2168–73.

112. Biswas T, Okunieff P, Schell MC, Smudzin T, Pilcher WH, Bakos RS, et al. Stereotactic radiosurgery for glioblastoma: retrospective analysis. Radiat Oncol. 2009;4:11. doi:10.1186/1748-717X-4-11.

113. Kong DS, Lee JI, Park K, Kim JH, Lim DH, Nam DH. Efficacy of stereotactic radiosurgery as a salvage treatment for recurrent malignant gliomas. Cancer. 2008;112:2046–51.

114. Patel M, Siddiqui F, Jin JY, Mikkelsen T, Rosenblum M, Movsas B, et al. Salvage reirradiation for recurrent glioblastoma with radiosurgery: radiographic response and improved survival. J Neurooncol. 2009;92:185–91. doi:10.1007/s11060-008-9752-9.

115. Sirin S, Oysul K, Surenkok S, Sager O, Dincoglan F, Dirican B, et al. Linear accelerator-based stereotactic radiosurgery in recurrent glioblastoma: a single center experience. Vojnosanit Pregl. 2011;68:961–6.

116. Elliott RE, Parker EC, Rush SC, Kalhorn SP, Moshel YA, Narayana A, et al. Efficacy of gamma-knife radiosurgery for small-volume recurrent malignant gliomas after initial radical resection. World Neurosurg. 2011;76:128–40.

117. Skeie BS, Enger PO, Brogger J, Ganz JC, Thorsen F, Heggdal JI, et al. Gamma knife surgery versus reoperation for recurrent glioblastoma multiforme. World Neurosurg. 2012;78:658–69. doi:10.1016/j.wneu.2012.03.024.

118. Lederman G, Wronski M, Arbit E, Odaimi M, Wertheim S, Lombardi E, et al. Treatment of recurrent glioblastoma multiforme using fractionated stereotactic radiosurgery and concurrent paclitaxel. Am J Clin Oncol. 2000;23:155–9.

119. Larson DA, Prados M, Lamborn KR, Smith V, Sneed PK, Chang S, et al. Phase II study of high central dose Gamma Knife radiosurgery and marimastat in patients with recurrent malignant glioma. Int J Radiat Oncol Biol Phys. 2002;54:1397–404.

120. Cuneo KC, Vredenburgh JJ, Sampson JH, Reardon DA, Desjardins A, Peters KB, et al. Safety and efficacy of stereotactic radiosurgery and adjuvant bevacizumab in patients with recurrent malignant gliomas. Int J Radiat Oncol Biol Phys. 2012;82:2018–24. doi:10.1016/j.ijrobp.2010.12.074.

121. Park KJ, Kano H, Iyer A, Liu X, Niranjan A, Flickinger JC, et al. Salvage gamma knife stereotactic radiosurgery followed by bevacizumab for recurrent glioblastoma multiforme: a case-control study. J Neurooncol. 2012;107:323–33. doi:10.1007/s11060-011-0744-9.

122. Niyazi M, Ganswindt U, Schwarz SB, Kreth FW, Tonn JC, Geisler J, et al. Irradiation and bevacizumab in high-grade glioma retreatment settings. Int J Radiat Oncol Biol Phys. 2012;82:67–76. doi:10.1016/j.ijrobp.2010.09.002.

123. Hundsberger T, Brugge D, Putora PM, Weder P, Weber J, Plasswilm L. Re-irradiation with and without bevacizumab as salvage therapy for recurrent or progressive high-grade gliomas. J Neurooncol. 2013;112:133–9. doi:10.1007/s11060-013-1044-3.

124. Kim B, Soisson E, Duma C, Chen P, Hafer R, Cox C, et al. Treatment of recurrent high grade gliomas with hypofractionated stereotactic image-guided helical tomotherapy. Clin Neurol Neurosurg. 2011;113:509–12. doi:10.1016/j.clineuro.2011.02.001.

125. Minniti G, Scaringi C, De Sanctis V, Lanzetta G, Falco T, Di Stefano D, et al. Hypofractionated stereotactic radiotherapy and continuous low-dose temozolomide in patients with recurrent or progressive malignant gliomas. J Neurooncol. 2013;111:187–94. doi:10.1007/s11060-012-0999-9.

126. Fogh SE, Andrews DW, Glass J, Curran W, Glass C, Champ C, et al. Hypofractionated stereotactic radiation therapy: an effective therapy for recurrent high-grade gliomas. J Clin Oncol. 2010;28:3048–53. doi:10.1200/JCO.2009.25.6941.

127. Gutin PH, Iwamoto FM, Beal K, Mohile NA, Karimi S, Hou BL, et al. Safety and efficacy of bevacizumab with hypofractionated stereotactic irradiation for recurrent malignant gliomas. Int J Radiat Oncol Biol Phys. 2009;75:156–63. doi:10.1016/j.ijrobp.2008.10.043.

128. Torcuator R, Zuniga R, Mohan YS, Rock J, Doyle T, Anderson J, et al. Initial experience with bevacizumab treatment for biopsy confirmed cerebral radiation necrosis. J Neurooncol. 2009;94:63–8. doi:10.1007/s11060-009-9801-z.

129. McKenzie JT, Guarnaschelli JN, Vagal AS, Warnick RE, Breneman JC, et al. Hypofractionated stereotactic radiotherapy for unifocal and multifocal recurrence of malignant gliomas. J Neurooncol. 2013;113:403–9. doi:10.1007/s11060-013-1126-2.

130. Cabrera AR, Cuneo KC, Desjardins A, Sampson JH, McSherry F, Herndon 2nd JE, et al. Concurrent stereotactic radiosurgery and bevacizumab in recurrent malignant gliomas: A prospective trial. Int J Radiat Oncol Biol Phys. 2013;86:873–9. doi:10.1016/j.ijrobp.2013.04.029.

131. Voynov G, Kaufman S, Hong T, Pinkerton A, Simon R, Dowsett R. Treatment of recurrent malignant gliomas with stereotactic intensity modulated radiation therapy. Am J Clin Oncol. 2002;25:606–11.

132. Larson DA, Suplica JM, Chang SM, Lamborn KR, McDermott MW, Sneed PK, et al. Permanent iodine 125 brachytherapy in patients with progressive or recurrent glioblastoma multiforme. Neuro Oncol. 2004;6:119–26.

133. Patel S, Breneman JC, Warnick RE, Albright Jr RE, Tobler WD, van Loveren HR, et al. Permanent iodine-125 interstitial implants for the treatment of recurrent glioblastoma multiforme. Neurosurgery. 2000;46:1123–8.

134. Gaspar LE, Zamorano LJ, Shamsa F, Fontanesi J, Ezzell GE, Yakar DA. Permanent 125iodine

implants for recurrent malignant gliomas. Int J Radiat Oncol Biol Phys. 1999;43:977–82.

135. Sneed PK, Stauffer PR, McDermott MW, Diederich CJ, Lamborn KR, Prados MD, et al. Survival benefit of hyperthermia in a prospective randomized trial of brachytherapy boost +/- hyperthermia for glioblastoma multiforme. Int J Radiat Oncol Biol Phys. 1998;40:287–95.

136. Yung WK, Albright RE, Olson J, Fredericks R, Fink K, Prados MD, et al. A phase II study of temozolomide vs. procarbazine in patients with glioblastoma multiforme at first relapse. Brit J Cancer. 2000;83(5):588–93.

137. Brada M, Hoang-Xuan K, Rampling R, Dietrich PY, Dirix LY, Macdonald D, et al. Multicenter phase II trial of temozolomide in patients with glioblastoma multiforme at first relapse. Ann Oncol. 2001;12(2):259–66.

138. Chang SM, Theodosopoulos P, Lamborn K, Malec M, Rabbitt J, Page M, et al. Temozolomide in the treatment of recurrent malignant glioma. Cancer. 2004;100(3):605–11.

139. Brada M, Stenning S, Gabe R, Thompson LC, Levy D, Rampling R, et al. Temozolomide versus procarbazine, lomustine, and vincristine in recurrent high-grade glioma. J Clin Oncol. 2010;28(30):4601–8. doi:10.1200/JCO.2009.27.1932.

140. Abacioglu U, Caglar HB, Yumuk PF, Akgun Z, Atasoy BM, Sengoz M. Efficacy of protracted dose-dense temozolomide in patients with recurrent high-grade glioma. J Neurooncol. 2011;103(3):585–93. doi:10.1007/s11060-010-0423-2.

141. Weller M, Tabatabai G, Reifenberger G, Wick W. et al. Dose-intensified rechallenge with temozolomide: one week on/one week off versus 3 weeks on/one week off in patients with progressive or recurrent glioblastoma. J Clin Oncol. 2010;28(Suppl 15): Abstract TPS154.

142. Franceschi E, Omuro AM, Lassman AB, Demopoulos A, Nolan C, Abrey LE. Salvage temozolomide for prior temozolomide responders. Cancer. 2005;104(11):2473–6.

143. Kong DS, Lee JI, Kim WS, Son MJ, Lim do H, Kim ST, et al. A pilot study of metronomic temozolomide treatment in patients with recurrent temozolomide-refractory glioblastoma. Oncol Rep. 2006;16(5):1117–21.

144. Berrocal A, Perez Segura P, Gil M, Balaña C, Garcia Lopez J, Yaya R, et al. Extended-schedule dose-dense temozolomide in refractory gliomas. J Neurooncol. 2010;96(3):417–22. doi:10.1007/s11060-009-9980-7.

145. Perry JR, Belanger K, Mason WP, Fulton D, Kavan P, Easaw J, et al. Phase II trial of continuous dose-intense temozolomide in recurrent malignant glioma: RESCUE study. J Clin Oncol. 2010;28(12):2051–7. doi:10.1200/JCO.2009.26.5520.

146. Kong DS, Lee JI, Kim JH, Kim ST, Kim WS, Suh YL, et al. Phase II trial of low-dose continuous (metronomic) treatment of temozolomide for recurrent glioblastoma. Neuro Oncol. 2010;12(3):289–96. doi:10.1093/neuonc/nop030.

147. Hammond A, Norden AD, Lesser GJ, et al. Phase II study of dose-intense temozolomide in recurrent glioblastoma. J Clin Oncol. 2011;29:2038.

148. Neyns B, Tosoni A, Hwu WJ, Reardon DA. Dose-dense temozolomide regimens: antitumor activity, toxicity, and immunomodulatory effects. Cancer. 2010;116(12):2868–77. doi:10.1002/cncr.25035.

149. Van den Bent MJ, Brandes AA, Rampling R, Kouwenhoven MC, Kros JM, Carpentier AF, et al. Randomized phase II trial of erlotinib versus temozolomide or carmustine in recurrent glioblastoma: EORTC Brain Tumor Group study 26034. J Clin Oncol. 2009;27(8):1268–74. doi:10.1200/JCO.2008.17.5984.

150. Brandes AA, Tosoni A, Amista P, Nicolardi L, Grosso D, Berti F, et al. How effective is BCNU in recurrent glioblastoma in the modern era? A phase II trial. Neurology. 2004;63(7):1281–4.

151. Reithmeier T, Graf E, Piroth T, Trippel M, Pinsker MO, Nikkhah G. BCNU for recurrent glioblastoma multiforme: efficacy, toxicity and prognostic factors. BMC Cancer. 2010;10:30. doi:10.1186/1471-2407-10-30.

152. Wick W, Puduvalli VK, Chamberlain MC, van den Bent MJ, Carpentier AF, Cher LM, et al. Phase III study of enzastaurin compared with lomustine in the treatment of recurrent intracranial glioblastoma. J Clin Oncol. 2010;28(7):1168–74. doi:10.1200/JCO.2009.23.2595.

153. Ahluwalia MS. 2010 Society for Neuro-Oncology Annual Meeting: a report of selected studies. Expert Rev Anticancer Ther. 2011;11(2):161–3. doi:10.1586/era.10.227.

154. Batchelor TT, Mulholland P, Neyns B, Nabors LB, Campone M, Wick A, et al. Phase III randomized trial comparing the efficacy of cediranib as monotherapy, and in combination with lomustine, versus lomustine alone in patients with recurrent glioblastoma. J Clin Oncol. 2013;31(26):3212–8. doi:10.1200/JCO.2012.47.2464.

155. Balana C, Villa S, Teixidor P. Evolution of care for patients with relapsed glioblastoma. Expert Rev Anticancer Ther. 2011;11(11):1719–29. doi:10.1586/era.11.152.

156. Brandes AA, Tosoni A, Franceschi E, Blatt V, Santoro A, Faedi M, et al. Fotemustine as second-line treatment for recurrent or progressive glioblastoma after concomitant and/or adjuvant temozolomide: a phase II trial of Gruppo Italiano Cooperativo di Neuro-Oncologia (GICNO). Cancer Chemother Pharmacol. 2009;64(4):769–75. doi:10.1007/s00280-009-0926-8.

157. Scoccianti S, Detti B, Sardaro A. Second-line chemotherapy with fotemustine in temozolomide-pretreated patients with relapsing glioblastoma: a single institution experience et al. Second-line

chemotherapy with fotemustine in temozolomide-pretreated patients with relapsing glioblastoma: a single institution experience. Anticancer Drugs. 2008;19(6):613–20. doi:10.1097/CAD.0b013e3283005075.

158. Addeo R, Caraglia M, De Santi MS, Montella L, Abbruzzese A, Parlato C, et al. A new schedule of fotemustine in temozolomide-pretreated patients with relapsing glioblastoma. J Neurooncol. 2011;102(3):417–24. doi:10.1007/s11060-010-0329-z.

159. Friedman HS, Prados MD, Wen PY, Mikkelsen T, Schiff D, Abrey LE, et al. Bevacizumab alone and in combination with irinotecan in recurrent glioblastoma. J Clin Oncol. 2009;27(28):4733–40. doi:10.1200/JCO.2008.19.8721.

160. Wong ET, Hess KR, Gleason MJ, Jaeckle KA, Kyritsis AP, Prados MD, et al. Outcomes and prognostic factors in recurrent glioma patients enrolled onto phase II clinical trials. J Clin Oncol. 1999;17(8):2572–8.

161. Ballman KV, Buckner JC, Brown PD, Giannini C, Flynn PJ, LaPlant BR, et al. The relationship between six-month progression-free survival and 12-month overall survival end points for phase II trials in patients with glioblastoma multiforme. Neuro Oncol. 2007;9(1):29–38.

162. Kreisl TN, Kim L, Moore K, Duic P, Royce C, Stroud I, et al. Phase II trial of single agent bevacizumab followed by bevacizumab plus irinotecan at tumor progression in recurrent glioblastoma. J Clin Oncol. 2009;27(5):740–5. doi:10.1200/JCO.2008.16.3055.

163. Chamberlain MC, Raizer J. Antiangiogenic therapy for high-grade gliomas. CNS Neurol Disord Drug Targets. 2009;8(3):184–94.

164. Vredenburgh JJ, Desjardins A, Herndon 2nd JE, Dowell JM, Reardon DA, Quinn JA, et al. Phase II trial of bevacizumab and irinotecan in recurrent malignant glioma. Clin Cancer Res. 2007;13(4):1253–9.

165. Chamberlain MC. Bevacizumab plus irinotecan in recurrent glioblastoma. J Clin Oncol. 2008;26(6):1012–3. doi:10.1200/JCO.2007.15.1605. author reply 1013.

166. Arcicasa M, Roncadin M, Bidoli E, Dedkov A, Gigante M, Trovo MG. Reirradiation and lomustine in patients with relapsed high-grade gliomas. Int J Radiat Oncol Biol Phys. 1999;43:789–93.

167. Glass J, Silverman CL, Axelrod R, Corn BW, Andrews DW. Fractionated stereotactic radiotherapy with cis-platinum radiosensitization in the treatment of recurrent, progressive, or persistent malignant astrocytoma. Am J Clin Oncol. 1997;20:226–9.

168. Wurm RE, Kuczer DA, Schlenger L, Matnjani G, Scheffler D, Cosgrove VP, et al. Hypofractionated stereotactic radiotherapy combined with topotecan in recurrent malignant glioma. Int J Radiat Oncol Biol Phys. 2006;66:S26–32.

169. Gay H. Role of the linear-quadratic model in high doses per fraction. Radiother Oncol. 2010;94:122–3. doi:10.1016/j.radonc.2009.08.039.

170. Courdi A. High doses per fraction and the linear-quadratic model. Radiother Oncol. 2010;94:121–2. doi:10.1016/j.radonc.2009.08.019.

171. Beauchesne PD, Bertrand S, Branche R, Linke SP, Revel R, Dore JF, et al. Human malignant glioma cell lines are sensitive to low radiation doses. Int J Cancer. 2003;105:33–40.

172. Chendil D, Oakes R, Alcock RA, Patel N, Mayhew C, Mohiuddin M, et al. Low dose fractionated radiation enhances the radiosensitization effect of paclitaxel in colorectal tumor cells with mutant p53. Cancer. 2000;89:1893–900.

173. Balducci M, Chiesa S, Diletto B, D'Agostino GR, Mangiola A, Manfrida S, et al. Low-dose fractionated radiotherapy and concomitant chemotherapy in glioblastoma multiforme with poor prognosis: a feasibility study. Neuro Oncol. 2012;14(1):79–86. doi:10.1093/neuonc/nor173.

174. Balducci M, Diletto B, Chiesa S, D'Agostino GR, Gambacorta MA, Ferro M, et al. Low-dose fractionated radiotherapy and concomitant chemotherapy for recurrent or progressive glioblastoma: final report of a pilot study. Strahlenther Onkol. 2014;190(4):370–6. doi:10.1007/s00066-013-0506-z.

175. Yovino S, Grossman SA. Treatment of glioblastoma in "elderly" patients. Curr Treat Options Oncol. 2011;12:253–62. doi:10.1007/s11864-011-0158-0.

176. Iwamoto FM, Reiner AS, Panageas KS, Elkin EB, Abrey LE. Patterns of care in elderly glioblastoma patients. Ann Neurol. 2008;64:628–34. doi:10.1002/ana.21521.

177. Kita D, Ciernik IF, Vaccarella S, Franceschi S, Kleihues P, Lütolf UM, et al. Age as a predictive factor in glioblastomas: population-based study. Neuroepidemiology. 2009;33:17–22. doi:10.1159/000210017.

178. Scott JG, Suh JH, Elson P, Barnett GH, Vogelbaum MA, Peereboom DM, et al. Aggressive treatment is appropriate for glioblastoma multiforme patients 70 years old or older; a retrospective review of 206 cases. Neuro Oncol. 2011;13:428–36. doi:10.1093/neuonc/nor005.

179. Keime-Guibert F, Chinot O, Taillandier L, Cartalat-Carel S, Frenay M, Kantor G, et al. Radiotherapy for glioblastoma in the elderly. N Engl J Med. 2007;356:1527–35.

180. Wick W, Platten M, Meisner C, Felsberg J, Tabatabai G, Simon M, et al. Temozolomide chemotherapy alone versus radiotherapy alone for malignant astrocytoma in the elderly: the NOA-08 randomised, phase 3 trial. Lancet Oncol. 2012;13:707–15. doi:10.1016/S1470-2045(12)70164-X.

181. Balducci M, Fiorentino A, De Bonis P, Chiesa S, Manfrida S, D'Agostino GR, et al. Impact of age and comorbidities in patients with newly diagnosed glioblastoma: pooled data analysis of three prospective mono-institutional phase II studies. Med Oncol. 2012;29(5):3478–83. doi:10.1007/s12032-012-0263-3.

182. Minniti G, Lanzetta G, Scaringi C, Caporello P, Salvati M, Arcella A, et al. Phase II study of short-course radiotherapy plus concomitant and adjuvant temozolomide in elderly patients with glioblastoma. Int J Radiat Oncol Biol Phys. 2012;83:93–9. doi:10.1016/j.ijrobp.2011.06.1992.

183. Perry JR, O'Callaghan CJ, Ding K, Roa W, Mason WP, Cairncross JG et al. A phase III randomized controlled trial of short-course radiotherapy with or without concomitant and adjuvant temozolomide in elderly patients with glioblastoma (NCIC CTG CE.6, EORTC 26062-22061, TROG 08.02, NCT00482677). J Clin Oncol 30, 2012 (suppl; abstr TPS2104)

184. Kirson ED, Gurvich Z, Schneiderman R, Dekel E, Itzhaki A, Wasserman Y, et al. Disruption of cancer cell replication by alternating electric fields. Cancer Res. 2004;64:3288–95.

185. Stupp R, Wong ET, Kanner AA, Steinberg D, Engelhard H, Heidecke V, et al. NovoTTF-100 A versus physician's choice chemotherapy in recurrent glioblastoma: a randomised phase III trial of a novel treatment modality. Eur J Cancer. 2012;48:2192–202. doi:10.1016/j.ejca.2012.04.011.

186. Marko NF, Weil RJ, Schroeder JL, Lang FF, Suki D, Sawaya RE. Extent of resection of Glioblastoma revisited: personalized survival modeling facilitates more accurate survival prediction and supports a maximum-safe-resection approach to surgery. J Clin Oncol. 2014;32(8):774–82. doi:10.1200/JCO.2013.51.8886.

# Clinical Evidence and Radiobiological Background of Particle Radiation Therapy

**5**

Walter Tinganelli, Marco Durante, and Alexander Helm

## Introduction

New technology, advanced imaging, rapid diagnosis and improvements in neurosurgical science have led to a better tumour delineation resulting in an increased number of patients considered tumour free, at least immediately following the treatment, while maintaining all neurological functions [1].

Radiotherapy, non-invasive and among the techniques used to fight cancer probably the safest one remains the most effective, both curative and palliative for almost 50 % of all patients suffering from solid tumours.

The application of modern technologies such as computer-controlled linear accelerators or 3D-tumour imaging as well as new techniques in the irradiation procedure, e.g. conformal radiation or the intensity modulated radiation therapy (IMRT) allows to reduce collateral damage to healthy tissue surrounding the tumour [2].

In conventional radiotherapy protocols, 60–70 Gy of high energetic X-rays are usually delivered to the tumour. To spare healthy tissue around, the dose is often given in 2 Gy of daily fractions for almost 7 weeks, providing the possibility for the normal tissue to recover between the fractions, thus reducing the collateral effects. The dose delivered depends on tumour type, localization and the patient's genetic background sensitivity to specific treatments [3].

However, even after the advantageous radiation therapy, tumours, especially those known to be radioresistant such as glioblastoma multiforme, may relapse a certain time following therapy. Recurrent tumours, apart from their radioresistance, are characterized by malignancy and aggressiveness of the primary tumour [4] pointing to a selection of resistant and invasive cells by the preceding treatment.

At very high dose, radiation is completely tumoricide; however, the delivery of such high doses in a target volume is impossible due to the inevitable increased dose deposited in the surrounding healthy tissues and/or organ at risk.

Charged particle therapy is considered as cutting edge technique in radio-oncology. Cancer patients are treated with a focused beam of accelerated ions targeted directly in the tumour instead of photons. Despite its various advantages, particle therapy per se and the constructions of centres to conduct it are relatively expensive. Nevertheless, the last 20 years of application of e.g. carbon ion therapy show that despite the high price to build a carbon ion facility the advantages of this treatment are indisputable [5].

W. Tinganelli (✉) • M. Durante • A. Helm
Helmholtzzentrum für Schwerionenforschung
GmbH (GSI), Darmstadt, Germany

Trento Institute for Fundamental Physics
and Applications (TIFPA), Italy
e-mail: w.tinganelli@gsi.de

© Springer International Publishing Switzerland 2016
L. Pirtoli et al. (eds.), *Radiobiology of Glioblastoma*, Current Clinical Pathology,
DOI 10.1007/978-3-319-28305-0_5

On the other hand, 50 centres for cancer treatment with protons are currently maintained in the world and more than 100,000 patients have been already treated.

Carbon ion centres instead are located in few countries, i.e. six centres in Asia (most of them in Japan) and two in Europe (Heidelberg Ion-Beam Therapy Center (HIT) in Heidelberg, Germany and Centro Nazionale di Adroterapia Oncologica (CNAO) in Pavia, Italy.)

The striking feature for charged particles in therapy as compared to conventional photon irradiation is the inverse dose-deposition distribution. While the photon irradiation releases most of the energy at their entrance in the tissue (entrance channel), charged particles release the maximum of their dose at the distal end of their path through the matter.

When a particle traverses the matter, it progressively decreases its kinetic energy and deposits a dose along the path by ionizing atoms. The dose deposition along the path is referred to as the linear energy transfer (LET) which increases with the deceleration of the particle. Almost at the end of its path, where its speed is rather low the particle releases the maximum of its energy, the maximum of the cross section resulting in the Bragg peak.

Although the energy deposition is very high at the end of the particle's path, the Bragg peak is rather narrow and thus a superimposition of many peaks, a so-called spread-out Bragg-peak (SOBP), is necessary to homogeneously distribute the dose in whole tumour volume (Fig. 5.1).

An SOBP is produced essentially in two different ways.

The passive scanning applies a beam with a fixed energy attenuated later by varying the thickness of a range shifter hence permitting the delivery of particles with different energies along the tumour (passive modulation, Fig. 5.2).

The second option, the active scanning comprises an SOBP produced by varying the initial energy the beam-extraction energy directly acting in the accelerated phase (active modulation, Fig. 5.3).

In the active modulation, a Dose Delivery System (DDS) is necessary. This system has to be implemented with the spot scanning technique.

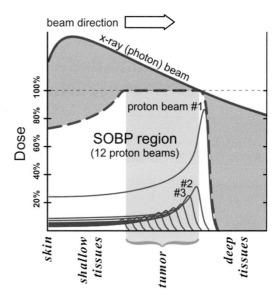

**Fig. 5.1** The superimposition of different single Bragg peaks (i.e. different ion beams of different energy) is necessary to produce an extended or spread-out Bragg-peak (SOBP) covering the whole tumour volume with a homogenously distributed dose. Reprinted by permission from Macmillan Publishers Ltd [7]

The treatment plan divides the target volume into slices that are intern subdivided into spots or voxels (volumetric pixel or volumetric picture elements). Every single voxel then is irradiated separately using a pencil beam for each spot, Fig. 5.3. The beam positioning is achieved using orthogonal magnets for the X and Y dimension [8]. Passive modulation was used from 1994 on at the National Institute of Radiological Sciences (NIRS) in Japan. At HIT, an active modulation beam is used since 2011. Pencil beam has been used also during the pilot project between 1997 and 2007 at the GSI Helmholtz Centre for Heavy Ion Research (GSI) in Germany and is still used in the National Centre of Oncological Hadrontherapy (CNAO) in Italy.

Particles at 75 % of the speed of light can penetrate up to 30 cm of tissue in a patient deviating from the target not more than 1 mm; one of the features making particle therapy extremely precise especially for the treatment of tumours with a complicated location in close proximity to highly radiation-sensitive or organs at risk. In the case of glioblastoma treatment the optic nerve displays such an organ at risk. Particle

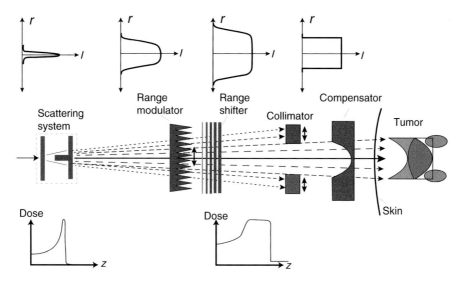

**Fig. 5.2** Passive scanning: ion beam energies are varied with range modulators that change the range in depth. Collimators subsequently provide the possibility to contour the target volume with permission of Springer [8]

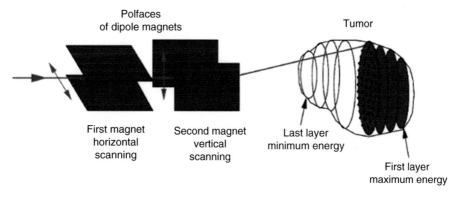

**Fig. 5.3** Active scanning: the target volume is divided in slices and voxel. Every voxel is treated sequentially. "In practice, 30–60 iso-energy layers are used filled with 5000–50,000 (all layers) pixels that are delivered with beam in 2–6 min" with permission of Springer [8]

therapy, due to its beneficial dose deposition in deep situated solid tumours and sparing healthy tissue and organs at risk, is nowadays considered an advanced method among the various types of cancer therapies.

## Biological Effects and Oxygen Enhancement Ratio

Despite the beneficial dose distribution, charged particles, particularly carbon ions, comprise further advantageous features as compared to the most advanced conventional X-rays therapies such as the IMRT.

Those advantages are due to the peculiar radiobiological effects of charged particles on tissues such as an increased relative biological effectiveness (RBE) as a result of the higher LET. Striking biological effects are, e.g. a reduced cell repair capacity and a decreased dependency on the cell cycle as compared to photon radiation [9]. Further putative advantages have been discovered just recently: carbon ion radiation suppresses metastasis and angiogenesis [10] and is discussed to trigger an immune response [11].

Apart from the above mentioned advantages, another crucial feature is that particle radiation compared to the conventional photons may overcome the strong radioresistance stemming from the oxygen lack in several tumours [12].

Solid tumours often include regions with a lack in oxygen and nutrition being related with an insufficient blood supply and the tumours' high rate of oxygen consumption. The outcome is generally correlated with a poor prognosis for the patients [13]. Besides the increased radioresistance, hypoxic regions are also regarded to serve as a cancer stem cell niche [14].

The radioresistance increase due to the oxygen lack is quantified by a parameter called oxygen enhancement ratio (OER). The OER is the ratio between the dose necessary in hypoxic and the dose necessary in normoxic conditions to produce the same biological effect. The microscopic reason of the increased sensitivity in the presence of oxygen mainly is the quenching of the DNA damage mechanism mediated by free radicals, the so-called indirect damage [15].

If enough oxygen molecules are present by the time of exposure, they may fix and stabilize the biological damage. However, the indirect damage depends on the radiation quality and on the LET. The DNA damage produced by high LET charged particles in contrast to low LET photons mainly comprises direct damage. The role of the indirect damage via the production of free radicals is negligible in that case.

Furthermore, at high density tracks, produced free radicals quench themselves due to close proximity [16].

High LET radiation thus provides the possibility to reduce the OER and subsequently to overcome the radioresistance due to oxygen [17]. Varying the distribution of the various LET values as well as the resulting doses when a tumour is irradiated thus displays a possible solution for the problem.

At the GSI Helmholtz Centre for Heavy Ion Research (GSI) in Darmstadt, Germany, a new semi-empirical model was implemented in the already existing treatment planning [18] applying data for the OER at different oxygenation condition and in dependence of different LET values [19] (Fig 5.4).

The idea is to implement in the system the OER value in order to generate a hypoxia-adapted

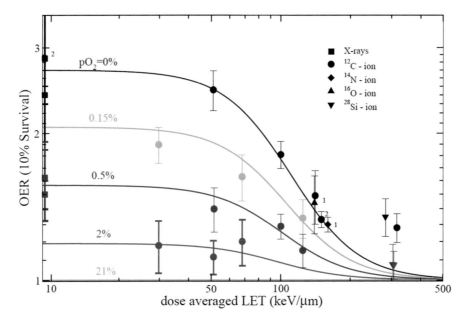

**Fig. 5.4** The solid lines represent the oxygen enhancement ratio as predicted by the model in dependence of oxygen concentration and dose averaged LET. The points represent experimental data corresponding to the respective conditions applying X-rays and various ion species as indicated by the symbols. Every experiment was repeated thrice unless indicated differently by the numbers close the data points [19]

treatment plan, which will be used for painting by voxel (*LET-painting*) the hypoxic tumours visualized by functional imaging, and to prescribe uniform cell killing across volumes with heterogeneous radiosensitivity .

At the present time, all particle therapy centres worldwide exclusively use proton and/or carbon ion beams. However, the idea to enlarge the spectrum of ions used for therapy is currently under investigation. Ions heavier than carbon are considered to target resistant tumour regions or ions heavier than protons such as lithium may serve to target sensitive tumours close to critical organs or paediatric tumours while increasing the effectiveness.

The spectrum of applicable ions is limited nevertheless due to other physical features bringing along disadvantages. A higher effectiveness is then opposed by an increased dose in the entrance channel, a fragmentation producing secondary particles and neutrons, changes in the shape of the SOBP and the dose painting and an increased dose beyond the distal end of the target volume. These issues restrict the application of heavier ions to a spectrum close to carbon.

Recent studies demonstrate that oxygen ions in some cases, especially for the highly resistant hypoxic tumours, display a suitable alternative to carbon.

Figure 5.5 demonstrates the computed relative decrease of the clinical hypoxia region due to the oxygen beam radiation compared with carbon.

Comparison of the computed carbon and oxygen ion OER along an extended target shows that oxygen may reduce the clinical hypoxic OER, decreasing subsequently the radioresistance, albeit keeping a lower dose compared to an equivalent carbon ion beam [19].

It is not clear yet how and if oxygen ions may really substitute carbon ions for particle therapy, but the data obtained so far indicate that it is worthwhile performing further studies and testing a putative application for the treatment of highly resistant tumours such as pancreatic ones.

Hypoxic regions of tumours are not only in the spotlight of research because of their high

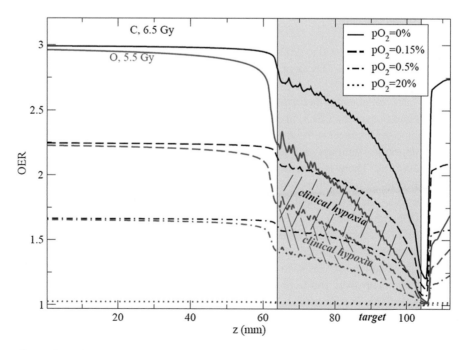

**Fig. 5.5** Comparison of computed carbon (*black*) and oxygen (*red*) OER along an extended target irradiation at different oxygen pressure (pO$_2$) levels. The hatched areas represent the clinical interesting regions for hypoxia (0.15 % < pO$_2$ < 0.5 %). Doses indicated are prescribed RBE-weighted doses in the target [19]

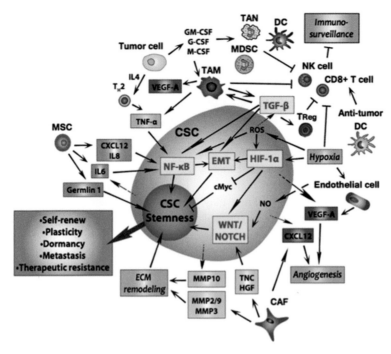

**Fig. 5.6** Glioma stem cells are regulated by microenvironment conditions such as hypoxia. In hypoxia CSCs stimulate blood vessels that themselves promote blood vessel formation. Those vessels create a vascular niche to help to maintain CSC population. It is a reciprocal relationship between CSCs and blood vessels that sustaines and quickens tumorigenesis. Reprinted from Cell Stem Cell, with permission from Elsevier [20]

radioresistance, but also discussed to promote so-called tumour initiating cells (TICs) or cancer stem cells (CSCs).

Those cells have the potential to form all cell types usually found in cancers. CSCs, in contrast to other non-tumorigenic cancer cells, are able to generate and persist in tumours and to cause relapse and metastasis. There is increasing evidence for those cells to reside in two different specific niches, i.e. the endothelial and the hypoxic niche (Fig. 5.6) [21–23].

The attention of much of the scientist now involved in cancer research is aimed to investigate the particular features of CSCs, to understand the mechanisms involved and to be able to target them preferentially in therapies.

The targeting and eradication of hypoxic regions using high LET radiation thus pose a promising tool for a therapy aiming at resistant CSCs, which may reduce the risk of tumour relapse and metastases.

# Radioimmunotherapy

Despite radio and immunotherapy are considered different branches of medicine, they can be overlapped provoking the immune system stimulation by radiation.

It is in fact demonstrated that sometime the tumour irradiation can trigger an immune-system response against the tumour itself and to the distal metastases, out of the irradiation field. This phenomenon is known as Ab-scopal effect.

Ab-scopal is the combination of the Latin word *Ab*, which means far, and the ancient Greek word *skopós*, which means target or aim. Ab-scopal is a distant goal or target (Fig. 5.7).

Radiation induces not only the cell death pathway, it increases and changes the antigen population on the cancer cells surface and the complex molecular patterns that lead to the dendritic cells (DC) maturation [24]. How this happens and the

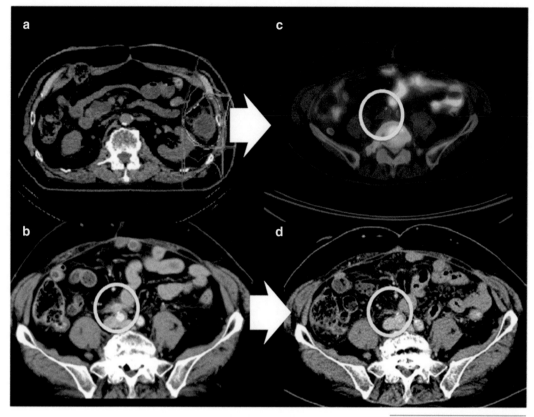

*TRENDS in Molecular Medicine*

**Fig. 5.7** The ab-scopal effect in a 77-year-old male patient at the National Institute of Radiological Sciences (NIRS) in Chiba, Japan. An abdominal lesion (**a**) was treated with 73.6 GyE C-ions (16 fractions) after resection of a sigmoid colon cancer. The paraaortic lymph node vis- ible in the computed tomography (CT) scan (**b**) had van- ished without treatment 6 months later (PET scan (**c**) and CT scan images (**d**)). Image courtesy of Dr Shigeru Yamada, NIRS Reprinted from [11] with permission of Elsevier

complete molecular pathways involved are still unknown although the complexity of this system begins to be traced [11].

Lymphocytes, CD8+ T cells, the high mobility group box 1 (HMGB1), the surface-membrane translocation of the endoplasmic reticulum resident protein 60, also known as calreticulin (CRT), are few of the factors necessary to activate an immune response.

Dendritic cells are antigen-presenting cells and their main function is to recognize the antigens on the cell surface and present them to the immune system T cells. After their contact with the antigens, DC migrate into the lymph nodes where they interact with the immune-system cells and contribute to the adaptive immune

response among which the cytotoxic T lymphocytes (CTLs). In Fig. 5.8 some aspects of the complex interaction between the various cells and molecules involved are displayed.

The final clonal expansions of the CTLs produce a specialized army that heads to the highly antigenic tumour clone cells and eliminate them through granzyme release and then caspase activation and mitochondrial membrane permeabilization (MOMP) [11]. Granzyme is a class of serine proteases released by cytotoxic T and natural killer (NK) cells through exocitated granules also containing the molecule perforin.

This process of elimination which often occurs in early tumour development is at some point attenuated. In this new phase, called

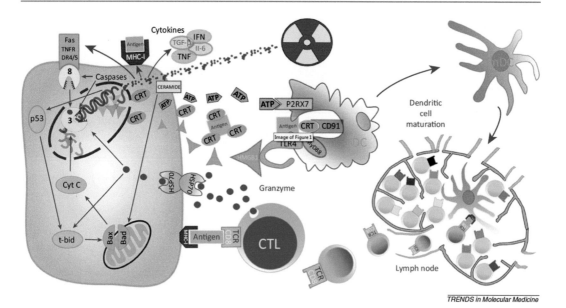

**Fig. 5.8** Illustration of the convergence of direct and immune-mediated effects of radiation treatment. *ATP* adenosine triphosphate, *Bad*, Bcl-2-associated death promoter, *CD8* T cell coreceptor (specific for MHC-I), *CD91* low-density lipoprotein receptor-related protein 1, *CRT* calreticulin, *CTL* cytotoxic T cell, *Cyt C* cytochrome c, *DC* dendritic cell, *Fas*, tumour necrosis factor receptor superfamily member 6 (CD95), *HMGB1* high-mobility group protein 1, *HSP70* heat shock protein 70, *IFN* interferon, *IL-6* interleukin 6, *mDC* mature dendritic cell, *MHC-I* major histocompatibility complex 1, *MyD88* myeloid differentiation primary response gene 88, *p53* protein 53, *P2RX7* P2 purinergic receptor 7, *t-bid* truncated BH3 interacting-domain death antagonist, *TCR* T cell receptor, *TGF-b* transforming growth factor-b, *TLR4* Toll-like receptor 4, *TNF* tumour necrosis factor, *TNFR* tumour necrosis factor receptor Reprinted from [11] with permission of Elsevier

of equilibrium, the immune system creates a growth-inhibitory environment and the antigenic tumour outgrowths are kept in check [25]. However this equilibrium tends to select a tumour cell subpopulation with a poor antigenic expression profile (a population of immunosuppressed cells), among them the Myeloid-derived suppressor cells (MDSCs) and the regulatory T cells. In this phase then, tumour becomes "invisible" to the immune surveillance and the cancer cells can escape, invade and migrate. This process is called immune editing [25]. Various drugs aim to shift the balance from escape and equilibrium to elimination.

Therefore the more in detail understanding of this process would give a combined radiation-drugs protocol that could train the patient immune system to engage the neoplasm and the distal metastases avoiding the major side effects due to high doses of not targeted chemotherapies and radiation.

In March 2012 after received immune adjuvant anti-cytotoxic T lymphocyte antigen 4 therapy for 1 year, a melanoma female patient had disease progression that required focal irradiation of her spinal metastasis with 28.5 Gy of 6 MV photons (IMRT) in three fractions [11].

No benefits 1 month after treatment [26] as expected from a highly radioresistant tumour [27, 28]. However, 4 months later, the multiple metastases outside the irradiation field had vanished. Checking at her value of cellular and molecular parameters, a clear immune response against tumour [26] was found.

Other cases of ab-scopal effects were then reported in protocols combining radiotherapy with Ipilimumab, a monoclonal antibody (anti-CTLA4).

A GBM patient study has been done and brought considerable success also with a vaccination approach using autologous tumour cells. The study reported a long-term surviving patient bearing CD8+ cells directed against a specific tumour antigen persisting even up to 3.5 years after vaccination [29].

Besides the CD8+T cells protocol, other method using the natural killer (NK) cell and the enhanced upregulation of surface antigen in the target cells due by radiation are now ongoing [30]. These protocols are effective especially in combination with adjuvant drugs that can knockdown particular molecules like TGF-beta and STAT3 and/or specific pathways [31]. Different drugs have been tested to draw a successful abscopal protocol. Important results were obtained using Sunitinib, a vascular endothelial growth factor (VEGF) inhibitor, combined with irradiation. TGF-beta seems to be an important inhibitor when vaccination is combined with radiation [11] while the STAT3 inhibition seems to be necessary for the glioblastoma multiforme (GBM) cells temozolomide treatment sensitization [32]. In a murine hind limb model, the drug (sunitinib)-radiation protocol was promising [11].

Also the c-Met inhibition was found to be an important tumour radiosensitizer [33].

In an immune-competent intracerebral murine GL261 glioma model [34] combining peripheral vaccination with irradiation [35], important results were obtaining.

The combined approaches drugs-radiation will trigger the immune response and will contribute to successful and lasting therapy success in glioma reducing the dose given to the patient.

In a very interesting study using an intracerebral rat glioma model, 5 Gy of gamma rays combined with a vaccination protocol were found to be superior, compared to 15 Gy alone in terms of reducing the tumour volume [11].

Considering the proven dependence of radiation treatment success on CD8+ cells [36], it could be instructive to determine whether this relies on direct tumour cell killing by CD8+ cells or cytokines, such as interferons, emitted by CD8+ cells [37], eventually stimulating NK cells [11, 31].

In conclusion, radiotherapy and immunology could be used together both to avoid toxicity and increase the success probability.

However to achieve this in a proper way, every patient should be analysed, even down at the DNA level to find the right and most appropriate individual protocol [11].

Glioblastoma multiforme (GBM) treatment with carbon ions has been ongoing in different ion therapy centres around the world. It is just in 2010 that different clinical trials started at HIT the Heidelberg ion therapy centre in Germany (see section "Carbon Beam Clinical Trials").

Recent studies seem to show that carbon ion irradiation is able to activate alone and without any adjuvant drug the ab-scopal effect in immune-competent C3H mice experiments.

The reason why, could be that in immunogenic cell death [38], both calreticulin exposure [39] and focused ER stress appear to depend on reactive oxygen species (ROS) [40].

The oxidative species are produced in different way comparing the high and low LET radiation. For high LET radiation ROS are produced in a focal manner along the particle track while low LET radiation increases the more sparsely ROS production [11].

Heavy ion irradiation is becoming then also the forefront of immune modulatory therapy regimens.

The current data suggest that charged particle therapy treatment may be optimally combined with immunotherapy in future clinical trials.

## Glioblastoma Multiforme Treatment

The standard treatment for patients suffering from glioblastoma multiforme was defined by Stupp [41] and intends to apply a combination of radiotherapy and the cytostatic drug temozolomide (TMZ). Prior to that, surgery is supposed to remove the main part of the tumour reducing the primary symptoms such as brain pressure. Subsequently, a total dose of 60 Gy is then delivered to the patient (30 daily fractions of 2 Gy), followed by adjuvant TMZ chemotherapy.

Glioblastoma multiforme typically features a high capacity to infiltrate normal surrounding tissue which is, together with the high radioresistance, the main reason for the poor prognosis for GBM [42]. Due to the infiltration a total removal of those TICs is nearly impossible, as physicians can resect the visible tumour but not the cells migrated in adjacent tissues developing metastasis.

After surgery then, where possible, radiotherapy is applied to reduce the surviving infiltrating cells irradiating the surrounding post-surgery zone. Chemotherapy is often applied concomitantly with radiation in order to antagonize metastasis and to kill distant infiltrating cells.

Glioblastoma multiforme is rather difficult to eradicate as well because of the delicate location in the brain, which has a limited capacity to repair itself. Additionally, most of the chemotherapeutics are not able to cross the blood–brain barrier and are then inefficient.

Few drugs have been found applicable in glioblastoma multiforme treatments, among them TMZ. TMZ, brand names Temodar, Temodal and Temcad, is an alkylating agent administered as an oral drug. At the physiological pH, it is activated and interferes with the DNA replication. Since tumour cells divide faster than normal cells, the compound preferentially provokes cell death of cancer cells. TMZ is effective to prolong the patients' overall life time prognosis but does not display a solution to the problem per se. Glioblastoma multiforme patients' median overall survival (OS) increases by 3 months after TMZ treatment. TMZ is most effective in tumours with a hypermethylated MGMT ($O^6$-methylguanine-DNA-methyltransferase) promoter [43] and was found more effective in combination with coadjutant drugs. The treatment of U87 (wild type p53) cells with a combination of TMZ and chloroquine (CQ), e.g. increases the apoptosis and decreases the proliferation rate of the cells. However, most of the effects of TMZ and CQ in glioma are via differential autophagy-associated mechanisms, and depend on the p53 status [44].

CQ may improve mid-term survival when administered in addition to conventional therapy for glioblastoma multiforme [45]. Procarbazine and vincristine improved the progression free survival but not the OS in anaplastic oligodendrogliomas and oligoastrocytomas [46].

## Proton Beam Clinical Trials

Surgery is the most important and whenever possible, the most recommended treatment for brain tumours and tumours in general. However, often its application is impossible or not suggested for the compliance which could result. Post-operative radiotherapy (PORT) is often suggested, however its advantages are not proven. In a low grade glioma protocol (LGG-EORTC 22845 trial), Mizumoto et al. found that the progression free survival (PFS) was better for patients that received PORT (54 Gy early, 30 fractions) compared to those that had no radiotherapy, but no increase of the OS resulted [47]. The PFS is a measure of the activity of a certain treatment on a particular disease. For its calculation, the first day of treatment or clinical trial and the date on which the disease progresses are taken into account (Guidance for Industry Clinical Trial Endpoints for the Approval of Cancer Drugs and Biologics. U.S. Department of Health and Human Services Food and Drug Administration; Centre for Drug Evaluation and Research (CDER); Centre for Biologics Evaluation and Research (CBER) 2007).

Radiotherapy is usually limited due to the tolerance of the healthy tissue around the tumour. Proton and carbon ion beam treatment are emerging as rather important for glioblastoma multiforme treatment because of their capacity to spare the healthy brain tissue surrounding the neoplasm. Namely, proton beam is considered low LET radiation and its RBE compared to photon irradiation is only 1.1. Due to this scarce relative biological advantage it is inconvenient considering also the elevated costs to build up a proton facility. Nevertheless, the dose distribution advantages and the high preciseness in the delineation of the tumour contours make this particle the most applied ion in any particle therapy centre worldwide.

This paragraph will present clinical trials comparing photon and proton irradiation.

As mentioned above, the conventional 60 Gy photon irradiation administered with the adjuvant drug TMZ is not sufficient for the improvement of the high-grade glioma (HGG) patients' prognosis. The median survival has been reported around 15 months while the 5 year survival is less than 10 % [48]. Increasing the dose to 90 Gy either with protons or photons improved the local control and the median survival of 23 glioblastoma patients to 20 months. For GBM patients, Tanaka et al. reported 38.4 % median survival times (MST) of 16.2, 12.4 and 24 months after 80–90 Gy of conformal high-dose X-ray and 11.4 % for patients treated with 60 Gy high-dose conformal X-ray radiotherapy.

Therefore the results of the clinical trial indicate that a total dose over 90 GyE is potentially able to control the GBM and to reduce tumour relapse. Most of the relapse cases were found in patients treated with 60–70 Gy while only one case reported recurrence in patients treated with 90 Gy [48].

Mizumoto et al. studied a clinical trial using a hypo-fractionated boost of proton beam and nimustine hydrochloride (N′-[(4-Amino-2-methyl-5-pyrimidinyl) methyl]-N-(2-chloroethyl)-N-nitrosourea) (ACNU). In this clinical trial, 20 glioblastoma patients were treated every day twice, morning and afternoon, with 6 h of distance between the two treatments. In the morning, patients were treated with 1.8 Gy (RBE) for tumour and surrounding oedema, in the afternoon 1.65 Gy (RBE) for the gross tumour on gadolinium-enhanced magnetic resonance imaging (MRI) over 28 days, for a total of 96.6 Gy (RBE) in 56 fractions. Among the 20 patients treated only one suffered from recurrence, the median survival of the patients was 21.6 months and PFS was 45.5 % in the first and 15.5 % in the second year. Radiation necrosis (RN) occurred in six cases, and a probable leukoencephalopathy was observed in one patient [49].

A second group of patients received 60 Gy and did not develop RN contrary to those patients that received higher doses [47].

The tumour relapse due to the cell infiltration in the surrounding tissues is still a problem but the use of methionine positron emission tomography would facilitate the evaluation of exact tumour invasion area.

In an another study, Mizumoto M et al. evaluated the characteristics of long-term survivors after post-operative hyper-fractionated concomitant boost X-ray and proton beam therapy (PBT). Among 81 patients only 23 had proper characteristics to be eligible for the clinical trial.

Those patients were treated with 28 fractions of 50.4 Gy X-ray and 28 fractions of protons up to 46.2 GyE in gadolinium-enhanced volumes after more than 6 h from the first X-ray exposure concurrent with nimustine hydrochloride or TMZ.

Treatment was completed in 43 days (median value) and the following results were obtained:

Six patients after 70.9 months developed necrosis but no tumour recurrence, five of these patients underwent necrotomy and two received bevacizumab after it.

The results suggest that proton therapy is useful to avoid tumour recurrence but it is necessary to cover the complete area of the tumour and to consider also the areas in which the infiltrated cells may be located. Necrosis is inevitable but the survival of patients was well preserved [50].

Matsuda et al. studied the effect of high doses of photon compared with high dose of proton irradiation in glioblastoma patients. The study has investigated a total of 67 patients (34 men and 33 women, aged 31–84 years, median: 59 years).

The first step was a surgical resection where possible. For 13 patients the resection was complete, partial for 47 patients and for seven patients only biopsy was taken (10 % of total number of patients). Forty-seven patients were then treated with chemotherapy, 32 patients with high doses of particle therapy (HDT) and 35 with fractionated photon radiotherapy (CRT). Successively all the patients, i.e. 67, received either photon or proton irradiation.

The 1 year survival of the patients was 67.2 % while the 2 year survival decreased to 33.7 %. The median OS was of 17.7 months. Patients treated with protons were found to have a longer OS (24.4 months) compared to patients treated with the conventional photon treated patients (14.2 months).

The OS for patients treated in the time between 1998 and 2007 increased from 15.2 months to 17.7 (95 % CI) months while the relative survival increased from 23.6 to 33.7 %. The reason may be due to the improvements of the surgical techniques, such as the introduction of fluorescence guidance in 1999 and of neuro-navigation in 2005 as well as the chemotherapeutic agents. Patients treated with particles had a better preoperative performance status (PS) and had likely a complete resection compared to photon irradiated patients.

Similarly, for patients that underwent a partial resection, the OS of those who received HDT increased versus those treated with CRT ($p = 0.005$).

The results of this study showed that patients treated with HDT lived longer than those treated with photon (CRT). However, randomized trials including strict criteria for patients need to be performed to demonstrate conclusively that prolonged survival is due to high dose radiotherapy [51].

In a clinical trial from 2009, conducted at the Proton Medical Research Centre at Tsukuba, Japan, by Yamamoto et al., 20 newly diagnosed glioblastomas were treated. The median OS was 21.6 % and the 1 and 2 year survival was 71.1 % and 45.3 %, respectively [52].

## Carbon Beam Clinical Trials

Surgery is not always possible and often a coadjutant treatment is necessary. Conventional radiotherapy with or without chemotherapy is often, especially for glioblastoma, not sufficient to increase the OS and free tumour recurrences. Protons, besides the advantages of a better and more precise dose distribution, have an RBE of only 1.1 and are thus less efficient in inactivating the most resistant hypoxic and cancer stem cells. Neither photons nor protons seem to be sufficient to completely eradicate the glioblastoma as described in the previous paragraph.

Three further directions are discussed for the future of radiotherapy:

- To expand the gap between tumour radiosensitivity and normal tissues

- To reduce the irradiated area with a more precise tumour-dose distribution
- To reduce the tumour resistance

The PBT and carbon beam therapy (CBT) are both considered potentially able to achieve a reduction of the irradiation field, in particular developing the intensity modulated particle therapy (IMPT).

Due to the high LET of carbon ions, it is possible to reduce the radioresistance of cancer cells to concentrate the maximum of the delivered dose in the tumour while sparing healthy tissues.

Carbon ions are discussed to be a good candidate for the HGG treatment. Figure 5.9 depicts a typical carbon ion treatment plan for a recurrent glioblastoma patient, clearly indicating the concentration of the applied dose in the target volume while the healthy tissue is almost not affected.

However, the best combination may be carbon ion beam treatment with chemotherapy. Carbon ions then should be concentrated on the tumour core while the drug should avoid recurrence killing the distal small metastases and sustain the tumour shrinkage. TMZ alone and/or in combination with different other drugs and carbon ion irradiation as a form of therapy is currently under investigation. The next paragraphs will focus on the different clinical trials applying carbon beam of the most involved centres around the world starting from the GSI Helmholtz Centre for Heavy Ion Research in Darmstadt, Germany, where more than 400 patients were treated in the first European pilot project which took place between 1997 and 2008.

## Germany: Pilot Project at GSI Helmholtz Centre for Heavy Ion Research

The project aimed at testing the efficiency of a carbon ion beam with active scanning for cancer treatment (Fig. 5.10). In this clinical trial 450 patients, mostly suffering from base-skull tumours were treated. The study was a collaboration of GSI, the Department of Radiology at the

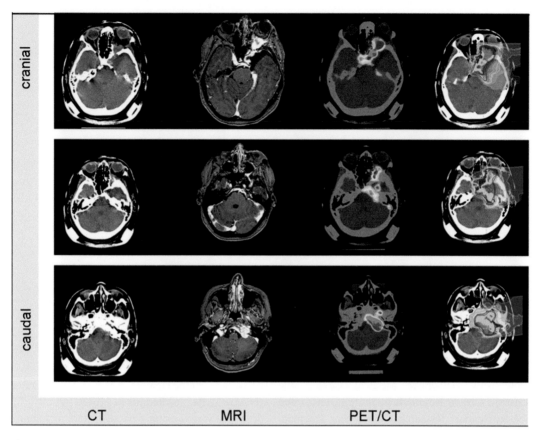

**Fig. 5.9** Carbon ion treatment plan. The dose is concentrated inside the tumour and most of the healthy tissue is spared [56]

**Fig. 5.10** A patient treated in the GSI pilot project is positioned in front of the beam exit (A. Zschau, GSI Helmholtzzentrum für Schwerionenforschung)

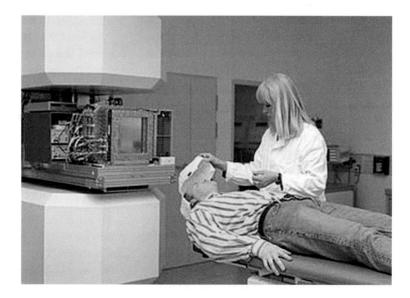

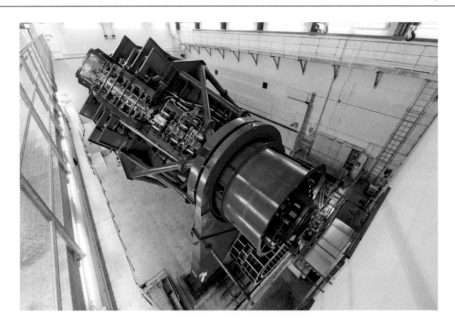

**Fig. 5.11** The HIT Heidelberg carbon ion gantry (Universitätsklinikum Heidelberg)

Heidelberg University Medical Center, the German Cancer Research Institute (DKFZ) and the Rossendorf Research Center near Dresden. The treatment was concentrated in 20 consecutive (30 min per exposure) days/fractions.

The local recurrence and survival was monitored for the following 5 years. In 75–90 % of the patients the tumour was stopped. In few cases only the patients suffered from side effect from the treatment. The results of the pilot project were promising and lead to an acceptance of that medical procedure as a new branch of radiotherapy.

## Japan: National Institute of Radiological Sciences

The NIRS in Chiba, Japan, is one of the most advanced radiological research institutes in the world. Starting in 1957, studies of clinical research, basic science and clinical radiation were performed at NIRS. Yet it was not before 1994 that the first patients were treated with the advanced particle beam therapy.

Currently, more than 8000 patients have been treated with high energy carbon ion radiation

produced in at the Heavy Ion Medical Accelerator (HIMAC), the accelerator of NIRS. Initially, the dose was varied using a passive beam technique. It is since few years, from 2011 on that patients can be treated also with a new, faster and advanced multiple-energy operation system three-dimensional raster scanning that gives the possibility to reduce drastically the total irradiation time (*Source*: NIRS webpage).

Moreover, NIRS as well as HIT (Germany) is equipped with the most advanced accelerator technology, the Gantry, as shown in Fig. 5.11.

A gantry is an ion treatment facility that allows for rotation of 360° around the patient. A treatment of patients in every angle is thus possible to the physicians to avoid the most sensitive entrance channels or organ at risk, where applicable.

### The NIRS/Tsukuba Glioblastoma Clinical Trials

Carbon ion irradiation showed favourable outcomes for patients with very resistant and recurrent tumours like the head and neck cancers. More than 800 patients, 11 % of the total number of patients have been treated at NIRS for head and neck cancer. A comparison between the local control of patients treated with a total dose of 57.6 GyE or 64.0 GyE for adenoid cystic carcinoma showed that patients treated with lower dose had a longer local control; yet, the reason remains to be elucidated.

Concerning the mucosal melanoma, the metastatic grade, usually very high, has been reduced using the chemotherapeutic DAV (daunomycin, cytarabine and vincristine). A phase I/II clinical trial has been conducted by Mizoe et al. Forty-eight patients with HGG (16 with anaplastic astrocytoma and 32 with GBM) were treated using photon and carbon ion therapy with nimustine hydrochloride (ACNU) (Table 5.1).

Patients were treated with XRT and chemotherapy first followed by a treatment with CRT.

Two field X-ray irradiation for a total of 2 Gy was delivered daily 5 days per week up to a total of 50 Gy. The targeted volume included the presumed infiltrated areas.

The chemotherapeutic agent ACNU was administered at the first, fourth or fifth week of X-ray treatment in a dose of 100 mg/m$^2$. After this first treatment CRT was then applied on 4 days per week with a total of eight fractions during 2 weeks. The total carbon dose was escalated from 16.8 to 24.8 Gy with a 10 % increment.

The results (Fig. 5.12) show that among the 32 patients divided in three groups according to the carbon dose, the OS for patients treated with high carbon ion dose 24.8 GyE was the highest.

The median m-PFS was:

- Four months for the four patients treated with 16.8 GyE
- Seven months for the 23 patients treated with 18.4, 20 or 22.4 GyE
- Fourteen months for the five patients treated with 24.8 GyE

The results demonstrated the effectiveness of carbon ion irradiation for the local control of glioblastoma. The combined treatment of X-rays, drugs and carbon ion irradiation hence seems to be promising for the cure of the glioblastoma.

CBT increases the local control and patient's survival (26 months). Moreover, CRT, due to the increased precision in dose distribution, reduces the damage to the brain tissue [58].

**Table 5.1** The characteristics of 48 patients who received combined therapy with X-ray radiotherapy (XRT), nimustine hydrochloride chemotherapy and carbon ion radiotherapy, according to Mizoe et al. Reprinted from [58] with permission of Elsevier, with minor modifications

| Total number | 48 |
|---|---|
| Histology (%) | |
| AA | 16 (33) |
| GBM | 32 (67) |
| Median age, years (%) | 53 (range, 18–78) |
| Age < 50 | 22 (46) |
| Age > 50 | 26 (54) |
| Sex (%) | |
| Male | 29 (60) |
| Female | 19 (40) |
| Extent of surgical resection (%) | |
| Gross total | 8 (17) |
| Subtotal | 8 (17) |
| Partial | 27 (56) |
| Biopsy | 5 (10) |
| Neurological function (%) | |
| Able to work | 29 (60) |
| Able to be at home | 19 (40) |
| Tumour location (%) | |
| Frontal | 22 (46) |
| Temporal | 10 (21) |
| Parietal | 5 (10) |
| Occipital | 6 (13) |
| Others | 5 (10) |
| KPS (%) | |
| 100 | 1 (2) |
| 90 | 26 (54) |
| 80 | 9 (19) |
| 70 | 4 (8) |
| 60 | 8 (17) |
| Mental status (%) | |
| Normal | 37 (77) |
| Not normal | 11 (23) |
| Symptom duration | |
| <3 months | 36 (75) |
| >or=3 months | 12 (25) |

*AA* anaplastic astrocytoma, *GBM* glioblastoma multiforme, *KPS* Karnofsky performance

## Germany: Heidelberg Ion Therapy Center (HIT)

The European centre for particle therapy HIT is a facility allowing for the treatment of patients with both protons and carbon ion using the first

**Fig. 5.12** Glioblastoma multiforme patients' survival after carbon ion irradiation at different doses. Median survival sorted by doses: low-dose group (16.8 GyE) median survival (MS) 7 months, middle-dose group (18.4–22.4 GyE) 19 months, high-dose group (24.8 GyE) 26 months. The differences were statistically significant ($p=0.0031$) Reprinted from [58] with permission of Elsevier

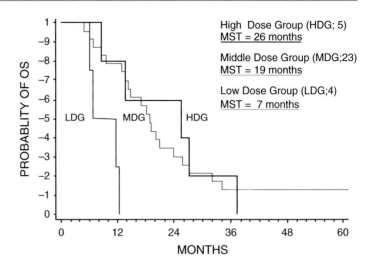

pencil beam raster scanning method in the world. In Fig. 5.13 a patient is positioned for the treatment at HIT with ions that are provided by the accelerator and the adjacent beam lines including the gantry.

Figure 5.14 depicts the Gantry treatment room at HIT.

The availability of both proton and carbon treatment in near future will provide the opportunity to compare the clinical trials applying photons in combination with protons or carbon. Despite the fact that recent studies point to carbon as an accepted particle for this new branch of radiotherapy, the research for alternative ions to be used in therapy is ongoing. Different ions, heavier and lighter than carbon, are now under investigation at GSI, HIT but also in other particle therapy and research centres such as the Trento Institute for Fundamental Physics and Applications (TIFPA) and the Proton Therapy Center in Trento, Italy.

## The Glioblastoma Clinical Trials at HIT

The radiochemotherapy, particularly the TMZ-radiotherapy combination, led to a significant increase of the survival of patients with glioblastoma multiforme but the results are still unsatisfactory.

In many patients, an increased expression of the epidermal growth factor receptor (EGFR) has been found in cancer biopsies. This muta-

tion provokes an overstimulation of the receptor that finally contributes to an uncontrolled cell division.

The addition of EGFR-inhibitors like the chemotherapeutic cetuximab together with TMZ to the conventional radiotherapy seems to be very promising.

- GERT is a one-armed single-centre phase I/II trial [59].

A dose escalation of TMZ from 50 to 75 mg/m$^2$ in combination with radiotherapy and cetuximab was applied.

Cetuximab was administered in the standard application dose of 400 mg/m$^2$ in the first week and then 250 mg/m$^2$ every following week. Forty-six patients were treated.

Feasibility, toxicity, the OS and the PFS were important endpoints to be studied.

The aim of the trial was to understand the safety and efficiency of the combined radiotherapy-immunotherapy with TMZ and cetuximab for primary glioblastoma patients [59].

Different are then nowadays the possibilities to fight glioblastoma multiforme:

Conventional radiotherapy, radiochemotherapy using TMZ alone or in combination with other drugs, and the most advanced particle therapies: proton and carbon ion beam.

The decades of experience at NIRS, Japan, suggest a higher efficiency of carbon ion treat-

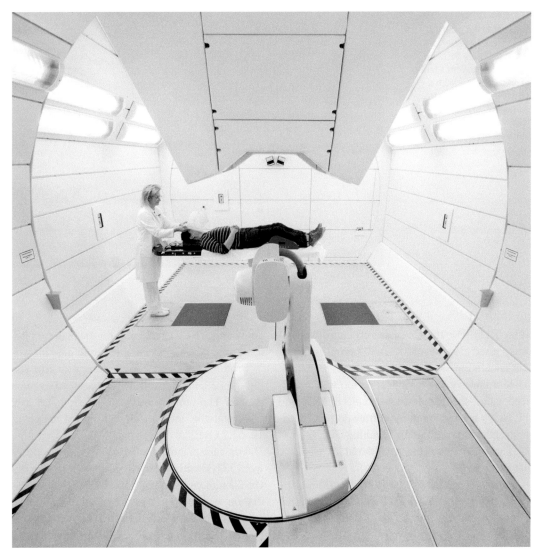

**Fig. 5.13** The HIT facility treatment room (Universitätsklinikum Heidelberg)

ment for glioblastoma and a lower toxicity compared with photon or proton irradiation.

At HIT clinical trials have been started to compare the effect of this different therapies. Currently, two different clinical trials are ongoing, being follow-ups of a previous study which included 33 patients (their characteristics are summarized in Table 5.2).

Thirty-three patients, 18 with glioblastoma with a median age of 42 years and three children, less than 18 years old, were treated. Thirty per

cent of the total number of patients was female and 70 % male.

The study aimed at the comparison between a carbon boost (6×3 GyE) and a proton boost (5×2 GyE) in glioma patients with a macroscopic tumour residue previously treated with 50 Gy of photons.

Two weeks prior to the treatment, patients' individual mask fixation was done using the thermoplastic-mask technique.

GBM patients' examination and treatment plan were performed with 18F-FET-PET/CT

**Fig. 5.14** Treatment room adjacent to the gantry at HIT. The possibility to rotate the beam delivery exit and the patient's table gives to the physician a virtually infinity possible number of irradiation field (Universitätsklinikum Heidelberg)

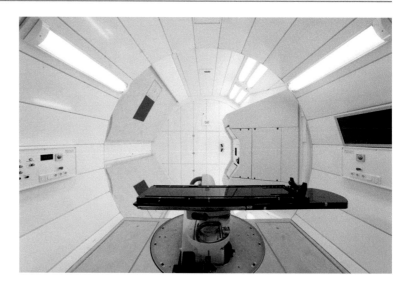

(Fig. 5.15). For the CT scan, no contrast agent was used to avoid any particle range miscalculation.

Morphology and tumour function was visualized using the gadolinium-enhanced MRI and PET/CTs tracing amino acid transporters in glioma and were fused to the planning CTs.

The treatment plans considered as well the areas at risk for infiltrating cells.

In this case, for the high-grade glioma, the clinical target volume (CTV) was calculated adding a 0.5 cm margin to the gross tumour volume ($CTV_{boost}$). The $CTV_{photons}$ instead was calculated taking into account 2–3 cm for the microscopic spread.

The definition of the clinical volume and the gross volume (GTV) is based on different clinical presentation like the performance status, neurological symptoms, images and others. Usually, for glioblastoma multiforme the GTV is considered the area of contrast enhancement observed on the CT scan or MRI. The CTV volume instead also takes in consideration the putative infiltrating cells and is therefore larger. For this reason, few centimetres of security margin are usually added to the GTV to reduce the risk of tumour relapse [60].

Subsequently, 3 mm of margin was included to generate the final particle therapy planning tar-

get volume (PTV) and 5 mm for the plan for photon irradiation.

Proton beam was chosen for paediatric and glioma patients as well as for one glioblastoma patient. The proton dose spanned from 1.8 to 2 GyE and the total dose was in the range of 10–57.2 GyE.

For carbon ion irradiation, the single doses were 3 GyE with a total dose range from 18 to 45 GyE. In all cases, a previous 50 Gy photon irradiation was done as initial requirement to be admitted to the clinical trial. From 33 patients treated, 17 received also TMZ in combination with radiotherapy at a concentration of 75 mg/m$^2$ on 7 days per week.

The resulting toxicity was moderate. One patient had a diminishing vision capacity, rapidly restored with an oral administration of corticosteroids, and another one suffered from diminishing hearing abilities. A total of 14.7 % of all patients had low-grade oedema and 24.2 % suffered from an increased fatigue during the day. Two patients had seizures.

TMZ as coadjutant drug did not increase the toxicity. In a single case only, a patient had a TMZ-related thrombocytopenia.

The median follow-up of the treatment was 4.5 months. The first tumour growth verification was performed 6 and 12 weeks after radiation

**Table 5.2** Details of 33 patients treated at HIT in a pilot study between November 2009 and January 2011. Modified from Rieken et al. [56]

| Patient characteristics | | |
|---|---|---|
| *Gender* | [*n*] | [%] |
| Male | 33 | 100 |
| Female | 10 | 30.3 |
| Age at RT | Years | |
| Median | 42 | |
| Range | 7–77 | |
| | [*n*] | [%] |
| Paediatric patients ≤18 years histology | 3 | 9.1 |
| Glioma | 26 | 100 |
| WHO II | 5 | 19.2 |
| WHO III | 3 | 11.5 |
| WHO IV | 18 | 69.2 |
| Meningioma | 7 | 100 |
| WHO I | 3 | 43 |
| WHO II | 3 | 43 |
| WHO III | 1 | 14 |
| | [*n*] | [%] |
| Radiotherapy | | |
| Mixed modality | 22 | 66.6 |
| [12C] only | 6 | 18.2 |
| [1H] only | 5 | 15.2 |
| | [*n*] | [%] |
| Particle reirradiation | 7 | 21.2 |
| | Gy | |
| Range carbon total dose | 18–45 | |
| Range proton total dose | 10–57.2 | |
| Range photon total dose | 50 | |
| | [*n*] | [%] |
| Relapse meningioma | 0 | 0 |
| Relapse glioma WHO II | 0 | 0 |
| Relapse glioma WHO III | 9 | 42.3 |

and no patient at that time had any statistically important improvements.

From the glioblastoma patients receiving particle therapy, 50 % showed an illness progression which led to a mortality of 44 %. A tumour recurrence was found for 27 % of them.

The OS and the PFS increased comparing radiotherapy alone to carbon ion irradiation and comparing radiotherapy to radiotherapy in combination with TMZ. The results suggest that particles are safe and their application feasible in patients with brain tumour, further-

more the treatment is associated with a low toxicity [56].

Another study has been done to compare radiotherapy, radiotherapy in combination with TMZ and carbon ion therapy.

Thirty-two glioblastoma multiforme patients have been treated.

Median OS was 9 months with radiotherapy (RT), 14 months with radiochemotherapy (RCHT), 18 months with a carbon boost (CB) and no significant differences between CB and RCHT were found. The median PFS instead was 5 months for RT patients, 6 months for RCHT patients, 8 months for the CB patients and here a significant difference was found between CB and RCHT [61].

Other two clinical trials currently taking place at the HIT are CINDERELLA and CLEOPATRA.

- The CINDERELLA trial compares carbon ion irradiation with fractionated stereotactic radiotherapy of patients with recurrent or progressive gliomas.
- The CLEOPATRA trial instead compares primary glioblastoma patients treated with a carbon ion boost or proton boost delivered after radiochemotherapy with TMZ.

CINDERELLA is treating recurrent or progressive glioblastoma patients including those with neurosurgical resection and those that already underwent chemotherapy or radiotherapy. Most of the patients in fact already received a full course of radiotherapy, for this reason a further reirradiation programme has to be applied cautiously [62].

Nowadays the modern precision photon techniques (FSRT) are used for a second course of radiotherapy due to their safeness and effectiveness. The patients' survival in this case is 22, 16 and 8 months for recurrent WHO grade II, III and IV tumours, respectively.

Within the first phase of the trial with carbon ions the recommended dose is determined in a dose escalation scheme. Following that, in the randomized phase II part, the radiation dose was evaluated in the experimental arm compared to the standard arm (FSRT, total dose of 36 Gy, sin-

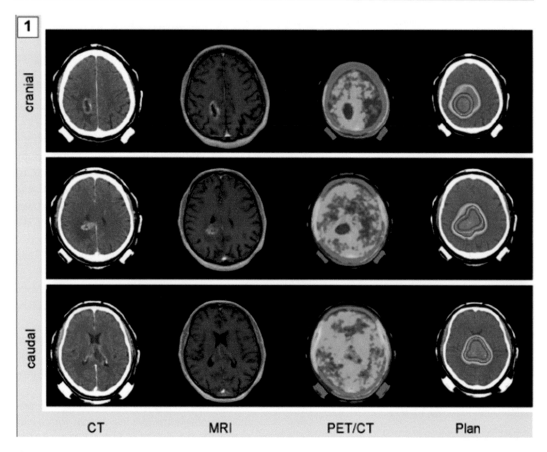

**Fig. 5.15** "Extensive glioblastoma multiforme in a 62-year-old man. Contrast agent-enhanced CT and MRI scan were fused with a FET-PET/CT examination and used to calculate a two beam carbon ion radiotherapy plan" [56]

gle fractionated dose of 2 Gy). Toxicity is the primary endpoint of phase I, for phase II instead it is the 12-months survival after reirradiation while the secondary endpoint is the PFS.

The most important inclusion criteria are the unifocal, supratentorial, recurrent glioma, the contrast enhancement on T1-weighted MRI and/or Amino-Acid-PET-positive high-grade tumour areas, indication for reirradiation, an age above 18 years and the Karnofsky performance score more or equal to 60 [62].

The Karnofsky performance score is a rating scale that allows evaluating the cancer patients' quality of life taking into account different parameters like the activity limitation, care of themselves and self-determination.

In the Karnofsky scale, a score of 60 corresponds to a patient that requires occasional assis-

tance, but is able to care for most of his personal needs.

The most important exclusion criteria are instead the multifocal glioma or glioblastoma cerebri, previous reirradiation or prior radiosurgery or treatment with interstitial radioactive seeds, time interval less than 6 months after primary radiotherapy.

CLEOPATRA compares carbon or proton boost treatment for patients with macroscopic glioblastoma already treated with a combined surgery-radiochemotherapy with TMZ. Radiation is delivered up to a total dose of 60 Gy using photons. Applying this treatment regimen, the OS could be extended significantly; however, the median OS is still about 15 months only.

In the experimental trial, the carbon boost up to 18 GyE is applied to the macroscopic tumour in six fractions at a single dose of 3 GyE. The standard protocol instead is applied using a proton boost up to 10 GyE in five single fractions of 2 GyE each. The endpoints are the OS as well as the PFS [62].

# References

1. Loeffler JS, Durante M. Charged particle therapy—optimization, challenges and future directions. Nat Rev Clin Oncol. 2013;10:411–24.
2. Gilbert MR. New treatments for malignant gliomas: careful evaluation and cautious optimism required. Ann Intern Med. 2006;144(5):371–3.
3. Durante M, Loeffler JS. Charged particles in radiation oncology. Nat Rev Clin Oncol. 2010;7(1):37–43.
4. Kamiya-Matsuoka C, Gilbert MR. Treating recurrent glioblastoma: an update. CNS Oncol. 2015;4(2): 91–104.
5. Kamada T, Tsujii H, Blakely EA, Debus J, De Neve W, Durante M, Jäkel O, Mayer R, Orecchia R, Pötter R, Vatnitsky S, Chu WT. Carbon ion radiotherapy in Japan: an assessment of 20 years of clinical experience. Lancet Oncol. 2015;16(2):e93–100.
6. Zhu X, El Fakhri G. Proton therapy verification with PET imaging. Theranostics. 2013;3(10):731–40.
7. Levin WP, Kooy H, Loeffler JS, DeLaney TF. Proton beam therapy. Br J Cancer. 2005;93(8):849–54.
8. Kraft G, Weber U. Tumor therapy with ion beams. In: Grupen C, Buvat I, editors. Handbook of particle detection and imaging. Berlin: Springer; 2012. p. 1179–205.
9. Schlaff CD, Krauze A, Belard A, O'Connell JJ, Camphausen KA. Bringing the heavy: carbon ion therapy in the radiobiological and clinical context. Radiat Oncol. 2014;9(1):88.
10. Akino Y, Teshima T, Kihara A, Kodera-Suzumoto Y, Inaoka M, Higashiyama S, Furusawa Y, Matsuura N. Carbon-ion beam irradiation effectively suppresses migration and invasion of human non-small-cell lung cancer cells. Int J Radiat Oncol Biol Phys. 2009;75(2):475–81.
11. Durante M, Reppingen N, Held KD. Immunologically augmented cancer treatment using modern radiotherapy. Trends Mol Med. 2013;19(9):565–82.
12. Shannon AM, Bouchier-Hayes DJ, Condron CM, Toomey D. Tumour hypoxia, chemotherapeutic resistance and hypoxia-related therapies. Cancer Treat Rev. 2003;29(4):297–307.
13. Bussink J, Kaanders JH, van der Kogel AJ. Tumor hypoxia at the micro-regional level: clinical relevance and predictive value of exogenous and endogenous hypoxic cell markers. Radiother Oncol. 2003;67(1): 3–15.
14. Collet G, El Hafny-Rahbi B, Nadim M, Tejchman A, Klimkiewicz K, Kieda C. Hypoxia-shaped vascular niche for cancer stem cells. Contemp Oncol (Pozn). 2015;19(1A):A39–43.
15. von Sonntag C. The basics of oxidants in water treatment. Part A: OH radical reactions. Water Sci Technol. 2007;55(12):19–23.
16. Meesungnoen J, Jay-Gerin JP. High-LET ion radiolysis of water: oxygen production in tracks. Radiat Res. 2009;171(3):379–86.
17. Tinganelli W, Ma NY, Von Neubeck C, Maier A, Schicker C, Kraft-Weyrather W, Durante M. Influence of acute hypoxia and radiation quality on cell survival. J Radiat Res. 2013;54 Suppl 1:i23–30.
18. Krämer M, Scholz M. Treatment planning for heavy-ion radiotherapy: calculation and optimization of biologically effective dose. Phys Med Biol. 2000; 45(11):3319–30.
19. Tinganelli W, Durante M, Hirayama R, Kraemer M, Maier A, Kraft-Weyrather W, Furusawa Y, Friedrich T, Scifoni E. Kill-painting of hypoxic tumours in charged particle therapy. Sci Rep. 2015;5:170–16.
20. Plaks V, Kong N, Werb Z. The cancer stem cell niche: how essential is the niche in regulating stemness of tumor cells? Cell Stem Cell. 2015;16(3):225–38.
21. Kunisaki Y. Cancer stem cells and the niches. Nihon Rinsho. 2015;73(5):739–44. Japanese.
22. Li L, Neaves WB. Normal stem cells and cancer stem cells: the niche matters. Cancer Res. 2006;66(9): 4553–7.
23. Saito S, Lin YC, Tsai MH, Lin CS, Murayama Y, Sato R, Yokoyama KK. Emerging roles of hypoxia-inducible factors and reactive oxygen species in cancer and pluripotent stem cells. Kaohsiung J Med Sci. 2015;31(6):279–86.
24. Bloy N, Pol J, Manic G, Vitale I, Eggermont A, Galon J, Tartour E, Zitvogel L, Kroemer G, Galluzzi L. Trial watch: radioimmunotherapy for oncological indications. Oncoimmunology. 2014;3(9):e954929.
25. Kalbasi A, June CH, Haas N, Vapiwala N. Radiation and immunotherapy: a synergistic combination. J Clin Invest. 2013;123(7):2756–63.
26. Postow MA, Callahan MK, Barker CA, Yamada Y, Yuan J, Kitano S, Mu Z, Rasalan T, Adamow M, Ritter E, Sedrak C, Jungbluth AA, Chua R, Yang AS, Roman RA, Rosner S, Benson B, Allison JP, Lesokhin AM, Gnjatic S, Wolchok JDN. Immunologic correlates of the abscopal effect in a patient with melanoma. Engl J Med. 2012;366:925–31.
27. Ivanov VN, Partridge MA, Huang SX, Hei TK. Suppression of the proinflammatory response of metastatic melanoma cells increases TRAIL-induced apoptosis. J Cell Biochem. 2011;112:463–75.
28. Kong LY, Gelbard A, Wei J, Reina-Ortiz C, Wang Y, Yang EC, Hailemichael Y, Fokt I, Jayakumar A, Qiao W, Fuller GN, Overwijk WW, Priebe W, Heimberger AB. Inhibition of p-STAT3 enhances IFN-a efficacy against metastatic melanoma in a murine model. Clin Cancer Res. 2010;16:2550–61.
29. Steiner HH, Bonsanto MM, Beckhove P, Brysch M, Geletneky K, Ahmadi R, Schuele-Freyer R, Kremer P, Ranaie G, Matejic D, Bauer H, Kiessling M, Kunze S, Schirrmacher V, Herold-Mende C. Antitumor vaccination of patients with glioblastoma multiforme: a

pilot study to assess feasibility, safety, and clinical benefit. J Clin Oncol. 2004;22:4272–81.

30. López-Larrea C, Suárez-Alvarez B, López-Soto A, López-Vázquez A, Gonzalez S. The NKG2D receptor: sensing stressed cells. Trends Mol Med. 2008;14:179–89.

31. Ogbomo H, Cinatl Jr J, Mody CH, Forsyth PA. Immunotherapy in gliomas: limitations and potential of natural killer (NK) cell therapy. Trends Mol Med. 2011;17:433–41.

32. Villalva C, Martin-Lannerée S, Cortes U, Dkhissi F, Wager M, Le Corf A, Tourani JM, Dusanter-Fourt I, Turhan AG, Karayan-Tapon L. STAT3 is essential for the maintenance of neurosphere-initiating tumor cells in patients with glioblastomas: a potential for targeted therapy? Int J Cancer. 2011;128:826–38.

33. Teulings HE, Tjin EP, Willemsen KJ, Krebbers G, van Noesel CJ, Kemp EH, Nieuweboer-Krobotova L, van der Veen JP, Luiten RM. Radiation-induced melanoma-associated leucoderma, systemic antimelanoma immunity and disease-free survival in a patient with advanced-stage melanoma: a case report and immunological analysis. Br J Dermatol. 2013;168: 733–8.

34. Maes W, Gool SW. Experimental immunotherapy for malignant glioma: lessons from two decades of research in the GL261 model. Cancer Immunol Immunother. 2011;60:153–60.

35. Newcomb EW, et al. The combination of ionizing radiation and peripheral vaccination produces long-term survival of mice bearing established invasive GL261 gliomas. Clin Cancer Res. 2006;12:4730–7.

36. Lee Y, Auh SL, Wang Y, Burnette B, Wang Y, Meng Y, Beckett M, Sharma R, Chin R, Tu T, Weichselbaum RR, Fu YX. Therapeutic effects of ablative radiation on local tumor require CD8+ T cells: changing strategies for cancer treatment. Blood. 2009;114: 589–95.

37. Demaria S, Formenti SC. Combining radiotherapy and cancer immunotherapy: a paradigm shift. J Natl Cancer Inst. 2013;105:256–65.

38. Krysko DV, Garg AD, Kaczmarek A, Krysko O, Agostinis P, Vandenabeele P. Immunogenic cell death and DAMPs in cancer therapy. Nat Rev Cancer. 2012;12:860–75.

39. Panaretakis T, Kepp O, Brockmeier U, Tesniere A, Bjorklund AC, Chapman DC, Durchschlag M, Joza N, Pierron G, van Endert P, Yuan J, Zitvogel L, Madeo F, Williams DB, Kroemer G. Mechanisms of pre-apoptotic calreticulin exposure in immunogenic cell death. EMBO J. 2009;28:578–90.

40. Garg AD, Krysko DV, Verfaillie T, Kaczmarek A, Ferreira GB, Marysael T, Rubio N, Firczuk M, Mathieu C, Roebroek AJ, Annaert W, Golab J, de Witte P, Vandenabeele P, Agostinis P. A novel pathway combining calreticulin exposure and ATP secretion in immunogenic cancer cell death. EMBO J. 2012;31:1062–79.

41. Stupp R, Mason WP, van den Bent MJ, Weller M, Fisher B, Taphoorn MJB, Belanger K, Brandes AA, Marosi C, Bogdahn U, Curschmann J, Samuel RCJ, Ludwin K, Gorlia T, Allgeier A, Lacombe D, Cairncross JG, Eisenhauer E, Mirimanoff RO. Radiotherapy plus concomitant and adjuvant temozolomide for glioblastoma. N Engl J Med. 2005;352:987–96.

42. Auffinger B, Spencer D, Pytel P, Ahmed AU, Lesniak MS. The role of glioma stem cells in chemotherapy resistance and glioblastoma multiforme recurrence. Expert Rev Neurother. 2015;31:1–12.

43. Thon N, Kreth S, Kreth FW. Personalized treatment strategies in glioblastoma: MGMT promoter methylation status. Onco Targets Ther. 2013;6:1363–72.

44. Lee SW, Kim HK, Lee NH, Yi HY, Kim HS, Hong SH, Hong YK. The synergistic effect of combination temozolomide and chloroquine treatment is dependent on autophagy formation and p53 status in glioma cells. Cancer Lett. 2015;360(2):195–204.

45. Sotelo J, Briceño E, López-González MA. Adding chloroquine to conventional treatment for glioblastoma multiforme: a randomized, double-blind, placebo-controlled trial. Ann Intern Med. 2006; 144(5):337–43.

46. van den Bent MJ, Carpentier AF, Brandes AA, Sanson M, Taphoorn MJ, Bernsen HJ, Frenay M, Tijssen CC, Grisold W, Sipos L, Haaxma-Reiche H, Kros JM, van Kouwenhoven MC, Vecht CJ, Allgeier A, Lacombe D, Gorlia T. Adjuvant procarbazine, lomustine, and vincristine improves progression-free survival but not overall survival in newly diagnosed anaplastic oligodendrogliomas and oligoastrocytomas: a randomized European Organisation for Research and Treatment of Cancer phase III trial. J Clin Oncol. 2006; 24(18):2715–22.

47. Mizumoto M, Oshiro Y, Tsuboi K. Proton beam therapy for intracranial and skull base tumors. Transl Cancer Res. 2013;2:2.

48. Fitzek MM, Thornton AF, Rabinov JD, Lev MH, Pardo FS, Munzenrider JE, Okunieff P, Bussiere M, Braun I, Hochberg FH, Hedley-Whyte ET, Liebsch NJ, Harsh 4th GR. Accelerated fractionated proton/photon irradiation to 90 cobalt gray equivalent for glioblastoma multiforme: results of a phase II prospective trial. J Neurosurg. 1999;91:251–60.

49. Mizumoto M, Tsuboi K, Igaki H. Phase I/II trial of hyperfractionated concomitant boost proton radiotherapy for supratentorial glioblastoma multiforme. Int J Radiat Oncol Biol Phys. 2010;77:98–105.

50. Mizumoto M, Yamamoto T, Takano S, Ishikawa E, Matsumura A, Ishikawa H, Okumura T, Sakurai H, Miyatake S, Tsuboi K. Long-term survival after treatment of glioblastoma multiforme with hyperfractionated concomitant boost proton beam therapy. Pract Radiat Oncol. 2015;5(1):e9–16.

51. Matsuda M, Yamamoto T, Ishikawa E, Nakai K, Zaboronok A, Takano S, Matsumura A. Prognostic factors in glioblastoma multiforme patients receiving high-dose particle radiotherapy or conventional radiotherapy. Br J Radiol. 2011;84(Spec Iss 1): S054–060.

52. Yamamoto T, Tsuboi K. Particle radiotherapy for malignant gliomas. Brain Nerve. 2009;61(7):855–66.

53. Fitzek MM, Thornton AF, Harsh 4th G, Rabinov JD, Munzenrider JE, Lev M, Ancukiewicz M, Bussiere M, Hedley-Whyte ET, Hochberg FH, Pardo FS. Dose-escalation with proton/photon irradiation for Daumas-Duport lower-grade glioma: results of an institutional phase I/II trial. Int J Radiat Oncol Biol Phys. 2001;51(1):131–7.

54. Hug EB, Muenter MW, Archambeau JO, DeVries A, Liwnicz B, Loredo LN, Grove RI, Slater JD. Conformal proton radiation therapy for pediatric low-grade astrocytomas. Strahlenther Onkol. 2002; 178(1):10–7.

55. Hauswald H, Rieken S, Ecker S, Kessel KA, Herfarth K, Debus J, Combs SE. First experiences in treatment of low-grade glioma grade I and II with proton therapy. Radiat Oncol. 2012;7:189.

56. Rieken S, Habermehl D, Haberer T, Jaekel O, Debus J, Combs SE. Proton and carbon ion radiotherapy for primary brain tumors delivered with active raster scanning at the Heidelberg Ion Therapy Center (HIT): early treatment results and study concepts. Radiat Oncol. 2012;7:41.

57. Freeman T. Treatments begin on HIT's heavy ion gantry. Medicalphysicsweb. 2012.

58. Mizoe JE, Tsujii H, Hasegawa A, Yanagi T, Takagi R, Kamada T, Tsuji H, Takakura K. Phase I/II clinical trial of carbon ion radiotherapy for malignant gliomas: combined X-ray radiotherapy, chemotherapy, and carbon ion radiotherapy. Int J Radiat Oncol Biol Phys. 2007;69(2):390–6.

59. Combs SE, Heeger S, Haselmann R, Edler L, Debus J, Schulz-Ertner D. Treatment of primary glioblastoma multiforme with cetuximab, radiotherapy and temozolomide (GERT)—phase I/II trial: study protocol. BMC Cancer. 2006;6:133.

60. Kantor G, Loiseau H, Vital A, Mazeron JJ. Gross tumor volume (GTV) and clinical target volume (CTV) in adult gliomas. Cancer Radiother. 2001;5(5):571–80.

61. Combs SE, Bruckner T, Mizoe JE, Kamada T, Tsujii H, Kieser M, Debus J. Comparison of carbon ion radiotherapy to photon radiation alone or in combination with temozolomide in patients with high-grade gliomas: explorative hypothesis-generating retrospective analysis. Radiother Oncol. 2013;108(1): 132–5.

62. Combs SE, Burkholder I, Edler L, Rieken S, Habermehl D, Jäkel O, Haberer T, Haselmann R, Unterberg A, Wick W, Debus J. Randomised phase I/II study to evaluate carbon ion radiotherapy versus fractionated stereotactic radiotherapy in patients with recurrent or progressive gliomas: the CINDERELLA trial. BMC Cancer. 2010;10:533.

# Mathematical Modelling of Radiobiological Parameters

**6**

Piernicola Pedicini, Lidia Strigari, Luigi Spiazzi,
Alba Fiorentino, Paolo Tini, and Luigi Pirtoli

## Introduction

All treatment strategies are studied at the preclinical and clinical level, and the related endpoints are used to extract radiobiological parameters in mathematical models. This chapter aims to provide an overview of these approaches based on clinical and cellular data.

P. Pedicini
I.R.C.C.S. Regional Cancer Hospital C.R.O.B.,
Rionero-in-Vulture, PZ, Italy

L. Strigari (✉)
Laboratory of medical physics and expert systems,
Regina Elena National Cancer Institute,
via E. Chianesi 53, Rome 00144, Italy
e-mail: strigari@ifo.it

L. Spiazzi
Physics Department, Spedali Civili Hospital,
Brescia, Italy

Λ. Fiorentino
Sacro Cuore Don Calabria Hospital, Negrar-Verona, Italy

P. Tini
Tuscany Tumor Institute, Florence, Italy

Unit of Radiation Oncology, University Hospital of
Siena (Azienda Ospedaliera-Universitaria Senese),
Viale Bracci 11, Siena, 53100, Italy

L. Pirtoli
Tuscany Tumor Institute, Florence, Italy

Unit of Radiation Oncology, Department of
Medicine, Surgery and Neurosciences, University of
Siena, Siena, Italy

As mentioned in the previous chapter, median survival of glioblastoma (GBM) patients is poor. In fact, the 1-year median survival rate of GBM patients is approximately 50 %, despite the use of aggressive standard treatments, i.e. macroscopic resection and radiochemotherapy followed by adjuvant temozolomide.

In particular, to date most patients die from disease progression, primarily local recurrence. In fact, the limited tolerance of normal tissues can lead to inadequate therapeutic radiation doses.

The use of modern treatment planning systems, combined with a multi-imaging modality and the possibility to use Image Guided Radiotherapy (IGRT) images in order to track dose deposits in the tumour, allows a reliable cumulated dose to be delivered to the tumour bed. One of the characteristics of this dose is, in many cases, the lack of homogeneity, due to the proximity of Organs at risk (OAR). Nevertheless, the dose grid dimension (8–12 mm$^3$ voxel volume) and imaging resolutions limit the dose delivery tracking to a cellular level. The use of inaccurate dosimetric data is one of the main flaws of model parameter estimations obtained from literature on clinical findings from the last decade.

In addition, when deriving model parameters from meta-analysis, the heterogeneity in investigated patient populations can lead to different values or produce contrasting results to those of individual studies. This is known as Simpson's paradox [1].

© Springer International Publishing Switzerland 2016
L. Pirtoli et al. (eds.), *Radiobiology of Glioblastoma*, Current Clinical Pathology,
DOI 10.1007/978-3-319-28305-0_6

The effect of tissue, or cell, irradiation depends on the dose but in general is not proportional (in probability or intensity) to the dose. The inherent stochastic nature of the interaction of radiation–matter, the cellular structure and the complexity of environmental interaction make it difficult to develop a simple and reliable model of cell killing [1–3].

The cumulative effect of dose delivery to tissue makes it impossible to derive the correct dose for each specific patient and cell type, which would maximize the benefit of irradiation in terms of probability of cure, severity of deterministic damage and probability of stochastic side effects [1].

Therefore, the necessity to define an adequate population based pattern of temporal and spatial dose delivery has seen the development of various models of cell killing and tumour control probability (TCP).

The first studies that involved the combined effect of dose per fraction and overall treatment time (OTT) were performed as early as the 30s [4, 5], but they were neglected in consequences of World War II. The first universally accepted model focused on the skin reaction was published in 1944 [6], accompanied by great uncertainty on energy and source to skin distance values limiting its application to modern radiotherapy.

The first model of lethal doses based on radiosensitivity of tumour cells and Poisson statistics was presented in 1961 [7].

In 1969, Ellis suggested a formula which related total dose, number of fractions and OTT to a quantity termed "Nominal Standard Dose". The authors intended, this quantity to represent "the biological effect of a given treatment regime" and enable the comparison of various treatment schedules (with different dose fraction, total dose and overall treatment times) [8]. Considering the poor prognosis for GBM patients in the late 70s, the scientific community paid greater attention to the dose effect for GBM [9] and the first attempts to correlate delivered dose and tissue damage by means of Computer Tomography scans were published [10].

In the past 20 years, an increased number of research projects aiming at simulating and formulating the mechanisms of tumour response to radiation treatment have been proposed. One of most simple and efficacious models for radiation response is the linear-quadratic (LQ) model proposed by Fowler [11, 12]. The LQ model describes cell survival after exposure to ionizing radiation and is expressed by a linear radiobiology parameter $\alpha$ (intrinsic whole tumour radiosensitivity) and a quadratic parameter $\beta$ (repair capability) with reference to two forms of DNA damage.

The LQ model determines the relative contribution of each selected dose schedule to the surviving fraction. However, it could be optimized by taking into account cell repopulation parameters, such as the kick-off time for tumour repopulation ($T_k$), the repopulation doubling time ($T_d$) and the effective tumour repopulation rate quantified by $\gamma = \ln2/T_d$ [3, 13–21].

## Cellular Dose Response Models

### Cell Killing

The basic assumption of the simple LQ model states that the surviving cell fraction after a homogeneous dose irradiation is [11]

$$S(D) = e^{-\left(\alpha D + \beta D^2\right)} \tag{6.1}$$

where D is the dose and Biological Effective Dose (BED) defined as

$$BED = D\left(1 + \frac{D}{\alpha/\beta}\right) \tag{6.2}$$

When assuming that more than a single fraction is delivered, each with a dose $d_i$, then (6.1) becomes

$$S(D) = e^{-\left(\alpha \sum_i d_i + \beta \sum_i d_i^2\right)} \tag{6.3}$$

If the dose $d$ is delivered in each fraction then (6.3) becomes

$$S(D) = e^{-n\left(\alpha d + \beta d^2\right)} \tag{6.4}$$

and (6.2) becomes

$$BED = nd\left(1 + \frac{d}{\alpha/\beta}\right) \tag{6.5}$$

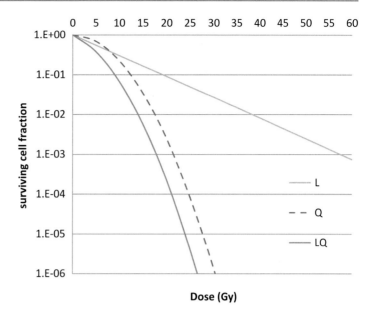

**Fig. 6.1** Cell survival against dose due to the linear (L), i.e. $\alpha D$, and quadratic (Q), i.e. $\beta D^2$ component. The combined effect is shown as LQ. The used parameters are $\alpha = 0.12/$ Gy and $\alpha/\beta = 8$ Gy

It is easier to describe BED in terms of equivalent dose given at 2 Gy per fraction [14, 22]

$$EQD_2 = D\frac{d + \alpha/\beta}{2\,Gy + \alpha/\beta} \qquad (6.6)$$

A graphical representation of the cell survival curve for the linear and quadratic component is shown in Fig. 6.1. The parameter $\alpha$ corresponds to the initial slope of the cell survival curve (i.e. the larger values of $\alpha$ correspond to the steeper initial slope) while $\beta$ determines the degree of downward curvature of the cell sur-vival curve (the larger value of $\beta$ corresponds to the more "bent" curve).

## Incomplete Repair

The LQ model as described in (6.1)–(6.6) cannot correctly estimate incomplete repair and OTT [23]. A formula that includes appropriate correction factors that link $EQD_2$ for a dose given within T days to one given in t is:

$$EQD_{2T} = D_t\frac{d(1 + H_m) + \alpha/\beta}{2\,Gy + \alpha/\beta} - (T - t)D_{prolif} \qquad (6.7)$$

where $H_m$ is the incomplete repair factor and the suffix m is equal to the fractions per day if it is assumed that there is a complete repair within the following day. $D_{prolif}$ is a parameter that gives the "lost" dose per day of delay. Some authors prefer to use a different symbol, $\lambda$ [24].

## Low-Dose Hypersensitivity

Although the LQ approach is widely used to describe tumour cell killing, at low doses (<1 Gy) the survival fraction does not monotonically decrease like the dose [25, 26]. In the range 10–30 cGy the surviving fraction is constant, while the radioresistance increases, reaching a maximum around 1 Gy and thereafter the curve shows a decreasing slope [25]. These results indicate a counter-intuitive effect, i.e. at low dose the cell surviving fraction increases with dose. Of note, the stated increased dose is not a subsequent irradiation, but a complete different irradiation with a different dose level.

Equation (6.1) can be corrected to take into account this effect [26]

$$S(D) = e^{-\left(\alpha_r D\left(1 + (\alpha_s/\alpha_r - 1)\exp[-D/D_C]\right) + \beta D^2\right)} \qquad (6.8)$$

## Genome-Dependent Radiation Sensitivity

Haas-Kogan et al. [27], using LQ and repair-saturation mathematical models, showed that p53 function influences the effect of fractionated radiotherapy on GBM tumours. They identified two distinct cellular responses to radiation, p53-independent apoptosis and p53-dependent G1-arrest, influencing radiobiological parameters that characterize the GBM radiation response. Some years later, a distinct genotype-dependent radiosensitivity group was identified in association with mutant ATM (ataxia telangiectasia mutated), wild-type TP53 (tumour protein 53) and mutant TP53 linked to intrinsic cellular radiosensitivity of GBM cell lines that grouped into four different radiosensitivity categories. This suggests the existence of multiple genotype-dependent mechanisms underlying the intrinsic cellular radiosensitivity [28, 29].

The coexistence of glioma-differentiated cancer cells (GDCC) and glioma-cancer stem cells (GCSCs) has been proposed to explain the intrinsic tumour heterogeneity to radiation response. The GCSCs have been reported to be less sensitive to radiation-induced damage through preferential activation of DNA damage checkpoint responses. Other authors [30, 31] have suggested that GCSCs can readily assume a quiescent state and later, following DNA repair, repopulate the tumour. DNA damage induced by radiotherapy treatment potently initiated activation of phosphorylation of the ATM, p53 and Chk2 checkpoint proteins. Phosphorylation of these checkpoint proteins resulted significantly higher in the GCSCs compared to GDCCs and could explain the reported intrinsic radiosensitivity difference [32, 33]. A model that simulates the coexistence of GCSC and GDCCs and their cell cycle phase in growth and radiation response has recently been proposed [34]. The authors integrated the LQ model, extended to take into account the effects of inter-fraction tumour repopulation and $\alpha$ and $\beta$ cell-specific radiosensitivity parameters, with the introduction of $\xi$ and $\lambda$ as radiation protection factors for quiescent cells and GCSCs, respectively. The simulations performed revealed that not only the higher intrinsic radioresistance of GCSCs but also the presence of a shift from asymmetric to symmetric division or a fast cycle of GCSCs after fractionated radiotherapy may contribute to the frequently observed accelerated repopulation after irradiation. The survival and increase of the GCSCs population during radiation therapy may be a leading cause of accelerated and more aggressive GBM recurrence after radiation therapy.

## Dual Compartment Tumour Survival, Mathematical Model

In an attempt to model subpopulation GCSCs, dual compartment tumour survival, a mathematical model has recently been proposed by Yu et al. [35]. The model assumes the radiation response as the sum of two subpopulations deriving from the coexistence of GCSCs and GDCCs, each with their distinctive LQ parameters. Thus, the dual compartment cell survival model is constructed as

$$S(D) = f \cdot e^{-\left(\alpha_1 D + \beta_1 D^2\right)} - (1-f) \cdot e^{-\left(\alpha_2 D + \beta_2 D^2\right)} \quad (6.9)$$

where f is the fraction of GCSCs, (1–f) is the fraction of GDCCs, while $\alpha_i$ and $\beta_i$ describe the radiobiological properties (intrinsic radiosensitivity and repair capacity) of each population. The increased radioresistance has been explained by the rapid regrowth of the GDCC compartment triggered by its depletion while a viable GCSC population is maintained.

Figure 6.2 illustrates the surviving fraction of two populations with $\alpha_1 = 0.12$/Gy (cell line#1), $\alpha_2 = 0.6$/Gy (cell line#2) and of a mixed population 50 % cell line#1 + 50 % cell line#2, with the same $\alpha_i/\beta_i$ ratio (i.e. 8 Gy).

The type of programmed cell death, as the response to treatment in glioma cells, has been widely debated in recent years, suggesting that cell autophagy is the main intracellular process involved and not apoptosis [36].

A dual compartment cell survival model has been proposed by Tini et al. [37] to explore the cell-autophagy role after in vitro irradiation of

**Fig. 6.2** The surviving fraction of two populations with $\alpha_1 = 0.12$/Gy (cell line#1), $\alpha_2 = 0.6$/Gy (cell line#2) and of a mixed population (50 % cell line#1 + 50 % cell line#2), assuming the same $\alpha_i/\beta_i$ ratio (i.e. 8 Gy)

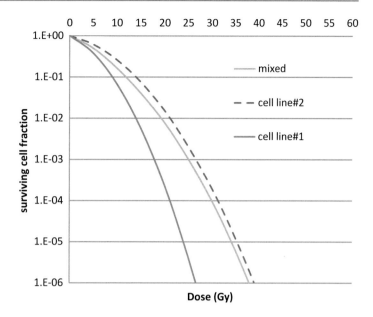

glioma cells (T98G, U373) integrating the low-dose hypersensitivity effect in its formulation. This model assumes radiation response in glioma cells derived by activation of cell autophagy involved in both the pro-survival mechanisms and direct programmed cell death (i.e. programmed autophagy-related cell death) [38]. This model that fits complex survival curves in T98G and U373 glioma cell lines in the presence of multi-modal response to radiation is formulated as

$$S(D) = A \cdot e^{-(\alpha_s D)} + (1-A) \cdot e^{-\left[(\alpha_r - \delta)D + \beta D^2\right]} \quad (6.10)$$

where the parameters represent

$A$ = effect of low-dose hypersensitivity
$\alpha_s$ = irreversible pro-death autophagy induced by DNA damage
$\alpha_r$ = not irreversible autophagy pro-death
$\delta$ = autophagy pro-survival
$\beta$ = repairable DNA damage

## TCP

Even in the simpler case of homogeneous irradiation the use of Poisson statistics to describe the probability that all clonogenic cells are killed has proven to be incorrect [39], this has led to the development of models based on cellular killing [24, 40–42]. All these models are based, more or less explicitly, on some assumptions [41]:

- Each tumour is made of a cluster of non-interactive clonogenic cells
- Radiosensitivity may vary between tumour (and patients)
- A tumour is controlled if all the clonogenic cells are inactivated
- Clonogenic cell inactivation is a mutually independent event

The combination of these assumptions allows the development of a statistical model based on the probability of inactivation of all clonogenic cells. The number of clonogenic tumour cells is critical in determining the TCP and some authors have based it on the initial tumour volume, as given by the following equation:

$$V = a \cdot N^b \quad (6.11)$$

where $a$ and $b$ are constant. Figure 6.3 illustrates the TCP against the dose when the number of

**Fig. 6.3** The TCP behaviour against the delivered dose when the number of clonogenic cells in the volume V increases from $10^6$ to $10^{10}$

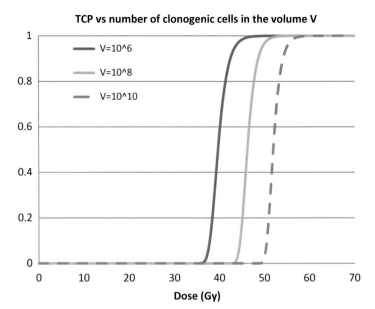

TCP vs number of clonogenic cells in the volume V

clonogenic cells in the volume V increases from $10^6$ to $10^{10}$.

$$TCP = \frac{1}{(2\pi)^{\frac{3}{2}}\sigma_{\ln k}\sigma_\alpha\sigma_\lambda}, \int\limits_{+\infty}^{-\infty} e^{-\exp(k'-\alpha'D-\beta D^2/N+\lambda'T)} e^{(k'-\ln(k))^2/(2\sigma_{\ln k}^2)} e^{(\alpha'-\alpha)^2/(2\sigma_\alpha^2)} e^{(\lambda'-\lambda)^2/(2\sigma_\lambda^2)} d\lambda' d\alpha' dk' \quad (6.12a)$$

where the parameters $\ln(k)$, $\alpha$ and $\lambda$ represent the clonogenic number, cellular sensitivity and repopulation rate, respectively [41].

$$TCP = \frac{1}{k}\sum_K^{i=1}\prod_M^{j=1} e^{-\rho_j v_i f_j \exp(-\alpha_i D_i - \beta_i D_i^2)} \quad (6.12b)$$

where in the original model [40] the quadratic term $\beta D_i^2$ was omitted for simplicity.

In (6.12b), $D_i$ is the dose received by a specific subunit and has to be considered fixed within the subunit, while $\rho_j$ is the variable clonogenic cell

These formulations are derived by statistical assumption as follows:

densities within the volume, each having a relative volume fraction $f_j$.

The third model uses a different $EQD_2$ formulation that considers the surviving fraction

$$S(d) = S(2Gy)^{\frac{d}{2Gy}\left(\frac{\alpha/\beta+d}{\alpha/\beta+2Gy}\right)} \quad (6.12c)$$

The TCP formulation includes radiosensitivity variability intra-patient (ind) and inter-patient (pop), assuming these variations can be described by the variability of S(2 Gy) [41].

$$TCP = \int G_{pop}\left(\overline{S(2Gy)}^{ind}, ,\overline{S(2Gy)}^{pop}, ,\sigma^{pop}\right)TCP_{ind} \, d\overline{S(2Gy)}^{ind} \quad (6.13)$$

where

$$TCP_{ind} = e^{-NC\sum_{NP}^{i=1}\left(v_i \overline{S(d_i)}\right)} \quad (6.14)$$

$$\overline{S(d_i)} = \int G_{ind}\left(S(2Gy)^{ind}, \overline{S(2Gy)}^{ind}, \sigma_{ind}\right)S(d_i) \, dS(2Gy)^{ind} \quad (6.15)$$

$$S(d_i) = S(2Gy)^{\sum_n^{k=1} \frac{d_k}{2Gy}\left(\frac{\alpha/\beta+d_k}{\alpha/\beta+2Gy}\right)} \quad (6.16)$$

where NP is the number of dose bins, NC is the number of clonogenic cells, n the number of

fractions and $\nu_i$ the volume corresponding to the i-th dose point. The probability density functions are expressed as follows [42]:

$$G_{pop}\left(\overline{S(2Gy)}^{ind},,\overline{S(2Gy)}^{pop},,\sigma^{pop}\right) = \frac{1}{\sqrt{2\pi}\sigma_{pop}}e^{-\left[\frac{\left(\overline{S(2Gy)}^{pop}-\overline{S(2Gy)}^{pop}\right)^2}{2\sigma_{pop}^2}\right]} \quad (6.17)$$

$$G_{ind}\left(S(2Gy)^{ind},\overline{S(2Gy)}^{ind},\sigma^{ind}\right) = \frac{1}{\sqrt{2\pi}\sigma_{ind}}e^{-\left[\frac{\left(S(2Gy)^{ind}-\overline{S(2Gy)}^{ind}\right)^2}{2\sigma_{ind}^2}\right]} \quad (6.18)$$

Models described above involve a wide number of parameters with statistical uncertainty. Notwithstanding this, the radiobiological models represent the only possible strategy to optimize treatment, compare rival plans or fractionation schemes or give an estimation of TCP at a given time after therapy.

Unfortunately, a radiobiological model able to overcome the poor GBM response to radiation is currently unavailable, due to the incomplete understanding of the underlying genetic and biomolecular alterations. Profiling studies based on gene or protein expression have revealed several altered, common, molecular pathways, resulting in the subclassification of distinct molecular subtypes (classical, mesenchymal, proneural, neural) that are different in terms of their prognosis and response to therapy [43]. This characterization is not currently in use in clinical practice. Furthermore, emerging evidence shows the existence of a stem like cell compartment in GBM, which demonstrates an increased resistance to ionizing radiation [16, 44, 45]. Due to the higher probability of killing radiosensitive cells with greater efficacy, all tumours during the course of treatment increase the mean radioresistance. GBM is characterized not only by an increase of the mean radioresistance, but also of the maximum.

There are other cellular models based on the possibility of a change in radioresistance during treatment [46] but their complexity is far beyond the aim of this chapter.

## Correlating Results of Cell-Culture SF with Clinical Empirical Data at Different Total Doses and Dose Per Fraction

The concept of *isoeffective doses* has been widely investigated in order to link the absorbed dose to the incidence of a specific biological effect attributable to irradiation. Survival curves have been obtained based on in vitro studies, providing some useful information on radiosensitivity of the investigated tumour and normal tissue cells. In particular, the $\alpha/\beta$ ratio has been derived to measure the sensitivity of the tumour or tissue to fractionation, i.e. to predict how the total dose for a given effect will change when the size of dose fraction is changed.

By using various treatment schedules for in vivo studies, the slope of the isoeffect curves has been determined, highlighting that they change according to the size of dose per fraction and depending on tissue type [47].

Also using in vivo data, the sensitivity to changes in fractionation schedule can be quantified by using the $\alpha/\beta$ ratio. A high $\alpha/\beta$ ratio (range, 7–20 Gy), as in acutely responding tissues and in tumours, indicates a more linear survival response of the target cells; a low $\alpha/\beta$ ratio (range, 0.5–6 Gy), as in late responding tissues, defines a significant curvature in the survival curve of the target cells. As a consequence, the effects of fractionation are relatively greater in the acutely responding than late responding tissues.

This suggests that acute responding tissues have flatter curves than late responding tissues, i.e. fractionation spares the late responding tissues. Of note $\alpha/\beta$ ratios could be different when calculated using (6.1) or (6.12b), as they are derived from different datasets with different weights to data, corresponding to low and high doses.

## Clinical Dose Response Models

### Poisson Hypothesis

In the clinical setting, TCP models derived from LQ based on the Poisson hypothesis have been used as a tool to estimate a radiobiological set of parameters from the available clinical outcome [47, 48].

The following equation predicts the progression-free survival based on the Poisson hypothesis

$$PFS = e^{-N \cdot e^{-D(\alpha+\beta d)+\frac{\ln 2}{T_d}(T-T_k)}} \tag{6.19}$$

A graphical method to estimate the radiobiological parameters in (6.19) by using a multiple step procedure has been proposed [48] and shown here in Fig. 6.4.

To combine the clinical outcomes from different published studies, different irradiation schedules need to be used. When comparing two fractionation regimens (e.g. a and b) (6.19) becomes:

$$\frac{\ln\left(PFS_a\right)}{\ln\left(PFS_b\right)} = e^{-N \cdot e^{\alpha(D_b-D_a)+\beta(D_b d_b-D_a D_a)+\frac{\ln 2}{T_d}(T-T_k)}} \tag{6.20}$$

In this formula, the dependence by cell number $N$ and $T_k$ disappeared. Moreover, (6.20) takes into account the different radiotherapy schedules and the related clinical outcome.

Therefore, when a sufficient number of different schedules and a large number of patients are enrolled (to reduce the stochastic fluctuations), an estimation of the cellular parameters ($\alpha$, $\beta$ and $T_d$) can be made by the following equation:

$$\frac{\alpha}{\beta} = \frac{d_b D_b - d_a D_a}{\frac{1}{\alpha}\left[C + \frac{\ln 2}{T_d}(T_b - T_a)\right] - (D_b - D_a)} \tag{6.21}$$

where

$$C = \ln\left(\frac{\ln\left(PFS_a\right)}{\ln\left(PFS_b\right)}\right) \tag{6.22}$$

and C is named "clinical efficacy factor".

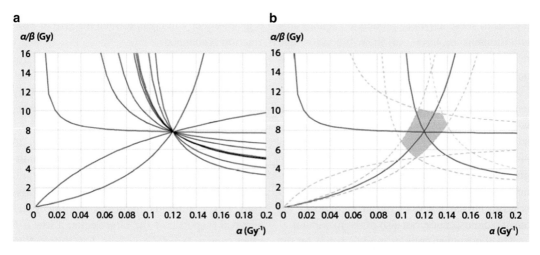

**Fig. 6.4** The relationship between $\alpha$ and $\alpha/\beta$ for glioblastoma multiforme. The black curves have been obtained from (6.19) using couples of clinical data and by varying $T_d$ value up to the coincidence for all curves. The intersec-tions of the curves represent the best estimate of $\alpha$, $\alpha/\beta$ and $T_d$ (**a**). The grey curves represent the 95 % confidence interval (only three curves shown) and the shaded area indicates the overall range of uncertainties (**b**)

Equation (6.21) establishes an independent relationship between $\alpha$ and $\alpha/\beta$ from which it is possible to include and compare studies with different clinical outcomes when $C \neq 0$.

The curves of different schedules are plotted in the $\alpha$ versus $\alpha/\beta$ graph. $T_d$ is varied until the coincidence of all curves is obtained, thus the intersection point provides an estimate of $\alpha$, $\alpha/\beta$ and $T_d$. This expedient allows the values of $N$ and $T_k$ and their uncertainties in subsequent steps to be calculated.

Moreover, (6.21) is also substantially independent from the impact of chemotherapy (i.e. temozolomide, TMZ, or bischloroethylnitrosourea, BCNU), which is unknown or indistinguishable when this approach is used, chemotherapy being generally adopted in all the investigated schedules or presenting limited differences in terms of radiosensitivity when different drugs are adopted.

Once the estimate of $\alpha$, $\beta$ and $T_d$ is made, an estimation of $D_{prolif}$, in fraction of 2 Gy, is obtained by the following equation:

$$D_{prolif} = \frac{\ln 2}{T_d \cdot (\alpha + 2\beta)} \quad (6.23)$$

Subsequently, an estimation of $T_k$ is obtained using the hypothesis of stem cells activation by the following equation [49]:

$$T_k = \frac{7\ln(N_0 / N_A)}{5d(\alpha + \beta d)} \quad (6.24)$$

Assuming that the process of stem cell activation for accelerated proliferation could begin when the tumour population has decreased to the order

**Table 6.1** Model parameters entracte from Pedicini et al. [47]

| Parameter | Best estimate | $CI_{95\%}$ |
|---|---|---|
| $\alpha(Gy^{-1})$ | 0.12 | 0.10–0.14 |
| $\beta$ ($Gy^{-2}$) | 0.015 | 0.013–0.020 |
| $\alpha/\beta$ (Gy) | 8 | 5.0–10.8 |
| $T_d$ (days) | 15.4 | 13.2–19.5 |
| $D_{prolif}$ (Gy) | 0.3 | 0.22–0.39 |
| $T_k$ (days) | 37 | 29–46 |
| $N$ (clonogens) | $9.1 \times 10^3$ | $4.0 \times 10^3$–$2.1 \times 10^4$ |

of a few thousand cells (e.g. $\ln(N_0/N_A)3000$), thus

$$T_k = \frac{11}{d(\alpha + \beta d)} \quad [49].$$

Finally, the estimation of $N$ is performed by using (6.19), in which $\alpha$, $\alpha/\beta$, $T_d$ and $T_k$ are fixed at the best values. All the above steps produce the best fit parameters useful to compare predicted TCP curves and experimental data.

The best estimate and the $CI_{95\%}$ for $\alpha$, $\alpha/\beta$, $T_d$, $N$, $T_k$ and $D_{prolif}$ are shown in Table 6.1.

## Multivariate Logistic Regression

In order to consider the combined effects (e.g. of drug delivery and radiotherapy approach, as well as patient age, and other variables), a multivariate logistic regression can be adopted to predict the TCP following preoperative CRT. The TCP can be expressed as:

$$P(z) = \frac{e^z}{1 + e^z} \quad (6.25)$$

where

$$z = a_0 + a_1 D + a_2 D \cdot d + a_3 OTT + a_4 \cdot age + a_5 \cdot 5FUdose + a_6 \cdot cisplatin dose + a_7 \cdot mitomycin C dose \quad (6.26)$$

In this approach, the LQ dose response model may incorporate not only the total radiotherapy dose and dose per fraction to estimate the $\alpha/\beta$ ratio [50], but also the other clinical and patient based covariates. Although they have no theoretical biological rationale, they nonetheless provide a useful numerical estimate of the true relationship for the range of values experienced in common practice. This model that in principle is applicable to GBM has so far only been applied to oesophageal cancer.

## Time-Dependent TCP

The survival of GBM patients, usually about 50 % at 1 year and decreasing over time, can be modelled [9] as follows including a time factor:

$$S'^{(D_j,\tau)} = e^{-N \cdot e^{-\left[aD + \beta GD^2 - \gamma(T - T_k)\right] \cdot e^{-a\tau}}} \quad (6.27)$$

where $\tau$ is the time after the treatment completion for the given dose $Dj$.

Here, the authors assumed that the survival rate depends exponentially on relapse time and the parameter a has been estimated using a fitting procedure for survival rate at 0.5, 1.0 and 1.5 years, using clinical data reported by Walker et al. [9] and by Salazar et al. [51, 52].

Finally, in the paper of Qi et colleagues, the $\alpha$ and $\alpha/\beta$ parameters have been provided for malignant gliomas with grade 3 or 4 [53] .

## Model Parameters

The selection of proper LQ parameters has been challenging particularly in the clinical setting for GBM. The repair half time for sublethal damage repair, T, is assumed to be 0.5 h [54].

An interpretation of the radiobiological parameters may help clinicians to identify an optimal fractionation schedule. In particular, an $\alpha/\beta$ of 8 Gy indicates high fractionation sensitivity while an $\alpha$ of 0.12 Gy$^{-1}$ supports a high intrinsic radiosensitivity of this tumour. Consequently, these parameters correspond to a low $\beta$ value (0.015 Gy$^{-2}$), which represents a high capability of GBM cells to repair the radiation damage. Moreover, based on the fit of clinical data, the $T_d$ shows a moderate value (15.4 days), together with a very long $T_k$ (37 days). This implies that the tumour radiation response with the OTT is substantially independent, thereby endorsing hypofractionation (doses greater than 2 Gy/fraction) or hyper-fractionation (doses less than 2 Gy/fraction with multiple daily sessions) schedules. This is supported by the outcome of hypofractionated studies that adopt a treatment of 25 Gy in which the reduction of OTT did not improve overall survival or progression-free survival, PFS (with a 1 PFS of 29.42 %) [55].

From another point of view, a higher value of $\gamma$ supports a strong dependence on OTT of the results can be explained by the selection of radioresistant stem cells, which are recruited during irradiation and tend to repopulate quickly [49, 56–59].

The best fit curve ($N = 9.1 \times 10^3$) and its confidence interval ($6.0 \times 10^3 - 1.4 \times 10^4$) indicate that a limited number of aggressive cells are able to repopulate tumour. Moreover, a long $T_k$ together with a moderate repopulation indicates substantial independence of the therapeutic results from the duration of the OTT. However, this mechanism appears to be negligible when compared to the mechanism of repair, which should be more pronounced in this cell type. This characteristic can be taken into account in favour of the time required by OAR in order to fully repair the radiation damage.

Model parameters indicate a strong dependence on total dose, thus an improvement of clinical results might be obtained with an increase in the total dose rather than with a reduction of the OTT. Based on the estimated radiobiological parameters, an increase of the total dose up to a BED of approximately 92 Gy (total dose, 74.8 Gy; dose per fraction, 2.2 Gy; 34 fractions) should lead to a TCP greater than 0.85. This result appears to be surprisingly higher than that obtained with standard fractionation (60 Gy × 30 fractions with a BED of approximately 74 Gy), which is approximately 0.3. This optimistic prediction by the model still requires mandatory confirmation. The fitted curve has $\gamma 50 = 3.31$, which is very close to the mean $\gamma 50$ of the clinically relevant range ($\gamma 50 = 3.20$) described in the literature [25, 60].

## Parallelism Between Classical and Biomolecular Modelling in Glioblastoma

Rockne and other authors included the effects of radiation therapy using the LQ radiobiological model in a tri-dimensional proliferation and infiltration (PI) model [61–65]. The PI model was developed in the early 1990s by Tracqui et al. [66] to describe the diffuse PI of glioma cells in the human brain. In this model, the rate of change of tumour cell density over time is equal to the net migration plus the net proliferation of tumour cells. The model uses partial differential equations with two parameters: net rate of migration ($D$, mm$^2$/year) and proliferation ($\rho$, year$-1$), which can be calculated using routine patient-specific clinical images. This model mimics a virtual *in silico* tumour response to treatment with the same growth kinetics of an individual patient, thus predicting the in vivo treatment response.

In recent years, these mathematical models have been integrated with bio-simulation methods to improve fitting and predictive ability in vivo in terms of treatment-related response. Starting from biomolecular evidence, some authors have developed multiscale models of GBM progression that cover processes from the cellular to the molecular scale. Antipas et al. [67] introduced the oxygen enhancement ratio (OER) in models, and Kim Y. et al. [68] proposed a multiscale mathematical model where cell migration and proliferation are controlled through an intracellular control system via microRNA-451 (miR-451)-AMPK complex in response to glucose availability and physical constraints in the microenvironment. Schuetzet al. [69] also proposed a model integrating the molecular interaction network (miR-451, LKB1 and AMPK) to cellular actions (e.g. chemotactic movement) to explain the regulation of GBM cell migration and proliferation. Swanson et al. [70] tried to integrate tumour-microenvironment interactions of normoxic glioma cells, hypoxic glioma cells, vascular endothelial cells, diffusible angiogenic factors and necrosis formation into a biologically based mathematical PI model for glioma. Specifically for radiotherapy treatment, Holdsworth et al. [71] included the patient-specific description of tumour growth and radiation response in the PI-RT model [64] to generate biologically guided treatment plans. Using an adaptive multi-objective evolutionary algorithm (MOEA), intensity modulated RT (IMRT) plans were optimized using clinical objectives to maximize normal tissue sparing and taking into account the reduction of tumour burden at various time points

in order to increase the TCP. Integrative biomolecular mathematical models of kinetics of tumour growth and response to radiotherapy via more complex "biomolecular-integrated" LQ models [72, 73] considering the dynamic instability of radioresistance of GBM (cellular subpopulations, kinetics growth and biomolecular alterations) could support better treatment management of the GBM patients as well as the design of more effective treatment strategies. These speculative investigations of alternative treatment strategies require further investigation before their introduction to clinical practice.

## Potential Confounding Factors

The contributions of several potentially confounding factors have not been fully taken into consideration in the currently proposed methods. These factors include: (1) data collection from institutes with different patient selection criteria and different treatment modalities; (2) the possible coexistence of different cell types within the target of enrolled patients, that may explain the variability of parameters and the need for more advanced models; (3) the different expression levels of molecular factors among patients, such as MGMT methylation and (4) other factors, such as hypoxia and reoxygenation that may influence the clinical outcome.

The role of molecular predictors is still under debate and might help in the design of new treatment strategies particularly in older patients with Recursive Partitioning Analysis $\geq 3$. Clinical data have been combined with other predictive factors to improve the recently proposed nomograms [74] with molecular and image-based classifiers.

Finally, the accelerated failure time model has been applied using data from 721 patients with glioblastoma to model factors affecting individualized survival after surgical resection [75]. An increased 2-years survival was associated with age, Karnofsky Performance status, the extension of resection of enhancing tumour on T1-postgadolinium magnetic resonance imaging and adjuvant therapy with external radiotherapy and/or temozolomide.

## Conclusion

In conclusion, mathematical models indicate that
moderately hypofractionated, high total dose
treatment schedules and use of TMZ deserve
consideration. Moreover, state-of-the-art modern
multimodality imaging techniques permit a better
tumour identification and contouring, as well as
modern innovative linear accelerator and on-board
imaging allow the delivery of high doses to the
tumours, sparing the surrounding healthy brain.

## References

1. AAPM TG 43. Quality assessment and improvement
of dose response models: some effects of study weak-
nesses on study findings. "C'est Magnifique?" AAPM
report 43, 1993
2. Joiner MC, Van der Kogel AJ, Steel GG. Introduction:
the significance of radiobiology and radiotherapy for
cancer treatment. In: Joiner MC, Van der Kogeleds A,
editors. Basic clinical radiobiology. 4th ed. London:
Hodder Arnold; 2009.
3. Los M, Rashedi I, Panigrahi S, Klonisch T, Schulze-
Osthoff K. Tumor growth and cell proliferation. In:
Molls M, Vaupel P, Nieder C, Anschereds MS, editors.
The impact of tumor biology on cancer treatment and
multidisciplinary strategies. Berlin: Springer; 2009.
4. Willers H, Beck-Bornholdt HP. Origins of radiotherapy and radiobiology: separation of the influence of
dose per fraction and overall treatment time on normal tissue damage by Reisner and Miescher in the
1930s. Radiother Oncol. 1996;38:171–3.
5. Bentzen SM. Quantitative clinical radiobiology. Acta
Oncol. 1993;32(3):259–75.
6. Strandquist M. A study of the cumulative effects of
fractionated X-ray treatment based on the experience
gained at radiumhemmet with the treatment of 280
cases of carcinoma of the skin and lip. Acta Radiol.
1944;55(Suppl):300–4.
7. Munro TR, Gilbert CW. The relation between tumour
lethal doses and the radiosensitivity of tumour cells.
Br J Radiol. 1961;34:246–51.
8. Ellis F. Dose, time and fractionation a clinical hypothesis. Clin Radiol. 1969;20(1):1–7.
9. Walker MD, Strikes TA, Sheline GE. An analysis of
dose-effect relationship in the radiotherapy of malignant glioma. Int J Radiat Oncol Biol Phys. 1979;5:
1725–31.
10. Mikhael MA. Radiation necrosis of the brain: correlation between computed tomography, pathology, and
dose distribution. J Comput Assist Tomogr. 1978;2(1):
71–80.
11. Fowler JF. The linear quadratic formula and progress
in fractionated radiotherapy. Br J Radiol. 1989;62:
679–94.
12. Fowler JF. Sensitivity analysis of parameters in linear-
quadratic radiobiologic modeling. Int J Radiat Oncol
Biol Phys. 2009;73(5):1532–7.
13. Kellerer AM. Studies of the dose-effect relation.
Experientia. 1989;45:13–21.
14. Joiner MC, Bentzen SM. Fractionation: the linear
quadratic approach. In: Joiner MC, Van der Kogeleds
A, editors. Basic clinical radiobiology. 4th ed.
London: Hodder Arnold; 2009.
15. Fowler JF. 21 years of biologically effective dose. Br
J Radiol. 2010;83:554–68.
16. Debus J, Abdollahi A. For the next trick: new discoveries in radiobiology applied to glioblastoma. Current
concepts and future perspective in radiotherapy of
glioblastoma. ASCO education book; 2014. e95–9.
17. Shahine BH, Ng CE, Raaphorst GP. Modelling of
continuous low dose rate and accelerated fractionated high dose rate irradiation treatments in a human
glioma cell line. Int J Radiat Biol. 1996;70(5):
555–61.
18. Williams JA, Williams JR, Yuan X, Dillehay
LE. Protracted exposure radiosensitization of experimental human malignant glioma. Radiat Oncol
Investig. 1998;6(6):255–63.
19. Cordes N, Plasswilm L, Sauer R. Interaction of paclitaxel (Taxol) and irradiation. In-vitro differences
between tumor and fibroblastic cells. Strahlenther
Onkol. 1999;175(4):175–81.
20. Nusser NN, Bartkowiak D, Röttinger EM. The influence of bromodeoxyuridine on the induction and
repair of DNA double-strand breaks in glioblastoma
cells. Strahlenther Onkol. 2002;178(9):504–9.
21. Garcia LM, Leblanc J, Wilkins D, Raaphorst
GP. Fitting the linear-quadratic model to detailed data
sets for different dose ranges. Phys Med Biol.
2006;51(11):2813–23.
22. Withers HR, Thames Jr HD, Peters LJ. A new isoeffect curve for change in dose per fraction. Radiother
Oncol. 1983;1:187–91.
23. Thames HD, Bentzen SM, Turesson I, Overgaard M,
van den Bogaert W. Time-dose factors in radiotherapy: a review of the human data. Radiother Oncol.
1990;19:219–35.
24. Roberts SA, Hendry JH. A realistic closed-form
radiobiological model of clinical tumor-control data
incorporating intertumor heterogeneity. Int J Radiat
Oncol Biol Phys. 1998;41(3):689–99.
25. Joiner MC, Marples B, Lambin P, Short SC, Turesson
I. Low-dose hypersensitivity: current status and possible mechanisms. Int J Radiat Oncol Biol Phys.
2001;49(2):379–89.
26. Joiner MC. Quantifying cell killing and cell survival.
In: Joiner MC, Van der Kogeleds A, editors. Basic
clinical radiobiology. 4th ed. London: HodderArnold;
2009.
27. Haas-Kogan DA, Yount G, Haas M, Levi D, Kogan
SS, Hu L, Vidair C, Deen DF, Dewey WC, Israel MA.
p53-dependent G1 arrest and p53-independent apoptosis influence the radiobiologic response of glioblastoma. Int J Radiat Oncol Biol Phys. 1996;36(1):
95–103.

28. Williams JR, Zhang Y, Russell J, Koch C, Little JB. Human tumor cells segregate into radiosensitivity groups that associate with ATM and TP53 status. Acta Oncol. 2007;46(5):628–38.

29. Williams JR, Zhang Y, Zhou H, Gridley DS, Koch CJ, Russell J, Slater JS, Little JB. A quantitative overview of radiosensitivity of human tumor cells across histological type and TP53 status. Int J Radiat Biol. 2008;84(4):253–64.

30. Mellor HR, Ferguson DJ, Callaghan R. A model of quiescent tumour microregions for evaluating multicellular resistance to chemotherapeutic drugs. Br J Cancer. 2005;93:302–9.

31. Scopelliti A, Cammareri P, Catalano V, Saladino V, Todaro M, Stassi G. Therapeutic implications of cancer initiating cells. Expert Opin Biol Ther. 2009;9:1005–16.

32. Bao S, Wu Q, McLendon RE, Hao Y, Shi Q, Hjelmeland AB, Dewhirst MW, Bigner DD, Rich JN. Glioma stem cells promote radioresistance by preferential activation of the DNA damage response. Nature. 2006;444:756–60.

33. Zhou W, Sun M, Li GH, Wu YZ, Wang Y, Jin F, Zhang YY, Yang L, Wang DL. Activation of the phosphorylation of ATM contributes to radioresistance of glioma stem cells. Oncol Rep. 2013;30(4):1793–801.

34. Gao X, McDonald JT, Hlatky L, Enderling H. Acute and fractionated irradiation differentially modulate glioma stem cell division kinetics. Cancer Res. 2013;73(5):1481–90.

35. Yu V, Nguyen D, Kupelian P, Kaprealian T, Selch M, Low D, Pajonk F, Sheng K. SU-C-BRE-03: dual compartment mathematical modeling of glioblastoma multiforme (GBM). Med Phys. 2014;41:94.

36. Palumbo S, Pirtoli L, Tini P, Cevenini G, Calderaro F, Toscano M, Miracco C, Comincini S. Different involvement of autophagy in human malignant glioma cell lines undergoing irradiation and temozolomide combined treatments. J Cell Biochem. 2012;113(7):2308–18.

37. Tini P, Palumbo S, Cevenini G., Miracco C., Comincini S., Pirtoli L. Autophagy as potential therapeutical target in glioblastoma. Acts of XXII Italian Congress AIRO. Rome November 17–20th 2012.

38. Palumbo S, Comincini S. Autophagy and ionizing radiation in tumors: the "survive or not survive" dilemma. J Cell Physiol. 2013;228(1):1–8.

39. Tucker SL, Thames HD, Taylor JMG. How well is the probability of tumor cure after fractionated irradiation described by Poisson statistics? Radiat Res. 1990;124:273–82.

40. Webb S, Nahum AE. A model for calculating tumour control probability in radiotherapy including the effects of inhomogeneous distribution of dose and clonogenic cell density. Phys Med Biol. 1993;38:653–66.

41. Niemierko A, Goitein M. Implementation of a model for estimating tumour control probability for an inhomogeneously irradiated tumor. Radiother Oncol. 1993;29:140–7.

42. Okunieff P, Morgan D, Niemierko A, et al. Radiation dose-response of human tumor. Int J Radiat Oncol Biol Phys. 1995;32:1227–37.

43. Verhaak RG, Hoadley KA, Purdom E, Wang V, Qi Y, Wilkerson MD, Miller CR, Ding L, Golub T, Mesirov JP, Alexe G, Lawrence M, O'Kelly M, Tamayo P, Weir BA, Gabriel S, Winckler W, Gupta S, Jakkula L, Feiler HS, Hodgson JG, James CD, Sarkaria JN, Brennan C, Kahn A, Spellman PT, Wilson RK, Speed TP, Gray JW, Meyerson M, Getz G, Perou CM, Hayes DN, Network CGAR. An integrated genomic analysis identifies clinically relevant subtypes of glioblastoma characterized by abnormalities in PDGFRA, IDH1, EGFR and NF1. Cancer Cell. 2010;17(1):98–110.

44. Vlashi E, McBride WH, Pajonk F. Radiation responses of cancer stem cells. J Cell Biochem. 2009;108(2):339–42.

45. Manninoa M, Chalmers AJ. Radioresistance of glioma stem cells: intrinsic characteristic or property of the 'microenvironment-stem cell unit'? Mol Oncol. 2011;5:374–86.

46. Wein LM, Cohen JE, Wu JT. Dynamic optimization of a linear-quadratic model with incomplete repair and volume-dependent sensitivity and repopulation. Int J Radiat Oncol Biol Phys. 2000;47(4):1073–83.

47. Thames Jr HD, Withers HR, Peters LJ, Fletcher GH. Changes in early and late radiation responses with altered dose fractionation: implications for dose-survival relationships. Int J Radiat Oncol Biol Phys. 1982;8(2):219–26.

48. Pedicini P, Fiorentino A, Simeon V, Tini P, Chiumento C, Pirtoli L, Salvatore M, Storto G. Clinical radiobiology of glioblastoma multiforme: estimation of tumor control probability from various radiotherapy fractionation schemes. Strahlenther Onkol. 2014;190(10):925–32. doi:10.1007/s00066-014-0638-9. Epub 2014 Apr 4.

49. Pedicini P. In regard to Pedicini et al. Int J Radiat Oncol Biol Phys. 2013;87(5):858.

50. Bentzen SM. Dose-response relationship in radiotherapy. In: Steel GG, editor. Basic clinical radiobiology. 2nd ed. London: Arnold; 1997. p. 78–86.

51. Salazar OM, Rubin P, Feldstein ML, et al. High dose radiation therapy in the treatment of malignant gliomas: final report. Int J Radiat Oncol Biol Phys. 1979;5:1733–40.

52. Salazar OM, Rubin P, McDonald JV, et al. High dose radiation therapy in the treatment of glioblastoma multiforme: a preliminary report. Int J Radiat Oncol Biol Phys. 1976;1:717–27.

53. Qi XS, Schultz CJ, Li XA. An estimation of radiobiologic parameters from clinical outcomes for radiation treatment planning of brain tumor. Int J Radiat Oncol Biol Phys. 2006;64(5):1570–80.

54. Brenner DJ, Hall EJ. Conditions for the equivalence of continuous to pulsed low dose rate brachytherapy. Int J Radiat Oncol Biol Phys. 1991;20:181–90.

55. Ciammella P, Galeandro M, D'Abbiero N, Podgornii A, Pisanello A, Botti A, Cagni E, Iori M, Iotti C. Hypo-fractionated IMRT for patients with newly

diagnosed glioblastoma multiforme: a 6 year single institutional experience. Clin Neurol Neurosurg. 2013;115(9):1609–14.

56. Pedicini P, Nappi A, Strigari L, Jereczek-Fossa BA, Alterio D, Cremonesi M, Botta F, Vischioni B, Caivano R, Fiorentino A, Improta G, Storto G, Benassi M, Orecchia R, Salvatore M. Correlation between EGFR expression and accelerated proliferation during radiotherapy of head and neck squamous cell carcinoma. Radiat Oncol. 2012;7:143.

57. Pedicini P, Caivano R, Strigari L, Benassi M, Fiorentino A, Fusco V. In regard to Miralbell et al. Re: dose-fractionation sensitivity of prostate cancer deduced from radiotherapy outcomes of 5969 patients in seven international institutional datasets: alpha/beta = 1.4 (0.9–2.2) Gy. Int J Radiat Oncol Biol Phys. 2013;85(1):10–1.

58. Pedicini P, Fiorentino A, Improta G, Nappi A, Salvatore M, Storto G. Estimate of the accelerated proliferation by protein tyrosine phosphatase (PTEN) over expression in postoperative radiotherapy of head and neck squamous cell carcinoma. Clin Transl Oncol. 2013;15(11):919–24.

59. Pedicini P, Strigari L, Benassi M. Estimation of a self-consistent set of radiobiological parameters from hypofractionated versus standard radiation therapy of prostate cancer. Int J Radiat Oncol Biol Phys. 2013;85(5):e231–7.

60. Daşu A, Toma-Daşu I, Fowler JF. Should single distributed parameters be used to explain the steepness of tumour control probability curves? Phys Med Biol. 2003;48:387–97.

61. Swanson KR, Rostomily RC, Alvord EC. A mathematical modelling tool for predicting survival of individual patients following resection of glioblastoma: a proof of principle. Br J Cancer. 2008;98: 113–9.

62. Rockne R, Alvord EC, Rockhill JK, Swanson KR. A mathematical model for brain tumor response to radiation therapy. J Math Biol. 2009;58:561–78.

63. Wang CH, Rockhill JK, Mrugala M, Peacock DL, Lai A, Jusenius K, et al. Prognostic significance of growth kinetics in newly diagnosed glioblastomas revealed by combining serial imaging with a novel biomathematical model. Cancer Res. 2009;69:9133–40.

64. Rockne R, Rockhill JK, Mrugala M, Spence AM, Kalet I, Hendrickson K, Lai A, Cloughesy T, Alvord Jr EC, Swanson KR. Predicting the efficacy of radiotherapy in individual glioblastoma patients in vivo: a mathematical modeling approach. Phys Med Biol. 2010;55(12):3271–85.

65. Roniotis A, Marias K, Sakkalis V, Manikis GC, Zervakis M. Simulating radiotherapy effect in high-grade glioma by using diffusive modeling and brain atlases. J Biomed Biotechnol. 2012;2012:715812.

66. Tracqui P, Cruywagen GC, Woodward DE, Bartoo GT, Murray JD, Alvord Jr EC. A mathematical model of glioma growth: the effect of chemotherapy on spatio-temporal growth. Cell Prolif. 1995;28(1): 17–31.

67. Antipas VP, Stamatakos GS, Uzunoglu NK, Dionysiou DD, Dale RG. A spatio-temporal simulation model of the response of solid tumours to radiotherapy in vivo: parametric validation concerning oxygen enhancement ratio and cell cycle duration. Phys Med Biol. 2004;49(8):1485–504.

68. Kim Y. Regulation of cell proliferation and migration in glioblastoma: new therapeutic approach. Front Oncol. 2013;3:53.

69. Schuetz TA, Becker S, Mang A, Toma A, Buzug TM. A computational multiscale model of glioblastoma growth: regulation of cell migration and proliferation via microRNA-451, LKB1 and AMPK. Conf Proc IEEE Eng Med Biol Soc. 2012;2012:6620–3.

70. Swanson KR, Rockne RC, Claridge J, Chaplain MA, Alvord Jr EC, Anderson AR. Quantifying the role of angiogenesis in malignant progression of gliomas: in silico modeling integrates imaging and histology. Cancer Res. 2011;71(24):7366–75.

71. Holdsworth CH, Corwin D, Stewart RD, Rockne R, Trister AD, Swanson KR, Phillips M. Adaptive IMRT using a multiobjective evolutionary algorithm integrated with a diffusion-invasion model of glioblastoma. Phys Med Biol. 2012;57(24):8271–83. doi:10.1088/0031-9155/57/24/8271. Epub 2012 Nov 29.

72. Leder K, Pitter K, Laplant Q, Hambardzumyan D, Ross BD, Chan TA, Holland EC, Michor F. Mathematical modeling of PDGF-driven glioblastoma reveals optimized radiation dosing schedules. Cell. 2014;156(3):603–16.

73. Jamali Nazari A, Sardari D, Vali AR, Maghooli K. Computer implementation of a new therapeutic model for GBM tumor. Comput Math Methods Med. 2014;2014:481935. Epub 2014 Aug 5.

74. Gorlia T, van den Bent MJ, Hegi ME, Mirimanoff RO, Weller M, Cairncross JG, Eisenhauer E, Belanger K, Brandes AA, Allgeier A, Lacombe D, Stupp R. Nomograms for predicting survival of patients with newly diagnosed glioblastoma: prognostic factor analysis of EORTC and NCIC trial 26981-22981/CE.3. Lancet Oncol. 2008;9(1):29–38. Epub 2007 Dec 21.

75. Marko NF, Weil RJ, Schroeder JL, Lang FF, Suki D, Sawaya RE. Extent of resection of glioblastoma revisited: personalized survival modeling facilitates more accurate survival prediction and supports a maximum-safe-resection approach to surgery. J Clin Oncol. 2014;32(8):774–82. doi:10.1200/JCO.2013.51.8886. Epub 2014 Feb 10.

# Clinical, Pathological, and Molecular Prognostic Parameters in Glioblastoma Patients Undergoing Chemo- and Radiotherapy

Paolo Tini, Clelia Miracco, Marzia Toscano, Silvia Palumbo, Sergio Comincini, Giovanni Luca Gravina, and Luigi Pirtoli

## Introduction: Prognostic Factors and Clinical Management of Glioblastoma

Glioblastoma (GB) accounts for about 55 % of primary brain tumors, with an incidence of five new cases/100,000 people/year. If untreated, median survival of GB is up to 3 months after diagnosis. The presently available literature uniformly reports the above data, and that multimodal treatment (surgery, radiotherapy—RT, chemotherapy—CHT) significantly improves median overall survival (OS), with about 40 %, 15 %, and 7–8 % outcomes, respectively at 1-, 2-, and 3-years [1–7]. Peak incidence of mortality occurs at the beginning of the second year after diagnosis, thereafter the risk of death halves at 2.5 years. Patients surviving more than 2 years after diagnosis, in fact, have a more favorable probability to survive afterwards, if compared to newly diagnosed cases. However, long-term survival remains poor with a 5-year OS rate barely reaching 5 %. The involvement of a multidisciplinary team in diagnosis, staging, and treatment of GB is mandatory for a correct management of GB. Postoperative RT is the mainstay of postsurgical management: a standard fractionated dose

P. Tini, M.D. (✉)
Tuscany Tumor Institute, Florence, Italy

Unit of Radiation Oncology, University Hospital of Siena (Azienda Ospedaliera-Universitaria Senese), Viale Bracci 11, Siena 53100, Italy
e-mail: paolo-tini@libero.it

C. Miracco
Tuscany Tumor Institute, Florence, Italy

Unit of Pathological Anatomy, Department of Medicine, Surgery and Neurosciences, University of Siena, Siena, Italy

M. Toscano • L. Pirtoli
Tuscany Tumor Institute, Florence, Italy

Unit of Radiation Oncology, Department of Medicine, Surgery and Neurosciences, University of Siena, Siena, Italy

S. Palumbo
Unit of Radiation Oncology, Department of Medicine, Surgery and Neurosciences, University of Siena, Siena, Italy

S. Comincini
Department of Technology and Biotechnology, University of Pavia, Italy

G.L. Gravina
Department of Radiological Sciences-Oncology and Pathological Anatomy, State University of Rome ("La Sapienza"), Rome, Italy

© Springer International Publishing Switzerland 2016
L. Pirtoli et al. (eds.), *Radiobiology of Glioblastoma*, Current Clinical Pathology,
DOI 10.1007/978-3-319-28305-0_7

of 60 Gy is recommended [8], even if altered fractionation schedules are also used, mainly consisting of short-course, hypofractionated RT in older patients. CHT has also acquired a key role in the management of this disease, and the alkylating agent Temozolomide (TMZ), delivered concurrently and sequentially with RT, is presently another standard of treatment [9]. The uncertainty in etiology of GB and the eventually fatal course, have driven research for many years towards an analytic approach of factors conditioning life expectancy. These efforts attempted to individuate both: parameters for a balanced treatment approach in terms of benefit/risk ratio; and characteristics of the natural history of this disease, possibly suitable for new and more effective therapeutic strategies. This contribution may give an overlook of prognostic parameters of GB of the present knowledge of these factors from a clinical point of view.

## Prognostic Parameters

Since the seventies of the past century, different prognostic factors were significantly associated with prognosis of GB, and generally classified as:

1. Patient-related
2. Treatment-related
3. Tumor-related

## Patient-Related Prognostic Parameters

Age at diagnosis, performance, and neurological status have a strong prognostic impact, according to large case-series published over more than 20 years [3, 4, 7, 10–23].

### Age

The Recursive Partitioning Analysis (RPA) by the Radiation Therapy Oncology Group (RTOG), combining the above factors with other patient- and treatment-related parameters for a comprehensive score system [10], indicates age as the best predictor of survival in high-grade gliomas:

patients aged 50 or older showed a shorter survival, if compared to younger ones. Old age may be associated with poor prognosis for several reasons. Less aggressive treatments for avoiding toxicity, due to presumably poor physiologic reserves, and comorbidities, may partly account for this evidence. However, phenotypically aggressive GBs occur in old patients, with characteristic molecular profiles [24]. GB, in fact, has two distinct modalities of development. The first one (representing the vast majority) is characteristic of the so-called primary GB, that arises de novo preferentially in old people; while in the second case, an evolution occurs from lower-grade gliomas, which is more frequently observed in younger patients (secondary GB). Oghaki and Kleihues [25, 26] correlated outcome with different biologic behaviors, and younger age of the affected subjects. Primary and secondary GBs, in fact, derive from precursor astrocytic cells through genetic pathways quite different from each other, including gene deletions, mutations, or amplifications [27], as addressed in a following section of this chapter. A SEER (the Surveillance, Epidemiology, and End Results program of the National Cancer Institute, USA) analysis of 34,664 patients affected by GB [28] confirmed the strong prognostic impact of age on survival. In that report, age behaves as a continuous variable in predicting survival, with the most significant decrease found in the group over 50 years, every additional year of age being associated with a significant decreased probability (hazard ratio—HR—1.037). Large series indicate that the mean age of long-term survivors is less than 50 years [29, 30], reported that only 2.2 % of 689 enrolled patients survived more than 3 years, and their mean age was 43.5 years.

### Performance Status

Patients' performance status (PS) represents a well-known quantitative prognostic indicator in GB [31], and some scoring systems are presently in use, taking into account the ability of performing the normal activities of the daily life. The Karnofsky Performance Status (KPS) scale is probably the more widely adopted tool, to this purpose. Karnofsky and Burchenal [32] realized the necessity for objective and standardized measurements of patients' performance, as a "*method of evaluating a therapeutic agent against cancer (…) in the absence of coincident and significant objective evidence of a therapeutic effect.*" Such a methodological approach could be appealing in tumors whose direct apparentness was not easily achievable, that is, the case of GB before the advent of CT and MRI. A growing body of evidence, in fact, subsequently confirmed the prognostic value of KPS in most oncologic settings, and particularly in GB. KPS describes a comprehensive 11-point scale, that quantifies—with 10 % progressive steps—the patient's functional status, with percentage values ranging from 100 % (normal activity, no symptoms) to 0 % (death). The evidence in favor of KPS as a prognostic factor in GB came from the original RTOG RPA classification analysis [10] comprehensive of 1578 patients, enrolled in the RTOG 74-01/ ECOG (Eastern Cooperative Oncology Group) 1374; RTOG 79-18; and RTOG 83-02 studies, and from the subsequent validation by the RTOG 90-06 analysis [30]. The prognostic watershed for survival was at the 70 % KPS score level, with a significantly better prognosis for patients showing values above this threshold, as compared to the other ones.

The ECOG PS evaluation, with a different score system, is used for the same purpose. This instrument, proposed by Oken et al. [33], known also as WHO or Zubrod score, is composed of five classes, depicting progressive impairments of clinical conditions from perfect health (score 0) to death (score 5). ECOG scale is probably more suitable for common practice due to the easy use, and to a correspondence with survival as reliable as that of the KPS system.

## Neurological Status

The early RTOG study quoted above significantly correlated the negative prognostic impact of an abnormal mental status on survival of GB patients [10]. Currently, clinicians mostly use the Mini-Mental Status Evaluation (MMSE) to quantify the impairment of mental status in high-grade gliomas [34], also in its "simplified" version, that is, the Folstein's test. It is a relatively short, stan-

dardized, and well-validated screening test devised for cognitive impairment and dementia [35]. It includes some easy questions and problems in different domains: the patient is required, for instance, to specify the actual time and place, to repeat lists of words, to address arithmetic issues, to show language use and understanding, and to exert motor skills. Any score greater than, or equal to, 27/30 points indicates a normal status. Scores below this value correspond to severe (≤9 points), moderate (10–18 points), or mild (19–24 points) cognitive impairment. A validation of MMSE score of 27 or higher as a favorable, independent predictor of survival came from a trial by the European Organization for Research and Treatment of Cancer (EORTC) and the National Cancer Institute of Canada (NCIC) [36]. Of notice, other authors reported similar findings in low-grade glioma [37].

## Treatment-Related Prognostic Factors

Resection of the tumor and the following RT and CHT [8] became more and more refined in the last decades, resulting in a progressive improvement of survival outcomes. The already quoted SEER database analysis [28], including 4664 GB patients, showed a progressive trend towards an increased median survival from 1973 to 2008. Patients diagnosed from 2005 to 2006 had a significantly improved survival, when compared to those accrued from 2000 to 2001. Other reports addressed the same subject with comparable results: a large cohort study (1059 patients treated in 18 radiotherapy centers in Italy) [7] also evidenced a significant difference in survival rate favoring patients recruited from 2002 to 2007, compared to those collected by the same study group from 1997 to 2001 in a previous patterns-of-care study [38]. Increased use of MRI imaging, more sophisticated neurosurgical techniques, 3-D conformal RT (3D-CRT) or Intensity-Modulated RT (IMRT), and TMZ CHT, together with an improved supportive management, may be the main factors for these better results, with respect to the past.

## Imaging

Magnetic resonance imaging (MRI) has been the standard of GB workup [39] in the pre- and the postoperative settings over the last two decades, and presently is adopted in current practice both for diagnosis and for therapy planning (surgery and RT). Standard MRI grounds most of the available data on prognosis of GB, in terms of progression-free survival (PFS). Clinical workup usually includes gadolinium-enhanced-T1 and T2 or FLAIR (Fluid Attenuation Inversion Recovery) sequences. In conventional T1-weighted MRI, gadolinium enhancement correlates with cell proliferation, expressed by Ki-67 nuclear staining of glioma cells, and with microvascular density, thus helping to some extent to differentiate high-grade from low-grade gliomas [40]. This sequence is used, in common practice, to drive the extension of surgical removal in GB. T2 and FLAIR sequences, depicts the overall extension of the tumor burden and the surrounding edema, and are used in RT planning, together with the T1 ring enhancement by gadolinium for boost volume contouring. Among the radiological findings, tumor necrosis, mass effect, and edema-surrounding tumor are associated with a significantly shorter survival time in many studies [41, 42]. However, most recent and advanced MRI methodologies may give further information, useful for GB diagnosis, treatment decision, patient outcome prediction, and follow-up monitoring. Diffusion-Weighted Imaging (DWI) evaluates cellular density, that is, a MRI technique providing a measure of the movement of free-water molecules: the higher is cell number in a given volume, the lower is water mobility, in that cell membranes hamper water diffusion. Thus, the Apparent Diffusion Coefficient (ADC) values are useful in differentiating on quantitative grounds, high-grade from low-grade gliomas [43]. Proton MR spectroscopy (MRS) measures brain and tumor metabolites in vivo. Specific GB metabolite MR spectral patterns are not fully univocal, but a significant correlation exists between GB cell proliferation (assessed by Ki-67 labeling index in GB sections) and the Choline/Creatinine–Phosphocreatinine ratio (Cho/Cr), and with the N-acetyl aspartate (NAA)/Cho ratio, out of the spectral peaks. This may be useful not only for the characterization of high-grade gliomas in respect of the normal brain, but also as a guide for biopsy, identifying areas of tumor-most representative of malignancy [44]. GB invasiveness may not be sufficiently evaluated by conventional MRI, in that peritumoral edema may obscure the presence of tumor cells, and is addressed by Diffusion Tensor Imaging (DTI), which measures water movements within the white matter tracts (DTI tractography), that can be displaced (in low-grade gliomas) or interrupted/infiltrated (in high-grade gliomas) by tumor [45]. The high angiogenesis activity, due to VEGF, is characteristic of GB and appears as microvascular density in Dynamic Susceptibility-weighted Contrast-enhanced (DSC) MRI: Microvascular density of Area (MVA) is the corresponding parameter that quantitatively correlates with prognosis [46]. MR-based perfusion studies and particularly tumor blood volume estimates have been shown to provide prognostic information on time to progression or survival [47–50]. Many other MRI methodologies and technical refinements were also developed in recent years, as exhaustively reviewed by some authors [44], and a large quantity of diagnostic features of GB, often related with "functional" parameters of tumor growth besides morphology, are presently achievable, that may help to establish diagnosis and extension of the disease. It is hard to assess the practical impact of these disclosures on the general management of GB, but their use in selected patients may substantially modify the therapeutic plan, for improving therapeutic outcome and limiting treatment-related damages. The same holds true for other functional diagnostic tools, such as radionuclide investigations. Recently, the results of C-Methionine (C-MET) Positron-Emission Tomography (PET) results seemed to show prognostic value for GB, dependent on the uptake by proliferative cells [51]. C-MET uptake highlights also a more extended active tumor volume, with respect to T1 gadolinium-enhanced RMI [52] in relapsing GBs. If confirmed in newly diagnosed cases, C-MET PET could have a relevant role in the preoperative imaging workup. To date, the widespread use of imaging assessment of GB extension (mainly MRI) may condition subsequent surgical resection and RT planning, thus might have an indirect prognostic role. Presently this assumption is difficult to substantiate, but as a suggestion by the results of the patterns-of-care studies on large series, quoted above [7, 38].

**Surgery**

The extension of tumor resection is case-dependent, due to tumor bulk, site, and patient medical conditions. A classification of the amount of removal is usually adopted for prognostic evaluation into three categories, as follows: gross total resection (GTR: in respect of preoperative imaging and intraoperative findings), subtotal resection (STR: a gross complete removal of the tumor is not achieved), and biopsy-only (BO: any attempt to ablative or even cytoreductive surgery is judged impossible or not advisable).

Upfront surgery in newly diagnosed GB patients consists of maximal safe resection, in fact, as a primary goal whenever feasible, in respect of tumor size, shape, proximity to blood vessels or functionally determinant (or "eloquent") brain regions. The anatomical localization of GB in the brain, in fact, may affect patient's survival, in that it may condition the surgical excision [41, 53, 54]. Frontal lobe tumors show better survival, as compared to those located in other sites [55, 56]. Prognosis of the rare cerebellar GBs, with respect to their supratentorial counterparts, was considered by several studies with nonunivocal results [57–59], and probably some favorable outcomes reported in this setting may be related to the young age of these patients [60–62]. Aggressiveness in surgical resection is also dependent on other factors, such as patient's age, KPS, and comorbidity status. The extent of tumor removal is balanced, in fact, considering the operative risk and neurologic dysfunctions. In our experience, 46 % of the patients had GTR, 40 % PR, 11.6 % BO [7]. Most related literature report comparable data. Intraoperative MRI and neuromonitoring have been associated with surgical protocols, for maximal safe resection. With respect to the use of intraoperative MRI, which is expensive and

labor consuming, 5-aminolevulinic acid (ALA) tumor-specific fluorescent vital staining helps surgeons to differentiate tumor and healthy brain tissue, with promising results. ALA was the first compound successfully employed to this purpose [63]. Sixty-five percent of ALA-driven resections achieved gross tumor removal vs. 36 % by conventional methods [64]. Sodium fluorescein is another fluorescent compound developed for the same purpose [65].

However, "radical" surgery for GB is an intrinsically abstract concept, given the well-documented infiltrative penetration of tumor cell far beyond contrast enhancement and surgical limits of resection [66]. Most neurooncological literature endorses the benefit or gross GB mass removal, howsoever, and a number of studies clearly indicate that the extensive surgical resection of GB is associated with a significant improvement of the survival outcomes [67]. Lacroix et al. [41] proposed a threshold of 98 % of resected tumor for a significant survival benefit. Sanai et al. [68] attempted a more detailed quantitative analysis of the impact of extent of resection on survival, out of 500 consecutive GB patients, with a significant advantage found after a minimal 78 % resection of the tumor mass, as evident by imaging contrast enhancement. Increasing amounts of resection, even up to the increment from 95 to 100 %, obtained further improvements in survival. Orringer et al. [69] showed that patients with more than 90 % tumor resection achieved an improved 1-year survival with respect to those with a lesser ablation. Chaichana et al. reported a similar finding [70] for every 5 % increment of tumor ablation, over a 70 % threshold of effectiveness of the resection.

Advanced age is a limiting factor for aggressive surgery in GB. Patients older than 65 years, in fact, may be unsuitable for tumor resection because of comorbidities. However, out of fitting cases, Oszvald et al. [71] reported that the overall survival of patients aged over 65 was significantly lower than in younger patients. Notably, the negative impact of age on survival was determinant only in patients undergoing BO, with no significant effect after tumor resection, and an effective role of surgery on survival was suggested in aged as well as in younger patients.

One can argue from a speculative point of view, whether extensive GB removal may be or not an independent variable in determining prognosis, as the possibility of extended resection may depend, in turn, on inherent tumor aggressiveness. No data are available to this regard from prospective random trials. Furthermore, at the present state-of-the-art, adjuvant RT and CHT have shown a significant effectiveness and this question might have some interest, in that hypothetically RT and CHT might compensate a less-than-optimal resection. These arguments are the subject of a recent study [72], based on a personalized survival model including extension of resection (EOR), age, KPS, and accomplishment of adjuvant RT and TMZ. This multivariate, continuous, no-threshold and nonlinear model provides for the first time an explicit evidence of the independent role of maximum-safe GB resection on prognosis. Further, it shows a significant superiority (20 %, i.e.: a predictive error of 4.7 months) in estimating survival effects by EOR over current methods for prediction of survival, based on thresholds and stepwise increments of effectiveness of tumor ablation. Further, the influence of adjuvant RT and TMZ administration on prognosis is also quantified on a personalized base: due to the nonlinear relationship between the percentage of resected tumor and survival, this study clearly showed that adjuvant therapy exerts a progressively greater effect, with increasing EOR. This holds true both for young and old patients, and for high- and low-KPS cases. Thus, a "cytoreductive" value of tumor debulking in GB, favoring the therapeutic effectiveness of adjuvant RT and CHT, seems to be demonstrated, that is, the same role that surgery may have in many other tumors.

## Radiotherapy

Radiation therapy has a consolidated role in the postsurgical, adjuvant treatment of GB, after the early studies quoted above, and its accomplishment is included in the RPA as a prognostic factor [10]. Postoperative RT is a principal element

in the treatment of patients with GB, as shown by different analysis from unselected series, demonstrating improved prognosis. As early as at the seventies of the last century, the addition of RT to surgery increased survival from 3–4 months to 7–12 months, after a random clinical trial [53]. Thumma et al. [28] confirmed the importance of RT in prolonging survival of patients with GB. In their analysis, they found that the "no-radiation" (HR: 3.45) and the "unknown radiation" groups (HR 2.50) showed a marked decreased survival, as compared to the "radiation" group of patients. Filippini et al. [4] showed that RT increased survival with a 39 % reduction in relative risk of dying. External-beam RT should begin within 8 weeks following surgical resection or biopsy. Conventional RT consists of 60 Gy, delivered through limited-field external-beam irradiation, with fractions of 2.0 Gy, 5 days per week, as stated by current guidelines [8]. However, 90 % of the tumors recur at the original site after RT, thus strategies to increase local radiation dose are the subject of clinical radiobiology research for improving patients' outcome. An RTOG–ECOG study randomized 253 patients to 60 Gy whole brain RT vs. 60 Gy plus 10 Gy boost to a limited volume, with no significant advantage on survival in the experimental arm [73]. The dose-escalation RTOG-98-03 phase-I trial failed to demonstrate survival advantage from 3D-CRT, with four dose increments from 64 up to 80 Gy, with 90 % GBs relapsing in the primary site and no advantage from higher doses [74]. Dose-escalation studies with IMRT seemed to show results slightly superior to those normally achievable with standard doses, with a reduction of in-field relapse [75]. However, a systematic, recent review of the studies addressing the subject of RT doses above 60 Gy in the TMZ era, concluded that high-dose treatments do not achieve any substantial prognostic improvement over that of standard dose schedules [76]. Other authors failed to demonstrate a benefit for doses >60 Gy using different RT strategies in newly diagnosed GBs, such as brachytherapy [77] or stereotactic radiosurgery (SRS) [78]. SRS as an initial boost followed by standard volume treatment was the subject of the prospective RTOG 93-05 trial, failing to show any superiority of this treatment over conventional RT in comparable cases [79]. Differently, Tanaka et al. retrospectively compared patient with GB who received conventional 60 Gy RT vs. 80–90 Gy 3D-CRT and found a survival benefit for high-dose 3D-CRT [80].

In conclusion, the vast majority of the available reports seem to show that RT is a prognostic factor just as a dichotomic parameter: the related survival advantage exists, as compared to surgery alone, but this is not dose-dependent according to a continuous dose-effectiveness function above 60 Gy, as normally happens in solid tumors. This observation poses an intriguing and still unresolved question, from a radiobiological point of view: the issue is widely addressed elsewhere in this book.

## Chemotherapy

Early studies on CHT of GB focused on drugs able to cross the Blood–brain Barrier (BBB) and particularly on nitrosoureas (alkylating agents with this capability) for clinical use, such as Carmustine (BCNU) or Semustine (MeCCNU). RT plus BCNU achieved a modest, not statistically significant improvement of long-term survival, as compared to RT alone, after a Brain Tumor Study Group random trial (BTSG 72-01) out of 358 "malignant glioma" patients [81]. Two independent meta-analyses also suggested that adjuvant nitrosoureas chemotherapy results in a modest increase in survival (from 6 to 10 %-increase in the 1-year survival rate) [82, 83]. Of note, this last study included a relevant percentage (37 %) of patients affected by gliomas of lower grade than GB.

Temozolomide is another alkylating agent able to cross the BBB, and early studies have shown a remarkable activity on recurrent GB [84]. EORTC and NCIC conducted a phase-III trial of RT alone (60 Gy over a period of 6 weeks) vs. concurrent RT-TMZ (75 mg/sm/day for 6 weeks) followed by adjuvant TMZ (150–200 mg mg/sm/day for 5 days, q. 28 days for six cycles), in patients with newly diagnosed GB [9]. Combined RT-TMZ had an acceptable side-effect profile and achieved a significant median survival increase (14.6 months vs. 12.1 months) and the 2-year survival rate was significantly greater, as compared to RT alone (26.5 % vs. 10.4 %), with a 37 % decreased risk of death. Presently, clinicians consider RT plus concurrent and adjuvant TMZ a standard of care for newly diagnosed GB. However, the inclusion of TMZ in postoperative therapy of GB patients is not an independent, favorable prognostic parameter, given that effectiveness of TMZ depends on the methylation status of the O6-methylguanine-DNA methyltransferase (MGMT) promoter. This was demonstrated out of the patients included in a EORTC–NCIC trial [85]. A significant median survival benefit was demonstrated, in fact, for patients undergoing RT-TMZ, whose GB showed a methylated MGMT promoter, as compared to those with the same feature undergoing RT only (21.7 vs. 15.3 months, respectively, $p=0.007$). Contrarily, the difference between the same treatment groups, out of non-methylated-MGMT GB patients, did not attain statistical significance. The MGMT activity in repairing the drug-induced DNA alkylation causes the lack of effectiveness of TMZ as an adjunct to RT in improving prognosis of GB in the postoperative setting, in fact, a situation prevented by the methylation of the MGMT promoter. This mechanism is the subject of a following section of this chapter, in that prognosis depends also on tumor-related factors, besides TMZ CHT accomplishment.

## Targeted Therapies

Novel perspectives derive in experimental studies from targeted therapies, either alone or combined with traditional RT and CHT [86, 87]. However, clinical trials, had not yet yielded significant results in terms of patient survival improvement. GB is a largely heterogeneous cancer, which partly justifies failure of its treatment [86, 88]. Large-scale omics analyses are unraveling GB pathobiological-altered pathways, which, in the future, might allow for a more comprehensive discovery of prognostic and predictive factors, as well as for novel targets for personalized therapies [88].

## Tumor-Related Prognostic Factors

### Pathology Classification of GB

Histological features of GB are pleomorphic cells, mitotic activity, intravascular microthrombi, necrosis with or without pseudopalisading, and microvascular proliferation, being the last two characteristics necessary for diagnosis. Different histological patterns are recognized, that is, small cell GB, giant cell GB, gliosarcoma, etc. However, these morphological features or categorizations may not have a reliable prognostic value, as life expectancy can be the same for all of them. On the other hand, the previously quoted distinction between "primary" and "secondary" GB, according to the evidence of a precursor lower-grade glioma in the latter, does not imply different morphology features, but has some impact on prognosis. The different aggressive behavior between these two entities is attributable to different genetic pathways in tumor evolution [89]: the former type of GB (95 % of the overall GBs, the most aggressive, arising *de novo* after a short clinical story) shows in many cases (70 %) LOH 10q, and—in 25–36 %—*EGFR* amplification, *p16$^{INK4a}$* deletion, *TP53* mutation and *PTEN* mutation. The latter (5 % of the cases) evolves over time, usually in younger patients, from grade II or grade III astrocytoma (with mutated *TP53* in 53–59 %) and mutated IDH1/2 trough one or two subsequent steps, eventually developing LOH 10q (63 %), *EGFR* amplification (8 %), *p16$^{INK4a}$* deletion (19 %), *TP53* mutation (65 %), and *PTEN* mutation (4 %) [27, 90]. *EGFR* amplification, IDH1/2 mutation, *TP53* mutation, and *PTEN* mutation rates are distinctive signatures between primary and secondary GBs.

WHO recognizes a "GBM-o" category of GB [91], which has areas of oligodendroglioma and corresponds to anaplastic oligoastrocytoma with mitosis and necrosis, with or without microvascular proliferation. GBM-o may have a better response to therapy and prognosis, as compared to standard GB. However, the identification of GBM-o requires molecular subtyping that discloses the genetic pathway of oligodendroglioma. Loss of heterozygosity 1p/19q correlates

with the morphology of oligodendroglioma, and is associated with *IDH* mutation, *MGMT* promoter methylation, G-CIMP phenotype, and a proneural phenotype (see below). Co-deletion of 1p/19q is mutually exclusive with *TP53* mutation. However, GBM-o shows low (≤30 %) rates of 1p/19q co-deletion and genetic heterogeneity, and this marker is useful for differentiation among anaplastic oligodendroglioma, mixed glioma or GBM-o [92].

The Cancer Genome Atlas Network (TCGA) catalogued recurrent genomic abnormalities in GB, which grounded a gene-expression molecular classification of GB into proneural, neural, classical, and mesenchymal subtypes [93]. An aggressive postsurgical therapy (that is, RT with >3 cycles of concurrent chemotherapy, versus a less intensive management), achieved a significantly reduced mortality in the classical (HR=0.45, $p$=0.02), and mesenchymal subtype (HR=0.54, $p$=0.002), a borderline impact on survival in the neural (HR=0.56, $p$=0.1), and no effect on the proneural subtype (HR=0.8, $p$=0.4). The proneural subtype is predominant in young age and in secondary GB.

### Biomolecular Factors

We consider henceforth the genetic and molecular signatures that have been most frequently associated with survival outcomes in GB on the grounds of analyses carried out of the pathological samples, taking into account both the prognostic parameters emerging independently from therapy, and those relevant for patients undergoing postoperative standard RT-CHT. We do not attempt here, to consider prognostic biomolecular factors in their relationship with therapy against molecular targets, due to the heterogeneity of data and a present general inconsistency of clinical results with respect to the biological premises. Furthermore, caution is necessary in interpreting the results reported hereafter, in that their significance may largely depend on methodological issues.

### MGMT-Methylation Status

The O6-methylguanine-DNA methyltransferase (*MGMT*) promoter methylation status is a prognostic biomarker in GB undergoing RT-TMZ [85], as outlined before, while its independent predictive power on survival is still uncertain. A meta-analysis study on 2018 high-grade glioma patients included in 20 reports showed that MGMT gene silencing was significantly associated with improved survival in patients undergoing RT-TMZ; this advantage was less significant in those receiving only RT, and null in those receiving neither TMZ nor RT [94, 95] randomly compared elder patients either to receive RT or TMZ: a survival benefit related to *MGMT*-methylation status was evident only for patients receiving TMZ. Contrarily, others demonstrated a better overall survival for high-grade gliomas showing methylation of the MGMT promoter, irrespective of therapy [96]. However, caution is necessary when interpreting all of these results, for several reasons.

First, most studies addressing the above issue, deal with high-grade gliomas in general. However, Anaplastic Astrocytoma (AA, or WHO grade-III glioma, that is included in the high-grade glioma category together with GB) does not show a significant survival advantage after TMZ therapy, in our experience [97]. Some authors evidenced, in fact, that MGMT promoter methylation status does not provide enough information about the sensitivity of AA to alkylating agents [98, 99], and that MGMT expression may be significantly lower in AA than in GB [100]. Thus, including AA in MGMT-methylation status evaluation as a factor for prognosis or response to therapy in GB may be inappropriate.

Second, the method of assessment of the methylation status was not the same in all studies addressed to this subject. Presently, in fact, methylation-specific PCR or pyrosequencing are considered the tests of choice to determine MGMT promoter methylation status, and immunohistochemistry for MGMT protein expression is not recommended [92].

Third, a sample classification according to the methylated and nonmethylated status for a gene, may be dependent on the relationship between the overall CpG island methylation, the CpG methylation at individual sites, and the effectiveness of gene silencing, that is dependent in turn on the location within the gene [101]. In conclusion, MGMT promoter methylation status is a reliable prognostic parameter only in GB patients undergoing a standard course RT-TMZ after surgery, whereas in other settings this role is an investigational subject.

## *IDH1/2* Mutations

Recent genomic studies have addressed Isocitrate Dehydrogenase 1 and 2 genes (*IDH1*, *IDH2*, and *IDH* as a whole) mutations as prognostic factors in GB [102]. These are common in secondary (73.4 %—[90]), but rare (≤10 %) in primary GB, and correlate with young age and longer survival, as compared to $IDH^{wt}$ patients. *IDH* mutation is mutually exclusive with *EGFR* amplification, whereas it is often associated with the methylation of the *MGMT* promoter.

A relatively large series of secondary GB (86 patients), in fact, was recently collected and analyzed [90] for the survival impact of the *IDH* mutation, together with 1p19q co-deletion, *p53* expression, and *MGMT*-methylation status. These authors confirmed that 1p19q co-deletion and *p53* expression were mutually exclusive, and showed that the *IDH* mutation was associated with both the *p53* expression and the methylation of the *MGMT* promoter. *IDH* mutation, 1p19q co-deletion, and *MGMT* promoter methylation were all significantly associated with increased overall and progression-free survival, whereas *p53* expression was not. After TMZ chemotherapy, GB patients with both the *IDH* mutation and the *MGMT* promoter methylation achieved the best survival result, those with no one of the two characteristics the worst, whereas those with the *IDH* mutation alone showed a result intermediate in between, with statistically significant differences. In conclusion, secondary GBs showing *IDH* mutation enjoy a better survival and response to TMZ as compared to the $IDH^{wt}$ counterpart, but whether the relationship between *IDH* mutation and *MGMT* promoter methylation is consequential, or depends on different epigenetic markers is not clarified, so far.

Recent data from the German Glioma Network [103] demonstrate that a high percentage (34 %) of 69 long-surviving (>36 months) primary GB patients have *IDH1/2* mutations, as compared to 4.3 % out of 257 controls (surviving ≤36 months). This might indicate a prognostic role for the rare *IDH* mutations in primary GB, as suggested also by studies addressing *IDH1* mutation at the clinical onset [104], failing however to show a highly significant correlation with a better clinical outcome at multivariate analysis, when considered in respect to other well-established prognostic factors.

## *PDGFRA* Amplification

Focal amplifications of the locus at 4q12 harboring Platelet-Derived Growth Factor Receptor Alpha (*PDGFRA*) are common in all types of GB, but with a high frequency in the proneural subtype, in which it is associated with high level of *PDGFRA* gene expression, that is, a characteristic signature [93]. However, *PDGFRA* amplification has a negative prognostic impact, when evaluated by FISH out of the rare IDH1-mutant adult de novo GBs [105]: overall median survival was 2179 days in 22 GBs with *IDH1*-mutant/*PDGFR*-no amplification, vs. 480 days in 16 cases with *IDH1*-mutant/*PDGFR*-amplification. This is a statistically significant difference both at the uni- and at the multivariate analysis (log-rank: $p=0.023$, Cox proportional HR: $p=0.01$, respectively).

## EGFR

### EGFR Expression

Epithelial Growth Factor Receptor (EGFR) gene amplification is present in 40–50 % of GBs, being more common in primary than in secondary type, and is a signature of the TGCA classical GB subtype [92]. In general, it has been associated with an aggressive behavior. *EGFR* amplification results in its overexpression [106, 107], in fact, and its downstream signaling pathways enhance many cellular activities, including growth, migration, and survival [108], promoting also resistance to both RT and CHT in clinical and preclinical studies [109, 110]. In other reports, low-*EGFR*-expressing GB patients had a worse response to TMZ-containing adjuvant therapeutic regimens, as compared to those showing either high expression or no expression at all [111].

However, in the clinical setting *EGFR* amplification/overexpression is reported to impact on survival with nonunivocal results: high levels have been associated with a longer median survival [106], or with a worse prognosis in younger patients, in respect of older ones [112, 113]. Some authors suppose a complex relationship between patient's age, *EGFR* amplification, *p53* expression, and survival in GB. The poor survival noted in young patients whose tumors overexpressed EFGR, in fact, correlated also with the co-existent expression of p53$^{wt}$ immunohistochemistry [112]. On the other hand, GB patients undergoing TMZ-containing therapy, showing EGFR amplification, maintenance of PTEN, p53$^{wt}$, and p16 had a relatively favorable prognosis [114]. Others found no significant correlation of EGFR amplification with survival [115].

The combined prognostic impact of *EGFR* expression and components of its downstream pathways, such as the PI3K-Akt-mTOR signaling mechanisms deserve consideration. Autophagy is one of the metabolic pathways inhibited by EGFR, which can act via mTOR or by direct inhibition of Beclin1, a cytoplasmic protein that induces autophagy by binding to the Vps34-Vps15 core [116, 117]. In our experience, low-EGFR and high-Beclin1 expressing GBs (24 patients) have a significantly better median survival (22 months), as compared to other ones (93 patients, median survival: 8 months) showing high-EGFR and both high- and low- Beclin1 expression ($p=0.001$), after standard RT-TMZ [118]. We also experimentally demonstrated that combined EGFR and autophagy modulation impact on IR and TMZ sensitivity in human GB cell lines [119]. In conclusion, probably the EGFR expression level is not a per se reliable prognostic parameter, at the present status of knowledge, but its role in the context of the survival prediction capability of other biological or clinical markers may deserve consideration for further research.

### EGFR Mutations

The most frequent mutant of *EGFR*, expressed in 30–50 % of GB, is the EGFR variant III (EGFRvIII). The deletion of exons 2–7, that is, the lack of the extracellular domain characterizes EGFRvIII, constitutively activate a high stimulation of the PI3K/Akt/mTOR pathway, and was found to inhibit therapy-induced apoptosis [120]. EGFRvIII enhances repair of DNA double-strand breaks, and is a cause of the resistance to gefitinib [121]. Other genetic alterations of EGFR, such as amplification, may affect both the extracellular domain, with activation of point mutations, and the cytoplasmic domain, with deletions [122]. GBs harboring EGFRvIII are more invasive, as compared to those with EGFR$^{wt}$ [123], but no data demonstrate so far a clear-cut impact on prognosis or on response to therapy.

### Loss of PTEN

Phosphatase and Tensin Homolog (*PTEN*) is a tumor suppressor gene that downregulates the PI3K/Akt/mTOR pathways, thus acting for reduced proliferation, apoptosis, and invasiveness [124]. Its mutation determined a shorter survival in GB patients, as compared to those harboring *PTEN*$^{wt}$ tumor, in early studies [106]. Presently, in the TMZ era, PTEN loss is not associated with poor survival in GBs undergoing current standard postoperative RT-TMZ [125]. These authors attributed their observation to a high effectiveness of TMZ in PTEN-deficient GB cells, due to their reduced homologous recombination repair activity of DSBs, and to the subsequent autophagy induction, on the ground of previous preclinical studies. In conclusion, loss of PTEN probably is an adverse prognostic marker only in GB patients not undergoing TMZ CHT.

### VEGF Expression

Vascular Endothelial Growth Factor (VEGF) is an angiogenic factor driving neovascularization, which is a hallmark of GB. However, high percentages of both Grade-III astrocytoma—or AA (66.7 %), and Grade IV astrocytoma—or GB (64.1 %) express VEGF, differently from Grade-II astrocytoma (36.8 %), out of a series of 162 cases of primary glial tumors [126]. This study demonstrated a strong correlation between VEGF expression and survival in the whole series, but not within any of the considered tumor grades. To date, no clear evidence exists of a

direct relationship between VEGF expression and survival outcome of GB patients, but great scientific efforts address, instead, the relationship of VEGF with GB stem cells, and targeting VEGF with antibodies and TK inhibitors in clinical prospective trials. As a marker of clinical outcome at the present state-of-the-art, VEGF is still "potentially prognostic" [127].

### Loss of Heterozygosity 10q

The allelic deletions on chromosome 10q are frequent in both primary and secondary GB, indicating that the loss of 10q tumor suppressor genes may be important in its tumorigenesis [128], such being also the case of PTEN (10q23), already dealt with. Loss of Heterozygosity (LOH) 10q significantly emerged as a poor prognostic marker in GB, after a study on 97 consecutive patients [129]. Furthermore, in a small patient series from India, LOH 10q was correlated both with a four-fold reduced 1-year survival (not attaining statistical significance), and with age ≥40 years ($p = 0.014$) [130].

### Telomerase mRNA Expression and Activity, and Alternative Lengthening of Telomeres

Telomerase messenger expression (human Telomerase Reverse Transcriptase (hTERT) mRNA) was evaluated by PCR, together with telomerase activity as assessed by Telomeric Repeat Amplification Control (TRAP), in their relationship with survival out of a series of 42 patients (33 GBs, 5 AAs, 4 differentiated astrocytoma, 1 oligoastrocytoma) [131]. Out of the whole series, both overall survival and disease-free interval were adversely affected by hTERT mRNA expression ($p = 0.046$ for both the survival parameters) and by telomerase activity ($p = 0.007$ and 0.008, respectively) at the Kaplan-Maier statistical analysis. The Cox proportional hazard model of overall survival confirmed a significant impact of hTERT mRNA expression and telomerase activity. These authors did not analyze results separately in GB patients. A more recent paper considered the same telomerase-associated parameters for survival [132] out of 100 GB patients, and only those aged ≤60 years, lacking both telomerase activation and hTERT positivity, showed a significantly better outcome, as compared to the other ones. Therefore, the role of telomerase activation as an independent prognostic factor in GB is not fully demonstrated so far, but deserves further study, taking into account the pathobiological features of GB in younger patients.

Relationship among telomerase activity, alternative lengthening of telomeres (ALT), and other oncogenes, is also worth of investigation. hTERT was found to promote cancer stemness through EGFR, thus inducing tumor progression [133]. In a previous study [134], we found high telomerase activity and reduced telomeres in a group of GB patients overexpressing EGFR, who were characterized by a low survival rate.

Alternative lengthening of telomeres (ALT), a presumed precursor to genomic instability, was found to be driven by mutation in ATRX (α-thalassemia/mental-retardation-syndrome-X-linked) in IDH1 mutant gliomas taking, together with the mutually exclusive del 1p,19q, a favorable prognostic impact [135, 136].

## MAPK and Akt Pathways Members, and *YKL40* Expression

Both Ras signaling pathways members, that is, the Raf/mitogen-activated protein (MAP) extracellular signal-regulated kinase (ERK)/MAP kinase (MAPK), and the phosphoinositide (PI3K)/Akt kinase/mTOR, have been shown as critical determinants of proliferation, invasiveness, and resistance of GB to ionizing radiation (revised by Pelloski et al. [137]). These authors demonstrated by immunohistochemistry, out of a series of 268 GB patients, that a high positive score for p-MAPK correlated with a significantly reduced survival probability ($p=0.003$), as well as many of the Akt cascade-activated members (p-Akt, $p=0.095$; p-mTOR, $p=0.021$; p-p70S6K, $p=0.013$). Low p-MAPK GBs showed a significantly better radiation response, as compared to those expressing high p-MAPK ($p=<0.001$). At multivariate analysis, only p-MAPK showed a significantly increased HR (1.5, range 1.1–2.2, $p=0.009$) as for survival, besides other well-known patient-related prognostic factors (age, PSK).

The aberrant initial Ras signaling has also a relevant interest for identification of prognostic factors in GB. However, Ras mutations are rare (2 %) in GB, according to the TGCA studies [138].

In vitro studies have shown that the chitinase 3-like protein (CHI3L1, or YKL40) may initiate the MAPK and the PI3K signaling cascades in human connective-tissue cells, by phosphorylation of ERK1/ERK2 and Akt, respectively [139]. YKL40 was expressed in 81 % of the cases reported by Pelloski et al., quoted above, and its expression exerted a strong negative impact on survival ($p=0.002$) [137], and is proposed as a possible candidate in regulation of the Ras-dependent pathways. YLK40 concentration can be detected in peripheral blood, as it is secreted both by tumor cells and by tumor-associated circulating macrophages: its concentration seems to correlate with an aggressive phenotype of GB, short survival, and resistance to RT (revised by Conçalves et al. [102]). However, assessment of the prognostic role of serum YLK40 level in GB is still investigational.

## Cytochrome *c* Oxidase

The enzyme Cytochrome *c* Oxidase (CcO) catalyzes the terminal transfer of electrons from cytochrome *c* to oxygen in the respiratory chain. Griguer et al. [140] have recently demonstrated by spectrophotometric determinations that a high CcO activity significantly correlates with reduced overall survival ($p=0.0001$) and progression-free survival ($p=0.0087$), out of a series of 58 primary GB patients, retrospectively evaluated. These authors extensively considered, in this regard, also previous data evidencing that CcO activity reduces Reactive Oxygen Species (ROS), thus facilitating chemoresistance to TMZ through suppression of apoptotic signaling. This series included also patients undergoing therapy before the advent of TMZ, and used for validation an external set of patients not undergoing TMZ CHT. Interestingly, the correlation between CcO activity and survival was not dependent on RT-TMZ treatment accomplishment, and the multivariate analysis indicated CcO activity as a prognostic parameter independent by age, gender, and MGMT promoter methylation status. CcO activity as a reliable, independent prognostic indicator in glioblastoma, and the hypotheses addressing its role in a mechanism of drug resistance, should be the subject of further research.

### *HOXA9* Gene Expression

Class I homeobox (HB) genes, encoding transcription factors playing a role both in normal development and in tumorigenesis, include *HOXA* genes, mainly activated in GB (revised by Conçalves et al. [102]). Among them, *HOXA9* expression—related to a transcriptional pathway of PI3K—is associated with enhanced cell proliferation, antiapoptotic function, and a worse prognosis in GB [141]: out of two different sets of GB patients, *HOXA9* positivity was significantly an independent factor, with worse overall and progression-free survival. This relationship was even more evident in methylated MGMT GBs, identifying a poor-prognosis set in this category of patients.

### MicroRNAs

Deregulation of some MicroRNAs (miRNAs or miRs) has been detected in GB and is the subject of a dedicated issue in this book, regarding preclinical investigations. A recent study, carried out of 480 GB samples of the TGCA dataset [142], addressed the prognostic role of specific miRNA interactions: high levels of miR-326/miR-130a and low levels of miR-323/miR-329/miR155/miR-210 were significantly associated with favorable OS, while high miR-326/miR-130a and low miR155/miR-210 were associated also with improved PFR. miR-323 and miR-329 were associated with long-term survival. McNamara et al. revised other data on prognostic role of miRNAs in GB patients [127].

### Glioma Stem Cell Markers

A great deal of evidence is growing of the role of GB cells showing stem characteristics (GSC) in tumor initiation and progression, and in conferring an increased resistance to therapy, as compared to their progeny: also this subject is thoroughly addressed elsewhere in this book. However, at the present status of knowledge, an extremely topical issue is whether suitable GSC markers exist that might be useful for identifying prognostic criteria also with respect to resistance to standard CHT and RT, as extensively reviewed in recent papers. Dahlrot et al. [143] have taken into account as many as 27 studies, published in the last decades, addressing also methodological issues: all of the revised papers included immunohistochemistry-based assessment of the investigated markers, and in many instances Western Blot, Confocal microscopy, Immunofluorescence, Immunoblotting, Northern Blot, Real-Time Polymerase Chain Reaction, and Gene-expression analyses. Grade II through IV (GB) cases are included, and the expression level of the CD133 membrane protein and of the filament marker Nestin resulted significantly increased with increasing grade of malignancy; their co-expression had even more influence for a dismal prognosis. Data also suggested trends for a prognostic impact for another surface marker (Podoplanine) and a RNA-binding protein (Musashi-1). Jackson et al. [144] addressed their analysis to the progressive enhancement and gain of GSCs during disease progression and GB recurrence after therapy, considering a possible relationship between GSC markers and the emergence of the more aggressive transcriptional subtype of GB (that is, mesenchymal GB) and of Gliosarcoma (GSM) in recurrences. According to these authors, CD133+ GSCs exhibit transcriptional profiles resembling the "better prognosis" proneural subtype, whereas CD133− GSCs may predominate in mesenchymal GB, and CD133 expression may be downregulated in GSM. Thus, correlating the CD133 expression with prognosis of GB may be misleading. The related literature, in fact, shows contradictory results, but methodological issues may be also determinant in this regard. The quantitative expression of CD133 stem cell antigen mRNA was assessed by RT-PCR in 48 primary GBs by Metellus et al. [145], and high CD133 mRNA expression was shown as a significantly ($p = 0.007$) adverse factor for overall and progression-free survival at multivariate analysis. Contrarily, the CD133 immunohistochemical expression was not a prognostic marker in an analysis out of 68 GB patients, which failed also in demonstrating a possible correlation between CD133 expression and MGMT protein expression or MGMT promoter methylation status [146].

A suitable approach for identifying useful GSC markers may be addressing the GSC-related gene-expression signatures out of large dataset analyses, such as TCGA. Kim et al. [147] identified stem-like cell-specific gene sets that could be used to divide the tumor samples into several groups, and showed a significantly ($p=0.0051$) improved 2-year overall survival for a group of genes (nestin, SOX2, and EZH2). Their downregulation corresponded to a significant ($p<0.003$) improvement in 2-year overall survival, that is, 34.3 % compared to 4.1 % for the group with overexpression of the same genes. Sandberg et al. [148] performed a genome-wide analysis of nine enriched populations of GSCs, in a comparison with five populations of stem cells from normal brain, using a functionally validated sphere-forming test. They identified a multiple-gene-expression signature that exists in GSCs, but not in normal brain stem cells, that significantly correlates with survival out of two publically available independent datasets of high-grade gliomas. In this report, the Wnt- and Hedgehog-pathways and the Notch-regulated targets showed altered expression in GSCs. In particular, they identified and characterized alterations of the Wnt-pathway, such as active β-catenin, which was present only in GSCs. Interestingly, a previous report of our group showed a negative impact of high β-catenin positive immunohistochemistry score on GB patients' prognosis, as well as of Gli-1 expression, which is a marker of the Hedgehog pathway activation [149].

In conclusion, at the present state-of-the-art, no GSC-related marker has a reliable role as a prognostic indicator in current clinical practice of GB, in spite of the great deal of preclinical research on this subject, showing intriguing perspectives.

## Conclusions

Present treatment modalities of GB in common practice are still based on the approach "one size fits all," that is, surgery, RT, and TMZ according to widely accepted guidelines, with a more or less grade of aggressiveness of each therapeutic agent resulting from tumor extension and expected patient tolerance. Survival outcomes were substantially stable over the last decade, in spite of substantial improvements in knowledge of the biology of this disease and of technological advances and medical procedure refinements. However, medical community is aware of the extreme complexity of GB since more than 30 years, and attempted to individuate suitable prognostic parameters, which may help to analyze therapeutic results and to drive therapeutic management. In particular, great expectations came from the recent assessment of the genomic landscape [150] and, in general, from the progressively improved understanding of the signal pathways of GB. The strikingly favorable impact of the tyrosine-kinase inhibitor imatinib on prognosis of chronic myeloid leukemia [151] and gastrointestinal stromal tumors (GIST) [152], in fact, has led to a diffuse hope that unveiling biologic prognostic markers of cancers may translate into effective target therapy. Unfortunately, this is not the case of GB so far: clinical research proceeded through prospective trials testing monoclonal antibodies, tyrosine-kinase inhibitors, or other "biological" agents directed against putative determinants of aggressiveness, on the grounds of preclinical results indicating inherent anticancer properties, or radiation- and/or chemotherapy enhancement, with no relevant outcome results [153, 154]. Possible hypotheses for explaining this discouraging scenario include: molecular signaling redundancy; clonal selection (or emergence) of resistant phenotypes under treatment; preclinical studies mainly addressed to tumor initiating or early-growth factors and not to late tumor progression mechanisms; difficulty in penetrating BBB by the drugs, etc. [153].

The trend towards a "personalized medicine" [155], which is more and more frequently implemented in other tumors, appears as presently impracticable in GB, due to its complexity. However, it is "*very reasonable to believe that in the era of individualized medicine, genomically and molecularly driven research in combination with multiple patients specific data (clinical, pathological, biological, proteomics, imaging,* etc.), *will ultimately be successful,"* as stated elsewhere in this book (Meldolesi E et al. Perspective of the Large Databases and Ontologic Models of Creation of Preclinical and Clinical Results). A shift towards new translational approaches is probably necessary. According to the above authors, observational studies can be implemented, grounded on large databases and heterogeneous data collection from multiple sources (i.e., clinical, imaging, laboratory, pathology, genomics, proteomics, other molecular biology data, etc.), without necessarily anticipating the possible study outcome, differently from prospective trials. Numerous information, ontology, and data standardization, "rapid-learning" machine techniques, advanced statistical methods, and external validation of the results, are necessary for this purpose. This approach could also include as a premise the yield of previous prospective trials (Evidence-Based Medicine, EBM), or also might produce hypotheses to be confirmed by random comparisons, but in general some limits of the prospective trials, e.g., selective patients, long time, reliability of results only within a restricted domain, might be overcome.

# References

1. Paszat L, Laperriere N, Groome P, et al. A population-based study of glioblastoma multiforme. Int J Radiat Oncol Biol Phys. 2001;51:100–7.
2. Grossman SA, O'Neill A, Grunnet M, et al. Phase III study comparing three cycles of infusional carmustine and cisplatin followed by radiation therapy with radiation therapy and concurrent carmustine in patients with newly diagnosed supratentorial glioblastoma multiforme: Eastern Cooperative Oncology Group Trial 2394. J Clin Oncol. 2003;21:1485–91.
3. Piroth MD, Gagel B, Pinkawa M, et al. Postoperative radiotherapy of glioblastoma multiforme: analysis and critical assessment of different treatment strategies and predictive factors. Strahlenther Onkol. 2007;183:695–702.
4. Filippini G, Falcone C, Boiardi A, et al. Prognostic factors for survival in 676 consecutive patients with newly diagnosed primary glioblastoma. Neuro-Oncology. 2008;10:79–87.
5. Tramacere F, Gianicolo E, Serinelli M, et al. Multivariate analysis of prognostic factors and survival in patients with "glioblastoma multiforme". Clin Ter. 2008;159:233–8.
6. Ma X, Lv Y, Liu J, Wang D, et al. Survival analysis of 205 patients with glioblastoma multiforme: clinical characteristics, treatment and prognosis in China. J Clin Neurosci. 2009;16:1595–8.
7. Scoccianti S, Magrini SM, Ricardi U, et al. Patterns of care and survival in a retrospective analysis of 1059 patients with glioblastoma multiforme treated between 2002 and 2007: a multicenter study by the Central Nervous System Study Group of Airo (Italian Association of Radiation Oncology). Neurosurgery. 2010;67:446–58.
8. Stupp R, Tonn JC, Brada M, et al., on behalf of the ESMO Guidelines Working Group. High-grade malignant glioma: ESMO clinical practice guidelines for diagnosis, treatment and follow-up. Ann Oncol. 2010;21:v190–3.
9. Stupp R, Mason WP, van den Bent MJ, et al. Radiotherapy plus concomitant and adjuvant temozolomide for glioblastoma. N Engl J Med. 2005;352:987–96.
10. Curran Jr WJ, Scott CB, Horton J, et al. Recursive partitioning analysis of prognostic factors in three Radiation Therapy Oncology Group malignant glioma trials. J Natl Cancer Inst. 1993;85:704–10.
11. Gamburg ES, Regine WF, Patchell RA, et al. The prognostic significance of midline shift at presentation on survival in patients with glioblastoma multiforme. Int J Radiat Oncol Biol Phys. 2000;48:1359–62.
12. Jeremic B, Milicic B, Grujicic D, et al. Multivariate analysis of clinical prognostic factors in patients with glioblastoma multiforme treated with a combined modality approach. J Cancer Res Clin Oncol. 2003;129:477–84.
13. Wasserfallen JB, Ostermann S, Pica A, et al. Can we afford to add chemotherapy to radiotherapy for glioblastoma multiforme? Cost identification analysis of concomitant and adjuvant treatment with temozolomide until patient death. Cancer. 2004;101:2098–105.
14. Stark AM, Nabavi A, Mehdorn HM, Blomer U. Glioblastoma multiforme-report of 267 cases treated at a single institution. Surg Neurol. 2005;63:162–9.
15. Adamson C, Kanu OO, Mehta AI, et al. Glioblastoma multiforme: a review of where we have been and where we are going. Expert Opin Investig Drugs. 2009;18:1061–83.
16. Li SW, Qiu XG, Chen BS, et al. Prognostic factors influencing clinical outcomes of glioblastoma multiforme. Chin Med J (Engl). 2009;122:1245–9.
17. Caloglu M, Yurut-Caloglu V, Karagol H, et al. Prognostic factors other than the performance status and age for glioblastoma multiforme: a single-institution experience. J BUON. 2009;14:211–8.
18. Chaichana K, Parker S, Olivi A, Quinones-Hinojosa A. A proposed classification system that projects outcomes based on preoperative variables for adult patients with glioblastoma multiforme. J Neurosurg. 2010;112:997–1004.
19. Helseth R, Helseth E, Johannesen TB, et al. Overall survival, prognostic factors, and repeated surgery in a consecutive series of 516 patients with glioblas-

toma multiforme. Acta Neurol Scand. 2010;122: 159–67.

20. Lai R, Hershman DL, Doan T, Neugut AI. The timing of cranial radiation in elderly patients with newly diagnosed glioblastoma multiforme. Neuro Oncol. 2010;12:190–8.

21. Ewelt C, Goeppert M, Rapp M, et al. Glioblastoma multiforme of the elderly: the prognostic effect of resection on survival. J Neurooncol. 2011;103:611–8.

22. Gerstein J, Franz K, Steinbach JP, et al. Radiochemotherapy with temozolomide for patients with glioblastoma. Prognostic factors and long-term outcome of unselected patients from a single institution. Strahlenther Onkol. 2011;187:722–8.

23. Siker ML, Wang M, Porter K, et al. Age as an independent prognostic factor in patients with glioblastoma: a Radiation Therapy Oncology Group and American College of Surgeons National Cancer Data Base comparison. J Neurooncol. 2011;104: 351–6.

24. Bozdag S, Li A, Riddick G, et al. Age-specific signatures of glioblastoma at the genomic, genetic, and epigenetic levels. PLoS One. 2013;29:8(4).

25. Ohgaki H, Kleihues P. Genetic pathways to primary and secondary glioblastoma. Am J Pathol. 2007;170:1445–53.

26. Ohgaki H, Kleihues P. Genetic alterations and signaling pathways in the evolution of gliomas. Cancer Sci. 2009;100:2235–41.

27. Brandes AA, Tosoni A, Franceschi E, et al. Glioblastoma in adults. Crit Rev Oncol Hematol. 2008;67:139–52.

28. Thumma SR, Fairbanks RK, Lamoreaux WT, et al. Effect of pretreatment clinical factors on overall survival in glioblastoma multiforme: a Surveillance Epidemiology and End Results (SEER) population analysis. World J Surg Oncol. 2012;10:176. doi:10.1186/1477-7819-10-176.

29. Chandler KL, Prados MD, Malec M, Wilson CB. Long-term survival in patients with glioblastoma multiforme. Neurosurgery. 1993;32:716–20.

30. Scott JN, Rewcastle NB, Brasher PM, et al. Which glioblastoma multiforme patient will become a long-term survivor? A population-based study. Ann Neurol. 1999;46:183–8.

31. Lamborn KR, Chang SM, Prados MD. Prognostic factors for survival of patients with glioblastoma: recursive partitioning analysis. Neuro Oncol. 2004;6:227–35.

32. Karnofsky DA, Burchenal JH. The clinical evaluation of chemotherapeutic agents in cancer. In: MacLeod CM, editor. Evaluation of chemotherapeutic agents. New York: Columbia University Press; 1949. p. 196.

33. Oken MM, Creech RH, Tormey DC, et al. Toxicity and response criteria of the Eastern Cooperative Oncology Group. Am J Clin Oncol. 1982;5(6):649–55.

34. Jeremic B, Milicic B, Grujicic D, et al. Clinical prognostic factors in patients treated with malignant glioma treated with combined modality approach. Am J Clin Oncol. 2004;27:195–204.

35. Folstein MF, McHugh PR. Mini-mental state. A practical method for grading the cognitive state of patients for the clinician. J Psychiatr Res. 1975; 12(3):189–98.

36. Gorlia T, van den Bent MJ, Hegi ME, et al. Nomograms for predicting survival of patients with newly diagnosed glioblastoma: prognostic factor analysis of EORTC and NCIC trial 26981-22981/ CE.3. Lancet Oncol. 2008;9(1):29–38.

37. Brown PD, Buckner JC, O'Fallon JR, et al. Importance of baseline mini-mental state examination as a prognostic factor for patients with low-grade glioma. Int J Radiat Oncol Biol Phys. 2004;58:117–25.

38. Magrini SM, Ricardi U, Santoni R, et al. Patterns of practice and survival in a retrospective analysis of 1722 adult astrocytoma patients treated between 1985 and 2001 in 12 Italian radiation oncology centers. Int J Radiat Oncol Biol Phys. 2006;65(3):788–99.

39. Carlsson SK, Brothers SP, Wahlestedt C. Emerging treatment strategies for glioblastoma multiforme. EMBO Mol Med. 2014;6:1359–70.

40. Tynninen O, Aronen HG, Ruhala M, et al. MRI enhancement and microvasularity density in gliomas: correlation with tumor cell proliferation. Invest Radiol. 1999;34:427–34.

41. Lacroix M, Abi-Said D, Fourney DR, et al. A multivariate analysis of 416 patients with glioblastoma multiforme: prognosis, extent of resection, and survival. J Neurosurg. 2001;95:190–8.

42. Schoenegger K, Oberndorfer S, Wuschitz B, et al. Peritumoral edema on MRI at initial diagnosis: an independent prognostic factor for glioblastoma? Eur J Neurol. 2009;16(7):874–8.

43. Kang Y, Choi H, Kim YJ, et al. Gliomas: Histogram analysis of apparent diffusion coefficient maps with standard- or high-b-value diffusion-weighted MR imaging—correlation with tumor grade. Radiology. 2005;261:882–90.

44. Kao H-W, Chiang S-W, Chung H-W. Advanced MR imaging of gliomas: an update. Biomed Res Int. 2013;2013:970586. http://dx.doi.org/10.1155/2013/ 970586:1-14.

45. Inoue T, Ogasawara K, Beppu T, et al. Diffusion tensor imaging for preoperative evaluation of tumor grade in gliomas. Clin Neurol Neurosurg. 2005;107:174–80.

46. Birner A, Piribauer M, Fisher I, et al. Vascular patterns in glioblastoma influence clinical outcome and associate with variable expression of angiogenic proteins: evidence for distinct angiogenic subtypes. Brain Pathol. 2003;13:133–43.

47. Law M, Oh S, Babb JS, et al. Low-grade gliomas: dynamic susceptibility-weighted contrast-enhanced perfusion MR imaging-prediction of patient clinical response. Radiology. 2006;238:658–67.

48. Mills SJ, Patankar TA, Haroon HA, et al. Do cerebral blood volume and contrast transfer coefficient predict prognosis in human glioma? AJNR Am J Neuroradiol. 2006;27:853–8.
49. Law M, Young RJ, Babb JS, et al. Gliomas: predicting time to progression or survival with cerebral blood volume measurements at dynamic susceptibility-weighted contrast enhanced perfusion MR imaging. Radiology. 2008;247:490–8.
50. Bisdas S, Kirkpatrick M, Giglio P, et al. Cerebral blood volume measurements by perfusion-weighted MR imaging in gliomas: ready for prime time in predicting short-term outcome and recurrent disease? AJNR Am J Neuroradiol. 2009;30:681–8.
51. Kim S, Chung JK, Im SH, et al. 11C-methionine PET as a prognostic marker in patients with glioma: comparison with 18F-FDG PET. Eur J Nucl Med Mol Imaging. 2005;32:52–9.
52. Galldikis N, Ullrich R, Schroeder M, et al. Volumetry of 11C-methionine PET uptake and MRI contrast enhancement in patients with recurrent glioblastoma multiforme. Eur J Nucl Med Mol Imaging. 2010;37:84–92.
53. Walker MD, Alexander Jr E, Hunt WE, et al. Evaluation of BCNU and/or radiotherapy in the treatment of anaplastic gliomas: a cooperative clinical trial. J Neurosurg. 1978;49:333–43.
54. Sawaya R, Hammoud M, Schoppa D, et al. Neurosurgical outcomes in a modern series of 400 craniotomies for treatment of parenchymal tumors. Neurosurgery. 1998;42:1044–56.
55. Simpson JR, Horton J, Scott C, et al. Influence of location and extent of surgical resection on survival of patients with glioblastoma multiforme: results of three consecutive Radiation Therapy Oncology Group (RTOG) clinical trials. Int J Radiat Oncol Biol Phys. 1993;26:239–44.
56. Jeremic B, Grujicic D, Antunovic V, et al. Influence of extent of surgery and tumor location on treatment outcome of patients with glioblastoma multiforme treated with combined modality approach. J Neurooncol. 1994;21:177–85.
57. Levine SA, McKeever PE, Greenberg HS. Primary cerebellar glioblastoma multiforme. J Neurooncol. 1987;5:231–6.
58. Djalilian HR, Hall WA. Malignant gliomas of the cerebellum: an analytic review. J Neurooncol. 1998;36:247–57.
59. Weber DC, Miller RC, Villa S, et al. Outcome and prognostic factors in cerebellar glioblastoma multiforme in adults: a retrospective study from the Rare Cancer Network. Int J Radiat Oncol Biol Phys. 2006;66:179–86.
60. Adams H, Chaichana KL, Avendano J, et al. Adult cerebellar glioblastoma: understanding survival and prognostic factors using a population-based database from 1973–2009. World Neurosurg. 2013;80(6):e237–43.
61. Jeswani S, Nuno M, Folkerts V, et al. Comparison of survival between cerebellar and supratentorial glioblastoma patients: surveillance, epidemiology, and end results (SEER) analysis. Neurosurgery. 2013;73:240–6.
62. Babu R, Sharma R, Karikari IO, et al. Outcome and prognostic factors in adult cerebellar glioblastoma. J Clin Neurosci. 2013;20:1117–21.
63. Stummer W, Novotny A, Stepp H, et al. Fluorescence-guided resection of glioblastoma multiforme by using 5-aminolevulinic acid-induced porphyrins: a prospective study in 52 consecutive patients. J Neurosurg. 2000;93:1003–13.
64. Stummer W, Pichlmeier U, Meinel T, et al. AL-GS Fluorescence-guided surgery with 5-aminolevulinic acid for resection of malignant glioma: a randomised controlled multicentre phase III trial. Lancet Oncol. 2006;7:392–401.
65. Schebesch KM, Proescholdt M, Hoemberger C, et al. Sodium fluorescein-guided resection under the YELLOW 560 nm surgical microscope filter in malignant brain tumor surgery. Acta Neurochir (Wien). 2013;155:693–9.
66. Claes A, Idema AJ, Wesseling P. Diffuse glioma growth: a guerrilla war. Acta Neuropathol. 2007;114:443–58.
67. Kuhnt D, Becker A, Ganslandt O, et al. Correlation of the extent of tumor volume resection and patient survival in surgery of glioblastoma multiforme with high-field intraoperative MRI guidance. Neuro Oncol. 2011;13:1339–48.
68. Sanai N, Polley MY, McDermott MW, et al. An extent of resection threshold for newly diagnosed glioblastoma. J Neurosurg. 2011;115:3–8.
69. Orringer D, Lau D, Khatri S, et al. Extent of resection in patients with glioblastoma: limiting factors, perception of resectability, and effect on survival. J Neurosurg. 2012;117:851–9.
70. Chaichana KL, Jusue-Torres J, Navarro-Ramirez R, et al. Establishing percent resection and residual volume thresholds affecting survival and recurrence for patients with newly diagnosed intracranial glioblastoma. Neuro Oncol. 2014;16:113–22.
71. Oszvald A, Guresir E, Setzer M, et al. Glioblastoma therapy in the elderly and the importance of the extent of resection regardless of age. J Neurosurg. 2012;116:357–64.
72. Marko NF, Weil RJ, Schroeder JL, et al. Extent of resection of glioblastoma revisited: personalized survival modeling facilitates more accurate survival prediction and supports a maximum-safe-resection approach to surgery. J Clin Oncol. 2014;32:774–82.
73. Nelson DF, Diener WM, Horton J, et al. Combined modality approach to malignant gliomas-reevaluation of RTOG7401/ECOG 1374 with long-term follow-up. NCI Monogr. 1988;6:279–84.
74. Tsien CI, Moughan J, Michalski JM, et al. Radiation Therapy Oncology Group trial 98-03. Phase I three-dimensional conformal radiation dose escalation study in newly diagnosed glioblastoma. Int J Radiat Oncol Biol Phys. 2009;73:699–708.

75. Tsien CI, Brown D, Normolle D, et al. Concurrent temozolomide and dose-escalated intensity-modulated radiation therapy in newly diagnosed glioblastoma. Clin Cancer Res. 2012;18:273–9.

76. Badiyan SN, Markovina S, Simpson JR, et al. Radiation therapy dose escalation for glioblastoma multiforme in the era of temozolomide. Int J Radiat Oncol Biol Phys. 2014;90:877–85.

77. Selker RG, Shapiro WR, Burger P, et al. The Brain Tumor Cooperative Group NIH Trial 87-01: a randomized comparison of surgery, external radiotherapy, and carmustine versus surgery, interstitial radiotherapy boost, external radiation therapy, and carmustine. Neurosurgery. 2002;51:343–55.

78. Tsao MN, Mehta MP, Whelan TJ, et al. The American Society for Therapeutic Radiology and Oncology (ASTRO) evidence based review of the role of radiosurgery for malignant glioma. Int J Radiat Oncol Biol Phys. 2005;63:47–55.

79. Souhami L, Seiferheld W, Brachman D, et al. Randomized comparison of stereotactic radiosurgery followed by conventional radiotherapy with carmustine to conventional radiotherapy with carmustine for patients with glioblastoma multiforme: report of Radiation Therapy Oncology Group 93-05 protocol. Int J Radiat Oncol Biol Phys. 2004;60:853–60.

80. Tanaka M, Ino Y, Nakagava K, et al. High dose conformal radiotherapy for supratentorial malignant glioma: a historical comparison. Lancet Oncol. 2005;6:953–60.

81. Walker MD, Green SB, Byar D, et al. Randomized comparison of radiotherapy and nitrosoureas for the treatment of malignant gliomas after surgery. N Engl J Med. 1980;303:1323–9.

82. Fine HA, Dear KB, Loeffler JS, et al. Meta-analysis of radiation therapy with and without adjuvant chemotherapy for malignant gliomas in adults. Cancer. 1993;71:2585–97.

83. Stewart LA. Chemotherapy in adult high-grade glioma: a systematic review and meta-analysis of individual patient data from 12 randomised trials. Lancet. 2002;359:1011–8.

84. Yung WK, Albright RE, Olson J, et al. A phase II study of temozolomide vs. procarbazine in patients with glioblastoma multiforme at first relapse. Br J Cancer. 2000;83:588–93.

85. Hegi ME, Diserens AC, Gorlia T, et al. MGMT gene silencing and benefit from temozolomide in glioblastoma. N Engl J Med. 2005;352:997–1003.

86. Ohka F, Natsume A, Wakabeyashi T. Current trends in targeted therapies for glioblastoma multiforme. Neurol Res Int. 2012;2012:878425. doi:10.1155/2012/878425. Epub 2012 Mar 5.

87. Mrugala MM. Advances and challenges in the treatment of glioblastoma: a clinician's perspective. Discov Med. 2013;15:221–30. http://discoverymedicine.com/Maciej-M-Mrugala/2013/04/25.

88. Cloughsey TF, Cavanee WK, Mischel PS. Glioblastoma: from molecular pathology to targeted treatment. Annu Rev Pathol. 2014;9:1–25.

doi:10.1146/annurev-pathol-011110-130324. Epub 2013 Aug 5.

89. Kleihues P, Louis DN, Scheithauer BW, et al. The WHO classification of the tumors of the central nervous system. J Neuropathol Exp Neurol. 2002;61: 215–25.

90. Song Tao Q, Lei Y, Si G, et al. IDH mutations predict longer survival and response to temozolomide in secondary glioblastoma. Cancer Sci. 2012;103: 269–73.

91. Louis DN, Ohgaki H, Wiestler OD, et al. WHO classification of tumors of the central nervous system. 4th ed. Lyon: IARC; 2007.

92. Olar A, Aldape KD. Using the molecular classification of glioblastoma to inform personalized treatment. J Pathol. 2014;232:165–77.

93. Verhaak RGW, Hoadley KA, Purdom E, et al. An integrated genomic analysis identifies clinically relevant subtypes of glioblastoma characterized by abnormalities in PDGFRA, IDH1, EGFR and NF1. Cancer Cell. 2010;17:98–110.

94. Olson R, Brastianos PK, Palma DA. Prognostic and predictive value of epigenetic silencing of MGMT in patients with high grade gliomas: a systematic review and meta-analysis. J Neurooncol. 2011;105: 325–35.

95. Wick W, Platten M, Meisner C, et al. Temozolomide chemotherapy alone versus radiotherapy alone for malignant astrocytoma in the elderly. The NOA-08 randomised, phase 3 trial. Lancet Oncol. 2012;13: 707–15.

96. Eoli M, Menghi F, Bruzzone MG, et al. Methylation of the O6-methylguanine-DNA methyltransferase and loss of heterozygosity on 19q and/or 17p are overlapping features of secondary glioblastoma with prolonged survival. Clin Cancer Res. 2007;13: 2606–13.

97. Scoccianti S, Magrini SM, Ricardi U, et al. Radiotherapy and temozolomide in anaplastic astrocytoma: a retrospective multicenter study by the Central Nervous System Study Group of AIRO (Italian Association of Radiation Oncology). Neuro Oncol. 2012;14:798–807.

98. Brell M, Tortosa A, Verger E, et al. Prognostic significance of O6-methylguanine-DNA methyltransferase determined by promoter hypermethylation and immunohistochemical expression in anaplastic glioma. Clin Cancer Res. 2005;11:5167–74.

99. Siker ML, ChakravartiA MMP. Should concomitant and adjuvant treatment with temozolomide be used as standard therapy in patients with anaplastic glioma? Crit Rev Oncol Hematol. 2006;60:99–111.

100. Capper D, Mittelbronn M, Meyermann R, Schittelhelm J. Pitfalls in the assessment of MGMT expression and in its correlation with survival in diffuse astrocytomas: proposal of a feasible immunohistochemical approach. Acta Neuropathol. 2008;115:249–59.

101. Van Vlodrop IJ, Niessen HE, Derks S, et al. Analysis of promoter CpG island hypermethylation in cancer:

location, location, location! Clin Cancer Res. 2011;17:4225–31.

102. Conçalves CS, Lourenço T, Xavier-Magalhães A, et al. Mechanisms of aggressiveness in glioblastoma : prognostic and potential therapeutic insights. In: Lichter T, editor. Evolution of the molecular biology of brain tumors and the therapeutic implication. Intech Open Science; 2013. p. 388–431. ISBN: 978-953-51-0989-1, doi:1010.5772/52361.

103. Hartmann C, Hentschel B, Simon M, et al. Long term survival in primary glioblastoma with *versus* without isocitrate dehydrogenase mutations. Clin Cancer Res. 2013;19:5146–57.

104. Yan W, Zhang W, You G, et al. Correlation of IDH mutation with clinicopathologic factors and prognosis in primary glioblastoma: a report of 118 patients from China. PLoS One. 2012;7(1-6), e30339. doi:10.1371/journal.pone.0030339.

105. Phillips JJ, Aranda D, Ellison DW, et al. *PDGFRA* amplification is common in pediatric and adult high-grade astrocytomas and identifies a poor prognostic group in IDH1 mutant glioblastoma. Brain Pathol. 2013;23:565–73.

106. Smith JS, Tachibana I, Passe SM, et al. PTEN mutation, EGFR amplification, and outcome in patients with anaplastic astrocytoma and glioblastoma multiforme. J Natl Cancer Inst. 2001;93:1246–56.

107. Aldape KD, Ballman K, Furth A, et al. Immunohistochemical detection of EGFRvIII in high malignancy grade astrocytomas and evaluation of prognostic significance. J Neuropathol Exp Neurol. 2004;63:700–7.

108. Nagane M, Coufal F, Lin H, et al. A common mutant epidermal growth factor receptor confers enhanced tumorigenicity on human glioblastoma cells by increasing proliferation and reducing apoptosis. Cancer Res. 1996;56:5079–86.

109. Barker 2nd FG, Simmons ML, Chang SM, et al. EGFR overexpression and radiation response in glioblastoma multiforme. Int J Radiat Oncol Biol Phys. 2001;51:410–8.

110. Hatampaa KJ, Burma S, Zhao D, Habib AA. Epidermal growth factor receptor in glioma: signal transduction, neuropathology, imaging, and radioresistance. Neoplasia. 2010;12:675–84.

111. Hobbs J, Nikiforova MN, Fardo DW, et al. Paradoxical relationship between the degree of EGFR amplification and outcome in glioblastomas. Am J Surg Pathol. 2012;36:1186–93.

112. Simmons ML, Lamborn KR, Takahashi M, et al. Analysis of complex relationships between age, p53, epidermal growth factor receptor, and survival in glioblastoma patients. Cancer Res. 2001;61:1122–8.

113. Batchelor TT, Betensky RA, Esposito JM, et al. Age-dependent prognostic effects of genetic alterations in glioblastoma. Clin Cancer Res. 2004; 10:228–33.

114. Ang C, Guiot MC, Ramanakumar AV, et al. Clinical significance of molecular biomarkers in glioblastoma. Can J Neurol Sci. 2010;37:625–30.

115. Quan AL, Barnett GH, Shih-Yuan L, et al. Epidermal growth factor receptor amplification does not have prognostic significance in patients with glioblastoma multiforme. Int J Radiat Oncol Biol Phys. 2005;63:695–703.

116. Kang R, Zeh HJ, Lotze MT, Tang D. The beclin1 network regulates autophagy and apoptosis. Cell Death Differ. 2011;18:571–80.

117. Wei Y, Zou Z, Becker N, et al. EGFR-mediated beclin1 phosphorylation in autophagy suppression, tumor progression, and tumor chemoresistance. Cell. 2013;154:1269–84.

118. Tini P, Belmonte G, Toscano M, et al. Combined epidermal growth factor receptor and beclin1 autophagic protein expression analysis identifies different clinical presentations, responses to chemo- and radiotherapy, and prognosis in glioblastoma. Bio Med Res Int. 2015;2015, 208076. http://dx.doi.org/10.1159/2015/208076.

119. Palumbo S, Tini P, Toscano M, et al. Combined EGFR and autophagy modulation impairs cell migration and enhances radiosensitivity in human glioblastoma cells. J Cell Physiol. 2014;229: 1863–73.

120. Nagane M, A. Levitzki, A. Gazit, et al. Drug resistance of human glioblastoma cells conferred by a tumor-specific mutant epidermal growth factor receptor through modulation of Bcl-XL and caspase-3-like proteases. Proc Natl Acad Sci U S A. 1998;95:5724–9.

121. Jutten B, Rouschop KMA. EGFR signaling and autophagy dependance for growth, survival, and therapy resistance. Cell Cycle. 2014;13:42–51.

122. TGCA – Cancer Genome Atlas Research Network. Comprehensive genomic characterization defines human glioblastoma genes and core pathways. Nature 2008;455:1061-8.

123. Fisher I, Aldape K. Molecular tools: biology, prognosis, and therapeutic triage. Neuroimaging Clin N Am. 2010;20:273–82.

124. Simpson L, Parsons R. PTEN: life as a tumor suppressor. Exp Cell Res. 2001;264:29–41.

125. Carico C, Nuño M, Mukherjee D, et al. Loss of PTEN is not associated with poor survival in newly diagnosed glioblastoma patients of the temozolomide era. PLoS One. 2012;7(3), e33684.

126. Oehring RD, Miletic M, Valter MM, et al. Vascular endothelial growth factor (VEGF) in astrocytic gliomas—a prognostic factor? J Neuro-Oncol. 1999;45:117–25.

127. McNamara MG, Sahebjan S, Mason WP. Emerging biomarkers in glioblastoma. Cancers (Basel). 2013;5:1103–19. doi:10.3390/cancers5031103.

128. Ohgaki H, Dessen B, Jourde B, et al. Genetic pathways to glioblastoma : a population-based study. Cancer Res. 2004;64:6892–9.

129. Schmidt MC, Antweiler S, Urban N, et al. Impact of genotype and morphology on the prognosis of glioblastoma. J Neuropathol Exp Neurol. 2002;61: 321–8.

130. Kakkar A, Suri V, Jha P, et al. Loss of heterozygosity on chromosome 10q in glioblastomas, and its association with other genetic alterations and survival in Indian patients. Neurol India. 2011;59:254–61.

131. Boldrini L, Pistolesi S, Gisfredi S, et al. Telomerase activity and hTERT mRNA expression in glial tumors. Int J Oncol. 2006;28:1555–60.

132. Lötsch D, Ghanim B, Laaber M, et al. Prognostic significance of telomerase-associated parameters in glioblastoma: effect of patient age. Neuro Oncol. 2013;15:423–32.

133. Beck S, Jin X, Sohn Y-W, et al. Telomerase activity-independent function of TERT allows glioma cells to attain cancer stem cells characteristics by inducing EGFR expression. Mol Cells. 2011;31:9–15.

134. Miracco C, De Santi MM, Luzi P, et al. *In situ* detection of telomeres by fluorescence *in situ* hybridization and telomerase activity in glioblastoma multiforme: correlation with p53 status, EGFR, c-myc, MIB1, and Topoisomerase IIα protein expression. Int J Oncol. 2003;23:1529–35.

135. Kannan K, Inagaki A, Silber J, et al. Whole-exome sequencing identifies ATRX mutation as a key molecular determinant in lower-grade glioma. Oncotarget. 2012;3:1194–203.

136. Wiestler B, Capper D, Holland-Letz T, et al. ATRX loss refines the classification of anaplastic gliomas and identifies a subgroup of IDH mutant astrocytic tumors with better prognosis. Acta Neuropathol. 2013;126:443–51.

137. Pelloski CE, Lin E, Zhang L, et al. Prognostic associations of activated mitogen-activated protein kinase and Akt pathways in glioblastoma. Clin Cancer Res. 2006;12:3935–41.

138. Network CGAR. Comprehensive genomic characterization defines human glioblastoma genes and core pathways. Nature. 2008;455:1061–8.

139. Recklies AD, White C, Ling H. The chitinase 3-like protein human cartilage glycoprotein 39 (HC-gp39) stimulates proliferation of human connective-tissue cells and activates both extracellular signal-regulated kinase- and protein kinase B-mediated signaling pathways. Biochem J. 2002;365:119–26.

140. Griguer CE, Cantor AB, Fathallah-Shaykh HM, et al. Prognostic relevance of cytochrome c oxidase in primary glioblastoma multiforme. PLoS One. 2013;8:e61035. doi:10.1371/journal.pone.0061035.

141. Costa BM, Smith JS, Chen Y, et al. Reversing HOXA9 oncogene activation by PI3K inhibition: epigenetic mechanism and prognostic significance in human glioblastoma. Cancer Res. 2010;70:453–63.

142. Qiu S, Lin S, Hu D, et al. Interaction of miR-323/miR-326/miR-329 and miR-130a/miR-155/mir-210 as prognostic indicators for clinical outcome of glioblastoma patients. J Transl Med. 2013;11:10. doi:10.1186/1479-5876-11-10.

143. Dahlrot RH, Hermansen SK, Hansen S, Kristensen BW. What is the clinical value of cancer stem cell markers in gliomas? Int J Clin Exp Pathol. 2013;6:334–48.

144. Jackson M, Hassiotou F, Nowak A. Glioblastoma stem-like cells: at the root of tumor recurrence and a therapeutic target. Carcinogenesis. 2014;36:177–85.

145. Metellus P, Nanni-Metellus I, Delfino C, et al. Prognostic impact of CD133 mRNA expression in 48 glioblastoma patients treated with concomitant radiochemotherapy: a prospective patient cohort at a single institution. Ann Surg Oncol. 2011;18:2937–45.

146. Melguizo C, Prados J, Gonzalez B, et al. MGMT promoter methylation status and MGMT and CD133 immunohistochemical expression as prognostic markers in glioblastoma patients treated with temozolomide plus radiotherapy. J Transl Med. 2012;10:250. doi:10.1186/1479-5876-10-250.

147. Kim Y-W, Kim SH, Kwon CH, et al. Identification of cancer stem-like cell signatures of glioblastoma based on the cancer genome atlas analysis. Neuro Oncol. 2011;13(Suppl 3):iii145–53 (Abst 16th annual meeting of the Society for Neuro-Oncology). doi:10.1093/neuronc/nor163.

148. Sandberg CJ, Altschuler G, Jeong J, et al. Comparison of glioma stem cells to neural stem cells from the adult human brain identifies dysregulated Wnt-signaling and a fingerprint associated with clinical outcome. Exp Cell Res. 2013;319:2230–43.

149. Rossi M, Magnoni L, Miracco C, et al. β-Catenin and Gli1 are prognostic markers in glioblastoma. Cancer Biol Ther. 2011;11:1–9.

150. Brennan C, Verhaak RGW, McKenna A, et al. The somatic genomic landscape of glioblastoma. Cell. 2013;155:462–77.

151. Druker BJ, Guilhot F, O'Brien SG, et al. Five-year follow-up of patients receiving imatinib for chronic myeloid leukemia. N Engl J Med. 2006;355:2408–17.

152. Blanke CD, Rankin C, Demetri GD, et al. Phase III randomized, intergroup trial assessing imatinib mesylate at two dose levels in patients with unresectable or metastatic gastrointestinal stromal tumors expressing the kit receptor tyrosinekinase. J Clin Oncol. 2008;26:626–32.

153. Bastien JIL, McNeill K, Fine HA. Molecular characterizations of glioblastoma, targeted therapy, and clinical results to date. Cancer. 2014;121:502–16.

154. Veliz I, Loo Y, Castillo O, et al. Advances and challenges in the molecular biology and treatment of glioblastoma—is there any hope for the future? Ann Transl Med. 2015;3(1):7. doi:10.3978/j.issn.2305-5839-2014.10.06.

155. NCI. NCI Dictionary of terms: personalized medicine (Internet). http://www.cancer.gov/dictionary?cdrid=561717.

# Radiation Tolerance of Normal Brain: QUANTEC 2010 and Beyond

**8**

Francesca De Felice, Vincenzo Tombolini, Michela Buglione, Daniela Musio, Luca Triggiani, and Stefano Maria Magrini

## Introduction

External beam radiation therapy (EBRT) plays a central role in the management of high-grade gliomas, both for curative and palliative intent. Advances in treatment strategies have improved patient survival; therefore neurotoxicity became a significant problem [1]. The use of ionizing radiations results in malignant cell damage and induces deterministic or stochastic side effects on normal tissues.

*The International Journal of Radiation Oncology Physics*, in a special issue, published the *Quantitative Analysis of Normal Tissue Effects in the Clinic* (QUANTEC) guidelines, a practice data collection—16 organ-specific clinical papers—aimed to summarize acute and late effects of EBRT and focused to better define dose recommendations to reduce the normal tissue toxicity for many organs at risks (OARs) [2].

The distinctive feature of QUANTEC, however, is not the inclusion of a series of summaries of organ radiation pathology or the update of the old "tolerance tables." The emphasis is on the clinic: the nature and severity of damage and all the clinical factors contributing to or limiting the risk of organ functional impairment are considered, along with the dose–volume–effect relationships. Moreover, the probability of each type of damage should be considered against the probability of tumor cure, for each dose level.

Radiotherapy technique optimization is therefore only an important starting point in order to limit the volume of OARs exposed and to preserve their architectural and functional component, without compromising the delivery of an optimal dose to the tumor target volume. In fact, a nonuniform dose distribution in normal tissues is a typical feature of the present day treatment planning and dose delivery techniques, especially in sites such as brain, where the tumor is often located in a normal functioning structure or in its close proximity. Nonuniform dose distributions add complexity to the task of defining dose limits for healthy tissues. Moreover, clinical/therapeutic factors (such as concomitant chemotherapy) may also greatly modify the dose-response curve for radiation damage.

F. De Felice • D. Musio
Department of Radiological, Oncological and Anatomo Pathological Sciences, University "Sapienza" of Rome, Rome, Italy

V. Tombolini
Department of Radiological, Oncological and Anatomo-Pathological Sciences, University "Sapienza" of Rome, Rome, Italy

Fondazione Eleonora Lorillard Spencer Cenci, Rome, Italy

M. Buglione • L. Triggiani • S.M. Magrini (✉)
Radiation Oncology Department, University and Spedali Civili - Brescia, Brescia, Italy
e-mail: magrini1954@gmail.com;
stefano.magrini@unibs.it

© Springer International Publishing Switzerland 2016
L. Pirtoli et al. (eds.), *Radiobiology of Glioblastoma*, Current Clinical Pathology,
DOI 10.1007/978-3-319-28305-0_8

Another important issue raised by the QUANTEC papers is therefore that of the organization of large perspective databases linking dosimetric data to clinical outcomes (both for toxicity and cancer control), to face these difficulties.

In this chapter an overview of normal tissue tolerance to EBRT is provided, with an emphasis on central nervous system (CNS) structures.

Topics covered include basic clinical radiobiology, a summary of physiopathology and clinical aspects of CNS toxicity, dose-volume limits, normal tissue complication probability, and future prospectives.

## Basic Clinical Radiobiology

*Normal tissue architecture*: Radiation injury to normal tissues is a complicated and progressive process. Tissue radiation tolerance depends on its architecture and its functional reserve. Each organ can be classified into "parallel" and "serial" and it is assumed to be composed of basic structures, defined functional subunits (FSUs) [3]. The spatial relationship between FSUs is not the same in all the tissues and it is essential to maintain organ integrity. In tissues with a *parallel organization*, each FSU performs the same function and the global functioning is the sum of the activities of the single FSUs. The organ dysfunction occurs when a critical number of FSUs is destroyed; the percentage of the entire organ volume exposed to a defined dose (e.g., V20 = the percentage of the organ that receives a dose of 20 Gy) is the main predictive factor of tissue complication probability. In contrast, in a *serial structure*, the damage suffered by only a single FSU is enough to determine the loss of function of the entire organ; therefore, the maximum absorbed dose results crucial to predict tissue tolerance [4].

The brain has a *mixed type* of organization. It is divided in several different anatomical regions, and, in the same region, any specific area controls a different physical or cognitive domain; in addition, we do not really know the function of many anatomical sites; finally, the structure of any

specific area may be predominantly parallel or serial in nature. Therefore, radiation brain damage, due to this anatomical and functional complexity, is very much influenced by the dose to the individual structure (and possibly by the volume thereof). The fraction of total brain volume exposed to radiation obviously matters, and data are available on the increasing risk of necrosis linked with the increase of the brain volume treated; but nowadays the advances in imaging and in dose computation techniques allow us to accumulate data on the radiation dose reaching the individual structure and on the selective sparing of the more functionally relevant ones.

*Predictive biologic models*: Different mathematical models have been considered to estimate probabilities of parallel and serial tissue complications. Detailed analysis of these models is beyond the aim of this chapter, and we will briefly describe only the Lyman-Kutcher-Burman (LKB) model, probably representing the most popular algorithm. It synthesizes the Lyman model [5] with the Kutcher-Burman dose-volume histogram (DVH) [6, 7], making easier the clinical evaluation in nonuniformly irradiated normal tissues. The LKB model permits physicians to apply the model of normal tissue response—in terms of complication probabilities, as developed by Emami [8]—under conditions of nonuniform irradiation, obtaining the so-called *generalized equivalent uniform dose* (gEUD). The gEUD is defined as the biologically equivalent dose that, if given uniformly, causes the same radiobiological effect as the actual inhomogeneous dose distribution [9]. In other words, with the concept of gEUD, a nonuniform dose distribution is converted into units representing the biologically equivalent homogeneous dose. The gEUD can be obtained directly from DVH and can be applied to specific complications deriving from damage to specific anatomic structures. Considering the DVH parameters, "parallel" type complications can be more easily related to mean absorbed dose, a better descriptor of the dose given to relatively large volumes, whereas "serial" type effects (that are more appropriately related to the value of the maximum absorbed dose) are associated to small volume dose hotspots. This predictive LKB model can only be cautiously used in daily clinical practice, along with the knowledge derived from the larger published series reporting the incidence of radiation-related damage in the different clinical settings. This is important, since the physician usually estimates complications risk deriving standard organ-specific dose-volume constraints.

## Toxicity in High-Grade Gliomas: Physiopathology and Summary of Clinical Aspects

During and after treatment, a spectrum of different radiation-induced toxicities is expected. Depending on the onset of symptoms, clinical response of the brain to EBRT is classified as acute (from the start up to 6 weeks at end of treatment), early delayed (from 6 weeks to 6 months after treatment) and late (6 months to years after treatment) toxicity. *Sequelae* depends on the tumor location; as already noticed, they are associated with EBRT dose, fraction size, and field size, and can be confounded by previous/concomitant therapies as well as comorbidity or tumor progression [10].

*Physiopathology*: Radiation therapy of high-grade gliomas is limited by the sensitivity of the normal tissue. The pathogenesis of radiation-induced brain toxicity is mainly explained by parenchymal and vascular cells damage. The *parenchymal theory* involves oligodendrocytes, which are the glial cells responsible for myelin production. Radiation induces oligodendrocyte death by a direct effect, p53-mediated, and by an indirect effect, releasing cytokines such as TNF-α. Oligodendrocytes loss is associated with demyelination and consequently with white matter necrosis. The *vascular hypothesis* claims that vascular endothelial damage causes ischemia and therefore tissue necrosis. Radiation-induced vascular alterations involve altered permeability, with platelet aggregation and thrombi formation; subsequently endothelial cell nuclear proliferation and deposits of fibrin in the vessel walls are observed. Moreover, radiation induces upregulation of several adhesion molecules, which medi-

ate inflammatory response, worsening vessel injury [11, 12].

*Acute toxicity*: Acute radiation toxicity includes fatigue, hair loss, headache, nausea associated or not to vomiting, otitis externa, skin erythema and, rarely, vertigo and seizures. All these symptoms are attributed to perilesional edema and impairment of the blood–brain barrier. Generally self-limiting, they are usually controlled by medications. Nausea and vomiting are especially associated to brainstem or posterior fossa irradiation, otitis externa is associated to ear irradiation, whereas alopecia depends on exit beam orientations.

*Early delayed toxicity*: Subacute toxicity is characterized by symptoms of somnolence, generalized fatigue, and headache. These symptoms may be tempered by administering steroids. Early delayed toxicity is probably a consequence of transient demyelination and changes in capillary permeability. *Late toxicity*: Late complications are possibly underestimated due to the poor prognosis of patients with high-grade gliomas. Late toxicity is considered to be secondary to focal or diffuse necrosis of the white matter. Radiation necrosis initially manifests itself with nonspecific symptoms and neurologic deficits. It is important to differentiate between radiation necrosis and recurrent disease. Metabolic and functional imaging techniques, such as magnetic resonance spectroscopy or positron emission tomography using the O-(2-18F-fluorethyl)-L-tyrosine [13], can be helpful in differential diagnosis. In a symptomatic patient, if feasible, the surgical resection and the institution of steroids-based therapy represent the optimal treatment. Radiation-induced leukoencephalopathy, due to diffuse necrosis, is a rare condition; it is especially associated to concomitant chemotherapy and not necessarily causes clinical symptoms.

Focal brain parenchyma damage may determine seizures or symptoms of increased intracranial pressure, as well as cranial nerves dysfunction. Hippocampus-dependent short-term learning and memory are influenced by the activity of neural stem cells. Progressive decline in these functions has been associated to long-term deletion of normal neurogenesis in the hippocampus, when the irradiation involves the temporal lobes [14].

Brain irradiation can also produce other long-term side effects. Decrease in visual acuity may follow irradiation of optic nerves/chiasm, generally within 3 years from EBRT. Optic nerve damage can cause monocular visual loss, whereas injury to the chiasm can result in bilateral vision loss. Eye irradiation may cause retinopathy, dry eye, and cataract formation; similarly, ototoxicity, especially hearing loss and vestibular damage, occurs if the ear is included in the irradiated volume. Neuroendocrine side effects, secondary to growth hormone deficiency, are documented if hypothalamic–pituitary axis is irradiated.

## Dose-Volume Constraints

In the 3D-conformal and intensity-modulated EBRT era, it is of paramount importance to accurately delineate all OARs volumes to contribute to the definition of a robust and detailed correlation between volume, absorbed dose, and normal tissue complication probability. Radiation-induced complications depend on dose distribution to the volume (in parallel tissues) and high-dose regions (in serial tissues).

## Constraints Evaluation

The dose constraints typically specify a fraction of some regions of interest (ROI) that must receive a dose lower than the defined one; in other words, they indicate the maximum dose and dose-volume limits for normal tissue structures. Constraints depend from the underlying biologic effects that regulate the clinical effects one would expect on normal tissues [15]. Ideally, if the dose values are within the tolerance limits, no side effects are expected. In daily practice the aim is to obtain an optimal balance between tumor coverage and OARs sparing. It is evident that the achievement of a dose level well below the tolerance dose guarantees a better normal tissue sparing. For some OARs, such as the spinal cord, a dose lower than that required meeting the

constraints, can be judged at a glance unnecessary; however, if this dose reduction does not worsen target volume coverage, it may constitute a "tolerance dose reserve" which may be advantageous in view of a further irradiation that could be needed. Moreover, for some other OARs, like parotids, further dose reduction beyond the tolerance limits could be per se a desirable goal, based on the evidence that functional damage is closely related to the extent of tissues exposed to much lower doses than the brain [16]. This concept could also be extended: when treating a target in the brain, uncertainties about the functional role of some anatomical areas might suggest keeping the dose to these areas as low as reasonably possible. Such an approach should be, however, balanced against the need of adequate target coverage and of an appropriate use of high tech, sometimes very costly resources.

To illustrate the difficulties intrinsic to dose-volume relationship evaluation, two examples of treatment plans of GBM have been used (Figs. 8.1 and 8.2). The figures refer to two cases where the clinical problem is that of giving a uniform dose of 60 Gy to the tumor, while sparing the optic nerve or chiasma and the brain stem. Clinicians should consider the DVHs for the PTV and for the OAR to decide if it is preferably a somewhat increased risk of optic neuropathy or brain stem damage to optimize PTV coverage or whether the toxicity is unacceptable and consequently PTV coverage should be sacrificed. The "acceptable" solutions could be slightly different, more or less precautionary, as in the cases shown, also according to the nature of the OAR: for example, in the case of chiasma, the maximum point dose could be more relevant than the medium dose.

Therefore, constraint evaluation relies yet on clinical judgment, also because multiple uncertainties in their definition are still to be solved.

## Causes of Uncertainty in Brain Tissue Constraint Definition

Several considerations can explain why the consensus on dose-volume constrains could not be

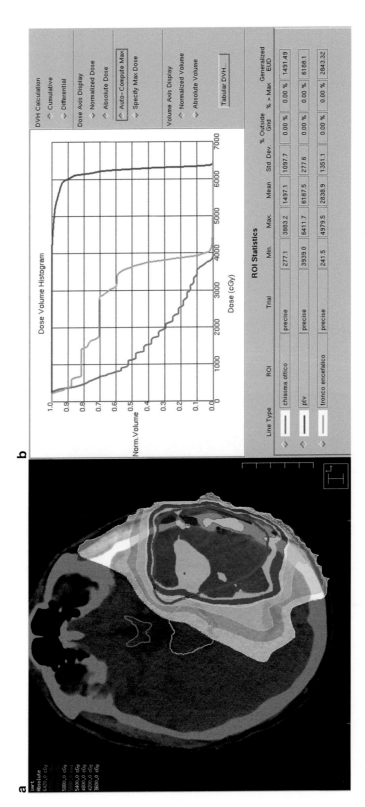

**Fig. 8.1** Treatment plan for a GBM tumor (60 Gy in 30 fractions prescription dose), with: isodose color-wash showing PTV (*red line*) and doses from 36 Gy (*light gray*) to 58 Gy (*green*) and 60 Gy (*dark orange*) (**a**) and DVHs for the chiasma (*green line*) brain stem (*yellow line*), and PTV (**b**)

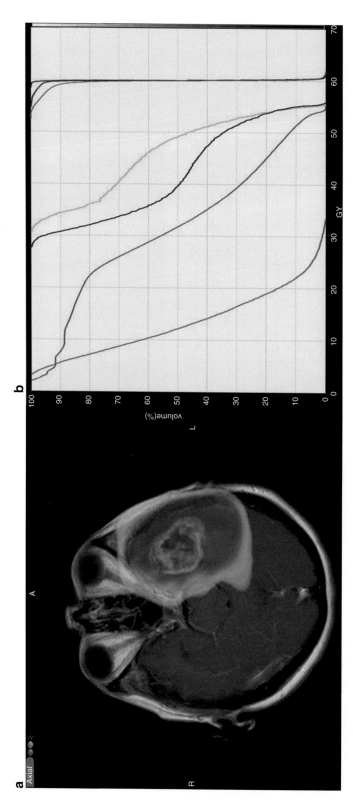

**Fig. 8.2** Treatment plan for a GBM tumor (60 Gy in 30 fractions prescription dose). Plan elaborated with a volumetric rotational IMRT. (**a**) Color-wash isodose distribution, isodose range 45–57 Gy. Isodoses are shown on the staging spin echo T1-weighted Magnetic resonance with contrast agent. The isodoses are calculated on the planning CT, and then propagated on the MR by means of the same rigid registration use for GTV delineation purpose. (**b**) DVHs of GTV, CTV, PTV, and left optic nerve (*green*), optical Chiasm (*blue*), brainstem (*orange*), and eye bulb (*light purple*)

optimal for the OARs involved in brain tumor treatment.

First, EBRT is often combined with chemo- or target-therapy, steroids, and antiepileptic agents. These are all potential causative agents of damage of both irradiated and un-irradiated tissue and confound the interpretation of EBRT toxicity, especially when questionable. The finding of neurologic and neurocognitive decline with nonspecific symptoms, such as personality changes and deficits in intelligence or dementia may in fact represent the results of multiple therapies [17]. Secondly, the development of hypofractionation schemes emphasizes the need for a more robust predictive model adjusted for dose per fraction. EBRT with doses of >2 Gy per day decreases the tolerance of the human brain [18, 19]. Lately, the increased use of a larger number of beam orientations, along with intensity-modulated radiation therapy, instead of the "old" parallel-opposed portals technique, results in a relatively large volume of potentially sensitive structures receiving a low cumulative dose. How this low dose "bath" would influence acute and late effects is still controversial; for organizational, social, and sometimes ethical reasons, prospective clinical trials, analyzing dose-

volume-response relationships for different treatment techniques, are indeed difficult to implement.

## Dose Tolerance Guidelines in the Central Nervous System

Table 8.1 summarizes dose and/or dose-volume parameters for the principal OARs involved in CNS tumor treatment, according to QUANTEC guidelines [18]. Individual dose constraints should however be decided according to physician experience and judgment and not merely applying a standard value.

*Brain*: The brain is considered a parallel tissue, although organ integrity may differ according to the localization of tumor, due to the complex functional anatomy of the organ. Brain consists of three major regions—cerebrum, cerebellum, and brainstem—each region is involved in many different functions and presents a different tolerance to radiation. Assuming that eloquent areas need tighter dose constraints, in general the entire brain is more sensitive to large fraction size (>2 Gy/fr). The initial estimate by Emami et al. [8] for a <5 % probability of necro-

**Table 8.1** QUANTEC guidelines for the principal organs at risk of central nervous system

| Organ | QUANTEC (Dose Gy) | | Risk (%) | Toxicity |
| | Standard fractionation | Single fraction | | |
|---|---|---|---|---|
| Brain | Mean <65 | | | |
| | Max 72 | | 5 | Necrosis |
| | Max 90 | | 10 | Necrosis |
| | | Max 12 (10 cm³) | >20 | Necrosis |
| Brainstem | Max 54 | | 5 | Necrosis/cranial neuropathy |
| | Max 59 (1–10 cm³) | | 5 | Necrosis/cranial neuropathy |
| | Max 64 (<1 cm³) | | 5 | Necrosis/cranial neuropathy |
| | | Max 12.5 | 5 | Necrosis/cranial neuropathy |
| Spinal cord | Max 50 | | 0.2 | Myelopathy |
| | Max 60 | | 6 | Myelopathy |
| | Max 69 | | 50 | Myelopathy |
| | | Max 13 | 1 | Myelopathy |
| Optic nerve/chiasm | Max <55 | | <3 | Optic neuropathy |
| | 55–60 | | 3–7 | Optic neuropathy |
| | >60 | | 8–20 | Optic neuropathy |
| | | Max 12 | <10 | Optic neuropathy |
| Cochlea | Mean ≤45 | | <30 | Hearing loss |

sis was of 60 Gy (for one-third of the brain), but it has been considered too conservative by QUANTEC authors.

For conventional fractionation, in fact, a maximal dose of 72 Gy is associated to a 5 % radiation necrosis risk, and a maximal dose of 90 Gy to a 10 % risk. However, there are few clinical situations in which a dose >60 Gy is needed.

For radiosurgery, the maximal dose depends on target diameter. It is >24 Gy for lesions of less than 2 cm in diameter, 18 Gy for tumor from 2 to 3 cm in diameters, and it is reduced at 15 Gy for lesion >3 cm in diameter. In a risk prediction analysis to evaluate radiation-induced tissue changes, Voges et al. [20] demonstrated that the V10 of surrounding normal brain tissue (excluding target volume) resulted more sensitive than the total volume (perilesional brain tissue plus target volume) covered by 10 Gy. In general terms, the risk of complications increases rapidly over 20 % if the volume of normal brain irradiated to >12 Gy is 5–10 cm³ [21]. A larger volume treated (at least for radiosurgery) and concomitant or previous use of methotrexate or other neurotoxic drugs seem to enhance the risk of radiation necrosis. Because of the marked heterogeneity of literature data regarding parameters like target volume, total dose and irradiation techniques, as well as tumor histology, high-level evidence for constraints values is lacking. Therefore, there is not yet a general consensus and the dose-volume limits should be used cautiously [21].

Brainstem: Brainstem can tolerate up to 54 Gy with a risk of radiation necrosis <5 %. Smaller volumes (1–10 cm³) may receive up to 59 Gy; a single point of the brainstem (<1 cm³) can tolerate up to 64 Gy. These constraints are referred to conventional fractionation, whereas for single fraction treatments, brainstem may be irradiated to a maximum dose of 12.5 Gy, with a risk of necrosis <5 %. Higher doses (range, 15–20 Gy) have been tested with relatively low morbidity in patients with brainstem metastasis. However, these higher tolerance doses need to be confirmed before recommending them [22, 23].

Cognitive effects: Cognitive effects in adults are poorly defined. Patients given EBRT for high-grade gliomas receive high radiation doses and could be at greater risk of damage, but there is a paucity of information on neurocognitive deterioration, due to their extremely poor prognosis, which precludes long-term follow-up. More data come from prospective studies evaluating dose-response effect of EBRT in noncentral nervous system cancers, like nasopharyngeal carcinoma, or in patients with CNS leukemia or treated for low-grade gliomas. Exposure of some brain areas may correspond to a significantly greater incidence of complications. Temporal lobe radionecrosis can affect cognitive functions, such as visual memory (right lobe lesion) and verbal ability (left lobe lesion). Temporal lobe necrosis correlates with hypofractionated EBRT schedules. Deleterious effects are increased in patients receiving a mean dose greater than 36 Gy or in patients in whom the V60 of temporal lobes is greater than 10 % [24]. Based on clinical data related to unresectable cerebral arteriovenous malformations treated by radiosurgery, symptomatic complications depend strongly on the location of tissue-induced changes. Centrally located lesion had a higher incidence of side effects than peripheral malformations [25]. Moreover, it has been proven that some cognitive functions, such as memory, are more vulnerable to decline than others [26].

Cognitive changes have been reported in children after doses ≥18 Gy to the entire brain, and exposure of supratentorial brain seems to be related to a more significant cognitive decline [27]. However, other factors may well contribute to the development of this complication: absence from school, altered social environment, hospitalization, surgery, and chemotherapy [28].

On the contrary, the effect of irradiation on the cognitive deterioration in adults is less well established [21]. Radiation-induced neurologic toxicity was first reported in the eighties in patients cured of brain metastasis who had received whole-brain RT given in daily fractions of 3–6 Gy [29]. The effects of brain RT have been often investigated, but its role as a cause of cognitive disturbance is still controversial. Several studies described improvement in neurocognitive function after RT, due to the induced tumor shrinkage [30–32]; other studies have suggested subsequent long-term cognitive disability, especially when high fraction doses (>2 Gy) were used [33]. Two studies indicated that whole-brain irradiation is more damaging than partial brain irradiation, although the number of patients in both studies was small [34, 35]. These results were not confirmed by a recent randomized controlled trial comparing whole-brain RT plus stereotactic radiosurgery with stereotactic radiosurgery alone [36]. However, in this study, the assessment of neurologic function was obtained with less sensitive measures and the follow-up period was short.

There is paucity of robust information derived from studies of neurocognitive function in GBM patients, due to their short life expectancy.

Patients with GBM tend to have global cognitive deficits, because the tumor itself and its accompanying syndromes, such as brain edema, neurological symptoms, and psychiatric disturbances adversely affect neurocognitive function [37]. Several studies showed that a progressive decline in cognitive function and quality of life over time is the result of the natural history of disease and of age, comorbidities, and psychological distress [38–41]. Talacchi et al. [42] showed that verbal and visuospatial memory and word fluency were impaired by tumor and the related edema. In a phase-III trial, patients were randomly assigned to receive RT plus supportive care or supportive care alone. Neurocognitive function or the quality of life was not altered by the addition of RT [43]. However, if one admits that neurologic decline could be in part related to normal brain tissue irradiation, recent studies demonstrating IMRT superiority in limiting the dose to the noninvolved brain and optic pathways might be more clinically relevant [44].

To conclude, insufficient data are available to clearly suggest that brain RT by itself causes severe neurocognitive function damage in adults and there is a need for a perspective collection of data taking into account not only dose/volume parameters, but also age, comorbid conditions, tumor size, etc.

*Cranial nerves*: With radiosurgical procedures, cranial neuropathy has been related to a brainstem maximum dose of 16 Gy. Effects on the III–VI cranial nerves when the cavernous sinus is included in the treated area are often associated to temporal lobe necrosis for radiosurgical treatments in the dose range of 10–40 Gy [45].

*Hypothalamic–pituitary axis*: The damage to the hypothalamic–pituitary axis (HPA) might cause GH deficiency (often subclinical) for doses >30 Gy; the incidence substantially increases for higher radiation doses (30–50 Gy). Thyroid-stimulating hormone and ACTH deficiency occur unfrequently for doses >50 Gy (3–6 %). Gonadotrophin deficiency and hyperprolactinemia are rare; however, gonadotrophin, ACTH, and TSH deficiencies occur more frequently after treatment of nasopharyngeal cancer with doses in excess of 60 Gy, and following conventional radiotherapy (30–50 Gy) for pituitary tumors [46]. Radiation-associated hypopituitarism is accurately reported after radiotherapy for pituitary adenomas, due to its long-term surveillance. Doses of 45–55 Gy, conventionally fractionated, have been historically used to treat these benign tumors. Partial or panhypopituitarism incidence increases with time from RT and it is not related to the technique. In patients with a normal pituitary function before RT, multiple hormonal deficiencies may occur in 20–40 % of cases after 10 years of follow-up and, in a few reports, this percentage increases to about 80 % by 15 years [47, 48]. However, this slow increase in the rate of hypopituitarism with time in patients treated for pituitary adenomas should be considered as multifactorial.

*Spinal cord*: Considering the possible occurrence of severe irreversible RT-induced injury, constraints are necessarily conservative, but when radiotherapy is the only curative option, thorough discussion with the patient is needed to explain the competitive risks of having cord damage from radiation or from the disease itself, before obtaining her/his informed consent. With conventional fractionation (2 Gy daily, 5 days a week) a maximum cord dose of 46–50 Gy should be respected. Myelopathy risk rates are estimated at 0.2 %, 6 %, and 50 % for a total dose of 50 Gy, 60 Gy, and 69 Gy, respectively [49]. If hypofractionated schedules are used, spinal cord should receive a lower dose; a maximum cord dose of 13 Gy in a single fraction or of 20 Gy in three fractions is associated with a <1 % of risk of damage [49].

*Optic structures*: Dose to the optic chiasm and optic nerve should be ≤54 Gy, with conventional fractionation of 2 Gy/die. If an OAR is very small and therefore difficult to be contoured, like the optic chiasm, it should be considered a serial-like organ "by default" and consequently dose constraints are referred to the maximum absorbed dose. A maximum dose <12 Gy appears safe in single fraction treatment.

Emami et al. [8] reported a 5 % and a 50 % risk of blindness for 50 Gy and 65 Gy, respectively, but tolerance may be greater: a total dose of 55–60 Gy is actually considered associated with a 3–7 % rate of radiation-induced optic neuropathy and the risk becomes 8–20 % for doses >60 Gy (conventional fractionation) [50]. After an accurate evaluation of competitive risks, also in this case, as for spinal cord, the patient may consent to disregard constraints.

The dose constraint for the whole retina is ≤50 Gy, whereas for smaller volumes a dose ≤60 Gy is accepted [51]. Dose to lens should be ≤12 Gy. Lacrimal gland should not receive more than 50 Gy to prevent the risk of atrophy, resulting in *keratoconjunctivitis sicca*; doses greater than 60 Gy result in permanent loss of secretion [52].

*Inner ear*: Damage to the cochlea may determine sensorineural hearing loss, whereas dysfunction of Eustachian tube may cause otitis media and tinnitus. The mean dose limit for sensorineural hearing loss equals ≤45 Gy; to minimize damage, it is preferable to keep the mean dose limit <35 Gy. With single fraction radiosurgery, a dose limit of ≤14 Gy is recommended. Radiation otitis tolerance doses have been set at 40 Gy (acute toxicity) and 65 Gy (chronic toxicity) [53, 54].

*Special situations*: Re-irradiation is an aggressive salvage treatment option for recurrent disease. The risk of brain necrosis seems more related to the cumulative total dose than to the time interval between treatments [55].

Retreatments are considered relatively safe if a total dose of 100 Gy, conventionally fractionated (or a biologically equivalent dose) is not exceeded.

## Normal Tissue Complications Assessment and Reporting: The QUANTEC Lesson

*Focus on assessment.* As strongly suggested by the QUANTEC papers, quantification of normal tissue complications requires a detailed assessment and a validated scoring system. Several of such systems have been established: RTOG/EORTC (*Radiation Therapy and Oncology Group and European Organization for Research and Treatment of Cancer*); CTCAE (*Common Terminology Criteria for Adverse Effects, National Cancer Institute*); WHO (*World Health Organization*). All these classifications are comparable even if emphasizing different aspects of damage. The CTCAE is a descriptive medical language used for reporting and grading side effects, considering different degrees of severity [56]. Table 8.2 shows the CTCAE descriptors for brain toxicity as an example.

In addition, to evaluate and compare late toxicity of EBRT on normal tissues, the SOMA/LENT scoring system (*Late Effects in Normal Tissues Subjective, Objective, Management, and Analytic Scales*) has been designed and validated by the RTOG/EORTC. It is a subjective (patient perception of damage) and objective (clinical evidence) data recording, created to standardize the reporting of toxic effects during follow-up [57].

The QUANTEC "system" represents actually an evolution of all those scoring systems and the attempt of reinforcing the attitude of clinicians for the prospective collection of clinically meaningful toxicity data.

*Focus on reporting.* It is however difficult to draw robust conclusions regarding specific normal tissue complications by literature data, due to small number of patients included in most series and to the different standards adopted to report clinical results. The QUANTEC papers underline

**Table 8.2** CTCAE v.4: main nervous system disorders

| Adverse event | Grade | | | | |
| --- | --- | --- | --- | --- | --- |
| | 1 | 2 | 3 | 4 | 5 |
| Amnesia | Mild; transient memory loss | Moderate; short-term memory loss; limiting instrumental ADL | Severe; long-term memory loss; limiting self-care ADL | | |
| Central nervous system necrosis | Asymptomatic; clinical or diagnostic observations only; intervention not indicated | Moderate symptoms; corticosteroids indicated | Severe symptoms; medical intervention indicated | Life-threatening consequences; urgent intervention indicated | Death |
| Headache | Mild pain | Moderate pain; limiting instrumental ADL | Severe pain; limiting self-care ADL | | |
| Leukoencephalopathy | Asymptomatic; small focal T2/FLAIR hyperintensities[a] | Moderate symptoms; focal T2/FLAIR hyperintensities[b] | Severe symptoms; extensive T2/FLAIR hyperintensities[c] | Life-threatening consequences; extensive T2/FLAIR hyperintensities[d] | Death |
| Memory impairment | Mild memory impairment | Moderate memory impairment; limiting instrumental ADL | Severe memory impairment; limiting self-care ADL | | |
| Seizure | Brief partial seizure; no loss of consciousness | Brief generalized seizure | Multiple seizures despite medical intervention | Life-threatening; prolonged repetitive seizures | Death |
| Somnolence | Mild but more than usual drowsiness or sleepiness | Moderate sedation; limiting instrumental ADL | Obtundation or stupor | Life-threatening consequences; urgent intervention indicated | Death |
| Nerve disorder | Asymptomatic; clinical or diagnostic observations only; intervention not indicated | Moderate symptoms; limiting instrumental ADL | Severe symptoms; limiting self-care ADL | | |

*ADL* activities of daily living

[a]Involving periventricular white matter or <1/3 of susceptible areas of cerebrum ± mild increase in subarachnoid space (SAS) and/or mild ventriculomegaly

[b]Involving periventricular white matter extending into centrum semiovale or involving 1/3 to 2/3 of susceptible areas of cerebrum ± moderate increase in SAS and/or moderate ventriculomegaly

[c]Involving periventricular white matter involving 2/3 or more of susceptible areas of cerebrum ± moderate-to-severe increase in SAS and/or moderate-to-severe ventriculomegaly

[d]Involving periventricular white matter involving most of susceptible areas of cerebrum ± moderate-to-severe increase in SAS and/or moderate-to-severe ventriculomegaly

that a proper understanding of the *anatomical correlates* of damage is very important [58]; such an information should therefore be collected within the *large databases* needed to achieve a better understanding of dose-volume correlations. We will briefly analyze those two points as far as glioma treatment is concerned.

The OARs to be considered consists of several CNS (and not properly CNS) structures: brain, brainstem, spinal cord; optic nerves and chiasm; cochlea; eyes and lens; pituitary gland. Each structure is independent of each other and has a peculiar functional status.

Accurate organ/function definition is critical to define potential irradiation damage. The utility of *segmenting each single structure in subregions*—such as thalamus, hippocampus, Broca area—has not been quantitatively established, yet [21]; but surely a relationship between the site involved and the severity of damage has been proven, at least for the more eloquent parts of the brain.

In fact, recent advances in stem cell neurobiology suggest that adult neurogenesis persists in subventricular zone (adjacent to lateral ventricles) and subgranular zone (adjacent to hippocampus). Therefore, these regions are responsible for normal brain tissue repair. This evidence reinforces the idea that radiation-induced dysfunction may be highly dependent on the dose received by some anatomical sites, affecting physiological proliferation of neural stem cells [59]. The clinical consequences of this information are controversial, since it is debated whether the periventricular area and the hippocampus harbor also glioma stem cells (GSCs). Preclinical studies indicate that subventricular and subgranular zones are also associated with GSCs proliferation [60]. The possible role of cancer stem cells in gliomagenesis implies several considerations. Because of their proven radio- and chemoresistance [61], GSCs may be involved in tumor progression and late recurrence. Evers et al. [62] showed that irradiation of the bilateral subventricular zones with a mean dose >43 Gy may lead to a progression-free survival advantage (15 versus 7.2 months; $p = 0.028$). Considering all the limitations of

this study—retrospective analysis, lack of O6-methylguanine-DNA-methyltransferase (MGMT) promoter methylation data, heterogeneity of salvage treatment—a prospective evaluation of this hypothesis is needed to definitely prove the clinical benefit.

Although anatomically distinct functional areas are generally not considered in the treatment planning process [21], the role of hippocampus and associated limbic system in memory formation has recently been emphasized, encouraging clinicians to spare these structures during brain irradiation [63, 64]. With improvement in radiation techniques, it is possible to minimize dose in uninvolved brain regions and it may contribute to preserve neurocognitive function, but there are several ethical controversies in terms of cost-effectiveness analysis. It is not clear, however, whether very costly RT technique can nowadays be considered a standard for these patients, since robust data are missing and results are usually hampered by their very gloomy prognosis [64].

The other main research priority raised by the QUANTEC papers is the *collection of large multi-institutional databases*. For the sake of clarity, we will directly quote the claim of the QUANTEC Authors for the adoption of a "data pooling" culture: "*Clinical studies of the dependence of normal tissue response on dose-volume factors are often confusingly inconsistent, as the QUANTEC reviews demonstrate. A key opportunity to accelerate progress is to begin storing high-quality datasets in repositories. Using available technology, multiple repositories could be conveniently queried, without divulging protected health information, to identify relevant sources of data for further analysis. After obtaining institutional approvals, data could then be pooled, greatly enhancing the capability to construct predictive models that are more widely applicable and better powered to accurately identify key predictive factors (whether dosimetric, image-based, clinical, socioeconomic, or biological). Data pooling has already been carried out effectively in a few normal tissue complication probability studies and should become a common strategy*" [65].

The collection of homogeneous data, based on standardization of reporting results, will probably be one of the most important steps also in GBM management [58]. The efforts spent in analytically contouring the different brain areas would hopefully populate large databases including individual patient-standardized data on volumes and subvolumes, absorbed doses to the different OARs and ROI, and clinical correlates. This could ultimately lead to a comprehensive understanding of dose-effect correlations easily applicable to the individual case.

## Overview

Although severe toxicity is uncommon with modern EBRT technique, functional deficits are increasingly studied, since they significantly impact on patient's quality of life. As patients with brain tumor survive longer, attention has focused on these issues and more accurate studies begin to be available. The QUANTEC review is an important critical collection of data, seminal to the development of any future effort to ameliorate the cost/benefit ratio for the treatment of gliomas (and other tumor types). To improve reliability and test the clinical utility of predictive models, good clinical prospective data must be collected. Multicenter studies and large databases are needed to ameliorate the knowledge of treatment tolerance, with the aim to achieve improved local control without compromising a better quality of life.

## References

1. Haberer S, Assouline A, Mazeron JJ. Normal tissue tolerance to external beam radiation therapy: brain and hypophysis. Cancer Radiother. 2010;14(4–5):263–8.
2. Marks LB, Ten Haken RK, Martel MK. Guest editor's introduction to QUANTEC: a user's guide. Int J Radiat Oncol Biol Phys. 2010;76(3 Suppl):S1–2.
3. Withers HR, Taylor JM, Maciejewski B. Treatment volume and tissue tolerance. Int J Radiat Oncol Biol Phys. 1988;14(4):751–9.
4. De Luca P, Jones D, Gahbauer R, Whitmore G, Wambersie A. The ICRU Report 83: prescribing, recording and reporting photon-beam intensity-modulated radiation therapy (IMRT). J ICRU. 2010;10(1):41–53.
5. Lyman JT. Complication probability as assessed from dose-volume histograms. Radiat Res Suppl. 1985; 8:S13–9.
6. Burman C, Kutcher GJ, Emami B, Goitein M. Fitting of normal tissue tolerance data to an analytic function. Int J Radiat Oncol Biol Phys. 1991;21(1):123–35.
7. Kutcher GJ, Burman C, Brewster L, Goitein M, Mohan R. Histogram reduction method for calculating complication probabilities for three-dimensional treatment planning evaluations. Int J Radiat Oncol Biol Phys. 1991;21(1):137–46.
8. Emami B, Lyman J, Brown A, Coia L, Goitein M, Munzenrider JE, Shank B, Solin LJ, Wesson M. Tolerance of normal tissue to therapeutic irradiation. Int J Radiat Oncol Biol Phys. 1991;21(1):109–22.
9. Niemierko A. Reporting and analyzing dose distributions: a concept of equivalent uniform dose. Med Phys. 1997;24(1):103–10.
10. Laack NN, Brown PD. Cognitive sequelae of brain radiation in adults. Semin Oncol. 2004;31(5):702–13.
11. Belka C, Budach W, Kortmann RD, Bamberg M. Radiation induced CNS toxicity—molecular and cellular mechanisms. Br J Cancer. 2001;85(9):1233–9.
12. Kim JH, Brown SL, Jenrow KA, Ryu S. Mechanisms of radiation-induced brain toxicity and implications for future clinical trials. J Neurooncol. 2008; 87(3):279–86.
13. Galldiks N, Rapp M, Stoffels G, Dunkl V, Sabel M, Langen KJ. Earlier diagnosis of progressive disease during bevacizumab treatment using O-(2-18F-fluoroethyl)-L-tyrosine positron emission tomography in comparison with magnetic resonance imaging. Mol Imaging. 2013;12(5):273–6.
14. Monje ML, Palmer T. Radiation injury and neurogenesis. Curr Opin Neurol. 2003;16(2):129–34.
15. Wu Q, Mohan R, Niemierko A, Schmidt-Ullrich R. Optimization of intensity-modulated radiotherapy plans based on the equivalent uniform dose. Int J Radiat Oncol Biol Phys. 2002;52(1):224–35.
16. Deasy JO, Moiseenko V, Marks L, Chao KS, Nam J, Eisbruch A. Radiotherapy dose-volume effects on salivary gland function. Int J Radiat Oncol Biol Phys. 2010;76(3 Suppl):S58–63.
17. Bentzen SM, Constine LS, Deasy JO, Eisbruch A, Jackson A, Marks LB, Ten Haken RK, Yorke ED. Quantitative Analyses of Normal Tissue Effects in the Clinic (QUANTEC): an introduction to the scientific issues. Int J Radiat Oncol Biol Phys. 2010;76(3 Suppl):S3–9.
18. Marks LB, Yorke ED, Jackson A, Ten Haken RK, Constine LS, Eisbruch A, Bentzen SM, Nam J, Deasy JO. Use of normal tissue complication probability models in the clinic. Int J Radiat Oncol Biol Phys. 2010;76(3 Suppl):S10–9.
19. Lee AW, Kwong DL, Leung SF, Tung SY, Sze WM, Sham JS, Teo PM, Leung TW, Wu PM, Chappell R, Peters LJ, Fowler JF. Factors affecting risk of symptomatic temporal lobe necrosis: significance of fractional

dose and treatment time. Int J Radiat Oncol Biol Phys. 2002;53(1):75–85.

20. Voges J, Treuer H, Sturm V, Büchner C, Lehrke R, Kocher M, Staar S, Kuchta J, Müller RP. Risk analysis of linear accelerator radiosurgery. Int J Radiat Oncol Biol Phys. 1996;36(5):1055–63.

21. Lawrence YR, Li XA, el Naqa I, Hahn CA, Marks LB, Merchant TE, Dicker AP. Radiation dose-volume effects in the brain. Int J Radiat Oncol Biol Phys. 2010;76(3 Suppl):S20–7.

22. Mayo C, Yorke E, Merchant TE. Radiation associated brainstem injury. Int J Radiat Oncol Biol Phys. 2010;76(3 Suppl):S36–41.

23. Kased N, Huang K, Nakamura JL, Sahgal A, Larson DA, McDermott MW, Sneed PK. Gamma knife radiosurgery for brainstem metastases: the UCSF experience. J Neurooncol. 2008;86(2):195–205.

24. Hsiao KY, Yeh SA, Chang CC, Tsai PC, Wu JM, Gau JS. Cognitive function before and after intensity-modulated radiation therapy in patients with nasopharyngeal carcinoma: a prospective study. Int J Radiat Oncol Biol Phys. 2010;77(3):722–6.

25. Karlsson B, Lax I, Söderman M. Factors influencing the risk for complications following Gamma Knife radiosurgery of cerebral arteriovenous malformations. Radiother Oncol. 1997;43(3):275–80.

26. Roman DD, Sperduto PW. Neuropsychological effects of cranial radiation: current knowledge and future directions. Int J Radiat Oncol Biol Phys. 1995;31(4):983–98.

27. Merchant TE, Kiehna EN, Li C, Shukla H, Sengupta S, Xiong X, Gajjar A, Mulhern RK. Modeling radiation dosimetry to predict cognitive outcomes in pediatric patients with CNS embryonal tumors including medulloblastoma. Int J Radiat Oncol Biol Phys. 2006;65(1):210–21.

28. Willard VW, Conklin HM, Wu S, Merchant TE. Prospective longitudinal evaluation of emotional and behavioral functioning in pediatric patients with low-grade glioma treated with conformal radiation therapy. J Neurooncol. 2015;122(1):161–8.

29. DeAngelis LM, Delattre JY, Posner JB. Radiation-induced dementia in patients cured of brain metastases. Neurology. 1989;39(6):789–96.

30. Steinvorth S, Wenz F, Wildermuth S, Essig M, Fuss M, Lohr F, Debus J, Wannenmacher M, Hacke W. Cognitive function in patients with cerebral arteriovenous malformations after radiosurgery: prospective long-term follow-up. Int J Radiat Oncol Biol Phys. 2002;54(5):1430–7.

31. Li J, Bentzen SM, Renschler M, Mehta MP. Regression after whole-brain radiation therapy for brain metastases correlates with survival and improved neurocognitive function. J Clin Oncol. 2007;25(10):1260–6.

32. Khuntia D, Brown P, Li J, Mehta MP. Whole-brain radiotherapy in the management of brain metastasis. J Clin Oncol. 2006;24(8):1295–304.

33. Klein M, Heimans JJ, Aaronson NK, van der Ploeg HM, Grit J, Muller M, Postma TJ, Mooij JJ, Boerman RH, Beute GN, Ossenkoppele GJ, van Imhoff GW, Dekker AW, Jolles J, Slotman BJ, Struikmans H, Taphoorn MJ. Effect of radiotherapy and other treatment-related factors on mid-term to long-term cognitive sequelae in low-grade gliomas: a comparative study. Lancet. 2002;360(9343):1361–8.

34. Kleinberg L, Wallner K, Malkin MG. Good performance status of long-term disease-free survivors of intracranial gliomas. Int J Radiat Oncol Biol Phys. 1993;26(1):129–33.

35. Gregor A, Cull A, Traynor E, Stewart M, Lander F, Love S. Neuropsychometric evaluation of long-term survivors of adult brain tumours: relationship with tumour and treatment parameters. Radiother Oncol. 1996;41(1):55–9.

36. Aoyama H, Shirato H, Tago M, Nakagawa K, Toyoda T, Hatano K, Kenjyo M, Oya N, Hirota S, Shioura H, Kunieda E, Inomata T, Hayakawa K, Katoh N, Kobashi G. Stereotactic radiosurgery plus whole-brain radiation therapy vs stereotactic radiosurgery alone for treatment of brain metastases: a randomized controlled trial. JAMA. 2006;295(21):2483–91.

37. Henriksson R, Asklund T, Poulsen HS. Impact of therapy on quality of life, neurocognitive function and their correlates in glioblastoma multiforme: a review. J Neurooncol. 2011;104(3):639–46.

38. Corn BW, Wang M, Fox S, Michalski J, Purdy J, Simpson J, Kresl J, Curran Jr WJ, Diaz A, Mehta M, Movsas B. Health related quality of life and cognitive status in patients with glioblastoma multiforme receiving escalating doses of conformal three dimensional radiation on RTOG 98-03. J Neurooncol. 2009;95(2):247–57.

39. Veilleux N, Goffaux P, Boudrias M, Mathieu D, Daigle K, Fortin D. Quality of life in neurooncology—age matters. J Neurosurg. 2010;113(2):325–32.

40. Klein M, Taphoorn MJ, Heimans JJ, van der Ploeg HM, Vandertop WP, Smit EF, Leenstra S, Tulleken CA, Boogerd W, Belderbos JS, Cleijne W, Aaronson NK. Neurobehavioral status and health-related quality of life in newly diagnosed high-grade glioma patients. J Clin Oncol. 2001;19(20):4037–47.

41. Yung WK, Albright RE, Olson J, Fredericks R, Fink K, Prados MD, Brada M, Spence A, Hohl RJ, Shapiro W, Glantz M, Greenberg H, Selker RG, Vick NA, Rampling R, Friedman H, Phillips P, Bruner J, Yue N, Osoba D, Zaknoen S, Levin VA. A phase II study of temozolomide vs. procarbazine in patients with glioblastoma multiforme at first relapse. Br J Cancer. 2000;83(5):588–93.

42. Talacchi A, Santini B, Savazzi S, Gerosa M. Cognitive effects of tumour and surgical treatment in glioma patients. J Neurooncol. 2011;103(3):541–9.

43. Keime-Guibert F, Chinot O, Taillandier L, Cartalat-Carel S, Frenay M, Kantor G, Guillamo JS, Jadaud E, Colin P, Bondiau PY, Meneï P, Loiseau H, Bernier V, Honnorat J, Barrié M, Mokhtari K, Mazeron JJ, Bissery A, Delattre JY, Association of French-Speaking Neuro-Oncologists. Radiotherapy for

glioblastoma in the elderly. N Engl J Med. 2007; 356(15):1527–35.

44. Aherne NJ, Benjamin LC, Horsley PJ, Silva T, Wilcox S, Amalaseelan J, Dwyer P, Tahir AM, Hill J, Last A, Hansen C, McLachlan CS, Lee YL, McKay MJ, Shakespeare TP. Improved outcomes with intensity modulated radiation therapy combined with temozolomide for newly diagnosed glioblastoma multiforme. Neurol Res Int. 2014;2014:945620.

45. Tishler RB, Loeffler JS, Lunsford LD, Duma C, Alexander 3rd E, Kooy HM, Flickinger JC. Tolerance of cranial nerves of the cavernous sinus to radiosurgery. Int J Radiat Oncol Biol Phys. 1993;27(2):215–21.

46. Darzy KH, Shalet SM. Hypopituitarism following radiotherapy. Pituitary. 2009;12(1):40–50.

47. Brada M, Ajithkumar TV, Minniti G. Radiosurgery for pituitary adenomas. Clin Endocrinol (Oxf). 2004;61(5):531–43.

48. Loeffler JS, Shih HA. Radiation therapy in the management of pituitary adenomas. J Clin Endocrinol Metab. 2011;96(7):1992–2003.

49. Kirkpatrick JP, van der Kogel AJ, Schultheiss TE. Radiation dose-volume effects in the spinal cord. Int J Radiat Oncol Biol Phys. 2010;76(3 Suppl):S42–9.

50. Mayo C, Martel MK, Marks LB, Flickinger J, Nam J, Kirkpatrick J. Radiation dose-volume effects of optic nerves and chiasm. Int J Radiat Oncol Biol Phys. 2010;76(3 Suppl):S28–35.

51. Monroe AT, Bhandare N, Morris CG, Mendenhall WM. Preventing radiation retinopathy with hyperfractionation. Int J Radiat Oncol Biol Phys. 2005;61(3):856–64.

52. Gordon KB, Char DH, Sagerman RH. Late effects of radiation on the eye and ocular adnexa. Int J Radiat Oncol Biol Phys. 1995;31(5):1123–39.

53. Chen WC, Jackson A, Budnick AS, Pfister DG, Kraus DH, Hunt MA, Stambuk H, Levegrun S, Wolden SL. Sensorineural hearing loss in combined modality treatment of nasopharyngeal carcinoma. Cancer. 2006;106(4):820–9.

54. Jereczek-Fossa BA, Zarowski A, Milani F, Orecchia R. Radiotherapy-induced ear toxicity. Cancer Treat Rev. 2003;29(5):417–30.

55. Mayer R, Sminia P. Reirradiation tolerance of the human brain. Int J Radiat Oncol Biol Phys. 2008;70(5):1350–60.

56. National Cancer Institute. Common terminology criteria for adverse events v4.0. http://evs.nci.nih.gov/ ftp1/CTCAE/CTCAE_4.03_2010-06-14_ QuickReference_5x7.pdf. Accessed 14 June 2010.

57. Pavy JJ, Denekamp J, Letschert J, Littbrand B, Mornex F, Bernier J, Gonzales-Gonzales D, Horiot JC, Bolla M, Bartelink H, EORTC Late Effects Working Group. Late effects toxicity scoring: the SOMA scale. Int J Radiat Oncol Biol Phys. 1995;31(5):1043–7.

58. Jackson A, Marks LB, Bentzen SM, Eisbruch A, Yorke ED, Ten Haken RK, Constine LS, Deasy JO. The lessons of QUANTEC: recommendations for reporting and gathering data on dose-volume dependencies of treatment outcome. Int J Radiat Oncol Biol Phys. 2010;76(3 Suppl):S155–60.

59. Barani IJ, Benedict SH, Lin PS. Neural stem cells: implications for the conventional radiotherapy of central nervous system malignancies. Int J Radiat Oncol Biol Phys. 2007;68(2):324–33.

60. Llaguno SA, Chen J, Kwon CH, Parada LF. Neural and cancer stem cells in tumor suppressor mouse models of malignant astrocytoma. Cold Spring Harb Symp Quant Biol. 2008;73:421–6.

61. Bao S, Wu Q, McLendon RE, Hao Y, Shi Q, Hjelmeland AB, Dewhirst MW, Bigner DD, Rich JN. Glioma stem cells promote radioresistance by preferential activation of the DNA damage response. Nature. 2006;444(7120):756–60.

62. Evers P, Lee PP, DeMarco J, Agazaryan N, Sayre JW, Selch M, Pajonk F. Irradiation of the potential cancer stem cell niches in the adult brain improves progression-free survival of patients with malignant glioma. BMC Cancer. 2010;10:384.

63. Kazda T, Jancalek R, Pospisil P, Sevela O, Prochazka T, Vrzal M, Burkon P, Slavik M, Hynkova L, Slampa P, Laack NN. Why and how to spare the hippocampus during brain radiotherapy: the developing role of hippocampal avoidance in cranial radiotherapy. Radiat Oncol. 2014;9:139.

64. Suh JH. Hippocampal avoidance whole-brain radiation therapy: a new standard for patients with brain metastases? J Clin Oncol. 2014;34:3789.

65. Deasy JO, Bentzen S, Jackson A, Ten Haken RD, Yorke ED, Constine LS, Sharma A, Marks LB. Improving normal tissue complication probability models: the need to adopt a "data-pooling" culture. Int J Radiat Oncol Biol Phys. 2010;76(3 Suppl):S151–4.

# Basic Knowledge of Glioblastoma Radiobiology

**9**

Monica Mangoni, Mariangela Sottili, Chiara Gerini, and Lorenzo Livi

## Introduction

Glioblastoma (GBM) is radioresistant tumors with an infaust prognosis. Local disease control is the main intent of treatment because of the high incidence of recurrence. Radiotherapy post surgical resection is the mainstay of the management of GBM; however, high dose treatments fail to improve survival. The addiction of temozolomide results in a statistically significant survival benefit [1].

Clinical research has been very active for 30 years, and has explored all the concepts developed in the laboratories of radiobiology. GBM is characterized by infiltrative growth and presence of central hypoxic regions. Main actors of invasion, angiogenesis, immune response, microenvironment, and cancer stem cells cooperate for chemo- and radioresistance. Moreover, interpatient and intratumor heterogeneity of tumor cells are responsible to heterogeneity of sensitivity to ionizing radiation (IR). Therefore, an improvement in our understanding of GBM radiobiology is necessary to give targets to clinical research.

M. Mangoni (✉) • M. Sottili • C. Gerini • L. Livi
Radiotherapy Unit, Department of Experimental and Clinical Biomedical Sciences, University of Florence, Largo Brambilla 3, 50134 Firenze, Italy
e-mail: monica.mangoni@unifi.it

## Basis of Radioresistance

### DNA Damage Response

Ionizing radiation can induce base damage, single-strand breaks, double-strand breaks (DSBs), sugar damage, and DNA–DNA and DNA–protein cross-links. DSBs are the most important damages as they are harder to repair than other DNA lesions. Mammalian cells have developed specialized pathways to sense, respond to, and repair these different types of damage. The DNA damage response (DDR) is a complex and coordinated system that determines the cellular outcome of DNA damage caused by radiation.

The DDR is not a single pathway, but rather a group of highly interrelated signaling pathways, each of which controls different effects on the cell. One of the earliest events known to occur in the DDR is the phosphorylation of a protein called histone H2AX. This phosphorylated form, known as gammaH2AX, is necessary for the recruitment of many of the other proteins involved in the DDR. Three related kinases have been shown to be able to phosphorylate H2AX at sites of DSBs: (1) ATM (ataxia telangiectasia mutated protein)/MRN; (2) DNA-PKcs-KU; (3) ATR-ATRIP. The phosphorylation occurs primarily by ATM. Activation of ATM, DNA-PKcs, and ATR leads to the phosphorylation not only of H2AX, but also of many other cellular proteins. Recent studies have shown that as many as 700 proteins are substrates for the ATM kinases in response to DNA damage [2]. Phosphorylation of these proteins acts as the signals to activate the various different downstream effectors of the DDR that are DNA repair, cell cycle checkpoints, and apoptosis (Fig. 9.1).

## ATM

ATM is a key DDR component and plays a central role in DSB repair and cell cycle checkpoints [3]. Following DNA damage, activation of ATM after irradiation can lead either directly to cell death (by phosphorylation of p53) or to a block in proliferation (by phosphorylation of p53 and the Chk1/2 kinases).

ATM status has been associated with intrinsic radiosensitivity [4]. ATM protein expression was correlated with radioresistance in primary glioblastoma cells in culture [5]. Increased radioresistance to X-rays as well as to carbon ions was observed in GBM cells exhibiting high levels of chromosomal instability and impaired ATM signaling. These results indicate the existence of highly radioresistant GBM cells, characterized by dysfunctional ATM signaling and high levels of intrinsic chromosomal instability [6]. Several studies demonstrated that inhibition of ATM kinase produced potent radiosensitization of GBM cells and of GBM cancer stem cells (CSCs) and effectively abrogated the enhanced DSB repair proficiency observed in GBM CSCs [7–9].

## DSB Pathways

There are two major DSB pathways engaged during DNA repair: nonhomologous end joining (NHEJ) and homologous recombination (HR).

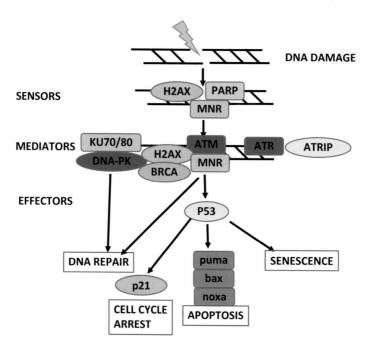

**Fig. 9.1** DNA damage response (DDR). The DDR is a complex and coordinated system that determines the cellular outcome of DNA damage caused by radiation. It is a group of highly interrelated signaling pathways, each of which controls different effects on the cell. Activation of ATM, DNA-PKcs, and ATR leads to the phosphorylation of H2AX and of many other cellular proteins that act as the signals to activate the various different downstream effectors of the DDR (apoptosis, cell cycle checkpoints, and DNA repair)

NHEJ is considered the major pathway for DSB repair and is initiated predominantly during the G1-phase of the cell cycle. NHEJ adheres broken DNA ends by ligases and excision repair enzymes. HR occurs during late S- and G2-phases and is an error-free method of repair using sister chromatids as templates to replace damaged DNA [10].

Cancer cells have enhanced DNA repair pathways than normal cells. A microarray analysis of temporal gene responses to ionizing radiation in glioblastoma cell lines showed upregulation of DNA repair genes. These genes included G22P1 (Ku70) and XRCC5 (Ku80) gene, known as important members of the NHEJ pathway [11]. Glioma stem cells contribute to radioresistance through preferential activation of the DNA damage checkpoint response and an increase in DNA repair capacity [12]. Glioma-initiating cells have a restricted DSB repair pathway involving predominantly HR associated with a lack of functional G1/S checkpoint arrest. This unusual behavior leads to less efficient NHEJ repair and overall slower DNA DSB repair kinetics. HR and cell cycle checkpoint abnormalities may contribute to the radioresistance of glioma-initiating cells [10, 13].

Spermidine/spermine-N1-acetyltransferase 1 (SAT1) is overexpressed almost uniformly in GBM tumor samples compared with normal brain. SAT1 catalyzes the acetylation of polyamines spermidine and spermine to form acetyl derivatives. Polyamine acetylation by SAT1 has a role in DSB repair through alteration of chromatin, and thereby contributes to radiation resistance. SAT1 increases acetylation of histone H3, increasing BRCA1 expression, and allowing activation of the HR pathway to repair DNA damage [14].

## P53

P53 is a tumor suppressor gene phosphorylated by ATM following DNA damage. P53 plays a major role in regulation of cellular stress responses. P53 regulates genes that control both programmed cell death through apoptosis and cell cycle checkpoints with delays in the movement of cells through the G1-, S-, and G2-phases of the cell cycle.

In nonmalignant cells, the p53 protein has a short half-life time and is expressed at low levels. After neoplastic transformation, the function of p53 is often altered or impaired due to mutations. Mutations in tumor suppressor p53 are the most common abnormality in GBM and play a complex role in promoting tumor formation [15, 16]. Different forms of p53 status in GBM cell lines (wildtype, mutant, abrogated, and null) have been correlated with radiation response [4, 17] and radiosensitivity [4].

## Cell Cycle Checkpoints

Cell cycle checkpoints are mechanisms that control the progression of the cell through the cell cycle. When defects on DNA replication or chromosome segregation are sensed, cell cycle checkpoints induce a cell cycle arrest until the defects are repaired. The main mechanisms of action of the cell cycle checkpoints are mediated by a family of protein kinases known as the cyclin-dependent kinases (CDKs), that form with cyclins specific cyclin-CDK complexes. These complexes activate different downstream targets to promote or prevent cell cycle progression [18]. There are three checkpoints: the G1 checkpoint, the G2/M checkpoint, and the metaphase checkpoint.

After exposure to IR, mammalian cells are arrested at G1 checkpoint and at G2/M checkpoint.

The halt at G1 checkpoint is regulated by p53 and is associated with upregulation of p21 which inhibits cell CDK2/Cyclin-E [19]. The halt at G2/M checkpoint is associated with activation of Chk1 and Chk2 checkpoint kinases which may phosphorylate Cdc25C to inhibit Cdc2/Cyclin-B and prevent entry into mitosis [20]. After irradiation, normal cell shows increased level of p53 and p21 expression.

GBM frequently loses the normal regulation of cell cycle progression. Homozygote loss or methylation of Retinoblastoma 1 (RB1) are among the most frequent alterations [14]. In different GBM cell lines, G1 arrest appears less pronounced or absent compared to normal cells and G2/M arrest plays a major role. This behavior can be due to impairment of p53 and other check-points related genes [21]. There is a correlation between G2/M block and radiosensitivity in some tumor cell lines. GBM cell lines harboring wild-type p53 show both G1 and G2/M blocks to limited degree, yielding a large amount of cell death. P53 null GBM cell lines demonstrate prominent G2/m block which may be responsible for the marked radioresistance [21].

After high LET irradiation, both wild-type p53 and null p53 GBM cell lines showed high yield of apoptosis. After high LET irradiation, p53 and G1 block seem to be less important to the yield of apoptosis, in contrast there is a marked G2/M block. These observations may indicate that high LET irradiation and molecular targeting focuses on modulation of G2/M checkpoint can increase radiosensitivity in GBM [21].

## Phosphatidylinositol 3-Kinase (PI3K)/ Akt Pathway

Phosphatidylinositol-3-kinases are a family of related intracellular signal transducer enzymes involved in important cellular functions such as cell growth, proliferation, differentiation, motility, survival, and intracellular trafficking (Fig. 9.2). PI 3-kinases are able to activate AKT (or protein kinase B-PKB), a protein kinase that plays a key role in multiple cellular processes such as glucose metabolism, apoptosis, cell proliferation, transcription, and cell migration. The PI3K/AKT pathway regulates mammalian target of rapamycin (mTOR) signaling pathway that serves as a central regulator of cell metabolism, growth, proliferation, and survival.

Several cancers show mutations of PI3K that cause a major activation of the kinase. Phosphatase and tensin homolog (PTEN) negatively regulates intracellular levels of phosphatidylinositol-3,4,5-trisphosphate in cells and functions as a tumor suppressor by negatively regulating Akt signaling pathway. The pathway is antagonized also by glycogen synthase kinase-3beta (GSK-3B).

Signaling through the PI3K/Akt survival pathway either induced by IR or due to constitutive activation of this pathway can play an important role in mediating resistance of cancer cells to radiotherapy. This PI3K/Akt medi-

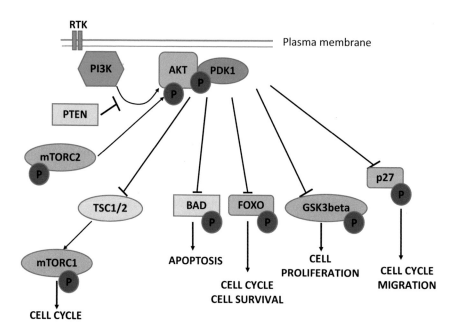

**Fig. 9.2** Phosphatidylinositol 3-kinase (PI3K)/Akt pathway. PI 3-kinases are able to activate AKT and the PI3K/AKT pathway regulates mTOR signaling pathway that serves as a central regulator of cell metabolism, growth, proliferation, and survival. PTEN negatively regulates intracellular levels of PI3K in cells and functions as a tumor suppressor by negatively regulating Akt signaling pathway

ated radioresistance has been demonstrated to be primarily due to induction of the repair of radiation-induced DNA-DSB most likely through the interaction of PI3K/Akt signaling with DNA-PKcs, a major enzyme of the NHEJ repair pathway [22]. DNA-PKcs moreover directly interacts the X-ray repair cross-complementing group 1 protein (XRCC1) involved in base excision repair (BER). Through stimulation of the PI3K/Akt pathway ionizing radiation can mediate phosphorylation of DNA-PKcs [23]. Deregulation of the phosphatidylinositol 3-kinase (PI3K)/Akt pathway is a frequent occurrence in GBM. Activation of the PI3K-Akt pathway results in disturbance of control of cell growth and cell survival, which contributes to a competitive growth advantage, metastatic competence as well as to therapy resistance [24]. Moreover, irradiation induces Akt activation in GBM cells and increases radioresistance, thus Akt may be a central player in a feedback loop [25]. Li et al. showed that inhibition of PI3K activation with specific inhibitors, or with inducible wild-type PTEN, inhibition of EGFR, as well as direct inhibition of Akt with Akt inhibitors during irradiation increased the radiosensitivity of GBM cells [25].

## Phosphatase and Tensin Homolog

PTEN is involved in regulating the PI3K/AKT/mTOR signaling pathway with a role in cell metabolism and in migration. In GBM are observed mutation, deletions or epigenetic silencing of PTEN [14] and are associated with poor patient survival [26]. Inactive PTEN leads to AKT hyperactivation, which in turn triggers cellular growth (through mTOR) and proliferation (through inhibition of GSK3-B) [26].

## Glycogen Synthase Kinase-3beta (GSK-3B)

GSK-3B is a protein kinase that acts as a regulator of cellular processes such as proliferation, migration, and invasion [27] GSK-3B phosphor-

ylates a multitude of metabolic and signaling proteins important for cell function, including acetyl-coenzyme-A carboxylase, cyclic adenosine monophosphate (AMP)-dependent protein kinase and pyruvate dehydrogenase. GSK-3B also controls the intracellular localization and degradation of cyclin D1 and beta-catenin [28]. GSK-3B is expressed in all tissues, but its highest expression is in the developing brain.

GSK-3B is implicated in various diseases including cancer. In glioblastoma, GSK-3B sustains invasion via the focal adhesion kinase, Rac1 and c-Jun N-terminal kinase-mediated pathway [29]. When its activation is dysregulated, GSK-3B is responsible of altered proliferation, migration, invasion, and maintenance of a stem cell-like cell fraction [28].

## Cell Death

Cell death is associated with several distinct morphologic processes named apoptosis, autophagic cell death, necrosis, and senescence. The pathways that control different kind of death are differentially activated in different tissues and are frequently altered in cancer.

Apoptosis is the so-called "type-I cell death." Apoptosis is a caspase-dependent programmed cell death that is morphologically characterized by chromatin condensation and nuclear fragmentation. Apoptosis is an important cellular defense against cancer development and loss of apoptotic sensitivity is recognized as an essential hallmark of cancer.

Autophagic cell death is the so-called "type-II cell death." Autophagy is considered to be an alternative mode of programmed cell death, which is characterized by increased number of autophagosomes in the cytoplasm [30] (Fig. 9.3). Autophagy means "self eating" and describes a process of digestion of part of the cell cytoplasm to remove superfluous or damaged organelles and to produce energy. The autophagosomes are double membrane structures that grow and inglobe part of cytoplasm, giving the cell a vacuolated appearance. The fusion of autophagosomes and lysosomes gives autolysosomes that are single

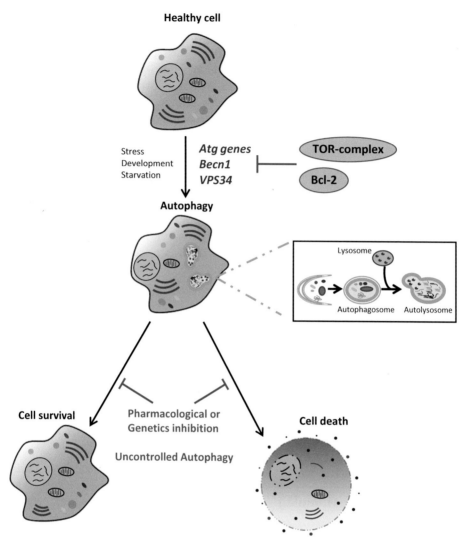

**Fig. 9.3** Autophagy. Autophagy is a cellular self-digestion mediated by fusion of autophagosomes with lysosomes. The mechanism of autophagy is highly regulated. ATG5/ATG7, Becn1, and VPS34 are some of the most important involved genes. The PI3K/AKT/mTOR exert an inhibitory control on autophagy. A complex regulatory network determines the cell fate between cell survival, by suppression of apoptosis, and cell death, either in collaboration with apoptosis or as a backup mechanism when apoptosis is defective

membrane that contains degenerating organelles that undergo degradation through the process of autophagy [31]. Autophagy is controlled by Atg proteins that initiate the production of the double membrane vesicles and it is activated in response to growth factors or nutrients depletion. mTOR is a sensor of the nutrition state of the cell and the pathway PI3K/AKT/mTOR has an important regulatory role in autophagy [32, 33]. Thus autophagy manifests a protective role in stressful conditions and might be involved in preventing several human diseases, such as cancer, some types of neurodegeneration, and muscular disorders [34]. These metabolic features make autophagy an effective mechanism for cell survival, but several evidences suggested that the stress-induced exacerbation of this process may also lead to a pro-death shift of the cellular fate [35, 36]. Thus in some cellular settings, autophagy can serve as a cell survival pathway, suppressing apoptosis, and in others, it can lead to death, either in collaboration with apoptosis or as a backup mechanism when apoptosis is defective [32]. In some cases, autophagy can act as tumor suppressor, and autophagy has been observed after some anticancer treatments as IR.

Necrosis is a passive form of unregulated process of cell destruction presenting marked cell swelling followed by release of intracellular components. Necrosis is observed also in tumors and can be induced by DNA-damaging treatments, including irradiation.

Senescence is a replicative death associated with the aging and observed when over time cells lose their ability to divide. Senescence is correlated with the shortening of telomeres at the ends of chromosomes. Senescence can be observed also after cell stress such as irradiation when cell enters a permanent cycle arrest (G0). This arrest may be associated with chromatin changes and morphological alteration of cytoplasm and granularity.

After irradiation, cell death can occur rapidly, within hours after irradiation, before cells reach the first mitosis. This type of death is called "interphase death" and is seen in a small minority of cell types, generally high proliferating cells and few kinds of tumors.

The majority of proliferating normal and tumor cells die at a relatively long time after irradiation, when cells attempt to divide. This is called reproductive or mitotic death and usually occurs some mitosis after the irradiation. The DDR repairs much of the initial radiation-induced damage, but is unable to completely restore the normal genome and cell eventually dies. The mitotic catastrophe prevents cells from aneuploidization [37]. Cells that experience catastrophic mitosis can die by apoptosis, autophagy, necrosis, or senescence.

In malignant brain tumors cell lines, it has been reported that rapid apoptosis is unlikely to occur after gamma irradiation [38]. GBM cells are resistant to apoptotic stimuli and thus to radiotherapy and conventional chemotherapy, because of the constitutive activation of several intracellular signaling pathways, such as PI3K, AKT, and mTOR [39]. Moreover, mutations in

GBMs often inactivate the apoptotic pathway, thus malignant glioblastomas are likely to be more sensitive to autophagic cell death as an alternative response to therapeutics [40].

Based on these findings, it is becoming clear that apoptosis does not play a significant role in the killing of GBM cells after IR at least with low-LET irradiation. In contrast, after high LET irradiation the incidence of apoptosis increases and high LET irradiation can give therapeutic gain [21].

In vitro and in vivo studies on GBM identified autophagy as the major non-apoptotic cell death type, also manifested following IR [41, 42] and TMZ [43] and it has been reported also that autophagy induction in glioma-initiating cells increased their radiosensitivity [39, 44]. Thus autophagy interfering agents may represent a new strategy to test in combination with chemoradiation [45–47].

## Telomere Profiling

A telomere is a region of repetitive nucleotide sequences at each end of a chromatid, which protects the end of the chromosome from deterioration or from fusion with neighboring chromosomes. Over time, due to each cell division, the telomere ends become shorter. As a cell becomes cancerous, it divides more often and its telomeres become shorter. If the telomeres become too short, the cell may die. Cancer cells can escape this fate by activating an enzyme called telomerase, which prevents the shortening of telomeres. Long telomeres and high telomerase activity have been widely associated with photon radioresistance in several cancers. The telomeric maintenance mechanism is determined by both telomere length and telomerase activity. Telomerase is restricted by the expression of its catalytic subunit hTERT (telomerase reverse transcriptase). HTERT overexpression induces telomeres elongation and inhibits irradiation-induced cell apoptosis. In contrast, telomerase inhibition leads to increased sensitivity toward photon irradiation together with telomere erosion [48].

TERT promoter mutations occur frequently in gliomas [49]. Telomerase activity and high levels of hTERT expression are demonstrated to be markers of poor prognosis in glioma [50, 51] and can be predictive markers of RT response in GBM. The shelterin protein complex (composed by TRF1, TRF2, TPP1, POT1, TIN2, and hRAP1) regulates telomeres protection, telomeres function, and telomeres length. In vitro, the cell response to photons is correlated with telomere length and with the POT1 basal level. In vivo, in GBM, both telomere length and the POT1 expression level were predictive of patient outcome. Cell response to carbon ions shows no correlation with these parameters, thus high LET irradiation can be useful in radioresistant patients [48].

## Growth Factors

Growth factors are signaling molecules that often promote cells maturation and differentiation. The cross-talks between the pathways of growth factors and their receptors contribute to the complexity of the biology of GBM and to high rate of relapse and radioresistance [52].

GBM shows a high expression of fibroblast growth factor (FGF-2) and its receptors (FGFR1, 2, 3, and 4). FGF2 is a mitogenic and angiogenic factor and its expression is a predictor of prognosis in high-grade gliomas [53, 54]. The 24 kDa FGF-2 isoform of FGF2 has a radioprotective role via increasing of DNA-PKcs, an enzyme involved in NHEJ [52, 55].

FGF-2 induced radioprotection is controlled by RhoB, that is activated by several stress condition, such as hypoxia [56]. Farnesylated RhoB inhibits radiation-induced mitotic cell death and controls radiation-induced centrosome over duplication [57]. It has been shown that the inhibition of Rho pathways induces radiosensitization and oxygenation in human glioblastoma xenografts. This effect is due to the improvement of the tumor oxygenation associated with a significant decrease of the vessel density and of the MMP2 expression [58].

Epidermal growth factor (EGF) is a potent mitogenic signaling molecule implicated in a variety of signaling pathways. The EGF receptor (EGFR) is frequently dysregulated in cancers and that leads to increased resistance to cancer therapy. Upregulation of wild type or expression of mutant EGFR is associated with tumor radioresistance and poor clinical outcome. Radioresistance is thought to be, at least in part, the result of a strong cytoprotective response powered by signaling via AKT and ERK, that is increased by radiation. This response may modulate DNA repair by enhancing DNA DSBs repair [26]. EGFR is the most commonly amplified gene in GBM. Amplification of EGFR results in upregulation of AKT and mitogen-activated protein kinase (MAPK) pathways. One of the most frequent mutations in malignant glioma is EGFR variant III (EGFRvIII). Expression of EGFRvIII promotes gamma-H2AX foci resolution and enhances DNA repair by DSBs repair [26]. Moreover, mutation of mutations is EGFRvIII results in constitutive upregulation of mitogenic signaling pathways as well as a loss of down-modulation by EGFR-targeted agents [15].

Platelet-derived growth factor receptor (PDGFR) is a membrane-bound receptor that modulates a variety of growth and proliferation signaling pathways. Overexpression or hyperactivity of PDGFR and their ligands platelet-derived growth factor (PDGF) are frequent events in human gliomas of all grades [15, 59] and their expression pattern in tumors suggests the presence of autocrine and paracrine stimulatory loops [59].

Vascular endothelial growth factor (VEGF) has pro-angiogenic functions and increases vascular permeability [60]. VEGF overexpression occurs in a variety of tumors including malignant brain tumors. The co-expression of VEGF and VEGF receptors (VEGFR) in some types of tumors suggests potential autocrine loop-signaling of VEGF within a tumor mass [60]. Moreover, it has been observed that serum VEGF levels are elevated in subsets of patients after radiotherapy [60, 61]. The autocrine VEGF-VEGFR2 interplay can be a factor contributing to GBM growth and radioresistance.

## Angiogenesis

Angiogenesis is the process of generation of new vessels from the local preexisting vessels. It is a prerequisite for all solid tumors to grow above 1 mm³. This process is regulated by inducers and inhibitors released from tumor cells, endothelial cells, and the extracellular matrix (ECM), and it is primarily mediated by VEGF. VEGF stimulates vessel formation by recruiting progenitor endothelial cells from the bone marrow and increases vascular permeability. VEGF-function is suggested to be primarily restricted to endothelial cells, because it binds to two endothelial cell tyrosine kinase receptors, VEGFR1 and VEGFR2 [62].

Radiotherapy was shown to exert direct antiangiogenic effects. However, radiation-induced endothelial cell damage and apoptosis can be evaded by paracrine release of angiogenic growth factor by tumor and stroma and by the upregulation of angiogenic receptors in the endothelium [63]. Thus it is very likely that the well-developed vascular system has an important role in tumor sustenance in GBM. A current hypothesis is that GBM-derived VEGF, elevated after irradiation, is a radioprotector for endothelial cells, thereby contributing to the radioresistance of GBM [62, 64].

## Hypoxia

Tumor hypoxia influences the outcome of anticancer treatments. After irradiation, $O_2$ participates in the chemical reactions that lead to the production of DNA damage because $O_2$ is an extremely electron-affinic molecule [65]. Cells that are anoxic during irradiation are about three times more resistant to radiation than cells that are well oxygenated at the time of irradiation [66].

High grade brain tumors show significant regions of hypoxia. The measure of oxygen pressure ($pO_2$) in brain tumors and in brain cortex demonstrated that intratumoral $pO_2$ values were significantly lower than that of $pO_2$ in brain cortex surrounding the tumor [67]. Results were confirmed by the measure of the oxygen status of human malignant brain tumors in vivo by the determination of the activities and expression of bioreductive enzymes in human brain tumor samples. These enzymes included DT-diaphorase, NADH cytochrome b5 reductase, and NADPH cytochrome P-450 reductase and were detected in all the tumors enzyme profiles analyzed [68]. The hypoxic areas in GBM can provoke an adaptive response leading to the selection for death resistance. Once tumor cells become adaptive to hypoxia, they are more resistant to apoptosis and less responsive to cancer therapy [69]. Carbon ions are less dependent on the oxygen enhancement ratio as compared with conventional photon irradiation and could therefore also eradicate hypoxic GBM cells.

In a panel of hypoxia-regulated genes, the mRNA of the ECM protein osteopontin (OPN) resulted consistently overexpressed in human malignant glioma samples [70, 71]. OPN plays an important role in tumor progression, including processes such as the decay of ECM, proliferation, apoptosis, migration, invasion, and metastasis [70, 72]. High OPN expression levels and the pattern of expression of splice variants have been associated with prognosis in GBM patients [69].

Recently it has been observed that ERKs, DNA-PKcs, and hypoxia-inducible factor 1 (HIF-1α) cooperate in radioresistance induced by hypoxia. MEK/ERK signal transduction pathway, through the sustained expression of DNA-PKcs, positively regulates expression and activity of HIF-1α protein, preserving GBM radioresistance in hypoxic condition [73].

Hypoxia can induce Livin upregulation. Livin is a member of the inhibitors of apoptosis proteins (IAP) family. IAP are involved in the negative regulation of apoptosis [68]. Livin can bind the endogenous IAP antagonist SMAC and caspase-3, caspase-7, and caspase-9 inhibiting apoptosis. The hypoxia-induced upregulation of Livin is responsible of apoptosis inhibition. Moreover, Livin increases resistance to cytotoxic therapies through a HIF1 α-dependent pathway [68].

## Cancer Stem Cells

The cancer stem cells (CSC) compartment represents the subpopulation of tumor cells with clonogenic potential and the ability to initiate new tumors. Besides self-renewal, one of their main features is their ability to differentiate into the variety of cells within the tumor with the potential to reconstitute the complete tumor phenotype [74]. The original model of CSC suggested a static intratumoral hierarchy, with a cancer stem cell population in the apex exhibiting high self-renewal and DNA-DSB repair capacities that consequently leads to their inherent resistance to conventional cancer therapies, such as radiotherapy. However, it is increasingly apparent that intratumoral hierarchies are more dynamic, and acquisition of tumor stem cell traits could be influenced by a number of niche factors, such as signaling induced by intratumoral hypoxia, or as a result of transition of tumor cells into the invasive state, or via intercellular communication. Based on the premise that recurrent GBM must be generated from few residual tumor cells post-surgery, the term "glioma-initiating cells" (GIC) seems to better describe this population [62]. CSC in glioma express CD 133. In xenograft transplantation assays, CD133-positive brain tumor cells have been shown to initiate tumor growth whereas the injection of marker-negative cells did not cause a tumor [75]. CD133-expressing glioma cells survive after irradiation in increased proportion relative to tumor cells without the surface marker in vitro and in vivo. Glioma stem cells preferentially activate the DNA damage checkpoints resulting in more effective repair of radiation-induced DNA damage than CD133-negative tumor cells. Thus CD133-positive glioma cells contribute to the radioresistance of glioblastoma [12, 76]. CSCs reside in and be supported by the tumor microvascular niches. Tumor microvascular endothelial cells (tMVECs) exhibit extreme resistance to radio- and chemotherapy, with the main response to irradiation being senescence. Even though permanently arrested, senescent tMVECs are still viable and able to support CSC growth with the same efficacy as non-senescent tMVECs.

Moreover, GBM CSCs themselves are capable of differentiating into cells with similar features as tMVECs that subsequently undergo senescence when exposed to radiation. This indicates that endothelial-like cells are therapy resistant and also that they support expansion of GBM cells and GBM CSCs [77].

## Extracellular Matrix

ECM is composed by extracellular molecules that provide support and adhesion to cells, separate cells and regulate intercellular communications. The main molecular components of ECM are proteoglycans, hyaluronic acid, and fibers.

Invasiveness and diffuse infiltration are among the GBM characteristics related to the rapid tumor recurrence. Important key molecules that enable cell invasion are ECM-degrading enzymes like matrix metalloproteinases (MMPs), cathepsin family proteases, and plasminogen activators. GBMs frequently show an elevation of various MMPs, in particular MMP-2 and MMP-9 have been shown to be critical for glioma cell invasion [78]. Moreover, irradiation was found to induce the catalytic activity and the synthesis of MMP-2 [79]. Integrins have an important role in cell invasiveness and migration. Integrins comprise a large group of at least 24 different heterodimeric transmembrane receptors that govern cell–ECM interactions [80]. In particular, $\alpha v\beta 3$-integrin is a binding receptor for ECM proteins and it serves as a receptor for MMP-2 on the cell surface, controlling both migration and proteolytic cleavage of ECM components [78]. It has been shown that irradiation induces a significant and dose-dependent increase in $\beta 1$- and $\beta 3$-integrin cell surface expression [78, 81]. Irradiation can activate $\alpha v\beta 3$-integrins and control radioresistance in several GBM cell lines by inhibition of radiation-induced mitotic dead. This regulation of glioma cell response to ionizing radiation is mediated through the integrin-linked kinase (ILK) and RhoB [82]. The inhibition of integrins by cilengitide is able to radiosensitize GBM cells. In xenograft studies, cotreatment with cilengitide and radiation dramatically amplified the effects of radiation, triggering an enhanced apoptotic response and suppression of tumor growth. These xenografted tumors showed activation of NFkB, a documented mediator of cellular response to radiation [83].

## Epithelial–Mesenchymal Transition

The epithelial–mesenchymal transition (EMT) is an important process that occurs during tumor invasion and metastasis, through which cancer cells acquire a more aggressive phenotype [84]. During EMT, epithelial cells typically lose their epithelial characteristics, including loss of cell polarity and cell–cell contact, and acquire a mesenchymal spindleshaped migrating phenotype.

The key event of EMT is the switch of E-cadherin (typical of epithelial cells) to N-cadherin (typical of mesenchymal cells), which renders the single cell more motile and invasive.

Tumor cells can also up-regulate other mesenchymal markers such as vimentin, fibronectin, and snail. Transcription factors such as snail and the basic helix-loop-helix protein TWIST1 are able to bind to E cadherin promoter and repress its transcription. Several receptor tyrosine kinases are able to induce EMT, such as the transforming growth factor β, EGF, FGF and Notch, that are associated with a more aggressive phenotype of cancer cells. Also hypoxia may induce EMT.

A mesenchymal phenotype is the hallmark of tumor aggressiveness in human malignant glioma. Several transcription factors have been identified as master regulators of ETM in high grade glioma: C/EBPβ, Stat3 [85], snail [86], and TWIST1 [87]. In GBM cell lines, upregulation of insulin like growth factor binding protein 4 (IGFBP4) was recently related to upregulation of molecules involved in EMT [88].

CXCR4 has also been demonstrated to be involved in the cell migration and lymph node metastasis of cancers. Activation of CXCR4 with SDF-1 triggers G protein signaling that activates a variety of intracellular signal transduction pathways and molecules regulating migration, chemotaxis, cell survival, proliferation, and adhesion.

SDF-1/CXCR4 contributes to tumor progression by induction of EMT. In GBM cell lines, EMT process can be triggered by the SDF-1/CXCR4 axis and eventually tumor cell invasion and proliferation are induced via activation of PI3K/AKT and ERK pathway [89]. Moreover, SDF-1 up-regulates survivin, an inhibitor of apoptosis proteins, via MEK/ERK and PI3K/AKT pathway, leading to cell cycle progression and EMT occurrence dependent on survivin [84].

Recently a gene signature study involving 31 genes related to cell cycle, cell junctions, and cell adhesion demonstrated that enrichment of EMT pathway was associated with radioresistant phenotype in glioma [90].

## MicroRNA

MicroRNAs represent an abundant class of endogenously expressed short nucleotide small noncoding RNA molecules that function to silence gene expression through a process of posttranscriptional modification. They exhibit varied functions during normal development and tissue homeostasis, and their dysregulation plays major roles in many cancer types [91].

Various studies have demonstrated the presence of microRNA aberrations in GBM and GBM CSCs. Aberrantly expressed microRNAs have widespread effects on tumorigenesis, including on critical GBM pathways such as receptor tyrosine kinase signaling, p53 signaling, and cell cycle control. Thus, microRNAs play a role in malignant transformation, progression, invasiveness, and response to therapeutic interventions. [91].

## Genomic Heterogeneity

Studies involving the use of microarray and DNA sequencing technology have evidenced distinct genomic subtypes of GBM, including the proneural, neural, mesenchymal, and classical genotypes. Different subtypes have different expression patterns and differences in clinical outcomes which can have important effects on prognosis and potential therapeutic targeting [14]. In addition, GBM can present loss of heterozygosity in multiple chromosomes and there are different patterns of dysregulated epidermal growth factor receptor, platelet-derived growth factor receptor, p53, phosphatase and tensin homolog, cell cycle proteins, and isocitrate dehydrogenase 1 [14]. Many GBM variants have been categorized by specific mutations, but these mutation patterns are often overlapping. Moreover, regional variation in chromosomal abnormalities, gene expression, and mutation can be found within a tumor mass and may account for mixed clinical responses to therapy.

## Conclusions

GBM is aggressive and radioresistant tumors. Biological therapies interfering with altered pathways as well as high LET radiation can increase response to radiation. A better knowledge of the biology and radiobiology of GBM is of primary importance in order to develop new strategies to improve outcome of patients.

## References

1. Stupp R, Mason W, Van der Bent M, Weller M, Fisher B, Taphoorn MJ, Belanger K, Brandes AA, Marosi C, Bogdahn U, Curschmann J, Janzer RC, Ludwin SK, Gorlia T, Allgeier A, Lacombe D, Cairncross JG, Eisenhauer E, Mirimanoff RO, European Organisation for Research and Treatment of Cancer Brain Tumor and Radiotherapy Groups, National Cancer Institute of Canada Clinical Trials Group. Radiotherapy plus concomitant and adjuvant Temozolomide for glioblastoma. N Engl J Med. 2005;352(10):987–96.
2. Matsuoka S, Ballif BA, Smogorzewska A, McDonald 3rd ER, Hurov KE, Luo J, Bakalarski CE, Zhao Z, Solimini N, Lerenthal Y, Shiloh Y, Gygi SP, Elledge SJ. ATM and ATR substrate analysis reveals extensive protein networks responsive to DNA damage. Science. 2007;316(5828):1160–6.
3. Shiloh Y, Ziv Y. The ATM protein kinase: regulating the cellular response to genotoxic stress, and more. Nat Rev Mol Cell Biol. 2013;14(4):197–210.
4. Williams JR, Zhang Y, Russell J, Koch C, Little JB. Human tumor cells segregate into radiosensitivity groups that associate with ATM and TP53 status. Acta Oncol. 2007;46(5):628–38.
5. Tribius S, Pidel A, Casper D. ATM protein expression correlates with radioresistance in primary glioblastoma cells in culture. Int J Radiat Oncol Biol Phys. 2001;50(2):511–23.
6. Dokic I, Mairani A, Brons S, Schoell B, Jauch A, Krunic D, Debus J, Régnier-Vigouroux A, Weber KJ. High resistance to X-rays and therapeutic carbon ions in glioblastoma cells bearing dysfunctional ATM associates with intrinsic chromosomal instability. Int J Radiat Biol. 2014;8:1–9.
7. Biddlestone-Thorpe L, Sajjad M, Rosenberg E, Beckta JM, Valerie NC, Tokarz M, Adams BR, Wagner AF, Khalil A, Gilfor D, Golding SE, Deb S, Temesi DG, Lau A, O'Connor MJ, Choe KS, Parada LF, Lim SK, Mukhopadhyay ND, Valerie K. ATM kinase inhibition preferentially sensitizes p53-mutant glioma to ionizing radiation. Clin Cancer Res. 2013;19(12):3189–200.
8. Carruthers R, Ahmed SU, Strathdee K, Gomez-Roman N, Amoah-Buahin E, Watts C, Chalmers AJ. Abrogation of radioresistance in glioblastoma stem-like cells by inhibition of ATM kinase. Mol Oncol. 2015;9(1):192–203.
9. Golding SE, Rosenberg E, Adams BR, Wignarajah S, Beckta JM, O'Connor MJ, Valerie K. Dynamic inhibition of ATM kinase provides a strategy for glioblastoma multiforme radiosensitization and growth control. Cell Cycle. 2012;11(6):1167–73.
10. Lim YC, Roberts TL, Day BW, Harding A, Kozlov S, Kijas AW, Ensbey KS, Walker DG, Lavin MF. A role for homologous recombination and abnormal cell-cycle progression in radioresistance of glioma-initiating cells. Mol Cancer Ther. 2012;11(9): 1863–72.
11. Otomo T, Hishii M, Arai H, Sato K, Sasai K. Microarray analysis of temporal gene responses to ionizing radiation in two glioblastoma cell lines: up-regulation of DNA repair genes. J Radiat Res. 2004;45(1):53–60.
12. Bao S, Wu Q, McLendon RE, Hao Y, Shi Q, Hjelmeland AB, Dewhirst MW, Bigner DD, Rich JN. Glioma stem cells promote radioresistance by preferential activation of the DNA damage response. Nature. 2006;444(7120):756–60.
13. Lim YC, Roberts TL, Day BW, Stringer BW, Kozlov S, Fazry S, Bruce ZC, Ensbey KS, Walker DG, Boyd AW, Lavin MF. Increased sensitivity to ionizing radiation by targeting the homologous recombination pathway in glioma initiating cells. Mol Oncol. 2014;8(8):1603–15.
14. Brett-Morris A, Wright BM, Seo Y, Pasupuleti V, Zhang J, Lu J, Spina R, Bar EE, Gujrati M, Schur R, Lu ZR, Welford SM. The polyamine catabolic enzyme SAT1 modulates tumorigenesis and radiation response in GBM. Cancer Res. 2014;74(23):6925–34.
15. Karsy M, Huang T, Kleinman G, Karpel-Massler G. Molecular, histopathological, and genomic variants of glioblastoma. Front Biosci. 2014;19:1065–87.
16. Rubner Y, Muth C, Strnad A, Derer A, Sieber R, Buslei R, Frey B, Fietkau R, Gaipl US. Fractionated

radiotherapy is the main stimulus for the induction of cell death and of Hsp70 release of p53 mutated glioblastoma cell lines. Radiat Oncol. 2014;9(1):89.

17. Kastan MB, Onyekwere O, Sidransky D, Vogelstein B, Craig RW. Participation of p53 protein in cellular response to DNA damage. Cancer Res. 1991;51(23 pt 1):6304–11.
18. Vermeulen K, Van Bockstaele DR, Berneman ZN. The cell cycle: a review of regulation, deregulation and therapeutic targets in cancer. Cell Prolif. 2003;36(3):131–49.
19. Hiyama H, Iavarone A, LaBaer J, Reeves SA. Regulated ectopic expression of cyclin D1 induces transcriptional activation of the cdk inhibitor p21 gene without altering cell cycle progression. Oncogene. 1997;14(21):2533–42.
20. Matsuoka S, Huang M, Elledge SJ. Linkage of ATM to cell cycle regulation by the Chk2 protein kinase. Science. 1998;282(5395):1893–7.
21. Tsuboi K, Moritake T, Tsuchida Y, Tokuuye K, Matsumura A, Ando K. Cell cycle checkpoint and apoptosis induction in glioblastoma cells and fibroblasts irradiated with carbon beam. J Radiat Res. 2007;48(4):317–25.
22. Toulany M, Schickfluss TA, Fattah KR, Lee KJ, Chen BP, Fehrenbacher B, Schaller M, Chen DJ, Rodemann HP. Function of erbB receptors and DNA-PKcs on phosphorylation of cytoplasmic and nuclear Akt at S473 induced by erbB1 ligand and ionizing radiation. Radiother Oncol. 2011;101(1):140–6.
23. Toulany M, Dittmann K, Fehrenbacher B, Schaller M, Baumann M, Rodemann HP. PI3K-Akt signaling regulates basal, but MAP-kinase signaling regulates radiation-induced XRCC1 expression in human tumor cells in vitro. DNA Repair (Amst). 2008;7(10):1746–56.
24. Narayan RS, Fedrigo CA, Stalpers LJ, Baumert BG, Sminia P. Targeting the Akt-pathway to improve radiosensitivity in glioblastoma. Curr Pharm Des. 2013;19(5):951–7.
25. Li HF, Kim JS, Waldman T. Radiation-induced Akt activation modulates radioresistance in human glioblastoma cells. Radiat Oncol. 2009;4:43.
26. Golding SE, Morgan RN, Adams BR, Hawkins AJ, Povirk LF, Valerie K. Pro-survival AKT and ERK signaling from EGFR and mutant EGFRvIII enhances DNA double-strand break repair in human glioma cells. Cancer Biol Ther. 2009;8(8):730–8.
27. Atkins RJ, Dimou J, Paradiso L, Morokoff AP, Kaye AH, Drummond KJ, Hovens CM. Regulation of glycogen synthase kinase-3 beta (GSK-3beta) by the Akt pathway in gliomas. J Clin Neurosci. 2012;19(11):1558–63.
28. Atkins RJ, Stylli SS, Luwor RB, Kaye AH, Hovens CM. Glycogen synthase kinase-3beta (GSK-3beta) and its dysregulation in glioblastoma multiforme. J Clin Neurosci. 2013;20(9):1185–92.
29. Chikano Y, Domoto T, Furuta T, Sabit H, Kitano-Tamura A, Pyko IV, Takino T, Sai Y, Hayashi Y, Sato H, Miyamoto KI, Nakada M, Minamoto

T. Glycogen synthase kinase 3beta sustains invasion of glioblastoma via the focal adhesion kinase, Rac1 and c-Jun N-terminal kinase-mediated pathway. Mol Cancer Ther. 2015;14:564–74.
30. Paglin S, Hollister T, Delohery T, Hackett N, McMahill M, Sphicas E, Domingo D, Yahalom J. A novel response of cancer cells to radiation involves autophagy and formation of acidic vesicles. Cancer Res. 2001;61(2):439–44.
31. Kroemer G, Levine B. Autophagic cell death: the story of a misnomer. Nat Rev Mol Cell Biol. 2008;9(12):1004–10.
32. Eisenberg-Lerner A, Bialik S, Simo HU, Kimchi A. Life and death partners: apoptosis, autophagy and the cross-talk between them. Cell Death Differ. 2009;16(7):966–75.
33. Meijer AJ, Codogno P. Signalling and autophagy regulation in health, aging and disease. Mol Aspects Med. 2006;27(5–6):411–25.
34. Yorimitsu T, Klionsky DJ. Eating the endoplasmic reticulum: quality control by autophagy. Trends Cell Biol. 2007;17(6):279–85.
35. Palumbo S, Tini P, Toscano M, Allavena G, Angeletti F, Manai F, Miracco C, Comincini S, Pirtoli L. Combined EGFR and autophagy modulation impairs cell migration and enhances radiosensitivity in human glioblastoma cells. J Cell Physiol. 2014;229(11):1863–73.
36. Wang N, Feng Y, Zhu M, Tsang CM, Man K, Tong Y, Tsao SW. Berberine induces autophagic cell death and mitochondrial apoptosis in liver cancer cells: the cellular mechanism. J Cell Biochem. 2010;111(6):1426–36.
37. Castedo M, Perfettini JL, Roumier T, Valent A, Raslova H, Yakushijin K, Horne D, Feunteun J, Lenoir G, Medema R, Vainchenker W, Kroemer G. Mitotic catastrophe constitutes a special case of apoptosis whose suppression entails aneuploidy. Oncogene. 2004;23:4362–70.
38. Stapper N, Stuschke M, Sak A, Stuben G. Radiation-induced apoptosis in human sarcoma and glioma cell lines. Int J Cancer. 1995;62(1):58–62.
39. Lefranc F, Kiss R. Autophagy, the Trojan horse to combat glioblastomas. Neurosurg Focus. 2006;20(4), E7.
40. Sharma K, Le N, Alotaibi M, Gewirtz DA. Cytotoxic autophagy in cancer therapy. Int J Mol Sci. 2014;15(6):10034–51.
41. Yao KC, Komata T, Kondo Y, Kanzawa T, Kondo S, Germano IM. Molecular response of human glioblastoma multiforme cells to ionizing radiation: cell cycle arrest, modulation of the expression of cyclin-dependent kinase inhibitors, and autophagy. J Neurosurg. 2003;98(2):378–84.
42. Zhuang W, Qin Z, Liang Z. The role of autophagy in sensitizing malignant glioma cells to radiation therapy. Acta Biochim Biophys Sin. 2009;41(5):341–51.
43. Kanzawa T, Zhang L, Xiao L, Germano IM, Kondo Y, Kondo S. Arsenic trioxide induces autophagic cell death in malignant glioma cells by upregulation of

mitochondrial cell death protein BNIP3. Oncogene. 2005;24(6):980–91.

44. Palumbo S, Pirtoli L, Tini P, Cevenini G, Calderaro F, Toscano M, Miracco C, Comincini S. Different involvement of autophagy in human malignant glioma cell lines undergoing irradiation and temozolomide combined treatments. J Cell Biochem. 2012; 113(7):2308–18.

45. Comincini S, Allavena G, Palumbo S, Morini M, Durando F, Angeletti F, Pirtoli L, Miracco C. MicroRNA-17 regulates the expression of ATG7 and modulates the autophagy process, improving the sensitivity to temozolomide and low-dose ionizing radiation treatments in human glioblastoma cells. Cancer Biol Ther. 2013;14(7):574–86.

46. Giatromanolaki A, Sivridis E, Mitrakas A, Kalamida D, Zois CE, Haider S, Piperidou C, Pappa A, Gatter KC, Harris AL, Koukourakis MI. Autophagy and lysosomal related protein expression patterns in human glioblastoma. Cancer Biol Ther. 2014;15(11): 1468–78.

47. Golden EB, Cho HY, Jahanian A, Hofman FM, Louie SG, Schönthal AH, Chen TC. Chloroquine enhances temozolomide cytotoxicity in malignant gliomas by blocking autophagy. Neurosurg Focus. 2014;37(6), E12.

48. Ferrandon S, Saultier P, Carras J, Battiston-Montagne P, Alphonse G, Beuve M, Malleval C, Honnorat J, Slatter T, Hung N, Royds J, Rodriguez-Lafrasse C, Poncet D. Telomere profiling: toward glioblastoma personalized medicine. Mol Neurobiol. 2013;47(1): 64–76.

49. Killela PJ, Reitman ZJ, Jiao Y, Bettegowda C, Agrawal N, Diaz LA, Friedman AH, Friedman H, Gallia GL, Giovanella BC, Grollman AP, He TC, He Y, Hruban RH, Jallo GI, Mandahl N, Meeker AK, Mertens F, Netto GJ, Rasheed BA, Riggins GJ, Rosenquist TA, Schiffman M, Shih IM, Theodorescu D, Torbenson MS, Torbenson MS, Velculescu VE, Wang TL, Wentzensen N, Wood LD, Zhang M, McLendon RE, McLendon RE, Bigner DD, Kinzler KW, Vogelstein B, Papadopoulos N, Yan H. TERT promoter mutations occur frequently in gliomas and a subset of tumors derived from cells with low rates of self-renewal. Proc Natl Acad Sci U S A. 2013;110: 6021–6.

50. Boldrini L, Pistolesi S, Gisfredi S, Ursino S, Ali G, Pieracci N, Basolo F, Parenti G, Fontanini G. Telomerase activity and hTERT mRNA expression in glial tumors. Int J Oncol. 2006;28(6):1555–60.

51. Lötsch D, Ghanim B, Laaber M, Wurm G, Weis S, Lenz S, Webersinke G, Pichler J, Berger W, Spiegl-Kreinecker S. Prognostic significance of telomerase-associated parameters in glioblastoma: effect of patient age. Neuro Oncol. 2013;15(4):423–32.

52. Cohen-Jonathan ME. From bench to bedside: experience of the glioblastoma model for the optimization of radiosensitization. Cancer Radiother. 2012;16(1):25–8.

53. Bredel M, Pollack IF, Campbell JW, Hamilton RL. Basic fibroblast growth factor expression as a predictor of prognosis in pediatric high-grade gliomas. Clin Cancer Res. 1997;3(11):2157–64.

54. Fukui S, Nawashiro H, Otani N, Ooigawa H, Nomura N, Yano A, Miyazawa T, Ohnuki A, Tsuzuki N, Katoh H, Ishihara S, Shima K. Nuclear accumulation of basic fibroblast growth factor in human astrocytic tumors. Cancer. 2003;97(12):3061–7.

55. Ader I, Muller C, Bonnet J, Favre G, Cohen-Jonathan E, Salles B, Toulas C. The radioprotective effect of the 24 kDa FGF-2 isoform in HeLa cells is related to an increased expression and activity of the DNA-dependent protein kinase (DNAPK) catalytic subunit. Oncogene. 2002;21(49):6471–9.

56. Skuli N, Monferran S, Delmas C, Lajoie-Mazenc I, Favre G, Toulas C, Cohen-Jonathan-Moyal E. Activation of RhoB by hypoxia controls hypoxia-inducible factor-1alpha stabilization through glycogen synthase kinase-3 in U87 glioblastoma cells. Cancer Res. 2006;66(1):482–9.

57. Milia J, Teyssier F, Dalenc F, Ader I, Delmas C, Pradines A, Lajoie-Mazenc I, Baron R, Bonnet J, Cohen-Jonathan E, Favre G, Toulas C. Farnesylated RhoB inhibits radiation-induced mitotic cell death and controls radiation-induced centrosome overduplication. Cell Death Differ. 2005;12(5):492–501.

58. Ader I, Delmas C, Bonnet J, Rochaix P, Favre G, Toulas C, Cohen-Jonathan-Moyal E. Inhibition of Rho pathways induces radiosensitization and oxygenation in human glioblastoma xenografts. Oncogene. 2003;22(55):8861–9.

59. Nazarenko I, Hede SM, He X, Hedrén A, Thompson J, Lindström MS, Nistér M. PDGF and PDGF receptors in glioma. Ups J Med Sci. 2012;117(2):99–112.

60. Knizetova P, Ehrmann J, Hlobilkova A, Vancova I, Kalita O, Kolar Z, Bartek J. Autocrine regulation of glioblastoma cell cycle progression, viability and radioresistance through the VEGF-VEGFR2 (KDR) interplay. Cell Cycle. 2008;7(16):2553–61.

61. Gridley DS, Loredo LN, Slater JD, Archambeau JO, Bedros AA, Andres ML, Slater JM. Pilot evaluation of cytokine levels in patients undergoing radiotherapy for brain tumours. Cancer Detect Prev. 1998;22: 20–9.

62. Donker M, Van Furth WR, Mulder-Van Der Kracht S, Hovinga KE, Verhoeff JJ, Stalpers LJ, van Bree C. Negligible radiation protection of endothelial cells by vascular endothelial growth factor. Oncol Rep. 2007; 18(3):709–14.

63. Debus J, Abdollahi A. For the next trick: new discoveries in radiobiology applied to glioblastoma. Am Soc Clin Oncol Educ Book. 2014;2014:e95–9.

64. Hovinga KE, Stalpers LJ, van Bree C, Donker M, Verhoeff JJ, Rodermond HM, Bosch DA, van Furth WR. Radiation-enhanced vascular endothelial growth factor (VEGF) secretion in glioblastoma multiforme cell lines—a clue to radioresistance? J Neurooncol. 2005;74(2):99–103.

65. Quintiliani M. The oxygen effect in radiation inactivation of DNA and enzymes. Int J Radiat Biol Relat Stud Phys Chem Med. 1986;50(4):573–94.

66. Rockwell S, Dobrucki IT, Kim EY, Marrison ST, Vu VT. Hypoxia and radiation therapy: past history, ongoing research, and future promise. Curr Mol Med. 2009;9(4):442–58.
67. Kayama T, Yoshimoto T, Fujimoto S, Sakurai Y. Intratumoral oxygen pressure in malignant brain tumor. J Neurosurg. 1991;74(1):55–9.
68. Rampling R, Cruickshank G, Lewis AD, Fitzsimmons SA, Workman P. Direct measurement of pO2 distribution and bioreductive enzymes in human malignant brain tumors. Int J Radiat Oncol Biol Phys. 1994; 29(3):427–31.
69. Hsieh CH, Lin YJ, Wu CP, Lee HT, Shyu WC, Wang CC. Livin contributes to tumor hypoxia-induced resistance to cytotoxic therapies in glioblastoma multiforme. Clin Cancer Res. 2015;21(2):460–70.
70. Güttler A, Giebler M, Cuno P, Wichmann H, Keßler J, Ostheimer C, Söling A, Strauss C, Illert J, Kappler M, Vordermark D, Bache M. Osteopontin and splice variant expression level in human malignant glioma: radiobiologic effects and prognosis after radiotherapy. Radiother Oncol. 2013;108(3):535–40.
71. Said HM, Hagemann C, Staab A, Stojic J, Kühnel S, Vince GH, Flentje M, Roosen K, Vordermark D. Expression patterns of the hypoxia-related genes osteopontin, CA9, erythropoietin, VEGF and HIF-1alpha in human glioma in vitro and in vivo. Radiother Oncol. 2007;83(3):398–405.
72. Rangaswami H, Bulbule A, Kundu GC. Osteopontin: role in cell signaling and cancer progression. Trends Cell Biol. 2006;16(2):79–87.
73. Marampon F, Gravina GL, Zani BM, Popov VM, Fratticci A, Cerasani M, Di Genova D, Mancini M, Ciccarelli C, Ficorella C, Di Cesare E, Festuccia C. Hypoxia sustains glioblastoma radioresistance through ERKs/DNA-PKcs/HIF-1α functional interplay. Int J Oncol. 2014;44(6):2121–31.
74. Borovski T, Vermeulen L, Sprick MR, Medema JP. One renegade cancer stem cell? Cell Cycle. 2009; 8(6):803–8.
75. Singh SK, Hawkins C, Clarke ID, Squire JA, Bayani J, Hide T, Henkelman RM, Cusimano MD, Dirks PB. Identification of human brain tumour initiating cells. Nature. 2004;432(7015):396–401.
76. Bütof R, Dubrovska A, Baumann M. Clinical perspectives of cancer stem cell research in radiation oncology. Radiother Oncol. 2013;108(3):388–96.
77. Borovski T, Beke P, van Tellingen O, Rodermond HM, Verhoeff JJ, Lascano V, Daalhuisen JB, Medema JP, Sprick MR. Therapy-resistant tumor microvascular endothelial cells contribute to treatment failure in glioblastoma multiforme. Oncogene. 2013;32(12): 1539–48.
78. Cordes N, Hansmeier B, Beinke C, Meineke V, van Beuningen D. Irradiation differentially affects substratum-dependent survival, adhesion, and invasion of glioblastoma cell lines. Br J Cancer. 2003; 89(11):2122–32.

79. Bauman GS, Fisher BJ, McDonald W, Amberger VR, Moore E, Del Maestro RF. Effects of radiation on a three-dimensional model of malignant glioma invasion. Int J Dev Neurosci. 1999;17(5–6):643–51.
80. Hynes RO. Integrins: bidirectional, allosteric signaling machines. Cell. 2002;110(6):673–87.
81. Wild-Bode C, Weller M, Rimner A, Dichgans J, Wick W. Sublethal irradiation promotes migration and invasiveness of glioma cells: implications for radiotherapy of human glioblastoma. Cancer Res. 2001;61: 2744–50.
82. Monferran S, Skuli N, Delmas C, Favre G, Bonnet J, Cohen-Jonathan-Moyal E, Toulas C. Alphavbeta3 and alphavbeta5 integrins control glioma cell response to ionising radiation through I.L.K and RhoB. Int J Cancer. 2008;123(2):357–64.
83. Mikkelsen T, Brodie C, Finniss S, Berens ME, Rennert JL, Nelson K, Lemke N, Brown SL, Hahn D, Neuteboom B, Goodman SL. Radiation sensitization of glioblastoma by cilengitide has unanticipated schedule-dependency. Int J Cancer. 2009;124(11):2719–27.
84. Liao A, Shi R, Jiang Y, Tian S, Li P, Song F, Qu Y, Li J, Yun H, Yang X. SDF-1/CXCR4 axis regulates cell cycle progression and epithelial-mesenchymal transition via up-regulation of survivin in glioblastoma. Mol Neurobiol. 2016;53:210–5.
85. Carro MS, Lim WK, Alvarez MJ, Bollo RJ, Zhao X, Snyder EY, Sulman EP, Anne SL, Doetsch F, Colman H, Lasorella A, Aldape K, Califano A, Iavarone A. The transcriptional network for mesenchymal transformation of brain tumours. Nature. 2010;463(7279):318–25.
86. Myung JK, Choi SA, Kim SK, Wang KC, Park SH. Snail plays an oncogenic role in glioblastoma by promoting epithelial mesenchymal transition. Int J Clin Exp Pathol. 2014;7(5):1977–87.
87. Mikheeva SA, Mikheev AM, Petit A, Beyer R, Oxford RG, Khorasani L, Maxwell JP, Glackin CA, Wakimoto H, González-Herrero I, Sánchez-García I, Silber JR, Horner PJ, Rostomily RC. TWIST1 promotes invasion through mesenchymal change in human glioblastoma. Mol Cancer. 2010;9:194.
88. Praveen Kumar VR, Sehgal P, Thota B, Patil S, Santosh V, Kondaiah P. Insulin like growth factor binding protein 4 promotes GBM progression and regulates key factors involved in EMT and invasion. J Neurooncol. 2014;116(3):455–64.
89. Lv B, Yang X, Lv S, Wang L, Fan K, Shi R, Wang F, Song H, Ma X, Tan X, Xu K, Xie J, Wang G, Feng M, Zhang L. CXCR4 signaling induced epithelial-mesenchymal transition by PI3K/AKT and ERK pathways in glioblastoma. Mol Neurobiol. 2015;52:1263–8.
90. Meng J, Li P, Zhang Q, Yang Z, Fu S. A radiosensitivity gene signature in predicting glioma prognostic via EMT pathway. Oncotarget. 2014;5(13):4683–93.
91. Brower JV, Clark PA, Lyon W, Kuo JS. MicroRNAs in cancer: glioblastoma and glioblastoma cancer stem cells. Neurochem Int. 2014;77:68–77.

# The Immune System and Its Contribution to the Radiotherapeutic Response of Glioblastoma

# 10

Benjamin Cooper, Ralph Vatner, Encouse Golden, Joshua Silverman, and Silvia Formenti

## Introduction

The immune system plays an important role in both counteracting and facilitating cancer development, and it contributes to the effects of standard cancer treatments. As such, the immune system is most certainly involved in the response of glioblastoma to radiotherapy; however, it is difficult to elucidate the specific role of immunity due to limitations in animal models and the difficulty in obtaining tissue to study molecular correlates of progression and response. Yet there is abundant evidence that leukocytes and other immune mediators recognize and respond to glioblastoma, and indirect evidence that they participate in the therapeutic response to radiation. After a brief introduction on the role of the innate and adaptive immune response to cancer, this chapter will review the effects of radiotherapy on the anti-tumor immune response, including inflammation, T-cell priming, and immune suppression. We will first introduce the concept of radiation induced immunogenic cell death, its application to the unique immunological landscape of the CNS, and

present available evidence that radiation induces an immune response against glioblastoma. We will then discuss some of the barriers of the brain/tumor microenvironment that may interfere with effective anti-tumor immunity, and conclude with suggested approaches to better harness the immune response in treatment of glioblastoma with radiotherapy.

## A Brief Overview of Anti-tumor Immunity

### Basic Elements and Structure of the Immune System

The immune system is a complex network of leukocytes, soluble elements, and epithelial barriers that cooperate to protect the host organism from exogenous pathogens and endogenous pathogenic processes by recognizing and responding to danger associated molecular patterns (DAMPs). A brief overview of the components of the immune system will be helpful for understanding its role in the response of glioblastoma to radiotherapy.

### Innate Immunity

The immune system can be broadly divided into the innate and adaptive arms. The innate immune system is the first line of defense against pathogens

B. Cooper (✉) • R. Vatner • E. Golden • J. Silverman
S. Formenti
Radiation Oncology, NYU Langone Medical Center,
New York, NY, USA
e-mail: Benjamin.cooper@nyumc.org

© Springer International Publishing Switzerland 2016
L. Pirtoli et al. (eds.), *Radiobiology of Glioblastoma*, Current Clinical Pathology,
DOI 10.1007/978-3-319-28305-0_10

and transformed cells. Comprising macrophages, dendritic cells (DCs), neutrophils, natural killer (NK) cells, basophils, eosinophils, and the complement system of soluble proteins, these elements have the germ-line encoded ability to recognize DAMPs and initiate inflammation. These DAMPs are often pathogen associated, such as the endotoxin components of bacterial cell walls or double stranded RNA produced in many viral infections. However, all cells both normal and transformed contain immune stimulatory molecules such as heat shock proteins (HSPs) [1, 2], high-motility protein group B1 (HMGB1) [3], and uric acid [4], all of which are danger signals when released from damaged and dying cells. Whether initiated by pathogens, or by the growth of transformed cells, cell turnover and death release antigens along with these DAMPs which are taken up by antigen presenting cells (APCs) such as DCs. In turn, DCs can activate adaptive immune responses by presenting antigen to lymphocytes in the context of the major histocompatibility complex (MHC) class I and class II molecules.

## Adaptive Immunity

The adaptive immune system is a more recent development in evolution, common only to vertebrates, and is characterized by specificity and memory. Lymphocytes, the effector cells of the adaptive immune system, come in two varieties, B-cells and T-cells. B-cells are responsible for making antibodies, soluble immunoglobulin proteins that form the basis for humoral immunity by opsonizing and neutralizing specific extracellular targets. T-cells come in many varieties, including the CD8[+] cytotoxic T-cells which target and kill intracellular pathogens and transformed cells, and the CD4[+] helper and regulatory T-cells that regulate the immune system through the production of cytokines and by facilitating the maturation of B-cells. The T-cell receptor (TCR) enables T-cells to recognize their specific targets, which are short peptide antigens presented by APCs in the context of MHC class I (for CD8[+] T-cells) or class II (for CD4[+] T-cells).

## Adaptive Immune Responses Must Be Primed

The baseline state of the adaptive immune system is anergic. In order to prevent autoimmunity, lymphocytes must first be primed by antigen presenting cells prior to responding to antigenic stimuli. The first signal needed for priming occurs when a naïve T-cell interacts with a DC presenting its cognate peptide antigen bound to MHC. Additional co-stimulatory signals are necessary to activate naïve T-cells, which are provided by DCs in response to activation by DAMPs through Toll-Like receptors (TLRs). These co-stimulatory signals are both protein ligands expressed on the DC surface membrane (e.g., CD80 and CD86) and soluble cytokines (such as IL-2) that act in a paracrine fashion on T-cells to induce activation and proliferation that define T-cell priming.

A system of immune checkpoints counterbalances this process, regulating primed T-cells by limiting their proliferative potential. It exists as an economy mechanism to return the immune system to its basal anergic state, and to prevent autoimmunity. One such checkpoint is the cytotoxic T-lymphocyte antigen-4 (CTLA-4) molecule that competes for binding with co-stimulatory receptors, sending anti-proliferative and pro-apoptotic signals to activated T-cells. Another example is the programmed death ligand 1 and 2 (PD-L1 and PD-L2), expressed by DCs in the lymph nodes and by other cells in the periphery, including tumor cells. These directly inhibit T-cells by signaling through the PD-1 receptor and triggering a feedback of T-cell apoptosis.

## Anti-tumor Immunity and Immunosurveillance of Cancer

There has long been a link between the immune system and cancer. As early as the middle of the nineteenth century, a correlation between inflammation and tumor rejection was observed in sarcoma patients who experienced tumor rejection after cutaneous streptococcal infection. Based on these observations, William Coley developed the first immunotherapy to cancer in the late nineteenth century [5]. These eponymously named Coley's Toxins were a concoction of thermally inactivated streptococcus and serratia bacteria that were injected into sarcomatous tumors, with reported anecdotal success. Even today there remains a reported link between inflammation and tumor protection in patients with glioblastoma who tend to have longer survival if they have postoperative infections [6].

Accumulating evidence that the immune system can recognize and eliminate tumors converged in the formal hypothesis proposed by Burnet and Thomas in the middle twentieth century that fighting cancer is one of the integral functions of the immune system. This was demonstrated experimentally by Schreiber and colleagues using a murine model of chemically induced sarcoma [7]. In this model, tumors that developed in immune-deficient mice were more immunogenic and were readily rejected by mice with a competent immune system. This is consistent with the observation that immunosuppressed humans have increased susceptibility to cancer [8]. Furthermore, recent advances in cancer immunotherapy demonstrate improved survival of patients with metastatic melanoma [9] and prostate cancer [10] in response to treatment with immunotherapy strategies aimed at recovering and amplifying T-cell responses.

## Tumors Develop in Immune-Competent Hosts by Evading the Immune System

Due to selective pressure imparted by the immune system, cancer can only progress once it develops a means to evade recognition and destruction by lymphocytes. One simple method of escape utilized by tumors and viruses alike is downregulation or inactivation of the cellular machinery responsible for MHC class I (MHC-I) antigen processing and presentation. If tumor peptide antigens are not presented by MHC-I, cytotoxic T-lymphocytes (CTLs) cannot recognize and eliminate transformed cells, although MHC downregulation does make tumors more susceptible to NK cell cytotoxicity. Tumors can also escape the immune system through interference

with CTL priming. One mechanism for this involves interactions between the tumor and intratumoral DCs [11–13]. Mediated by the tumor microenvironment [14], intratumoral DCs often have an immature or regulatory phenotype characterized by the presentation of tumor antigens without co-stimulation. This mechanism results in cross-tolerance and anergy of T-cells [15–17]. The importance of this immunosuppressive mechanism is highlighted by the close temporal correlation of antigen specific tolerance of CD4$^+$ and CD8$^+$ tumor specific T-cells with accelerated tumor growth [18, 19]. Additionally, regulatory DCs (regDCs) can facilitate tumor immune escape, as adoptive transfer of regDCs into tumor bearing mice is sufficient for promoting tumor growth and metastasis [20, 21].

One of the most effective means of disrupting anti-tumor immunity is by inhibiting the effector function of CTLs. In their evolving cross-talk with the host's immune system, tumors recruit Tregs and myeloid elements—mainly tumor associated macrophages (TAMs) and myeloid derived suppressor cells (MDSCs)—that upregulate the immunosuppressive cytokines transforming growth factor-β (TGF-β) and IL-10 [22–25]. These anti-inflammatory cytokines hinder anti-tumor immunity by blunting the cytotoxic activity of CTLs. Moreover, TAMs and MDSCs modify the tumor microenvironment by producing arginase and nitric oxide synthase that deplete L-arginine, an essential nutrient for proper T-cell function [26, 27]. Furthermore, these immune-suppressive myeloid cells produce reactive oxygen and nitrogen species that modify the chemokine and antigen receptors on CTLs, both locally and systemically, impairing their tumor homing and cytotoxic ability [28].

## The Immune System and Glioblastoma

### CNS Immunity and Immune Privilege

The CNS is commonly thought to be an immune privileged site, with the widespread misconception that tumors within the CNS are not accessible to immune regulation and destruction. This idea largely originates from experiments by Medawar et al. demonstrating that allogeneic tissues transplanted into the CNS are not quickly and vigorously rejected in the same manner as tissues transplanted to other parts of the body [29]. Historically, there are three observations that have been invoked to support this notion of CNS immune privilege: (1) The blood brain barrier (BBB) prevents passive diffusion of leukocytes and antibodies into the CNS, (2) there is no lymphoid tissue in the CNS to mediate T-cell priming, and (3) there are few lymphocytes in the CNS under baseline physiologic conditions.

However, there is mounting evidence that while different from other sites, the CNS is not truly immune privileged [30]. The BBB prevents passive diffusion of soluble molecules into the CNS, but does not exclude lymphocytes. Furthermore, inflammation in the brain potentiates trafficking of primed lymphocytes, partially by breaking down the BBB, making it "leaky" and exposing T-cells to chemokines that mediate recruitment of primed T-cells to sites of inflammation. One of the hallmarks of glioblastoma is abnormal vasculature, which is supported by the radiographic finding of gadolinium contrast extravasation causing enhancement on magnetic resonance imaging (MRI). Given this glioma associated breakdown in the blood brain barrier, the BBB is unlikely to prevent elements of the immune system from infiltrating into glioblastoma, and there is evidence that T-cells can enter the CNS and detect recurrent glioblastoma in patients [31]. Adoptively transferred T-cells specific for glioblastoma can also home to tumors, again supporting the potential role for the immune system in the anti-glioma response to radiotherapy.

Despite the anatomical structure and absence of traditional lymphoid tissue in the CNS, functional lymphatic vessels lining the dural sinuses have been identified which are capable of transporting both fluid and immune cells from the CSF to the deep cervical lymph nodes [32]. Immune priming can still occur in the CNS, although the specific mechanism of T-cell priming is an active area of research. One possible site for priming is in the cervical lymph nodes. Intracranial injection of soluble antigen drains through the cribriform plate and can be detected in the cervical lymph nodes [33], and exogenous DCs introduced into the CNS migrate to the cervical lymph nodes through the same route and can prime effective immune responses against antigens in the CNS. There is a question regarding the nature of the APC responsible for T-cell priming against CNS antigenic targets such as epitopes associated with glioblastoma since there are few DCs in the CNS, and microglia and other endogenous APCs have not been identified in the cervical lymph nodes draining the CNS. However, once T-cells are primed they readily circulate from the peripheral blood into the CNS. While relatively sparse, there are lymphocytes in the brain, and these have effector function. Multiple sclerosis is an apt example of an autoimmune disease mediated by T-cells penetrating into the CNS, a phenomenon well characterized in the experimental autoimmune encephalomyelitis model of MS in which anti-neuronal T-cells are induced by peripheral vaccination, demonstrating that the CNS is not impervious to immune infiltration and attack [34].

## Evidence for an Anti-glioma Immune Response

Even in the absence of treatment, there is evidence for a spontaneous immune response to glioblastoma. Histopathological analysis of gliomas demonstrate a T-cell infiltrate [34] recruited by the activated endothelium in tumor vasculature. Even in the absence of treatment, an inflammatory signature characterized by the invasion of tumors by lymphocytes portends a more favorable clinical outcome, suggesting that the immune system does respond to glioblastoma [35, 36]. Additional evidence of an anti-glioma response comes from vaccination trials targeting *EGFRvIII* that demonstrated the generation of *EGFRvIII* specific T-cells that could recognize and kill glioblastoma cells. Many of these patients went on to develop recurrent tumors, and pathological analysis revealed an absence of *EGFRvIII* expression, which is consistent with specific immune mediated destruction of *EGFRvIII* tumor cells [37].

## Evidence for Glioma Induced Immune Evasion

GBM cell lines secrete soluble factors that lead to an enrichment of Tregs [38], contributing to poor outcome. Unlike many other tumor pathologies, increasing CD8+ T-cell numbers do not correlate with an improved prognosis in glioblastoma, possibly due to immunoregulatory elements of the tumor microenvironment [39]. Patients with intracranial neoplasms also tend to have fewer peripheral CD4+ T-cells and defective TCR mediated signaling that may lead to cellular immune dysfunction [40, 41]. Most intratumoral DCs are recruited from peripheral monocytes which differentiate into DCs within the tumor; however, this differentiation is actively inhibited in glioblastoma [42, 43]. Moreover, glioma cells express low levels of MHC-I [44] making them difficult to detect by T-cells, and downregulation of MHC correlates with tumor cell invasion [45]. Glioma cells can even inhibit T-cell function directly by expression of immune checkpoint inhibitors such as PD-L1 [46, 47].

The immune infiltrate in glioma is generally not directed against the tumor; rather it tends to actively participate in immune evasion (Fig. 10.1). Analogous to the situation in peripheral tumors, many of these infiltrating leukocytes are immunosuppressive, preventing an effective anti-tumor immune response. Macrophages and microglia form the majority of these infiltrating leukocytes, up to 30 % of the tumor cell mass. Glioma associated macrophages (GAMs) are actively recruited by the tumor via a complex chemo-attraction process involving chemokines, cytokines, and matrix proteins [48–52]. The chemokines CXCL1 and tumor necrosis factor of mouse embryo (TROY) secreted by glioma cells participate in GAM recruitment [50, 53]. GAMs and glioma cells then exist in symbiosis

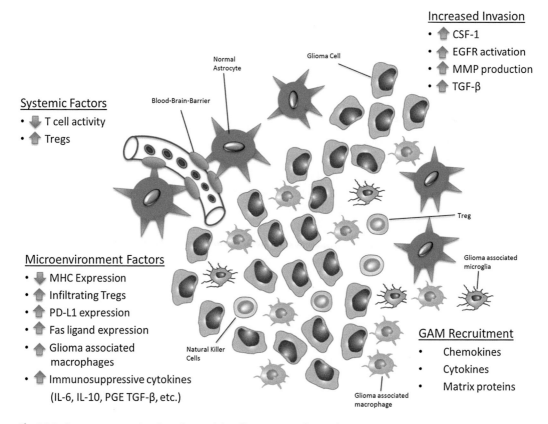

**Fig. 10.1**  Immunosuppression, invasion, and the glioma tumor microenvironment

through an elaborate paracrine network sustained by mediators such as colony stimulating factor-1 (CSF-1), a powerful chemokine for microglial recruitment. This invasive stimulus is reciprocated by GAMs through epidermal growth factor receptor activation (EGFR) and matrix metalloprotease (MMP) 2, 9, and 14 production [49, 50]. Experiments with CD11b-HSVTK mouse models, which specifically deplete microglia and macrophages, result in an 80 % reduction in glioma volume, demonstrating the importance and necessity of GAMs in the growth and development of glioblastoma [54]. Both glioma cells and tumor associated macrophages secrete immunosuppressive cytokines such as TGF-β1, β2, and β3 [55–57], as well as IL-6 [58, 59], IL-10 [60], prostaglandin E [61], and gangliosides.

Pretreatment immune parameters are prognostic in many disease processes. Elevation of one such factor, the pretreatment neutrophil-lymphocyte (NL) ratio, has been shown to correlate with poor outcomes in cancer of the bladder [62], colon [63], prostate [64], and GBM [65]. While the exact mechanism is not known, NL ratio correlates with levels of MDSCs which can promote tumor growth and invasion as well as inhibit T-cell responses both peripherally and in the tumor. The threshold of significance for the NL ratio varies with investigator and disease site, but a cut-off of 4 was selected in a study of 84 patients with GBM. Patients with a pre-corticosteroid NL ratio greater than 4 had a median survival of 7.5 versus 11.2 months, which was significant on both univariate and multivariate analysis, highlighting the importance of host immunity and lymphocytes in GBM outcome [65].

## GAMs Induce Growth and Invasion of GBM

In vitro studies have demonstrated the ability of tumor cells to recruit microglia to the tumor site and transform these leukocytes into tumor-supportive cells [66]. Both microglia and tumor cells release cytokines, including TGF-β1 which promote tumor invasion and progression in addition to suppressing the local anti-tumor immune responses [67, 68]. CD133+ glioma stem cells also stimulate this tumor growth and invasion through production of TGF-β1 [69]. Tumor cells, stem cells, microglia, and macrophages also make proteases such as MMP-9 which enzymatically degrade extracellular matrix facilitating tumor invasion [70]. Pro-inflammatory cytokines such as IL-1 also increase the migratory capacity of glioma cells [71, 72].

## Effects of Radiation Therapy on the Glioma Immune Response

Classical radiobiology attributes the therapeutic effect of radiotherapy to the cytotoxic effect of radiotherapy-induced DNA damage in tumor cells. However, emerging evidence points to additional mechanisms wherein radiotherapy influences the immune system and, hence, tumor immunity [73]. The effect of radiotherapy on the immune system is complex, with the induction of mechanisms that both suppress and stimulate anti-tumor immune responses [74].

The following section will discuss the various effects of radiotherapy on the immune system. The first aspect involves the direct effects on lymphocytes, including leukopenia and immunogenic cell death [75]. Following this, an examination of the evidence in non-glioma and glioblastoma model systems will highlight the experimental evidence demonstrating how radiotherapy influences the immune system and its effects on glioblastoma. Radiotherapy can also affect the blood–brain barrier (BBB), angiogenesis, lymphocyte recruitment, and normal microglia (which play a role in the CNS immune system) and these effects on tumor immunity will be described. An understanding of the various mechanisms by which radiotherapy affects tumor immunity may enable selective therapeutic promotion of anti-tumor effects and inhibition of pro-tumor effects in order to improve the efficacy of RT in treating glioblastoma.

## Radiation Induced Leukopenia

The most direct action of RT on the immune system is through depletion of lymphocytes by radiation induced apoptosis [76]. Lymphocytes are exquisitely sensitive to radiation and are readily eliminated by exposure to doses of even a single fraction of 1.8–2 Gy [77], the fractionated dose routinely used in the treatment of GBM. Effectively all lymphocytes circulating through the intracranial vasculature are exposed to radiation throughout the 6–7 week course of partial brain radiotherapy routinely prescribed for GBM. This results in lymphopenia, an effect compounded by temozolomide and other chemotherapeutics administered to patients concurrently with radiotherapy. This effect has been demonstrated in patients undergoing extracorporeal blood irradiation, a process that results in no dose delivered to bone marrow or lymphatic tissue. After this treatment the systemic lymphocyte concentration dropped by 50% in response to even modest doses of less than 60 cGy [78]. Models of radiation exposure to circulating leukocytes from a typical GBM treatment plan estimates that a single 2 Gy fraction results in exposure of 5 % of the circulating blood volume to a lymphotoxic dose of greater than 0.5 Gy. Upon completion of a standard 60 Gy course of fractionated radiation, 99 % of the blood volume is exposed to a potentially lymphotoxic dose [79]. This immunosuppressive effect of radiation on the immune system must be considered when combining RT and immunotherapies.

## Chemotherapy Induced Immunosuppression

In addition to radiotherapy, standard treatments including chemotherapy and corticosteroids can contribute to immune suppression, making the immunomodulatory effects of RT difficult to isolate from the effects of other medical therapies. Temozolomide, the most common chemotherapeutic agent used to treat GBM, can cause leukopenia and resultant immune suppression [80–82]. Corticosteroids used for managing cerebral edema can also contribute to immunosuppression by inducing apoptosis of T-cells and thymocytes [83–85], resulting in an increased risk for opportunistic infections [86].

## RT Induces Immunogenic Cell Death

In contrast to its immunosuppressive effects, radiotherapy can potentiate anti-tumor immunity by inducing immunogenic death of cancer cells [87]. The destruction of tumor cells by RT and the subsequent release of tumor antigens and immune adjuvants facilitate the priming of anti-tumor CTLs [88]. Radiation facilitates the transfer of tumor antigens from dying cancer cells to APCs by inducing the translocation of calreticulin (CRT) to the cell membrane, an "eat me" signal for receptor mediated endocytosis by APCs. As discussed above RT also releases ATP and other DAMPs such as HSPs [1, 2], HMGB1 [3], and uric acid [4], which act as endogenous adjuvants. These stimulate APCs to express pro-inflammatory cytokines and membrane bound co-stimulatory molecules that mediate T-cell priming. Radiation induced immunogenic cell death has been modeled in vitro, and depends on both dose and fractionation [89–91]. Preclinical evidence for radiation induced immunogenic cell death abounds in many tumor models, including breast cancer, prostate cancer, and melanoma, and there is some evidence gathered in vitro for glioma. For example, single fractions of up to 20 Gy induce apoptosis as well as the expression and release of the endogenous adjuvant HSP70 from the U87 glioma cell line [92].

## Immunogenic Cell Death and T-cell Priming in Non-glioma Models

There is evidence from both humans and mice that radiotherapy can induce a specific anti-tumor immune response. By experimental necessity, much of this evidence comes from murine tumor lines (primarily melanoma) which allow for measurement of specific CTL responses against known peptide epitopes. Studies of ionizing radiation in murine melanoma show that both single doses of 15–20 Gy and fractionated RT induce cross-presentation of tumor associated antigens [93], and this results in cross-priming of CTLs detected in the tumor and tumor draining lymph nodes [94], and is dependent on TLR4 signaling [3]. There is some correlation between the number of CTLs primed and the dose of single fraction radiation, but fractionated treatment results in the same number of primed CTLs, irrespective of RT dose [95]. Conversely, when combined with anti-CTLA-4 blockade, fractionated, but not single dose radiation, appeared to optimally induce anti-tumor responses in breast and colorectal syngeneic tumor models [96].

## Combinations of Radiotherapy and Immunotherapy in Glioblastoma Models

Since radiotherapy alone is rarely a curative treatment, combinations of radiotherapy with immune modulators have been a focus of study in order to improve treatment efficacy. The combination of immune checkpoint blockade and radiation is an effective strategy for inducing anti-tumor immunity in murine glioma models, seen for both CTLA-4 antagonists in combination with IL-12 [99] as well as PD-1 blockade with a systemically administered monoclonal antibody [98]. Mice were implanted with GL261 glioma cells intracranially and then treated with the small animal radiation research platform, which allows for stereotactic radiation delivery. Median survival was approximately doubled ($p < 0.05$) in the combined radiation and anti-PD-1 arm when compared to the untreated control group or either treatment modality alone. More importantly, there were more cytotoxic T-cells and less Tregs observed in the combined treatment arm compared to the control arms [98]. Alternatively, mice harboring poorly immunogenic GL261 tumors implanted and grown orthotopically and then treated with stimulatory antibodies directed at 4-1BB combined with 8 Gy of cranial RT delivered in two fractions results in complete tumor rejection in two-thirds of mice, with 5 of 6 long term survivors rejecting future tumor challenge. Antitumor immunity was associated with increased glioma-specific production of interferon-γ with an increased number of tumor-infiltrating lymphocytes [99].

Combinations of these immunostimulatory approaches are even more effective at producing clinically relevant anti-tumor immunity in murine models. Using the GL261 intracranial model of glioblastoma, focal radiotherapy (10 Gy) combined with both CTLA-4 blockade (shutting off the brake) and activation of 4-1BB (stepping on the gas) results in an extension of mouse median survival to 67 days compared with 24 days with RT alone [100]. Some prolongation in survival was seen in RT combined with CTLA-4 blockade compared to focal RT alone but not seen in RT combined with 4-1BB compared to RT alone. Furthermore, treatment with triple therapy resulted in a higher density of CD4+ and CD8+ tumor infiltrating lymphocytes, and depletion of CD4+ cells, but not CD8+ cells, had a detrimental effect on tumor control, calling into question the benefit of CD8+ CTLs in this anti-glioma response. These promising preclinical results have led to clinical studies now accruing testing the effects of anti-PD-1 (Pidilizumab—NCT01952769; Nivolumab—NCT02017717) and anti-PD-L1 (MEDI4736—NCT02336165) clinical trials.

## RT Induces Humoral Immune Responses to GBM

In addition to cellular mediated immunity discussed above, there is evidence that radiation can promote priming of B-cells resulting in glioma specific antibody formation. In a clinical study involving 24 patients with newly diagnosed glioblastoma, glioma-expressed antigen 2 (GLEA2) seroreactivity was measured prior to, during, and after RT, and these levels were compared to healthy controls and patients with lung cancer. Radiotherapy induced a transient increase in GLEA2 specific antibodies during the course of RT [101]. Importantly, development of glioma specific antibodies such as GLEA2 and PDH-finger protein 3 (PHF3) correlate with improved survival in patients treated for GBM, suggesting a role for an anti-tumor humoral immune response in the treatment response to radiotherapy [102].

## RT Improves Antigen Presentation by GBM and Stimulates Anti-tumor Immunity

Not only does radiotherapy facilitate the priming of glioma specific T-cells through the induction of immunogenic cell death, RT also induces expression of MHC-I on glioblasts making them better targets for CTL killing. Antigen presentation by MHC-I is crucial for anti-tumor immunity through interactions with the T-cell receptor of tumor specific CTLs [103], and one mechanism by which GBM evades immune destruction is through the downregulation of antigen presentation [45]. In adenocarcinoma, radiotherapy counteracts this mechanism for immune escape by upregulating antigen processing and presentation by tumor cells [104]. A similar effect has been observed in GL261 gliomas in mice treated with whole brain RT (WBRT; 8 Gy in two fractions), vaccination with irradiated GL261 cells injected peripherally, or both WBRT and vaccination. Upregulation of MHC-I was observed after WBRT, and there was an associated increase in CD4+ and CD8+ T-cell infiltration; however, RT or vaccination alone did not confer a significant survival advantage. Combined treatment increased long-term survival in the range of 40–80 % compared to 0–10 % in mice treated with vaccination alone. Furthermore, surviving mice demonstrated antitumor immunity by rejecting rechallenge with GL261 cells, suggesting the generation of a protective immune response from treatment with radiotherapy combined with vaccination [105].

## Induction of Pro-inflammatory Cytokines by RT

Radiation therapy can have an inflammatory effect on the glioma microenvironment through upregulation of specific cytokines. Cytokines are a diverse group of small soluble proteins that include chemokines, colony-stimulating factors, interleukins (IL), interferons, and tumor necrosis factors (TNF). They act in an autocrine and paracrine fashion to induce the differentiation,

proliferation, and migration of leukocytes and neural precursors [106]. Radiation has been shown to promote the upregulation of the pro-inflammatory cytokines TNF-$\alpha$ and IL-1$\beta$, and the chemokine monocyte chemoattractant protein-1 (MCP-1) in rats treated with WBRT using a single dose of 10 Gy [107]. The potent pro-inflammatory cytokines IL-1$\beta$ and IL-6 were also shown to be increased in glioblastoma cell lines exposed to radiation [108]. TNF-$\alpha$, a cytokine that can induce inflammation and apoptosis, is induced in astrocytes and microglia grown in cell culture and treated with multiple 2 Gy RT doses, an effect that may contribute to an anti-tumor immune response against GBM [109]. This was confirmed in mice treated with either single dose or fractionated WBRT up to 40 Gy with an over twofold increase of TNF-$\alpha$ mRNA [110].

Radiotherapy has a similar pro-inflammatory effect when delivered internally using nanoparticle bound Rhenium-188 which delivers beta particle radiation directly to intracranial tumors in the 9L Fisher rat glioma model. Using this method, two fractions of 8 Gy increased peripheral levels of IL-2 and interferon-$\gamma$ and resulted in recruitment and activation of immune cells to the tumor. These recruited leukocytes have not been rigorously defined, but include CD11b/c+ amoeboid cells resembling monocytes, macrophages, and microglia with increased expression of MHC-I and MHC-II. NK cells, DCs, CD4+, and CD8+ cells were also recruited. Furthermore, 83 % of rats treated with these radioactive nanoparticles were often cured of their tumors, which were universally fatal in all control rats. Surviving animals were resistant to rechallenge with 9L glioma cells, suggesting protective immunological memory [111].

Some pro-inflammatory cytokines induced by RT can have effects on the tumor microenvironment that promote the growth and invasion of gliomas. For example, IL-1$\beta$ is upregulated in response to RT, and this induces hypoxia-inducible factor 1$\alpha$ (HIF-1$\alpha$) through the Ras pathway. HIF-1$\alpha$ is a critical cytokine in angiogenesis that promotes blood vessel development as well as tumor invasion and progression in patients with GBM [112]. Radiation induced

HIF-1α could lead to angiogenesis even under normoxic conditions [113].

Not all effects of radiotherapy promote antitumor immunity. Radiation can also induce regulatory cytokines that can suppress inflammation and the anti-tumor immune response. Radiation delivered both in vitro and in vivo induces TGF-β production by glioma cells [114–117]. This increase in TGF-β is thought to promote self-renewal and effective DNA damage repair in glioblastoma stem cells (GSC) leading to radiation resistance [14, 118]. Promising preclinical research involving LY36947, a small molecule inhibitor of the TGF-β1 receptor kinase, in combination with radiation in GBM cell lines demonstrated a decrease in DNA damage response and a 75 % reduction in neurosphere formation [119]. Further understanding of the cytokine response to RT will drive novel drug development and hopefully provide an effective tool to combat radioresistance of GBM.

The effect of RT on glioma and normal brain is complex, inducing a combination of pro-inflammatory and anti-inflammatory cytokines. This is supported by cytokine mRNA induction in the brains of Fischer rats treated with WBRT in a single fraction of 15 Gy. Four hours after treatment there is a spike in IL-1β and TGF-β1 expression, as well as an early increase in phospholipase $A_2$ and COX-2, indicating a mixed pro- and anti-inflammatory state after RT. In addition to inducing inflammation, there was enhanced glioma cell infiltration observed after F98 glioma cells were introduced intracranially after WBRT [120].

## RT Breaks Down the BBB

The brain parenchyma is unique in regards to the rest of the body due to the unique biologic interface known as the blood-brain barrier (BBB) that isolates the CNS from the rest of the systemic circulation. The BBB is created by tight junctions between capillary endothelial cells in the brain and is crucial for brain homeostasis [121]. Integrity of the BBB also isolates the CNS from many immune active substances including immunoglobulins. Breakdown of the BBB is enhanced

by RT in a dose dependent manner. There is evidence that RT at low doses (18–24 Gy) given to children with acute leukemia does not disrupt the BBB. In a study of 23 patients who had CSF and plasma levels of Ara-C measured before, during, and after prophylactic cranial irradiation, there was not a significant change in the CSF:plasma ratio, implying lack of BBB breakdown due to radiation delivered at these low doses [122]. A study of 14 patients with primary brain tumors injected systemically with $^{99M}$Tc-glucoheptonate and then radiated with 30–40 Gy in 2 Gy per fraction demonstrated the contribution to BBB breakdown by the tumor and radiation individually, as well as the combined tumor and treatment effect on the BBB. The area of the brain containing the tumor had a pretreatment enhancement that was 22 % higher than the uninvolved brain. The uninvolved, but radiated brain enhanced 25 % above background and the treated brain containing tumor enhanced 75 % over the pretreatment uninvolved brain demonstrating the marked BBB destruction caused by the combination of local tumor and RT effects [123]. This breakdown of the BBB by radiation likely facilitates treatment by allowing immunoglobulins, complement, leukocytes, and chemotherapeutics access to the tumor microenvironment.

## RT Enhances Macrophage and Monocyte Recruitment

As gliomas grow, they become heavily infiltrated with glioma associated microglia and macrophages (GAMs) that can make up as much as one-third of the tumor mass [124], and this recruitment is further enhanced by radiotherapy [125]. This is demonstrated in an autopsy study of patients with brain tumors treated with I-125 implants to a mean dose of 62.3 Gy, with brain tissue obtained at time points ranging from 0.75 to 60 months after radiotherapy [126]. Immunohistochemistry revealed an acute influx of migrating macrophages, apparently concerned with the elimination of necrotic debris, with microglial accumulation in the region directly adjacent to the necrotic center.

## Glioma and Microglia Promoted Angiogenesis

Another important hallmark of malignancy in gliomas is angiogenesis, the development of blood vessels in order to meet the metabolic demands of the growing tumor [127]. While much of the work on GBM has been focused on the tumor cells ability to drive angiogenesis [128], there is increasing evidence that the microglia may be a major driver of blood vessel formation. GAMs express Flt-1, a tyrosine kinase inhibitor that binds to VEGF, and is a positive regulator of angiogenesis [129]. When combined with glioma cells, Flt-1 knockout cells led to tumors of decreased volume and vascularity, suggesting the importance of GAMs in angiogenesis [130].

A different in vivo technique was employed in order to study the effects of radiation on the normal brain parenchyma [131]. Their main focus was to look at a process termed vasculogenesis, the development of tumor vasculature by colonizing of circulating endothelial cells from the bone marrow. They had previously reported on the importance of GAMs in vasculogenesis by implanting tumor cells in preirradiated MMP-9 knockout mice and controls to demonstrate the lack of tumor growth or vasculogenesis in the tumors without MMP-9 support from the surrounding microenvironment [132]. They first used an orthotopic tumor model of U251 GBM cells implanted intracranially and the mice were given whole brain RT. Growth and regression was confirmed in a radiation dose dependent manner by histology and MRI. The irradiated cells demonstrated vascular damage and increased HIF-1 leading to increased recruitment of GAMs. Irradiated, hypoxic tumors also demonstrated increased levels of SDF-1 which has been shown to phosphorylate CXCR4 [133] and lead to revascularization. The addition of drug AMD3100, which blocks the SDF-1/CXCR4 interaction, prevented the return of blood flow in irradiated tumors thus preventing tumor recurrence. These promising results have led to clinical trials including AMD3100 in the treatment regimen of high grade glioma in conjunction with radiation (clinicaltrials.gov identifiers: NCT01977677, NCT01339039).

## Clinical Experience Targeting the Immune System After Chemoradiation

There have been a number of efforts recently to combine immunotherapy with radiotherapy to augment the anti-tumor immune effects of radiotherapy (Table 10.1). A strategy to increase both the likelihood and duration of anti-tumor immunity in response to immunotherapy is to add radiotherapy as an adjunct to bolster the immune response [134, 135]. When combined with radiotherapy, immunotherapeutic approaches can be broadly separated into (1) the promotion of cross-priming of tumor specific CTLs, (2) the stimulation of immune effector function of CTLs primed by RT, and (3) neutralization of the immunosuppressive effects of the tumor microenvironment. Essentially all current clinical approaches fall into the first two categories, with the third category primarily in the preclinical stage.

## TLR Agonists

TLR-3 is the receptor for poly-ICLC, a double stranded RNA shown to increase the antibody response to antigen, and augment the activation of natural killer cells, macrophages, and T-cells [136–140]. The North American Brain Tumor Consortium conducted a single-arm phase II trial of poly-ICLC in conjunction with radiation in patients with newly diagnosed supratentorial glioblastoma [141]. Poly-ICLC was administered intramuscularly three times per week at 20 mcg/kg, and radiation was delivered 5 days per week to a total dose of 60 Gy in 2 Gy within 1 week of starting poly-ICLC. The combined treatment was followed by poly-ICLC for up to 1 year, or until the tumor progressed. Thirty eligible patients demonstrated a 1 year overall survival of 69 %

**Table 10.1** Prospective trials highlighting immunotherapeutic strategies for gliomas

| Immunotherapeutic approach | Class | Representative therapeutic | Setting | Design/primary endpoint |
|---|---|---|---|---|
| Cellular | Adoptive T-cell transfer | Activated T-cells | [143]—PG/RG | [143, 144]—Phase I/safety |
| | | | [144]—PG | |
| Vaccination | Tumor-associated antigen vaccine | Dendritic cells pulsed with tumor-associated antigen | [145]—RG | [145]—Phase I/II |
| | | | [146]—PG/RG | [146]—Phase I/immunogenicity |
| | | | [147]—PG | [147]—Randomized phase II/efficacy |
| | Tumor-specific antigen vaccine | Vaccine targeted to EGFRvIII (Rindopepimut) | [149]—PG | [149]—Phase I/safety |
| | | | [150]—PG | [150]—Phase II/efficacy |
| | | | [151]—PG | [151]—Phase II/efficacy |
| | Whole tumor lysate | DCVax | [152]—PG | [152]—Phase I/safety |
| | | | [153]—PG/RG | [153]—Phase I/safety |
| | | | [154]—PG/RG | [154]—Phase I/dose escalation |
| | | | [155]—RG | [155]—Phase I/II |
| | | | [156]—RG | [156]—Phase I/safety |
| | | | [157]—PG/RG | [157]—Phase II/efficacy |
| | | | [158]—PG | [158]—Pilot/feasibility |
| | | | [159]—PG | [159]—Phase I/safety |
| | | | [160]—PG | [160]—Phase I/dose escalation |
| | | | [161]—PG | [161]—Phase I/II |
| | | | [162]—PG | [162]—Phase I/dose escalation[a] |
| | | | [163]—PG | [163]—Randomized phase II/efficacy |
| | Heat shock proteins | HSPPC-96 | [165]—RG | [165]—Phase I/dose escalation |
| | | | [166]—RG | [166]—Phase II/efficacy |
| | Glioma stem cells | Dendritic cells transfected with mRNA from GSCs | [167]—PG | [167]—Phase I/II |

*PG* primary glioma, *RG* recurrent glioma, *GSC* glioma stem cells
[a]Manuscript describing patients from both whole tumor lysate and tumor-associated antigen protocols NCT00068510 and NCT0061200

which compares favorably to RT alone but is comparable to the current standard of care, radiation with concurrent temozolomide [82].

## Adoptive Cell Transfer

Adoptive cell transfer is a type of immunotherapy that involves the isolation of autologous blood-borne or tumor-infiltrating lymphocytes followed by their selection, expansion, and activation ex vivo and subsequent reinfusion into the host [142]. In a phase I study, patients with progressive primary or recurrent malignant glioma, previously treated with standard radiotherapy, were inoculated intradermally with irradiated autologous tumor cells and granulocyte macrophage-colony stimulating factor as an

adjuvant. Cells from surgically removed inguinal lymph nodes were then removed, expanded, and reintroduced intravenously. There were no Grade 3 or 4 toxicities and 3 of 10 patients demonstrated regression or stable disease [143]. A subsequent phase I trial from this group demonstrated similar results with 4/12 patients glioma patients treated in the upfront setting demonstrating partial regression [144].

## Dendritic Cell Based Vaccines

Active immunotherapy utilizing DCs has the advantage of eliciting a specific de novo immune response against selected tumor antigens. Another vaccination method employed to combat the inherent heterogeneity of glioma cells was to target glioma-associated antigen (GAA) in the hopes of generating a more potent cytotoxic anti-tumor immune response. In a phase I/II trial, 22 patients with recurrent glioblastoma underwent treatment with autologous dendritic cells loaded with synthetic GAA and poly-ICLC. The treatment was well tolerated with 9/22 patients demonstrating progression free status for at least 1 year [145]. A separate phase I trial was recently reported from the Cedars-Sinai group that tested a similar strategy in 17 newly diagnosed and three recurrent GBM patients, as well as one brainstem glioma patient. The median overall survival in the newly diagnosed cohort was an impressive 38 months [146]. The highest level of evidence supporting this approach to treatment, currently only published in abstract form, is a randomized, double-blinded, placebo controlled trial evaluating the addition of a tumor-associated antigen loaded DC vaccine (ICT-107) to standard radiotherapy and temozolamide. This trial randomized 124 patients after 6 weeks of concurrent chemoradiation in a 2:1 ratio to vaccine or placebo and demonstrated a statistically significant 2 month advantage in progression-free survival in the ICT-107 vaccine group. There was no difference in overall survival at the time of abstract reporting, but the patients in the study continue to be followed [147].

In a different vaccine study, DCs were loaded with synthetic antigenic peptides from *EGFRvIII*, a common driver mutation in GBM [148, 149]. Twelve patients were treated with intradermal injection of DCs pulsed with an *EGFRvIII*-specific peptide. The injections were given in three equal doses, 2 weeks apart, without further intervention until clinical or radiographic progression. This therapy was well tolerated, and 83 % of the patients demonstrated an immune response with an impressive overall median survival of 22.8 months. This success led to a phase II multi-institutional trial [150, 151] using a similar DC based therapy after concurrent chemoradiation that demonstrated median overall survival of 26 months which was significantly longer when compared to a group of matched controls (HR 5.3; $p = .0013$; $n = 17$). Interestingly, 82 % of patients lost *EGFRvIII* expression at progression, which is indirect evidence that vaccination led to

specific anti-tumor immunity, immunoediting, and immune escape. This immunotherapeutic strategy warrants further investigation in a randomized, controlled trial.

Since it is not known which antigenic peptides will produce the most robust immune response, another approach to vaccination is to load DCs with antigens derived from each patient's individual tumor, creating a personalized vaccine specific for each patient. This was tested in a phase I study [152] in which patients with recurrent GBM received autologous DCs pulsed with lysate prepared from each patient's tumor and then re-introduced in three injections. Evidence of specific cellular immunity was observed in 57 % of patients, and 50 % of patients who underwent re-operation had a significant CD8+ T-cell infiltrate. This treatment was well tolerated with no significant adverse or autoimmune effects reported. A subsequent trial demonstrated similar results in a cohort of 14 patients [153], and multiple other groups performed phase I or phase I/II trials in the primary or recurrent glioma setting with comparable results [154–162]. Perhaps the most provocative trial employing whole tumor lysate is the randomized phase II trial by a group in Taiwan. This trial randomized 34 patients with newly diagnosed GBM between chemoradiation (60 Gy + temozolomide) and chemoradiation with the addition of a tumor lysate DC vaccine. With a median follow-up of 33 months the overall survival in the vaccination group was 32 months versus 15 months in the control group ($p < .002$) [163]. A multi-institutional phase III trial is warranted to confirm these compelling preliminary data.

## Vaccination: Heat Shock Proteins

Heat shock proteins are another form of personalized autologous vaccine that has been tested in clinical trials after chemoradiation. HSPs are molecular chaperones that are thought to participate in the processing and presentation of peptide antigens on MHC-I. HSPs purified from tumor cells are associated with tumor specific peptide antigens, and these HSP-peptide complexes induce tumor specific immunity that can result in tumor rejection [164]. This approach has been utilized in a phase I dose escalation trial involving 12 patients with recurrent GBM treated with the HSP gp96 purified from surgically resected tumor. Eleven of the 12 patients treated demonstrated a tumor specific peripheral immune response. The median survival was 47 weeks in the 11 immune responders compared to 16 weeks in the single non-responder [165]. These results led to a multi-center phase II trial evaluating 41 patients previously treated with standard partial brain irradiation to 60 Gy with concurrent temozolamide and presented with operable, recurrent GBM. The median survival was similar in this expanded cohort of patients at 43 weeks [166]. An interesting finding that certainly warrants further examination was the significant negative correlation between pre-vaccination lymphopenia and survival, highlighting the importance of an intact immune system pretreatment. These exciting results have led to a RTOG 1470 phase II randomized trial comparing bevacizumab and gp96 vaccination with bevacizumab alone in patients with resectable, recurrent GBM.

## Conclusions

We are entering an exciting time in the treatment of what has historically been a universally fatal disease. While there have been many advances in the past decade there is still much work to be done. There are many trials currently open and accruing (Table 10.2) and many more are ongoing.

**Table 10.2** Trials actively recruiting studying immunotherapy in brain tumors

| Immunotherapeutic approach | Class | Therapeutic | Clinicaltrial.gov identifier |
|---|---|---|---|
| Cellular | Chimeric antigen receptor (CAR)—engineered T-cells | • Genetically modified HER2/CAR CMV-specific CTLs | • NCT01109095 |
| | | • Anti-EGFRvIII CAR transduced PBL | • NCT01454596 |
| Vaccination | Dendritic cell vaccine | • Tumor lysate<br>• Dendritic Cell Vaccine in combination with Imiquimod cream<br>• Tumor specific peptide | • NCT01808820,<br>NCT01204684,<br>NCT02010606,<br>NCT01635283,<br>NCT01957956,<br>NCT00045968 |
| | | • ICT-121 DC vaccine | • NCT01792505,<br>NCT01678352,<br>NCT01902771<br>NCT01400672 (with RT) |
| | | • ADU-623 | • NCT02193347,<br>NCT02078648,<br>NCT02149225,<br>NCT01920191,<br>NCT01498328 |
| | | | • NCT02049489 |
| | | | • NCT01967758 |
| | Virus | • Live attenuated, oral (Sabin) serotype 1 poliovirus vaccine (PVSRIPO) | • NCT01491893 |
| | | • Measles Virus Derivative Producing CEA (MV-CEA) | • NCT00390299 |
| | Heat shock proteins | • NCT00390299gp96 vaccination | • NCT02122822 |
| | | • NCT00390299HSPPC-96 | • NCT01814813 |
| Immunomodulation | IDO inhibitor | • Indoximod | • NCT02052648 |
| | Anti-PD1 | • CT-011 | • NCT01952769 |
| | Anti-CLTA-4 and Anti-PD1 | • Ipilumimab and Nivolumab | • NCT02017717 |
| | Anti-PD-L1 | • MEDI4736 | • NCT02336165 |

Future studies will need to take a careful look at pretreatment immune competence as well as investigate how to best incorporate radiation therapy with regards to timing, total dose, and fractionation. Checkpoint inhibitors and agonists need to be studied both alone and in combination with radiation to ensure the maximum efficacy. Overall survival remains the most reliable measure of treatment outcome rather than tumor response.

A concerted effort in both understanding the cross talk of GBM with the host's immune system and in testing immunotherapy in this disease will significantly contribute to win the battle against a disease that is so devastating to patients of all ages in all walks of life.

# References

1. Srivastava P. Roles of heat-shock proteins in innate and adaptive immunity. Nat Rev Immunol. 2002; 2(3):185–94.
2. Pasi F, Paolini A. Effects of single or combined treatments with radiation and chemotherapy on survival and danger signals expression in glioblastoma cell lines. BioMed Res Int. 2014;2014:453497.
3. Apetoh L, Ghiringhelli F, Tesniere A, Obeid M, Ortiz C, Criollo A, et al. Toll-like receptor 4-dependent contribution of the immune system to anticancer chemotherapy and radiotherapy. Nat Med. 2007;13(9):1050–9.
4. Shi Y, Evans JE, Rock KL. Molecular identification of a danger signal that alerts the immune system to dying cells. Nature. 2003;425(6957):516–21.
5. Coley II WB. Contribution to the knowledge of sarcoma. Ann Surg. 1891;14(3):199–220.
6. De Bonis P, Albanese A, Lofrese G, de Waure C, Mangiola A, Pettorini BL, et al. Postoperative infection may influence survival in patients with glioblastoma: simply a myth? Neurosurgery. 2011; 69(4):864–8; discussion 8–9.
7. Dunn GP, Old LJ, Schreiber RD. The immunobiology of cancer immunosurveillance and immunoediting. Immunity. 2004;21(2):137–48.
8. Serraino D, Piselli P, Busnach G, Burra P, Citterio F, Arbustini E, et al. Risk of cancer following immunosuppression in organ transplant recipients and in HIV-positive individuals in southern Europe. Eur J Cancer. 2007;43(14):2117–23.
9. Robert C, Long GV, Brady B, Dutriaux C, Maio M, Mortier L, et al. Nivolumab in previously untreated melanoma without BRAF mutation. N Engl J Med. 2015;372(4):320–30.
10. Kantoff PW, Higano CS, Shore ND, Berger ER, Small EJ, Penson DF, et al. Sipuleucel-T immuno-

11. Burnet M. Cancer; a biological approach. I. The processes of control. Br Med J. 1957;1(5022):779–86.
12. Gabrilovich D. Mechanisms and functional significance of tumour-induced dendritic-cell defects. Nat Rev Immunol. 2004;4(12):941–52.
13. Seliger B, Massa C. The dark side of dendritic cells: development and exploitation of tolerogenic activity that favor tumor outgrowth and immune escape. Front Immunol. 2013;4:419.
14. Bouquet F, Pal A, Pilones KA, Demaria S, Hann B, Akhurst RJ, et al. TGFbeta1 inhibition increases the radiosensitivity of breast cancer cells in vitro and promotes tumor control by radiation in vivo. Clin Cancer Res. 2011;17(21):6754–65.
15. Sotomayor EM, Borrello I, Rattis FM, Cuenca AG, Abrams J, Staveley-O'Carroll K, et al. Cross-presentation of tumor antigens by bone marrow-derived antigen-presenting cells is the dominant mechanism in the induction of T-cell tolerance during B-cell lymphoma progression. Blood. 2001; 98(4):1070–7.
16. Cuenca A, Cheng F, Wang H, Brayer J, Horna P, Gu L, et al. Extra-lymphatic solid tumor growth is not immunologically ignored and results in early induction of antigen-specific T-cell anergy: dominant role of cross-tolerance to tumor antigens. Cancer Res. 2003;63(24):9007–15.
17. Perrot I, Blanchard D, Freymond N, Isaac S, Guibert B, Pacheco Y, et al. Dendritic cells infiltrating human non-small cell lung cancer are blocked at immature stage. J Immunol. 2007;178(5):2763–9.
18. Dunn GP, Bruce AT, Ikeda H, Old LJ, Schreiber RD. Cancer immunoediting: from immunosurveillance to tumor escape. Nat Immunol. 2002;3(11): 991–8.
19. Willimsky G, Blankenstein T. Sporadic immunogenic tumours avoid destruction by inducing T-cell tolerance. Nature. 2005;437(7055):141–6.
20. Koebel CM, Vermi W, Swann JB, Zerafa N, Rodig SJ, Old LJ, et al. Adaptive immunity maintains occult cancer in an equilibrium state. Nature. 2007;450(7171):903–7.
21. Zhong H, Gutkin DW, Han B, Ma Y, Keskinov AA, Shurin MR, et al. Origin and pharmacological modulation of tumor-associated regulatory dendritic cells. Int J Cancer. 2014;134(11):2633–45.
22. Gajewski TF, Meng Y, Blank C, Brown I, Kacha A, Kline J, et al. Immune resistance orchestrated by the tumor microenvironment. Immunol Rev. 2006; 213:131–45.
23. Sica A, Mantovani A. Macrophage plasticity and polarization: in vivo veritas. J Clin Invest. 2012;122(3):787–95.
24. Ostrand-Rosenberg S, Sinha P, Beury DW, Clements VK. Cross-talk between myeloid-derived suppressor cells (MDSC), macrophages, and dendritic cells enhances tumor-induced immune suppression. Semin Cancer Biol. 2012;22(4):275–81.

therapy for castration-resistant prostate cancer. N Engl J Med. 2010;363(5):411–22.

25. Gajewski TF, Schreiber H, Fu YX. Innate and adaptive immune cells in the tumor microenvironment. Nat Immunol. 2013;14(10):1014–22.

26. Rodriguez PC, Quiceno DG, Zabaleta J, Ortiz B, Zea AH, Piazuelo MB, et al. Arginase I production in the tumor microenvironment by mature myeloid cells inhibits T-cell receptor expression and antigen-specific T-cell responses. Cancer Res. 2004;64(16): 5839–49.

27. Rodriguez PC, Ochoa AC. Arginine regulation by myeloid derived suppressor cells and tolerance in cancer: mechanisms and therapeutic perspectives. Immunol Rev. 2008;222:180–91.

28. Gabrilovich DI, Ostrand-Rosenberg S, Bronte V. Coordinated regulation of myeloid cells by tumours. Nat Rev Immunol. 2012;12(4):253–68.

29. Medawar PB. Immunity to homologous grafted skin; the fate of skin homografts transplanted to the brain, to subcutaneous tissue, and to the anterior chamber of the eye. Br J Exp Pathol. 1948;29(1):58–69.

30. Xie L, Yang SH. Interaction of astrocytes and T cells in physiological and pathological conditions. Brain Res. 2015;1623:63–73.

31. Arbab AS. Cytotoxic T-cells as imaging probes for detecting glioma. World J Clin Oncol. 2010; 1(1):3–11.

32. Louveau A, et al. (2015). Structural and functional features of central nervous system lymphatic vessels. Nature 523(7560):337–341.

33. Goldmann J, Kwidzinski E, Brandt C, Mahlo J, Richter D, Bechmann I. T cells traffic from brain to cervical lymph nodes via the cribroid plate and the nasal mucosa. J Leukoc Biol. 2006;80(4):797–801.

34. Handel AE, Lincoln MR, Ramagopalan SV. Of mice and men: experimental autoimmune encephalitis and multiple sclerosis. Eur J Clin Invest. 2011; 41(11):1254–8.

35. Pitroda SP, Zhou T, Sweis RF, Filippo M, Labay E, Beckett MA, et al. Tumor endothelial inflammation predicts clinical outcome in diverse human cancers. PLoS One. 2012;7(10), e46104.

36. Gousias K, Voulgaris S, Vartholomatos G, Voulgari P, Kyritsis AP, Markou M. Prognostic value of the preoperative immunological profile in patients with glioblastoma. Surg Neurol Int. 2014;5:89.

37. Choi BD, Gedeon PC, Sanchez-Perez L, Bigner DD, Sampson JH. Regulatory T cells are redirected to kill glioblastoma by an EGFRvIII-targeted bispecific antibody. Oncoimmunology. 2013;2(12), e26757.

38. Crane CA, Ahn BJ, Han SJ, Parsa AT. Soluble factors secreted by glioblastoma cell lines facilitate recruitment, survival, and expansion of regulatory T cells: implications for immunotherapy. Neuro Oncol. 2012;14(5):584–95.

39. Yue Q, Zhang X, Ye HX, Wang Y, Du ZG, Yao Y, et al. The prognostic value of Foxp3+ tumor-infiltrating lymphocytes in patients with glioblastoma. J Neurooncol. 2014;116(2):251–9.

40. Fecci PE, Mitchell DA, Whitesides JF, Xie W, Friedman AH, Archer GE, et al. Increased regulatory T-cell fraction amidst a diminished CD4 compartment explains cellular immune defects in patients with malignant glioma. Cancer Res. 2006;66(6):3294–302.

41. Morford LA, Elliott LH, Carlson SL, Brooks WH, Roszman TL. T cell receptor-mediated signaling is defective in T cells obtained from patients with primary intracranial tumors. J Immunol. 1997;159(9):4415–25.

42. Zou JP, Morford LA, Chougnet C, Dix AR, Brooks AG, Torres N, et al. Human glioma-induced immunosuppression involves soluble factor(s) that alters monocyte cytokine profile and surface markers. J Immunol. 1999;162(8):4882–92.

43. Ogden AT, Horgan D, Waziri A, Anderson D, Louca J, McKhann GM, et al. Defective receptor expression and dendritic cell differentiation of monocytes in glioblastomas. Neurosurgery. 2006;59(4):902–9; discussion 9–10.

44. Lampson LA, Hickey WF. Monoclonal antibody analysis of MHC expression in human brain biopsies: tissue ranging from "histologically normal" to that showing different levels of glial tumor involvement. J Immunol. 1986;136(11):4054–62.

45. Zagzag D, Salnikow K, Chiriboga L, Yee H, Lan L, Ali MA, et al. Downregulation of major histocompatibility complex antigens in invading glioma cells: stealth invasion of the brain. Lab Invest. 2005; 85(3):328–41.

46. Wintterle S, Schreiner B, Mitsdoerffer M, Schneider D, Chen L, Meyermann R, et al. Expression of the B7-related molecule B7-H1 by glioma cells: a potential mechanism of immune paralysis. Cancer Res. 2003;63(21):7462–7.

47. Berghoff AS, Kiesel B, Widhalm G, Rajky O, Ricken G, Wohrer A, et al. Programmed death ligand 1 expression and tumor-infiltrating lymphocytes in glioblastoma. Neuro Oncol. 2015;17: 1064–75.

48. Badie B, Schartner J, Klaver J, Vorpahl J. In vitro modulation of microglia motility by glioma cells is mediated by hepatocyte growth factor/scatter factor. Neurosurgery. 1999;44(5):1077–82; discussion 82–3.

49. Coniglio SJ, Eugenin E, Dobrenis K, Stanley ER, West BL, Symons MH, et al. Microglial stimulation of glioblastoma invasion involves epidermal growth factor receptor (EGFR) and colony stimulating factor 1 receptor (CSF-1R) signaling. Mol Med. 2012;18:519–27.

50. Held-Feindt J, Hattermann K, Muerkoster SS, Wedderkopp H, Knerlich-Lukoschus F, Ungefroren H, et al. CX3CR1 promotes recruitment of human glioma-infiltrating microglia/macrophages (GIMs). Exp Cell Res. 2010;316(9):1553–66.

51. Okada M, Saio M, Kito Y, Ohe N, Yano H, Yoshimura S, et al. Tumor-associated macrophage/microglia infiltration in human gliomas is correlated with MCP-3, but not MCP-1. Int J Oncol. 2009;34(6):1621–7.

52. Eibinger G, Fauler G, Bernhart E, Frank S, Hammer A, Wintersperger A, et al. On the role of

25-hydroxycholesterol synthesis by glioblastoma cell lines. Implications for chemotactic monocyte recruitment. Exp Cell Res. 2013;319(12): 1828–38.

53. Jacobs VL, Liu Y, De Leo JA. Propentofylline targets TROY, a novel microglial signaling pathway. PLoS One. 2012;7(5), e37955.

54. Markovic DS, Vinnakota K, Chirasani S, Synowitz M, Raguet H, Stock K, et al. Gliomas induce and exploit microglial MT1-MMP expression for tumor expansion. Proc Natl Acad Sci U S A. 2009;106(30): 12530–5.

55. Munz C, Naumann U, Grimmel C, Rammensee HG, Weller M. TGF-beta-independent induction of immunogenicity by decorin gene transfer in human malignant glioma cells. Eur J Immunol. 1999;29(3): 1032–40.

56. Siepl C, Bodmer S, Frei K, MacDonald HR, De Martin R, Hofer E, et al. The glioblastoma-derived T cell suppressor factor/transforming growth factor-beta 2 inhibits T cell growth without affecting the interaction of interleukin 2 with its receptor. Eur J Immunol. 1988;18(4):593–600.

57. Bodmer S, Strommer K, Frei K, Siepl C, de Tribolet N, Heid I, et al. Immunosuppression and transforming growth factor-beta in glioblastoma. Preferential production of transforming growth factor-beta 2. J Immunol. 1989;143(10):3222–9.

58. Schneider J, Hofman FM, Apuzzo ML, Hinton DR. Cytokines and immunoregulatory molecules in malignant glial neoplasms. J Neurosurg. 1992; 77(2):265–73.

59. Lichtor T, Libermann TA. Coexpression of interleukin-1 beta and interleukin-6 in human brain tumors. Neurosurgery. 1994;34(4):669–72; discussion 72–3.

60. Huettner C, Paulus W, Roggendorf W. Messenger RNA expression of the immunosuppressive cytokine IL-10 in human gliomas. Am J Pathol. 1995;146(2): 317–22.

61. Fontana A, Kristensen F, Dubs R, Gemsa D, Weber E. Production of prostaglandin E and an interleukin-1 like factor by cultured astrocytes and C6 glioma cells. J Immunol. 1982;129(6):2413–9.

62. Gondo T, Nakashima J, Ohno Y, Choichiro O, Horiguchi Y, Namiki K, et al. Prognostic value of neutrophil-to-lymphocyte ratio and establishment of novel preoperative risk stratification model in bladder cancer patients treated with radical cystectomy. Urology. 2012;79(5):1085–91.

63. Walsh SR, Cook EJ, Goulder F, Justin TA, Keeling NJ. Neutrophil-lymphocyte ratio as a prognostic factor in colorectal cancer. J Surg Oncol. 2005;91(3):181–4.

64. Keizman D, Gottfried M, Ish-Shalom M, Maimon N, Peer A, Neumann A, et al. Pretreatment neutrophil-to-lymphocyte ratio in metastatic castration-resistant prostate cancer patients treated with ketoconazole:

association with outcome and predictive nomogram. Oncologist. 2012;17(12):1508–14.

65. Bambury RM, Teo MY, Power DG, Yusuf A, Murray S, Battley JE, et al. The association of pretreatment neutrophil to lymphocyte ratio with overall survival in patients with glioblastoma multiforme. J Neurooncol. 2013;114(1):149–54.

66. Badie B, Schartner J. Role of microglia in glioma biology. Microsc Res Tech. 2001;54(2):106–13.

67. Watters JJ, Schartner JM, Badie B. Microglia function in brain tumors. J Neurosci Res. 2005;81(3):447–55.

68. Wesolowska A, Kwiatkowska A, Slomnicki L, Dembinski M, Master A, Sliwa M, et al. Microglia-derived TGF-beta as an important regulator of glioblastoma invasion—an inhibition of TGF-beta-dependent effects by shRNA against human TGF-beta type II receptor. Oncogene. 2008;27(7):918–30.

69. Ye XZ, Xu SL, Xin YH, Yu SC, Ping YF, Chen L, et al. Tumor-associated microglia/macrophages enhance the invasion of glioma stem-like cells via TGF-beta1 signaling pathway. J Immunol. 2012; 189(1):444–53.

70. Hu F, Ku MC, Markovic D, ADzaye OD, Lehnardt S, Synowitz M, et al. Glioma-associated microglial MMP9 expression is upregulated by TLR2 signaling and sensitive to minocycline. Int J Cancer. 2014;135(11):2569–78.

71. Rajaraman P, Brenner AV, Butler MA, Wang SS, Pfeiffer RM, Ruder AM, et al. Common variation in genes related to innate immunity and risk of adult glioma. Cancer Epidemiol Biomarkers Prev. 2009; 18(5):1651–8.

72. Basu A, Krady JK, Levison SW. Interleukin-1: a master regulator of neuroinflammation. J Neurosci Res. 2004;78(2):151–6.

73. Golden EB, Formenti SC. Is tumor (R)ejection by the immune system the "5th R" of radiobiology? Oncoimmunology. 2014;3(1), e28133.

74. Formenti SC, Demaria S. Combining radiotherapy and cancer immunotherapy: a paradigm shift. J Natl Cancer Inst. 2013;105(4):256–65.

75. Golden EB, Formenti SC. Radiation therapy and immunotherapy: growing pains. Int J Radiat Oncol Biol Phys. 2015;91(2):252–4.

76. Shohan J. Some theoretical considerations on the present status of roentgen therapy. Boston Med Surg J. 1916;175(10):321–7.

77. Sellins KS, Cohen JJ. Gene induction by gamma-irradiation leads to DNA fragmentation in lymphocytes. J Immunol. 1987;139(10):3199–206.

78. Weeke E. The development of lymphopenia in uremic patients undergoing extracorporeal irradiation of the blood with portable beta units. Radiat Res. 1973;56(3):554–9.

79. Yovino S, Kleinberg L, Grossman SA, Narayanan M, Ford E. The etiology of treatment-related lymphopenia in patients with malignant gliomas: modeling radiation dose to circulating lymphocytes

explains clinical observations and suggests methods of modifying the impact of radiation on immune cells. Cancer Invest. 2013;31(2):140–4.

80. Brock CS, Newlands ES, Wedge SR, Bower M, Evans H, Colquhoun I, et al. Phase I trial of temozolomide using an extended continuous oral schedule. Cancer Res. 1998;58(19):4363–7.

81. Alvino E, Pepponi R, Pagani E, Lacal PM, Nunziata C, Bonmassar E, et al. O(6)-benzylguanine enhances the in vitro immunotoxic activity of temozolomide on natural or antigen-dependent immunity. J Pharmacol Exp Ther. 1999;291(3):1292–300.

82. Stupp R, Mason WP, van den Bent MJ, Weller M, Fisher B, Taphoorn MJ, et al. Radiotherapy plus concomitant and adjuvant temozolomide for glioblastoma. N Engl J Med. 2005;352(10):987–96.

83. Cifone MG, Migliorati G, Parroni R, Marchetti C, Millimaggi D, Santoni A, et al. Dexamethasone-induced thymocyte apoptosis: apoptotic signal involves the sequential activation of phosphoinositide-specific phospholipase C, acidic sphingomyelinase, and caspases. Blood. 1999;93(7):2282–96.

84. Cohen O, Ish-Shalom E, Kfir-Erenfeld S, Herr I, Yefenof E. Nitric oxide and glucocorticoids synergize in inducing apoptosis of CD4(+)8(+) thymocytes: implications for 'Death by Neglect' and T-cell function. Int Immunol. 2012;24(12):783–91.

85. Herold MJ, McPherson KG, Reichardt HM. Glucocorticoids in T cell apoptosis and function. Cell Mol Life Sci. 2006;63(1):60–72.

86. Schiff D. Pneumocystis pneumonia in brain tumor patients: risk factors and clinical features. J Neurooncol. 1996;27(3):235–40.

87. Rubner Y, Muth C, Strnad A, Derer A, Sieber R, Buslei R, et al. Fractionated radiotherapy is the main stimulus for the induction of cell death and of Hsp70 release of p53 mutated glioblastoma cell lines. Radiat Oncol. 2014;9(1):89.

88. Shi Y, Rock KL. Cell death releases endogenous adjuvants that selectively enhance immune surveillance of particulate antigens. Eur J Immunol. 2002;32(1):155–62.

89. Golden EB, Apetoh L. Radiotherapy and immunogenic cell death. Semin Radiat Oncol. 2015;25(1):11–7.

90. Golden EB, Frances D, Pellicciotta I, Demaria S, Helen Barcellos-Hoff M, Formenti SC. Radiation fosters dose-dependent and chemotherapy-induced immunogenic cell death. Oncoimmunology. 2014;3, e28518.

91. Golden EB, Pellicciotta I, Demaria S, Barcellos-Hoff MH, Formenti SC. The convergence of radiation and immunogenic cell death signaling pathways. Fronti Oncol. 2012;2:88.

92. Paolini A, Pasi F, Facoetti A, Mazzini G, Corbella F, Di Liberto R, et al. Cell death forms and HSP70 expression in U87 cells after ionizing radiation and/or chemotherapy. Anticancer Res. 2011;31(11):3727–31.

93. Lee Y, Auh SL, Wang Y, Burnette B, Wang Y, Meng Y, et al. Therapeutic effects of ablative radiation on

local tumor require CD8+ T cells: changing strategies for cancer treatment. Blood. 2009;114(3):589–95.

94. Lugade AA, Moran JP, Gerber SA, Rose RC, Frelinger JG, Lord EM. Local radiation therapy of B16 melanoma tumors increases the generation of tumor antigen-specific effector cells that traffic to the tumor. J Immunol. 2005;174(12):7516–23.

95. Schaue D, Ratikan JA, Iwamoto KS, McBride WH. Maximizing tumor immunity with fractionated radiation. Int J Radiat Oncol Biol Phys. 2012; 83(4):1306–10.

96. Dewan MZ, Galloway AE, Kawashima N, Dewyngaert JK, Babb JS, Formenti SC, et al. Fractionated but not single-dose radiotherapy induces an immune-mediated abscopal effect when combined with anti-CTLA-4 antibody. Clin Cancer Res. 2009;15(17):5379–88.

97. Vom Berg J, Vrohlings M, Haller S, Haimovici A, Kulig P, Sledzinska A, et al. Intratumoral IL-12 combined with CTLA-4 blockade elicits T cell-mediated glioma rejection. J Exp Med. 2013;210(13):2803–11.

98. Zeng J, See AP, Phallen J, Jackson CM, Belcaid Z, Ruzevick J, et al. Anti-PD-1 blockade and stereotactic radiation produce long-term survival in mice with intracranial gliomas. Int J Radiat Oncol Biol Phys. 2013;86(2):343–9.

99. Newcomb EW, Lukyanov Y, Kawashima N, Alonso-Basanta M, Wang SC, Liu M, et al. Radiotherapy enhances antitumor effect of anti-CD137 therapy in a mouse Glioma model. Radiat Res. 2010;173(4):426–32.

100. Belcaid Z, Phallen JA, Zeng J, See AP, Mathios D, Gottschalk C, et al. Focal radiation therapy combined with 4-1BB activation and CTLA-4 blockade yields long-term survival and a protective antigen-specific memory response in a murine glioma model. PLoS One. 2014;9(7), e101764.

101. Heisel SM, Ketter R, Keller A, Klein V, Pallasch CP, Lenhof HP, et al. Increased seroreactivity to glioma-expressed antigen 2 in brain tumor patients under radiation. PLoS One. 2008;3(5), e2164.

102. Pallasch CP, Struss AK, Munnia A, Konig J, Steudel WI, Fischer U, et al. Autoantibodies against GLEA2 and PHF3 in glioblastoma: tumor-associated autoantibodies correlated with prolonged survival. Int J Cancer. 2005;117(3):456–9.

103. Weidle UH, Georges G, Tiefenthaler G. TCR-MHC/peptide interaction: prospects for new anti-tumoral agents. Cancer Genomics Proteomics. 2014;11(6):267–77.

104. Reits EA, Hodge JW, Herberts CA, Groothuis TA, Chakraborty M, Wansley EK, et al. Radiation modulates the peptide repertoire, enhances MHC class I expression, and induces successful antitumor immunotherapy. J Exp Med. 2006;203(5):1259–71.

105. Newcomb EW, Demaria S, Lukyanov Y, Shao Y, Schnee T, Kawashima N, et al. The combination of ionizing radiation and peripheral vaccination produces long-term survival of mice bearing estab-

lished invasive GL261 gliomas. Clin Cancer Res. 2006;12(15):4730–7.

106. Ip NY. The neurotrophins and neuropoietic cytokines: two families of growth factors acting on neural and hematopoietic cells. Ann N Y Acad Sci. 1998; 840:97–106.

107. Lee WH, Sonntag WE, Mitschelen M, Yan H, Lee YW. Irradiation induces regionally specific alterations in pro-inflammatory environments in rat brain. Int J Radiat Biol. 2010;86(2):132–44.

108. Ross HJ, Canada AL, Antoniono RJ, Redpath JL. High and low dose rate irradiation have opposing effects on cytokine gene expression in human glioblastoma cell lines. Eur J Cancer. 1997;33(1):144–52.

109. Chiang CS, McBride WH. Radiation enhances tumor necrosis factor alpha production by murine brain cells. Brain Res. 1991;566(1-2):265–9.

110. Gaber MW, Sabek OM, Fukatsu K, Wilcox HG, Kiani MF, Merchant TE. Differences in ICAM-1 and TNF-alpha expression between large single fraction and fractionated irradiation in mouse brain. Int J Radiat Biol. 2003;79(5):359–66.

111. Vanpouille-Box C, Lacoeuille F, Belloche C, Lepareur N, Lemaire L, LeJeune JJ, et al. Tumor eradication in rat glioma and bypass of immunosuppressive barriers using internal radiation with (188)Re-lipid nanocapsules. Biomaterials. 2011;32(28):|6781–90.

112. Zagzag D, Zhong H, Scalzitti JM, Laughner E, Simons JW, Semenza GL. Expression of hypoxia-inducible factor 1alpha in brain tumors: association with angiogenesis, invasion, and progression. Cancer. 2000;88(11):2606–18.

113. Sharma V, Dixit D, Koul N, Mehta VS, Sen E. Ras regulates interleukin-1beta-induced HIF-1alpha transcriptional activity in glioblastoma. J Mol Med. 2011;89(2):123–36.

114. Barcellos-Hoff MH. Radiation-induced transforming growth factor beta and subsequent extracellular matrix reorganization in murine mammary gland. Cancer Res. 1993;53(17):3880–6.

115. Ehrhart EJ, Segarini P, Tsang ML, Carroll AG, Barcellos-Hoff MH. Latent transforming growth factor beta1 activation in situ: quantitative and functional evidence after low-dose gamma-irradiation. FASEB J. 1997;11(12):991–1002.

116. Wang J, Zheng H, Sung CC, Richter KK, Hauer-Jensen M. Cellular sources of transforming growth factor-beta isoforms in early and chronic radiation enteropathy. Am J Pathol. 1998;153(5):1531–40.

117. Satoh E, Naganuma H, Sasaki A, Nagasaka M, Ogata H, Nukui H. Effect of irradiation on transforming growth factor-beta secretion by malignant glioma cells. J Neurooncol. 1997;33(3):195–200.

118. Kirshner J, Jobling MF, Pajares MJ, Ravani SA, Glick AB, Lavin MJ, et al. Inhibition of transforming growth factor-beta1 signaling attenuates ataxia telangiectasia mutated activity in response to genotoxic stress. Cancer Res. 2006;66(22):10861–9.

119. Hardee ME, Marciscano AE, Medina-Ramirez CM, Zagzag D, Narayana A, Lonning SM, et al. Resistance of glioblastoma-initiating cells to radiation mediated by the tumor microenvironment can be abolished by inhibiting transforming growth factor-beta. Cancer Res. 2012;72(16):4119–29.

120. Desmarais G, Fortin D, Bujold R, Wagner R, Mathieu D, Paquette B. Infiltration of glioma cells in brain parenchyma stimulated by radiation in the F98/Fischer rat model. Int J Radiat Biol. 2012;88(8):565–74.

121. Rubin LL, Staddon JM. The cell biology of the blood-brain barrier. Annu Rev Neurosci. 1999;22:11–28.

122. Riccardi R, Riccardi A, Lasorella A, Servidei T, Mastrangelo S. Cranial irradiation and permeability of blood-brain barrier to cytosine arabinoside in children with acute leukemia. Clin Cancer Res. 1998;4(1):69–73.

123. Qin DX, Zheng R, Tang J, Li JX, Hu YH. Influence of radiation on the blood-brain barrier and optimum time of chemotherapy. Int J Radiat Oncol Biol Phys. 1990;19(6):1507–10.

124. Badie B, Schartner JM. Flow cytometric characterization of tumor-associated macrophages in experimental gliomas. Neurosurgery. 2000;46(4):957–61. discussion 61-2.

125. Vatner RE, Formenti SC. Myeloid-derived cells in tumors: effects of radiation. Semin Radiat Oncol. 2015;25(1):18–27.

126. Julow J, Szeifert GT, Balint K, Nyary I, Nemes Z. The role of microglia/macrophage system in the tissue response to I-125 interstitial brachytherapy of cerebral gliomas. Neurol Res. 2007;29(3):233–8.

127. Mongiardi MP. Angiogenesis and hypoxia in glioblastoma: a focus on cancer stem cells. CNS Neurol Disord Drug Targets. 2012;11(7):878–83.

128. Folkman J. What is the evidence that tumors are angiogenesis dependent? J Natl Cancer Inst. 1990;82(1):4–6.

129. Shalaby F, Rossant J, Yamaguchi TP, Gertsenstein M, Wu XF, Breitman ML, et al. Failure of blood-island formation and vasculogenesis in Flk-1-deficient mice. Nature. 1995;376(6535):62–6.

130. Kerber M, Reiss Y, Wickersheim A, Jugold M, Kiessling F, Heil M, et al. Flt-1 signaling in macrophages promotes glioma growth in vivo. Cancer Res. 2008;68(18):7342–51.

131. Kioi M, Vogel H, Schultz G, Hoffman RM, Harsh GR, Brown JM. Inhibition of vasculogenesis, but not angiogenesis, prevents the recurrence of glioblastoma after irradiation in mice. J Clin Invest. 2010;120(3):694–705.

132. Ahn GO, Brown JM. Matrix metalloproteinase-9 is required for tumor vasculogenesis but not for angiogenesis: role of bone marrow-derived myelomonocytic cells. Cancer Cell. 2008;13(3):193–205.

133. Jin DK, Shido K, Kopp HG, Petit I, Shmelkov SV, Young LM, et al. Cytokine-mediated deployment of

SDF-1 induces revascularization through recruitment of CXCR4+ hemangiocytes. Nat Med. 2006;12(5):557–67.

134. Formenti SC, Demaria S. Radiation therapy to convert the tumor into an in situ vaccine. Int J Radiat Oncol Biol Phys. 2012;84(4):879–80.

135. Demaria S, Formenti SC. Radiotherapy effects on anti-tumor immunity: implications for cancer treatment. Front Oncol. 2013;3:128.

136. Talmadge JE, Adams J, Phillips H, Collins M, Lenz B, Schneider M, et al. Immunomodulatory effects in mice of polyinosinic-polycytidylic acid complexed with poly-L-lysine and carboxymethylcellulose. Cancer Res. 1985;45(3):1058–65.

137. Levy HB, Lvovsky E, Riley F, Harrington D, Anderson A, Moe J, et al. Immune modulating effects of poly ICLC. Ann N Y Acad Sci. 1980; 350:33–41.

138. Hubbell HR, Liu RS, Maxwell BL. Independent sensitivity of human tumor cell lines to interferon and double-stranded RNA. Cancer Res. 1984;44(8):3252–7.

139. Dick RS, Hubbell HR. Sensitivities of human glioma cell lines to interferons and double-stranded RNAs individually and in synergistic combinations. J Neurooncol. 1987;5(4):331–8.

140. Strayer DR, Weisband J, Carter WA, Black P, Nidzgorski F, Cook AW. Growth of astrocytomas in the human tumor clonogenic assay and sensitivity to mismatched dsRNA and interferons. Am J Clin Oncol. 1987;10(4):281–4.

141. Butowski N, Chang SM, Junck L, DeAngelis LM, Abrey L, Fink K, et al. A phase II clinical trial of poly-ICLC with radiation for adult patients with newly diagnosed supratentorial glioblastoma: a North American Brain Tumor Consortium (NABTC01-05). J Neurooncol. 2009;91(2):175–82.

142. Maus MV, Fraietta JA, Levine BL, Kalos M, Zhao Y, June CH. Adoptive immunotherapy for cancer or viruses. Annu Rev Immunol. 2014;32:189–225.

143. Plautz GE, Barnett GH, Miller DW, Cohen BH, Prayson RA, Krauss JC, et al. Systemic T cell adoptive immunotherapy of malignant gliomas. J Neurosurg. 1998;89(1):42–51.

144. Plautz GE, Miller DW, Barnett GH, Stevens GH, Maffett S, Kim J, et al. T cell adoptive immunotherapy of newly diagnosed gliomas. Clin Cancer Res. 2000;6(6):2209–18.

145. Okada H, Kalinski P, Ueda R, Hoji A, Kohanbash G, Donegan TE, et al. Induction of CD8+ T-cell responses against novel glioma-associated antigen peptides and clinical activity by vaccinations with {alpha}-type 1 polarized dendritic cells and polyinosinic-polycytidylic acid stabilized by lysine and carboxymethylcellulose in patients with recurrent malignant glioma. J Clin Oncol. 2011;29(3):330–6.

146. Phuphanich S, Wheeler CJ, Rudnick JD, Mazer M, Wang H, Nuno MA, et al. Phase I trial of a multi-epitope-pulsed dendritic cell vaccine for patients with newly diagnosed glioblastoma. Cancer Immunol Immunother. 2013;62(1):125–35.

147. Wen PY, Reardon DA, Phuphanich S, Aiken R, Landolfi JC, Curry WT, Zhu JJ, Glantz MJ, Peereboom DM, Markert J, LaRocca RV, O'Rourke D, Fink KL, Kim LJ, Gruber ML, Lesser GJ, Pan E, Kesari S, Hawkins ES, Yu J. A randomized, double-blind, placebocontrolled phase 2 trial of dendritic cell (DC) vaccination with ICT-107 in newly diagnosed glioblastoma (GBM) patients. J Clin Oncol. 2014;32:5s.

148. Frederick L, Wang XY, Eley G, James CD. Diversity and frequency of epidermal growth factor receptor mutations in human glioblastomas. Cancer Res. 2000;60(5):1383–7.

149. Sampson JH, Archer GE, Mitchell DA, Heimberger AB, Herndon 2nd JE, Lally-Goss D, et al. An epidermal growth factor receptor variant III-targeted vaccine is safe and immunogenic in patients with glioblastoma multiforme. Mol Cancer Ther. 2009;8(10):2773–9.

150. Sampson JH, Heimberger AB, Archer GE, Aldape KD, Friedman AH, Friedman HS, et al. Immunologic escape after prolonged progression-free survival with epidermal growth factor receptor variant III peptide vaccination in patients with newly diagnosed glioblastoma. J Clin Oncol. 2010;28(31):4722–9.

151. Sampson JH, Aldape KD, Archer GE, Coan A, Desjardins A, Friedman AH, et al. Greater chemotherapy-induced lymphopenia enhances tumor-specific immune responses that eliminate EGFRvIII-expressing tumor cells in patients with glioblastoma. Neuro Oncol. 2011;13(3):324–33.

152. Yu JS, Wheeler CJ, Zeltzer PM, Ying H, Finger DN, Lee PK, et al. Vaccination of malignant glioma patients with peptide-pulsed dendritic cells elicits systemic cytotoxicity and intracranial T-cell infiltration. Cancer Res. 2001;61(3):842–7.

153. Yu JS, Liu G, Ying H, Yong WH, Black KL, Wheeler CJ. Vaccination with tumor lysate-pulsed dendritic cells elicits antigen-specific, cytotoxic T-cells in patients with malignant glioma. Cancer Res. 2004;64(14):4973–9.

154. Liau LM, Prins RM, Kiertscher SM, Odesa SK, Kremen TJ, Giovannone AJ, et al. Dendritic cell vaccination in glioblastoma patients induces systemic and intracranial T-cell responses modulated by the local central nervous system tumor microenvironment. Clin Cancer Res. 2005;11(15):5515–25.

155. Yamanaka R, Homma J, Yajima N, Tsuchiya N, Sano M, Kobayashi T, et al. Clinical evaluation of dendritic cell vaccination for patients with recurrent glioma: results of a clinical phase I/II trial. Clin Cancer Res. 2005;11(11):4160–7.

156. De Vleeschouwer S, Fieuws S, Rutkowski S, Van Calenbergh F, Van Loon J, Goffin J, et al. Postoperative adjuvant dendritic cell-based immunotherapy in patients with relapsed glioblastoma multiforme. Clin Cancer Res. 2008;14(10):3098–104.

157. Wheeler CJ, Black KL, Liu G, Mazer M, Zhang XX, Pepkowitz S, et al. Vaccination elicits correlated immune and clinical responses in glioblastoma multiforme patients. Cancer Res. 2008;68(14):5955–64.

158. Ardon H, Van Gool S, Lopes IS, Maes W, Sciot R, Wilms G, et al. Integration of autologous dendritic cell-based immunotherapy in the primary treatment for patients with newly diagnosed glioblastoma multiforme: a pilot study. J Neurooncol. 2010;99(2): 261–72.

159. Fadul CE, Fisher JL, Hampton TH, Lallana EC, Li Z, Gui J, et al. Immune response in patients with newly diagnosed glioblastoma multiforme treated with intranodal autologous tumor lysate-dendritic cell vaccination after radiation chemotherapy. J Immunother. 2011;34(4):382–9.

160. Prins RM, Soto H, Konkankit V, Odesa SK, Eskin A, Yong WH, et al. Gene expression profile correlates with T-cell infiltration and relative survival in glioblastoma patients vaccinated with dendritic cell immunotherapy. Clin Cancer Res. 2011;17(6):1603–15.

161. Ardon H, Van Gool SW, Verschuere T, Maes W, Fieuws S, Sciot R, et al. Integration of autologous dendritic cell-based immunotherapy in the standard of care treatment for patients with newly diagnosed glioblastoma: results of the HGG-2006 phase I/II trial. Cancer Immunol Immunother. 2012;61(11):2033–44.

162. Prins RM, Wang X, Soto H, Young E, Lisiero DN, Fong B, et al. Comparison of glioma-associated antigen peptide-loaded versus autologous tumor lysate-loaded dendritic cell vaccination in malignant glioma patients. J Immunother. 2013;36(2): 152–7.

163. Cho DY, Yang WK, Lee HC, Hsu DM, Lin HL, Lin SZ, et al. Adjuvant immunotherapy with whole-cell lysate dendritic cells vaccine for glioblastoma multiforme: a phase II clinical trial. World Neurosurg. 2012;77(5–6):736–44.

164. Binder RJ, Han DK, Srivastava PK. CD91: a receptor for heat shock protein gp96. Nat Immunol. 2000;1(2):151–5.

165. Crane CA, Han SJ, Ahn B, Oehlke J, Kivett V, Fedoroff A, et al. Individual patient-specific immunity against high-grade glioma after vaccination with autologous tumor derived peptides bound to the 96 KD chaperone protein. Clin Cancer Res. 2013;19(1):205–14.

166. Bloch O, Crane CA, Fuks Y, Kaur R, Aghi MK, Berger MS, et al. Heat-shock protein peptide complex-96 vaccination for recurrent glioblastoma: a phase II, single-arm trial. Neuro Oncol. 2014;16(2):274–9.

167. Vik-Mo EO, Nyakas M, Mikkelsen BV, Moe MC, Due-Tonnesen P, Suso EM, et al. Therapeutic vaccination against autologous cancer stem cells with mRNA-transfected dendritic cells in patients with glioblastoma. Cancer Immunol Immunother. 2013; 62(9):1499–509.

# Genetic and Epigenetic Determinants in Tumor Initiation and Progression of Glioblastoma

# 11

A. Cimini, A. Fidoamore, M. d'Angelo,
A. Antonosante, L. Cristiano, E. Benedetti,
and Antonio Giordano

Malignant gliomas are the most common tumors of the Central Nervous System (CNS). The incidence rates were higher in more developed countries than in less developed ones [1]. The evidence that the incidence is constant worldwide suggests that environmental, geographical, and nutritional factors have not a specific role in this cancer, where genetic and epigenetic factors more probably account for its etiology [2]. The World Health Organization (WHO) classifies astrocytomas on histologic type, with tumor grade depending on the degree of nuclear atypia, mitotic activity, microvascular proliferation, and necrosis, with increased anaplasia corresponding to higher tumor grade. Grades are low-grade, or WHO grade I (pilocytic astrocytoma) and grade II (diffuse astrocytoma) and high-grade, or WHO grade III (anaplastic astrocytoma) and grade IV (glioblastoma, GB) [3, 4]. The most common, biologically aggressive and lethal subtype of brain tumors is glioblastoma (GB, WHO grade IV) which is characterized by high cellular proliferation, infiltration, necrosis, angiogenesis, resistance to apoptosis, genomic instability and by high cell density and atypia [5, 6].

The age represents one of the most important prognostic factors [7]. The peak incidence is between 45 and 70 years, average age at diagnosis is 64 years for glioblastomas and 45 years in the case of anaplastic gliomas [8]. Patients suffering from GB have a median survival of 15 months [9, 10], only 5 % survive more than 5 years despite aggressive therapies [11]; therefore, this makes it a considerable public health issue [2].

A. Cimini (✉)
Department of Life, Health and Environmental Sciences, University of L'Aquila, L'Aquila, Italy

Sbarro Institute for Cancer Research and Molecular Medicine and Center for Biotechnology, Temple University, Philadelphia, PA, USA
e-mail: annamaria.cimini@univaq.it

A. Fidoamore • M. d'Angelo • A. Antonosante
L. Cristiano, • E. Benedetti
Department of Life, Health and Environmental Sciences, University of L'Aquila, L'Aquila, Italy

A. Giordano
Sbarro Institute for Cancer Research and Molecular Medicine and Center for Biotechnology, Temple University, Philadelphia, PA, USA

Department of Medicine, Surgery and Neuroscience, University of Siena, Siena, Italy

## Risk Factors and Etiology

Risk factors for developing gliomas are poorly identified, thus prevention does not really exist. Many environmental, dietary, and lifestyle factors were investigated but unequivocal evidences were not found so far [12]. Most GB appear to be sporadic, although several genetic disorders have been associated with increased incidence, such as tuberous sclerosis, neurofibromatosis type 1 and type 2, von Hippel Lindau disease, Turcot and

© Springer International Publishing Switzerland 2016
L. Pirtoli et al. (eds.), *Radiobiology of Glioblastoma*, Current Clinical Pathology,
DOI 10.1007/978-3-319-28305-0_11

Li-Fraumeni syndromes [2]. Adults affected by more benign brain tumors such as meningiomas or low grade gliomas that received radiotherapy as initial treatment also exhibited higher risk for developing GB [12]. It appears that for the majority of cases of malignant gliomas, there is no a specific known cause. What is now considered a new challenge is the definition of the molecular epidemiology of malignant gliomas, by the genome-wide association studies, genomic and epigenetic expression arrays, and all the possible methods able to match population controls. These studies are related to single nucleotide polymorphisms of genes associated with DNA repair, cell cycle control, metabolism, inflammation. However, despite all these studies, that included large cooperative studies, so far why patients may develop malignant gliomas is not known. Moreover, the role/s of the individual genomic susceptibility associated with gliomagenesis is still not completely elucidated [13].

## Genetic Pattern

The study performed by The Cancer Genome Atlas (TCGA) project sequenced 601 cancer-related candidate genes in more than 200 human GB samples. The study also analyzed genome-wide DNA copy number changes, DNA methylation status, and protein-coding and noncoding RNA expression [14]. Another study considered 20,661 protein-encoding genes in 22 GB samples and allineated the genetic alteration with DNA copy number and profiles of gene expression [15].

These studies provided an exhaustive view of the complex genomic profile of GB, evidentiating a set of crucial signaling pathways commonly mutated in GB controlling cellular proliferation, survival (apoptosis and necrosis), invasion, and angiogenesis [5, 14–16].

Many oncogenes have been indicated overexpressed/amplified and/or activated:

1. Epidermal growth factor receptor (EGFR), involved in the control of cell proliferation, is amplified and overexpressed in more than one-third of glioblastomas, sometimes in a truncated and rearranged form. The most common alteration is the deletion of exons 2–7 from the extracellular domain, resulting in a truncated mutant receptor, with the variant 3 (EGFRvIII) being the more frequent observed EGFRvIII enhanced tumorigenicity by increasing proliferation and reducing apoptosis, probably through the Ras-Shc-Grb2 pathway [17].

2. Platelet-derived growth factor (PDGFR) is one of the major mitogen in the connective tissue cells and glia; it is a dimer of A and B chains. The ligands are recognized by two types of cell surface receptors, PDGFR-α and PDGFR-β, which belong to the tyrosine kinase family of receptors. In both low- and high-grade astrocytomas overexpression of PDGFR-α was reported, indicating that PDGFR-α is involved in tumor cell proliferation in both early and late stages of gliomagenesis. In contrast, amplification of the PDGFR-β gene was detected only in a small fraction (16 %) of glioblastomas [17].

3. MDM2 (Mouse double minute 2) contains a TP53 DNA-binding site. It forms a complex with TP53, thereby abolishing its transcriptional activity. Thus, in normal cells, this autoregulatory feedback modulates both the activity of the TP53 protein and the expression of the MDM2 gene. An increase of TP53 levels blocks the entry into the cycle in the G 1 phase; at the same time, TP53 induces the expression of MDM2, resulting in a TP53–MDM2 complex formation that may overcome the G 1 checkpoint and allows the entry into the S-phase of the cell cycle. Therefore, MDM2 amplification/overexpression constitutes an alternative mechanism to escape from TP53-regulated control of cell cycle [17].

GB is also characterized by mutations leading to loss of function of key tumor suppressor genes:

1. PTEN (Phosphatase and tensin homolog) on chromosome 10 encodes a central domain with homology to the catalytic region of protein tyrosine phosphatases, which is crucial

for the protein phosphatase and 3′-phosphoinositol phosphatase activities. The amino terminal domain of PTEN is fundamental for the regulation of cell migration and invasion by dephosphorylating focal adhesion kinase. The PTEN gene is mutated in 15–40 % of glioblastomas [18].

2. p53 on chromosome 17 is the guardian of the genoma preventing the propagation of cells with unstable genomes, by arresting the cell cycle in the G1 phase or inducing apoptosis, through its function as a transcription factor, binding and regulating at transcriptional level the promoters of >2500 potential effector genes. The best known of these effectors is the transcriptional target CDNK1A, which encodes the protein for the CDK2 inhibitor p21. This gene is not altered in gliomas but its expression is generally abrogated by functional inactivity of p53 or by mitogenic signals through the PI3K and MAPK pathways [5].

3. Rb (Retinoblastoma tumor suppressor gene).

   In quiescent cells, hypophosphorylated Rb blocks cell proliferation by sequestering the E2F transcription factors, which prevents the transactivation of genes essential for the progression of the cell cycle. Mitogenic stimuli trigger the activation of the MAPK cascade leading to the induction of cyclin D1 and its association with the cyclin-dependent kinases CDK4 and CDK6. These CDK complexes in turn phosphorylate Rb, triggering E2F transactivation of transcriptional targets, determining S-phase entry and progression. In Gliomas Rb-mediated cell cycle control is generally abrogated through different genetic alterations [5].

4. p16/INK4A (Tumor suppressor) is encoded by the CDKN2A controlling cell growth by the inhibition of the cyclin-dependent kinases CDK4 and CDK6, by reducing their capacity to phosphorylate the Rb protein, and thus allowing G1/S-phase transition of the cell cycle. Thus, the loss of cell cycle control may be derived from the altered expression of any of the following genes: loss of CDKN2A (p16) expression, overexpression/

amplification of CDK genes, or loss of RB function [17].

5. p19$^{Arf}$. The CDKN2A (p16 or INK4a) locus codes for two gene products (p16 and p19 $^{Arf}$). The putative tumor suppressor p19 $^{Arf}$ blocks MDM2-induced degradation and silencing of p53 [17].

6. Loss of heterozygosity (LOH) on large regions at 10q, 10q23, and 10q25-26 loci or loss of the entire copy of chromosome 10 are the most frequent genetic alterations in glioblastomas [17].

7. DCC (deleted in colorectal cancer) gene located at 18q21. It encodes a 1447-amino acid transmembrane domain protein belonging to a family of neural cell adhesion molecules and is preferentially expressed in the nervous system. DCC immunohistochemistry reveals that loss of expression increases during progression from low-grade astrocytoma (7 %) to glioblastoma (47 %) [17].

Recently it was report as, on 291GB, the 46 % of case had at least one somatic mutation in gene involved in epigenetic events. In particular, these mutations determined the alteration of DNA methylation, histone modification, and nucleosome positioning, and were generally related to altered gene expression [19]. The genes are those involved in DNA methylation (isocitrate dehydrogenase [IDH] 1, IDH2), histone modification (mixed lineage leukemia 2 [MLL2], MLL3, MLL4, Enhancer of zeste 2 [EZH2], and histone deacetylase 2 [HDAC2]), and chromatin remodeling (a-thalassaemia /mental retardation syndrome X-linked [ATRX], death-domain associated protein [DAXX], CREB binding protein [CREBBP] and SWI / SNF-related matrix-associated, actin-dependent regulator of chromatin A2 [SMARCA2]) [20].

## Primary and Secondary Glioblastoma

Glioblastomas may be primary or secondary with respect to their clinical history and there is a great difference in the age distribution of patients.

Primary glioblastomas, also termed de novo, are more common in older patients, aged >50 years [18], occurring from the acquisition of multiple genetic alterations resulting in an acute de novo appearance with no evidence of previous symptoms or antecedent lower grade pathology [18]. Secondary glioblastomas are less frequent and tend to occur in younger patients, aged below 45 years; they develop through the progression from lower grade astrocytoma (WHO grade II) towards higher malignancy grades. About 70 % of grade II gliomas progress into grade III/IV within 5–10 year from diagnosis. It is worth noting that, in spite of their different clinical histories, primary and secondary GB are morphologically and clinically indistinguishable and characterized by an equally poor prognosis. However, although these GB subtypes reach a common phenotypic endpoint, recent genomic studies have revealed different genetic profiles between primary and secondary GB as well as new glioma subclasses within each category [5].

Recently a large-scale genomic and epigenomic profiling studies, such as The Cancer Genome Atlas, have produced new data that have allowed a better insight into gliomagenesis [21]. In this study it was identified a CpG island methylator phenotype (G-CIMP) in gliomas and this phenotype was associated with *IDH1* mutation. The authors showed as G-CIMP patients were younger at diagnosis and display improved survival, moreover G-CIMP was distinctive of secondary GB, because G-CIMP was more prevalent among low- and intermediate-grade gliomas.

The genetic pathway to primary and secondary glioblastomas at a population level is summarized in Fig. 11.1.

## Epigenetic Determinants

The hallmarks of cancer and also of GB consists of epigenetically deregulated genes able to increase survival, proliferation, insensitivity to inhibitory signals, angiogenesis, and metastatic and invasion potential (Fig. 11.2) [22]. Epigenetic determinants, like DNA methylation and histone modifications, can affect the transcription of mRNA and microRNA (miRs) that in turn regulate the expression of several key cellular proteins [23, 24].

The transcriptome analysis studies recently performed have evidentiated that about 90 % of the human genome is transcribed and transcription is not occurring only for protein-coding

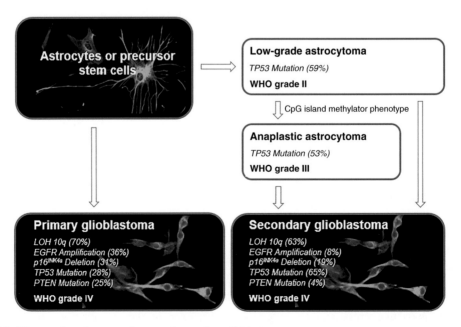

**Fig. 11.1** The genetic pathway to primary and secondary glioblastomas

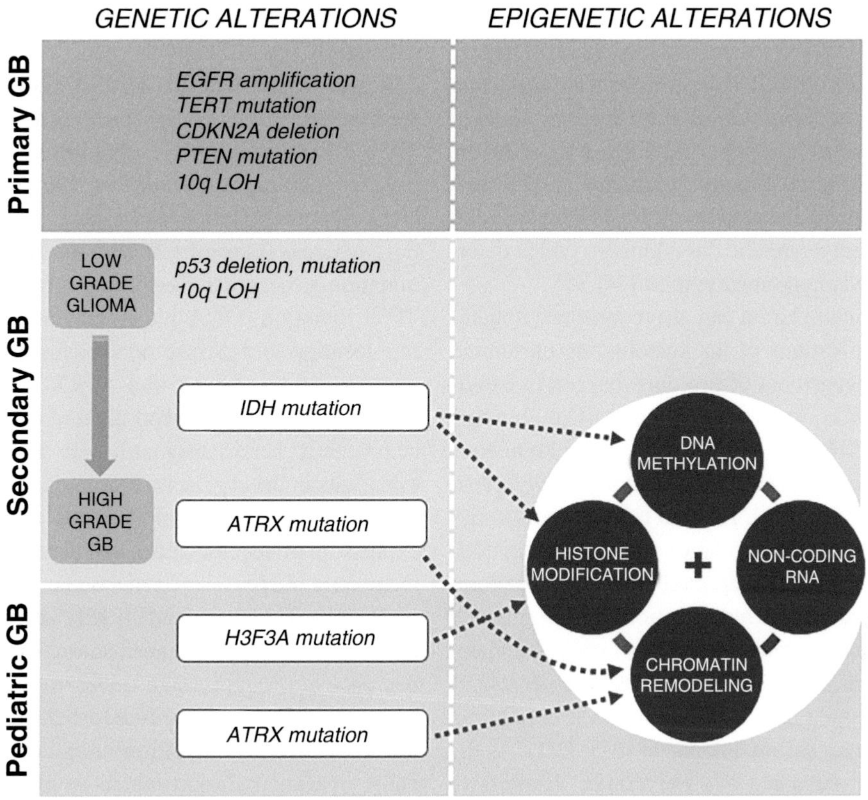

**Fig. 11.2** Genetic and epigenetic determinants in human glioblastoma

regions [25]. The expression of significant numbers of noncoding RNA (ncRNA) is regulated during development for each specific cell-type and these RNA, named microRNA (miR) and long noncoding RNA (lncRNA), are associated with different cell functions [26]. Previous studies have reported that ncRNA, other than being considered key regulators of cellular differentiation and proliferation, may also be considered as tumor suppressive or have oncogenic activities in many types of cancer [27]. Recent findings seem to indicate miRs, particularly miR-29, as controller of epigenetic regulatory enzymes [23]. miR-29c was significantly downregulated in glioma cell lines and human primary glioma tissues. In addition the overexpression of miR-29c reduced the proliferation and arrested the cell cycle, suggesting that miR-29c may be a tumor suppressor involved in the progression of glioma [28].

The chromosomal structure stability and the control of gene expression are known to be regulated by an appropriate maintenance of DNA methylation [29].

CpG islands (CGIs), that are sites of transcription initiation, 1000 base pairs (bp) long, show a frequent absence of DNA methylation, an elevated G+C base composition and little CpG depletion. Silencing of CGI promoters is achieved through dense CpG methylation or polycomb recruitment [30]. It has been proposed that altered DNA methylation profiles may result in the development and progression of gliomas [21, 31]. Cancer cells often have simultaneously both global hypomethylation and regional hypermethylation, with the latter occurring particularly at select gene-associated CpG islands that are generally unmethylated [32].

The glioma CpG island methylator phenotype (G-CIMP) tumors are often reported in secondary GB, which presents a grade progression from low-grade glioma to high-grade GB [33]. Moreover G-CIMP are distinguished by both mutations in IDH1 or IDH2 and hypermethylation of DNA (proneural type) [21]. IDH are NAD+ and NADP+-dependent enzymes that catalyze the third step of the tricarboxylic acid (TCA) cycle. Mutations in IDH1 trigger to the accumulation of 2-hydroxyglutarate (2-HG) that in turn impairs the activity of 10–11 translocation (TET) methylcytosine dioxygenase, which determines DNA hypermethylation [34, 35].

DNA methylation can also coordinate epigenetic modifications of the surrounding chromatin by the engagement of proteins that bind methylated CpG sequences (methyl-CpG-binding domain [MBD] proteins) connected with histone deacetylases (HDACs) and histone methyltransferase (HMTs) [36]. Histone modifications functionally affect the regulation of transcription [19] and it has been reported that the enzymes involved in histone modifications are deregulated in gliomas. Particularly, the most studied epigenetic enzymes, Ezh2, a lysine methyltransferase, is overexpressed in glioblastoma and it is required for GB stem cell maintenance [37]. EZH2 is the catalytic subunit of Polycomb Repressive Complex 2 (PRC2), and has a substrate specificity for the lysine 27 of histone 3 (H3K27) and produces dimethylated H3K27 (H3K27me2) or H3K27me3 [38]. Trimethylation of histone H3 lysine 27 (H3K27me3) has been reported as crucial epigenetic modification during development, including neural cell differentiation. Aberrant H3K 27me3 is generally reported in many types of cancer [38], and many studies have shown that H3K27me3-mediated gene silencing is a mechanism different from gene silencing triggered by DNA methylation [39]. In fact, H3K27me3 and DNA methylation are generally not simultaneously present in CpG islands in genome-wide analysis [40].

The pattern of gene silencing mediated by H3K27me3 can vary during differentiation due to the presence of H3K27 methylases (EZH2 and EZH1) and demethylases (UTX and JMJD3) [41].

A previous study reported, in infant and adolescent GB, that frequent heterozygous mutations in H3F3A, which encodes the replication-independent histone H3 variant H3.3, determine amino acid substitutions at two crucial positions within the histone tail (K27M, G34R/G34V) [42, 43].

Cases of GB with the H3F3A G34 mutation are characterized by high rates of mutation in TP53, ATRX, and DAXX, high levels of alternative lengthening of telomeres (ALT) activity, DNA hypomethylation and a hemispheric location, whereas cases of GB with the H3F3A K27 mutation are characterize by high frequencies of TP53 mutation, DNA hypomethylation, a midline location and diffuse pontine location, and a poor prognosis. Given that ATRX and DAXX are essential for the incorporation of H3.3 at pericentromeric heterochromatin and at telomeres, mutations in these genes are strongly related with alternative lengthening of telomeres and with the expression of specific genes that determines gliomagenesis [42].

Histone H3.3 mutated in K27 operates in a dominant-negative manner leading to a general decrease of the repressive H3K27me3 [44]. The reduced levels of H3K27me3 might also affect the total DNA methylation status determining DNA hypomethylation which in turn activates gene expression. The K27 mutant and the consequent decrease of H3K27me3 have the same effect of the loss of EZH2 function, which indicates that EZH2 might exert as tumor suppressor. However, these evidences are not in agreement with the finding that high EZH2 activity increases the level of H3K27me3 and that EZH2 may operate as an oncogene by repressioning of tumor suppressor genes [45–48]). Ezh2 mRNA is regulated by miRNA-101, a microRNA downregulated in GB [49]. The possible dual role of EZH2 as oncogene or tumor suppressor in human cancers indicates that signals outcoming downstream of altered EZH2 activity depend on the context.

It is worth noting that mutations in H3F3A take place exclusively with mutations in IDH1 [50]. As mentioned, IDH1 mutations determines the accumulation of 2-HG, that operates as inhibitor of multiple α-ketoglutarate (α-KG)-dependent dioxygenases, that includes histone demethylases and the TET protein family [34, 51, 52]. This inhibition determines particular changes in the patterns of histone and DNA methylation. The different mutations are correlated with GB with clear clinical characters, due to distinct molecular profiles that involved differences in gene expression and DNA methylation profiles.

## Role of Hypoxia in Epigenetic Regulation of Gene Expression

Hypoxia represents a negative prognostic factor for several cancers, including those of the brain [53]. Hypoxia is mostly present in high-grade gliomas [54, 55] and the level of oxygen concentrations in GB ranges between 2.5 and 0.5 % for mild hypoxia and 0.5–0.1 % for moderate/severe hypoxia [56]. Severe hypoxia is less frequent but commonly found in surrounding areas of extensive cellular necrosis [57], which are a histopathological feature of GB and consist of foci of micronecrosis encircled by pseudopalisading hypercellular neoplastic cells [58].

These hypoxic microenvironments maintain glioblastoma stem cells (GSCs) and promotes reprogramming towards a cancer stem cell phenotype [59, 60]. Cellular hypoxia is toxic, mainly when severe hypoxia leads to cell death; however cancer cells have developed adaptive mechanisms through epigenetic modifications which allow them to survive and even grow in hypoxic conditions [61, 62]. It is widely known that the transcriptional responses, which are crucial for cell adaptation to hypoxic conditions, are predominantly controlled by the hypoxia-induced transcription factor (HIF) family, the master regulator of oxygen homeostasis [63]. The HIF transcriptional complex is a heterodimer composed of one of three oxygen sensitive $\alpha$-subunits (HIF-$1\alpha$, HIF-$2\alpha$, or HIF-$3\alpha$) and a constitutively expressed $\beta$-subunit, HIF-$1\beta$ [64]. In the presence of oxygen (normoxic condition), HIF-$\alpha$ is hydroxylated by prolyl hydroxylase enzymes (PHD1, PHD2, and PHD3) enabling interaction with the Von Hippel Lindau (VHL) protein and subsequent ubiquitination and proteasomal degradation. In the absence of oxygen (hypoxic condition), PHD activity is inhibited, which leads to stabilization and nuclear translocation of the HIF-$\alpha$ subunits enabling them to bind to nuclear HIF-$1\beta$ and form transcriptionally active heterodimer, involved in the transcription and upregulation of over 100 genes involved in tumorigenesis [63].

The most important result of HIF activation is a metabolic shift in aerobic glycolysis known as Warburg effect, through the regulation of the expression of glucose transporters (GLUTs) and metabolic enzymes such as pyruvate kinase (PK), particularly the embryonic isoform M2, hexokinase II (HK2), lactate dehydrogenase (LDH), pyruvate dehydrogenasekinase (PDK) [63–66].

However, the hypoxia-induced transcription factors require the cooperation of epigenetic events in order to meet the activation of hypoxic response pathways [67]. Particularly, epigenetic modifications both at the DNA and histone level are able to regulate the HIF binding to target gene promoters. Hypoxia itself has the ability to induce epigenetic modifications, resulting in transcriptional changes and chromosomal remodeling and further instability by changing DNA methylation histone modifications, and microRNAs [68–71].

Epigenetics and hypoxia can interact each other in different ways:

1. HIF stabilization is influenced by the epigenetically controlled expression of VHL and PHD3.
2. Epigenetic mechanisms regulate HIF binding by maintaining a transcriptionally active chromatin conformation within and around HIF binding site regions. This may occur through the action of the HIF-$1\alpha$ coactivation complex or through direct modifications of the HRE binding sites which prevent HIF binding.
3. Many histone demethylase enzymes are HIF-1 target genes and as a consequence, they have a role in the regulation of transcription during the hypoxic response.
4. Significative changes in histone modifications and DNA methylation occur in response to hypoxic exposure [68].

Several studies suggest that the hypoxic response depend on the cooperation of epigenetics since, when studying the HIF-$1\alpha$ coactivation complex, several epigenetic modifying enzymes have been found in direct contact with HIF-1α during the initial cellular response to hypoxia [68]. In fact, it is known that the histone acetyltransferase enzyme CBP/p300 is associate with HIF-1α and is involved in the coactivation of a series hypoxia-inducible genes. This interaction can be abolished by factor-inhibiting HIF (FIH) hydroxylation or the oxygen-dependent binding of VHL protein, which inhibits HIF-1α transactivation through the recruitment of histone deacetylase (HDAC) enzymes. Other members of the HIF-1α coactivation complex SRC-1 and TIF2 have also been found to have histone acetyltransferase activity which enhances the hypoxia-inducible activity of HIF-1α both independently and in synergy with CBP/p300 [68].

Histone deacetylase enzymes such as HDAC1, 3, and 7 have also been involved in the actions of HIF-1α [68]. A range of global histone modifications are observed in hypoxia, determining gene transcription activation and repression. Particularly, it has been shown that hypoxia increased H3K4me3 (associated with activation of gene transcription) and decreased levels of H3K27me3 (a repressor of transcription) in both activated and repressed hypoxia-responsive genes studied [68, 72], suggesting that this event may determine a more adaptable chromatin response to hypoxia.

There are few studies which have investigated the DNA methylation changes occurring during hypoxia. It has been proposed that chronic hypoxia can lead to hypomethylation and consequent increase of genomic instability and aneuploidy which is generally observed in tumorigenesis [62, 69, 73].

In addition, it has been reported that the HIFs demand epigenetic-modifying proteins to promote tumor malignancy in GB. In fact, it was demonstrated that the histone methyltransferase mixed-lineage leukemia 1 (MLL1) is induced by hypoxia and it increases the hypoxic responses. Loss of MLL1 downregulates the expression of HIF2α and target genes and reduced the self-renewal, growth, and tumorigenicity of GSCs which expressed higher levels of MLL1 in hypoxia than matched non-stem tumor cells [74].

Moreover, hypoxia can impact on the regulation of a subset of Jumonji proteins that have histone demethylase properties, specifically at lysine and arginine residues and contain a common catalytic Jumonji C domain. In fact, it has been reported that HIF-1α is implicated in the transactivation of Jumonji proteins in a hypoxic environment, both in vitro and in vivo. Jumonji proteins as JMJD1A, JMJD2B, JMJ2C, and JARD1A are direct targets of HIF, and their expression is induced upon HIF binding in response to hypoxia. In particular, it has been shown that JMJD1A is upregulated by hypoxia in breast cancer cell MCF7 and glioblastoma cell U87 [75–78].

## Conclusions

Malignant gliomas are the most common primary brain tumor in adults, but the prognosis for patients with these tumors remains poor despite advances in diagnosis and standard therapies such as surgery, radiation therapy, and chemotherapy. Progress in the treatment of gliomas now depends to a great extent on the understanding of the complex interplay between genetic and epigenetic determinants in the different subclasses of gliomas.

Patient personalized therapies will not only improve the effectiveness of the therapeutic scheme by inhibiting specific signaling pathways but also may also overcome the problem of drug/radio-resistance. By aiming at multiple targets at once, the new treatment will limit the tumor's ability to overcome drug resistance by affecting different pathways simultaneously and therefore limiting their proliferative capacity and their resistance.

## References

1. Ferlay J, Shin HR, Bray F, Forman D, Mathers C, Parkin DM. Estimates of worldwide burden of cancer in 2008: GLOBOCAN. Int J Cancer. 2010;127(12):2893–917.
2. Jacob G, Dinca EB. Current data and strategy in glioblastoma multiforme. J Med Life. 2009;2(4):386–93.

3. Kleihues P, Louis DN, Scheithauer BW, Rorke LB, Reifenberger G, Burger PC, et al. The WHO classification of tumors of the nervous system. J Neuropathol Exp Neurol. 2002;61(3):215–25.
4. Louis DN, Ohgaki H, Wiestler OD, Cavenee WK, Burger PC, Jouvet A, et al. The 2007 WHO classification of tumours of the central nervous system. Acta Neuropathol. 2007;114(2):97–109.
5. Furnari FB, Fenton T, Bachoo RM, Mukasa A, Stommel JM, Stegh A, et al. Malignant astrocytic glioma: genetics, biology, and paths to treatment. Genes Dev. 2007;21(21):2683–710.
6. Westphal M, Lamszus K. The neurobiology of gliomas: from cell biology to the development of therapeutic approaches. Nat Rev Neurosci. 2011;12(9):495–508.
7. Schwartzbaum JA, Fisher JL, Aldape KD, Wrensch M. Epidemiology and molecular pathology of glioma. Nat Clin Pract Neurol. 2006;2(9):494–503.
8. Fisher JL, Schwartzbaum JA, Wrensch M, Wiemels JL. Epidemiology of brain tumors. Neurol Clin. 2007;25(4):867–90 [Review].
9. Chen J, Li Y, Yu TS, McKay RM, Burns DK, Kernie SG, et al. A restricted cell population propagates glioblastoma growth after chemotherapy. Nature. 2012;488:522–6.
10. Westermark B. Glioblastoma—a moving target. Ups J Med Sci. 2012;117(2):251–6.
11. Central Brain Tumor Registry of the United States. Statistical report: primary brain and central nervous system tumors diagnosed in the United States in 2004–2007. Hinsdale: Central Brain Tumor Registry of the United States: 2011.
12. Mrugala MM. Advances and challenges in the treatment of glioblastoma: a clinician's perspective. Discov Med. 2013;15(83):221–30.
13. Rajaraman P, Melin BS, Wang Z, McKean-Cowdin R, Michaud DS, Wang SS, et al. Genome-wide association study of glioma and meta-analysis. Hum Genet. 2012;131(12):1877–88.
14. TCGA (The Cancer Genome Atlas Research Network). Comprehensive genomic characterization defines human glioblastoma genes and core pathways. Nature. 2008;455:1061–8.
15. Parsons DW, Jones S, Zhang X, Lin JC, Leary RJ, Angenendt P, et al. An integrated genomic analysis of human glioblastoma multiforme. Science. 2008;321(5897):1807–12.
16. Chen J, McKay RM, Parada LF. Malignant glioma: lessons from genomics, mouse models, and stem cells. Cell. 2012;149(1):36–47.
17. Kleihues P, Ohgaki H. Primary and secondary glioblastomas: from concept to clinical diagnosis. Neuro Oncol. 1999;1(1):44–51.
18. Ohgaki H, Kleihues P. Genetic pathways to primary and secondary glioblastoma. Am J Pathol. 2007;170(5):1445–53.
19. Dawson MA, Kouzarides T. Cancer epigenetics: from mechanism to therapy. Cell. 2012;150(1):12–27.
20. Brennan CW, Verhaak RG, McKenna A, Campos B, Noushmehr H, Salama SR, et al. TCGA Research Network. The somatic genomic landscape of glioblastoma. Cell. 2013;155(2):462–77.
21. Noushmehr H, Weisenberger DJ, Diefes K, Phillips HS, Pujara K, Berman BP, et al. Identification of a CpG island methylator phenotype that defines a distinct subgroup of glioma. Cancer Cell. 2010;17(5):510–22.
22. Esteller M. Epigenetics in cancer. N Engl J Med. 2008;358(11):1148–59.
23. Guil S, Esteller M. DNA methylomes, histone codes and miRNAs: Tying it all together. Int J Biochem Cell Biol. 2009;41(1):87–95.
24. Nelson KM, Weiss GJ. MicroRNAs and cancer: past, present, and potential future. Mol Cancer Ther. 2008;7(12):3655–60.
25. Birney E, Stamatoyannopoulos JA, Dutta A, Guigó R, Gingeras TR, Margulies EH, et al. Identification and analysis of functional elements in 1% of the human genome by the ENCODE pilot project. Nature. 2007;447(7146):799–816.
26. Kapranov P, Willingham AT, Gingeras TR. Genome-wide transcription and the implications for genomic organization. Nat Rev Genet. 2007;8(6):413–23.
27. Esteller M. Non-coding RNAs in human disease. Nat Rev Genet. 2011;12(12):861–74.
28. Fan YC, Mei PJ, Chen C, Miao FA, Zhang H, Li ZL. MiR-29c inhibits glioma cell proliferation, migration, invasion and angiogenesis. J Neurooncol. 2013;115(2):179–88.
29. Bernstein BE, Meissner A, Lander ES. The mammalian epigenome. Cell. 2007;128(4):669–81.
30. Deaton AM, Bird A. CpG islands and the regulation of transcription. Genes Dev. 2011;25(10):1010–22 [Review].
31. Natsume A, Kondo Y, Ito M, Motomura K, Wakabayashi T, Yoshida J. Epigenetic aberrations and therapeutic implications in gliomas. Cancer Sci. 2010;101(6):1331–6.
32. Kondo Y, Katsushima K, Ohka F, Natsume A, Shinjo K. Epigenetic dysregulation in glioma. Cancer Sci. 2014;105(4):363–9 [Review].
33. Lai A, Kharbanda S, Pope WB, Tran A, Solis OE, Peale F, et al. Evidence for sequenced molecular evolution of IDH1 mutant glioblastoma from a distinct cell of origin. J Clin Oncol. 2011;29(34):4482–90.
34. Figueroa ME, Abdel-Wahab O, Lu C, Ward PS, Patel J, Shih A, et al. Leukemic IDH1 and IDH2 mutations result in a hypermethylation phenotype, disrupt TET2 function, and impair hematopoietic differentiation. Cancer Cell. 2010;18(6):553–67.
35. Dang L, White DW, Gross S, Bennett BD, Bittinger MA, Driggers EM, et al. Cancer-associated IDH1 mutations produce 2-hydroxyglutarate. Nature. 2009;462(7274):739–44.
36. Esteller M. Cancer epigenomics: DNA methylomes and histone modification maps. Nat Rev Genet. 2007;8(4):286–98.

37. Suvà ML, Riggi N, Janiszewska M, Radovanovic I, Provero P, Stehle JC, et al. EZH2 is essential for glioblastoma cancer stem cell maintenance. Cancer Res. 2009;69:9211–8.

38. Margueron R, Reinberg D. The Polycomb complex PRC2 and its mark in life. Nature. 2011;469(7330): 343–9.

39. Gal-Yam EN, Egger G, Iniguez L, Holster H, Einarsson S, Zhang X, et al. Frequent switching of Polycomb repressive marks and DNA hypermethylation in the PC3 prostate cancer cell line. Proc Natl Acad Sci U S A. 2008;105(35):12979–84.

40. Brinkman AB, Gu H, Bartels SJ, Zhang Y, Matarese F, Simmer F, et al. Sequential ChIP-bisulfite sequencing enables direct genome-scale investigation of chromatin and DNA methylation cross-talk. Genome Res. 2012;22(6):1128–38.

41. Kondo Y, Shen L, Issa JP. Critical role of histone methylation in tumor suppressor gene silencing in colorectal cancer. Mol Cell Biol. 2003;23(1):206–15.

42. Schwartzentruber J, Korshunov A, Liu XY, Jones DT, Pfaff E, Jacob K, et al. Driver mutations in histone H3.3 and chromatin remodelling genes in paediatric glioblastoma. Nature. 2012;482(7384):226–31.

43. Wu G, Broniscer A, McEachron TA, Lu C, Paugh BS, Becksfort J, et al. Somatic histoneH3 alterations in pediatric diffuse intrinsic pontine gliomas and nonbrainstem glioblastomas. Nat Genet. 2012;44(3): 251–3.

44. Bender S, Tang Y, Lindroth AM, Hovestadt V, Jones DT, Kool M, et al. Reduced H3K27me3 and DNA hypomethylation are major drivers of gene expression in K27M mutant pediatric high-grade gliomas. Cancer Cell. 2013;24(5):660–72.

45. Varambally S, Dhanasekaran SM, Zhou M, Barrette TR, Kumar-Sinha C, Sanda MG, et al. The polycomb group protein EZH2 is involved in progression of prostate cancer. Nature. 2002;419(6907):624–9.

46. Tanaka S, Miyagi S, Sashida G, Chiba T, Yuan J, Mochizuki-Kashio M, et al. Ezh2 augments leukemogenicity by reinforcing differentiation blockage in acute myeloid leukemia. Blood. 2012;120(5):1107–17.

47. Mallen-St Clair J, Soydaner-Azeloglu R, Lee KE, Taylor L, Livanos A, Pylayeva-Gupta Y, et al. EZH2 couples pancreatic regeneration to neoplastic progression. Genes Dev. 2012;26(5):439–44.

48. Neff T, Sinha AU, Kluk MJ, Zhu N, Khattab MH, Stein L, et al. Polycomb repressive complex 2 is required for MLL-AF9 leukemia. Proc Natl Acad Sci U S A. 2012;109(13):5028–33.

49. Varambally S, Cao Q, Mani RS, Shankar S, Wang X, Ateeq B, et al. Genomic loss of microRNA-101 leads to overexpression of histone methyltransferase EZH2 in cancer. Science. 2008;322:1695–9.

50. Sturm D, Witt H, Hovestadt V, Khuong-Quang DA, Jones DT, Konermann C, et al. Hotspot mutations in H3F3A and IDH1 define distinct epigenetic and biological subgroups of glioblastoma. Cancer Cell. 2012;22(4):425–37.

51. Xu W, Yang H, Liu Y, Yang Y, Wang P, Kim SH, et al. Oncometabolite 2-hydroxyglutarate is a competitive inhibitor of α-ketoglutarate-dependent dioxygenases. Cancer Cell. 2011;19(1):17–30.

52. Lu C, Ward PS, Kapoor GS, Rohle D, Turcan S, Abdel-Wahab O, et al. IDH mutation impairs histone demethylation and results in a block to cell differentiation. Nature. 2012;483(34):474–8.

53. Melillo G. Inhibiting hypoxia-inducible factor 1 for cancer therapy. Mol Cancer Res. 2006;4(9):601–5.

54. Evans SM, Judy KD, Dunphy I, Jenkins WT, Hwang WT, Nelson PT, et al. Hypoxia is important in the biology and aggression of human glial brain tumors. Clin Cancer Res. 2004;10:8177–84.

55. Singh SK, Vartanian A, Burrell K, Zadeh G. A microRNA link to glioblastoma heterogeneity. Cancers. 2012;4(3):846–72.

56. Evans SM, Judy KD, Dunphy I, Jenkins WT, Nelson PT, Collins R, et al. Comparative measurements of hypoxia in human brain tumors using needle electrodes and EF5 binding. Cancer Res. 2004;64:1886–92.

57. Heddleston JM, Li Z, Lathia JD, Bao S, Hjelmeland AB, Rich JN. Hypoxia inducible factor in cancer stem cells. Br J Cancer. 2010;102(5):789–95.

58. Brat DJ, Kaur B, Van Meir EG. Genetic modulation of Hypoxia induced gene expression and angiogenesis: relevance to brain tumours. Front Biosci. 2003;8:d100–16.

59. Heddleston JM, Li Z, McLendon RE, Hjelmeland AB, Rich JN. The hypoxic microenvironment maintains glioblastoma stem cells and promotes reprogramming towards a cancer stem cell phenotype. Cell Cycle. 2009;8(20):3274–84.

60. Seidel S, Garvalov BK, Wirta V, Von Stechow L, Schanzer A, Meletis K, et al. A hypoxic niche regulates glioblastoma stem cells through hypoxia inducible factor 2α. Brain. 2010;133:983–95.

61. Harris AL. Hypoxia—a key regulatory factor in tumour growth. Nat Rev Cancer. 2002;2(1):38–47.

62. Thirlwell C, Schulz LKE, Dibra HK, Beck S. Suffocating cancer: hypoxia-associated epimutations as targets for cancer therapy. Clin Epigenetics. 2011;3:1–9.

63. Semenza GL. HIF-1 mediates metabolic responses to intratumoral hypoxia and oncogenic mutations. J Clin Invest. 2013;123(9):3664–71.

64. Lin Q, Cong X, Yun Z. Differential hypoxic regulation of hypoxia-inducible factors 1α and 2α. Mol Cancer Res. 2011;9(6):757–65.

65. Tennant DA, Duràn RV, Boulahbel H, Gottlieb E. Metabolic transformation in cancer. Carcinogenesis. 2009;30(8):1269–80.

66. Christofk HR, Vander Heiden MG, Harris MH, Ramanathan A, Gerszten RE, Wei R, et al. The M2 splice isoform of pyruvate kinase is important for cancer metabolism and tumour growth. Nature. 2008;452:230–3.

67. Watson JA, Watson CJ, McCrohan AM, Woodfine K, Tosetto M, McDaid J, et al. Generation of an epigenetic signature by chronic hypoxia in prostate cells. Hum Mol Genet. 2009;18:3594–604.

68. Watson JA, Watson CJ, McCann A, Baugh J. Epigenetics, the epicenter of the hypoxic response. Epigenetics. 2010;5(4):293–6.
69. Pal A, Srivastava T, Sharma MK, Mehndiratta M, Das P, Sinha S, et al. Aberrant methylation and associated transcriptional mobilization of Alu elements contributes to genomic instability in hypoxia. J Cell Mol Med. 2010;14(11):2646–54.
70. Xia X, Lemieux ME, Li W, Carroll JS, Brown M, Liu XS, et al. Integrative analysis of HIF binding and transactivation reveals its role in maintaining histone methylation homeostasis. Proc Natl Acad Sci U S A. 2009;106(11):4260–5.
71. Cortez MA, Ivan C, Zhou P, Wu X, Ivan M, Calin GA. MicroRNAs in cancer: from bench to bedside. Adv Cancer Res. 2010;108:113–57.
72. Johnson AB, Denko N, Barton MC. Hypoxia induces a novel signature of chromatin modifications and global repression of transcription. Mutat Res. 2008; 640(1–2):174–9.
73. Shahrzad S, Bertrand K, Minhas K, Coomber BL. Induction of DNA hypomethylation by tumor hypoxia. Epigenetics. 2007;2(2):119–25.
74. Heddleston JM, Wu Q, Rivera M, Minhas S, Lathia JD, Sloan AE, et al. Hypoxia-induced mixed-lineage leukemia 1 regulates glioma stem cell tumorigenic potential. Cell Death Differ. 2012;19: 428–39.
75. Beyer S, Kristensen MM, Jensen KS, Johansen JV, Staller P. The histone demethylases JMJD1A and JMJD2B are transcriptional targets of hypoxia-inducible factor HIF. J Biol Chem. 2008;283(52): 36542–52.
76. Wellmann S, Bettkober M, Zelmer A, Seeger K, Faigle M, Eltzschig HK, et al. Hypoxia upregulates the histone demethylase JMJD1A via HIF-1. Biochem Biophys Res Commun. 2008;372(4):892–7.
77. Pollard PJ, Loenarz C, Mole DR, McDonough MA, Gleadle JM, Schofield CJ, et al. Regulation of Jumonjidomain-containing histone demethylases by hypoxiainducible factor (HIF)-1alpha. Biochem J. 2008;416(3):387–94.
78. Yang J, Ledaki I, Turley H, Gatter KC, Montero JCM, Li JL. Role of hypoxia-inducible factors in epigenetic regulation via histone demethylases. Ann N Y Acad Sci. 2009;1177:185–97.

# Tumor Microenvironment, Hypoxia, and Stem Cell-Related Radiation Resistance

## 12

Mariangela Sottili, Chiara Gerini, Isacco Desideri,
Mauro Loi, Lorenzo Livi, and Monica Mangoni

## Introduction

Glioblastoma is among the most prevalent and lethal primary tumor of the brain [1–3]. Despite the aggressive therapeutic options, the prognosis for patients with glioblastoma remains extremely poor, with a median survival slightly above 1 year [4]. The major problems with this malignancy are the highly infiltrative nature and the resistance to therapy of tumor cells [2, 3].

Radiotherapy is the most effective nonsurgical therapeutic treatment for glioblastoma, because it can conform to highly irregular target volumes [5, 6], but tumor recurrence is yet almost inevitable [7]. Since tumor recurrence usually occurs in the initial treated tissues/areas and local control is not improved even by an increase in radiation dose [8], this tumor is considered to be radioresistant [5, 6].

Resistance to therapy is attributable to the cellular and phenotypical heterogeneity that characterizes this tumor [9]. Indeed, glioblastoma is a highly heterogeneous tumor, with distinctive histopathological and molecular features [10].

M. Sottili • C. Gerini • I. Desideri • M. Loi • L. Livi
M. Mangoni (✉)
Radiotherapy Unit, Department of Experimental and
Clinical Biomedical Sciences, University of Florence,
Largo Brambilla 3, Firenze 50134, Italy
e-mail: monica.mangoni@unifi.it

Increasing evidence supports the hypothesis that the intratumoral heterogeneity derives from a combination of genetic/epigenetic events (that lead to coexisting genetically distinct clones) and of a cellular hierarchy dominated by a subpopulation of cells exhibiting stem cell properties, named glioblastoma stem cells (GSCs) [1]. In addition, multiple interactions between tumor cells and microenvironment contribute to tumor progression.

## Tumor Microenvironment

The bulk of tumors is composed of a variety of cell types: tumor cells, cancer stem cells, and several other nonmalignant host cells, including fibroblasts, stromal cells, glial cells, immunitary system cells, and blood and lymphatic vessels. All these cells are embedded in an extracellular matrix. It has become increasingly evident that not only the genetic aberrations in malignant cells, but also the interaction among cancer cells, nonmalignant cells, soluble factors, and other elements of the tumor microenvironment are critical in the pathophysiology of cancer. Complex multilevel communication and interaction between tumor cells and nonmalignant cells have the ability to adapt tumor cells to the microenvironment and to change it to their own advantage [11]. Microenvironment cells can secrete a number of factors, such as growth factors, neuro-

© Springer International Publishing Switzerland 2016
L. Pirtoli et al. (eds.), *Radiobiology of Glioblastoma*, Current Clinical Pathology,
DOI 10.1007/978-3-319-28305-0_12

trophic factors, and chemokines, that play a vital role in controlling the course of pathology [12]. Different cell types from the tumor microenvironment can communicate also by transferring of bioactive molecules, including microRNAs, that contribute to tumor progression [11]. In addition, the tumor-vasculature not only nourishes glioblastomas, but also provides a specialized niche for cancer stem cells [13]. Recent studies showing that glioblastoma cells grown as orthotopic xenografts are more radioresistant than the same cells grown in vitro have suggested that the brain microenvironment, besides its pivotal role in tumor maintenance, is also implicated in radioresistance [14].

The tumor microenvironment is abnormal and these abnormalities can fuel tumor progression and treatment resistance. Normalization of the microenvironment can improve treatment outcome in mice and patients with malignant and nonmalignant diseases [15–19].

## Glioblastoma Stem Cells

While ambiguity remains over the precise origin of GSCs, several reports supported the implication of GSCs in initiation, progression, and regrowth of the tumor after therapy [1, 9, 20]. In fact, GSCs have a high tumorigenic capacity [21, 22], a highly migratory nature [23], and display many of the properties of normal neural stem cells, that render them relatively insensitive to radiotherapy [24–27].

The definitions of GSCs are various, but it is generally accepted that they possess clonal self-renewal, and multilineage differentiation potential. In addition, when injected in immunodeficient mice, GSCs are able to reconstitute glioblastoma tumors phenotypically similar to the disease originally present in the patient from which they are derived [7, 20, 22, 24, 28].

Like normal stem cells, GSCs are dependent on cues from the surrounding microenvironment and are located in specialized regions called "niches," most notably the perivascular and hypoxic niches [1]. These niches are composed of several tumor-associated stromal cells (i.e.,

vascular and immune cells, neural precursor cells, microglia, myofibroblasts) and extracellular components, and provide GSCs with molecular signals that promote the stem cell phenotype [29–33].

GSCs living in perivascular and hypoxic niches express the surface marker CD133/prominin-1 that has been the first and most widely used antigen for the enrichment of GSCs and has been validated in fresh patient's specimens [22, 25]. The association between the expression of CD133 and the clinical outcome of glioblastoma patients has been demonstrated in several clinical studies [34–36].

However, more recently some doubts on the assumption that CD133 is a universal marker for GSCs have been raised, since experimental evidence showed the existence of both CD133+ CD133− populations in GSCs and demonstrated that also CD133− cells were able to form tumors [37].

These reports have suggested that a single marker is insufficient to identify the GSC population. The search for more robust GSCs surface markers has led to the identification of other molecules, such as CD15/SSEA-1 [38], CD44, inhibitors of DNA-binding protein(Id)-1 [39], CD90 [40], L1CAM, integrin α6, A2B5, and Musashi homolog 1 (MSI1) [22, 41–44].

Interestingly, the identification of GSCs has provided new explanations of glioblastoma radiation resistance [45]. Indeed, in in vitro and in vivo studies Bao and colleagues [25] showed that after ionizing radiation glioblastoma tumor cells became extremely enriched for GSCs and that irradiated GSCs were more radioresistant as compared to the non-stem cells population and were able to repopulate both in vitro and in vivo. These data suggested that GSCs may play a pivotal role in glioblastoma radioresistance and tumor aggressiveness [28].

Radiation therapy targets the proliferative potential of the tumors by killing rapidly dividing cells within the bulk of the tumor, but cancer stem cells remain unaffected. Thus, the therapeutic treatment leads to the selection of the more aggressive GSCs, resulting later in recurrence of the tumor, which becomes also resistant to further conventional therapy [24].

## Mechanisms of GSCs Radiation Resistance

### Enhanced DNA Repair

Ionizing radiation therapeutic effect relays on its capability to produce unrepairable DNA damages, mostly double-strand breaks, within tumor cells [46]. In addition to these lethal DNA damages, also radiation-induced sublethal damages contribute to tumor lethality [26]. DNA lesions triggered by irradiation activate the DNA damage checkpoint signaling, a complex signal transduction pathway that includes several proteins, such as Chk1/2 kinases, ataxia telangiectasia mutated (ATM), MRE11-RAD50-NBS1 (MRN) complex, DNA-dependent protein kinase catalytic subunit (DNA-PKcs), ATM and Rad3 related (ATR), Rad17, and other checkpoint proteins [26, 47, 48]. The activation of the DNA damage checkpoint induces cell-cycle arrest to allow the cells to repair DNA, or triggers a pro-apoptotic signal to eliminate those cells where the DNA damage is irreparable [49, 50]. Interestingly, GSCs have been reported to be more efficient in repairing damaged DNA and more resistant to radiation-induced apoptosis as compared to non-stem glioma cells both in vitro and in vivo [25].

Indeed, CD133+ cells show an enhanced basal activation of ATM, Chk1, Chk2, and Rad17, that may be further upregulated in response to DNA damage, resulting in an increased survival of GSCs after irradiation [51, 52]. Accordingly, CD133+ glioma cells radiosensitivity is partially restored by treatment with specific inhibitors of Chk1/2 [25] and ATM kinases [51].

A recent study showed that the protein poly (ADP-ribose) polymerase (PARP)-1, involved in single-strand break repair, plays a pivotal role in the constitutive activation of the DNA repair machinery and the subsequent radioresistance of GSCs [53]. PARP inhibitors, such as veliparib and olaparib, have been shown to radiosensitize glioblastoma cells both in vitro and in vivo [54, 55] and are tested in clinical trials for glioblastoma and brain tumors (http://clinicaltrials.gov, NCT01390571, NCT00994071, NCT00687765).

Moreover, the DNA damage response machinery is activated also by BMI-1, a polycomb complex protein shown to be enriched in GSC and required for maintaining GSC self-renewal [28]. BMI-1 has been suggested to increase GSCs radioresistance since it is rapidly recruited to sites of DNA damage in CD133+ GSCs after irradiation, colocalized with ATM kinase and the histone gamma-H2AX and preferentially copurified with non-homologous end joining (NHEJ) proteins [56]. Loss of BMI-1 leads to weakened DNA repair and increases sensitivity to radiation, and results in inhibition of glioblastoma proliferation [57].

### Evasion of Cell Death Pathways

Radioresistance of GSCs has been suggested to derive also from the activation of anti-apoptotic factors. Indeed, it has been observed that GSCs express several anti-apoptotic genes (i.e., BCL-2, BCL2L1a, and MCL1) to a higher extent as compared to differentiated cells [58, 59]. Moreover, increased levels of ATF5, a transcription factor that promotes cell survival by stimulating the transcription of the anti-apoptotic protein MCL1 [60], have been observed in glioblastoma.

Specific inhibitors of the 26S proteasome, a protease complex involved in cell death, such as MG132, saquinavir, and bortezomib, have shown to induce cell death and to increase glioma cell radiosensitivity [61–63].

Although conflicting results have been obtained in clinical studies evaluating bortezomib as a single agent or in combination with established therapeutic regimens [64], a phase I trial using bortezomib and concurrent temozolomide and radiotherapy demonstrated that bortezomib is effective in the treatment of central nervous system malignancies, with a tolerable toxicity profile [65]. Furthermore, bortezomib, in association with temozolomide and radiation therapy, is now undergoing a phase II study for the treatment of patients with newly diagnosed glioblastoma multiforme or gliosarcoma (http://clinicaltrials.gov, NCT00998010).

As described in Chap. 9, ionizing radiation may also affect alternative forms of programmed cell death, such as autophagy [66].

## Quiescence

It is well known that cells change their sensitivity to radiation all along the cell cycle, ranging from greatest sensitivity while in mitosis to extreme resistance in late S-phase [67]. Cellular quiescence may be involved in the acquired or constitutive resistance of cancer stem cells to radio-chemotherapy [68]. Indeed, Liu et al. observed that CD133+ GSCs derived from treatment-refractory recurrent glioblastoma tumors showed a quiescent phenotype distinct from the differentiated cells within the majority of tumor mass [23]. Radioresistant clones of GSCs exhibit a decreased glucose uptake and preferentially activate the fatty acid oxidation pathway, thus using lipid metabolism and autophagy for energy production [69]. This metabolic adaptation allows radioresistant GSCs to retain their quiescent status, and therefore strengthens their repair abilities against radiation-induced DNA damage.

Surviving cells reenter cell cycle division after radiation treatment, thus the fractionation of the radiation treatment could be able to kill also radioresistant GSCs.

## Hypoxia

Tumor hypoxia has been linked to resistance to radiation treatment, recurrence of cancer and poor prognosis of glioblastoma patients [70–72]. Hypoxia and hypoxia-related factors have been shown to play a pivotal role in supporting the survival and maintaining the intrinsic cellular features of GSCs, rendering them more resistant to radiation treatment, and thus driving glioblastoma initiation and progression [73–76]. Experimental evidence also suggested that hypoxia may be able to reprogram CD133– GSCs to become CD133+ [77]. McGee et al. demonstrated that glioblastoma radiosensitivity was improved by increasing the intratumoral oxygenation through the normalization of the vasculature [78].

Tumor hypoxia exists in two principal forms: (a) chronic hypoxia, derived from a limitation of oxygen diffusion due to tumor expansion and (b) acute or cycling hypoxia, caused by intermittent blood flow due to altered structure or function of the blood vessels within the tumor, that provokes cycling changes in tumor oxygenation [79]. Previous reports highlighted only the role of chronic hypoxia on cancer cells radiosensitivity [80, 81], but the observation that, following radiotherapy, tumor commonly recurred in regions with numerous intermittent vascular stasis [82] led the researchers to investigate also cycling hypoxia effects [83, 84]. Hsieh et al. [5, 6] showed that cycling hypoxia induced more radioresistance in glioma cells as compared to non-interrupted hypoxia, thus concluding that cyclically hypoxic cells are the utmost resistant to radiation and could therefore be responsible for tumor relapse.

Hypoxia stimulates the synthesis of the hypoxia inducible factors (HIFs), a family of transcription factors that regulate the expression of a number of genes critical for tumor progression, angiogenesis, resistance to therapy and cancer stem cells phenotype maintenance, thus allowing GSCs to survive [58, 59, 85–87]. The expression of HIFs correlates with tumor radiotherapy response [88, 89]. The main HIFs isoforms in cancer are HIF-1$\alpha$, mostly regulating acute hypoxic responses, and HIF-2$\alpha$, that controls prolonged hypoxic gene activation [26, 90]. Both HIF-1$\alpha$ and HIF-2$\alpha$ appeared to promote a stem-like phenotype in GSCs, by inducing the expression of CD133 through the activation of Sox2, Oct4, and Notch, transcription factors associated with the control of stem cells self-renewal and multipotency [31–33, 75]. While HIF-1$\alpha$ was expressed both in GSCs than in non-stem cells and was stabilized only in acute low oxygen conditions, HIF-2$\alpha$ was specifically present in GSCs and worked both on low and physiological oxygen levels. This result suggested differential roles of the two isoforms in GSCs, with HIF-2$\alpha$ having the dominant role in GSCs. Moreover, HIF-1$\alpha$ has been demonstrated to recruit endothelial and pericyte progenitor cells, thus promoting angiogenesis and tumor cell invasiveness in glioblastoma [91]. For that reasons, both HIFs isoforms have been proposed as targets for glioblastoma treatment [31–33, 92–94].

## Angiogenesis and Vasculogenesis

Tumor response to radiation therapy depends on tissue vascularity [95, 96]. Interestingly, GSCs have been described to play a pivotal role in tumor angiogenesis promotion [45, 95]. GSCs-derived tumors have been shown to exhibit a greater vascularity than tumors originated by non-stem tumor cells, partly because of the significantly higher VEGF expression levels found in GSCs as compared to non-stem glioblastoma cells [95]. This enhanced VEGF production induced an increase in endothelial cell migration and vessel formation both in vitro [95] and in vivo [97]. Moreover, it has been reported that GSCs were able to directly differentiate in cells of the endothelial lineage and that a significant portion of the newly formed vessels were of glioma stem cells origin [98–100]. Accordingly, the direct targeting of endothelial cells led to a reduction of the tumor bulk.

## Extracellular Matrix Components

Increasing evidence support the hypothesis that the interactions between GSCs and extracellular matrix (ECM) components within the tumor may influence GSCs response to radiotherapy in several ways [101]. First, they may operate as a deposit for growth factors with a modulatory role in radiation responses, such as epidermal growth factor (EGF) and fibroblast growth factor (FGF), which appear to decrease radiation-induced GSCs apoptosis in vitro [25]. In addition, the observation that expression and activation of integrins b1 [102], avb3, and avb5 [103] was associated with an enhanced radioresistance of glioma cells in vitro led to hypothesize that the ECM components could act as a milieu for the initiation of integrin-induced prosurvival signals in GSCs after radiotherapy. Furthermore, it has been suggested that the vicinity of GSCs to ECM components could promote GSCs survival and proliferation following irradiation. This hypothesis is sustained by some studies, reporting that the ECM glycoprotein tenascin C is mainly expressed in the stem-like cells in glioblastoma,

participates in the generation of an environmental niche for neural stem cell development, and may contribute to glioblastoma progression and metastasis [104, 105]. In addition, the observed correlation between tenascin C expression and glioblastoma patients' poor survival [106] suggests that tenascin C may exert a radioprotective effect on GSCs, likely through the stimulation of the growth of cells survived to ionizing radiation.

## Nitric Oxide and Reactive Oxygen Species

Recent studies have supported the potential role of nitric oxide (NO) in glioblastoma resistance to radiation therapy. Charles et al. [107] observed that endothelial nitric oxide synthase (eNOS) was expressed in tumor endothelial cells, which were in proximity of the NO receptor-expressing GSCs. NO produced from the endothelial cells activated the Notch pathway in GSCs, enhancing tumor formation and progression. Since GSCs radiosensitivity has been demonstrated to be increased by the inhibition of the Notch pathway [99, 100], it has been speculated that NO increases GSCs radioresistance through the activation of the Notch pathway in the perivascular niche [101].

Since lower levels of reactive oxygen species (ROS) have been observed in stem cells of the central nervous system, an increased expression of ROS scavengers has been suggested as a further mechanism underlying GSCs radioresistance [108, 109]. In fact, a higher activity of free radical scavenging pathways could spare stem cells from DNA damage following radiotherapy [26].

## Signaling Pathways Involved in Radiation Resistance

Accumulating evidence suggests that multiple signaling pathways may be involved in the protection of GSCs from radiation-induced injury [110] (see Fig. 12.1).

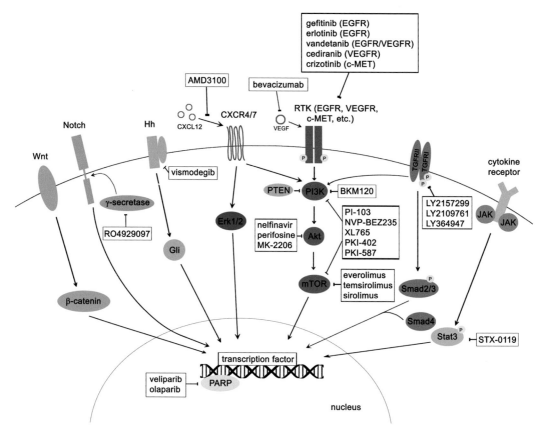

**Fig. 12.1** Main signaling pathways involved in GSCs radioresistance. *Hh* Hedgehog Homolog, *Gli* Gli transcription factors, *RTK* receptor tyrosine kinase, *PI3K* phosphatidylinositol 3-kinase, *Akt* also known as Protein Kinase B (PKB), *mTOR* mammalian target of rapamycin, *JAK* Janus kinase, *STAT* signal transducer and activator of transcription, *PARP* poly ADP ribose polymerase, *SMAD* small mother against decapentaplegic, *TGFR* transforming growth factor receptor

## Wnt/β-Catenin

The Wnt/β-catenin signaling pathway is a pivotal developmental pathway reported to contribute to stem cell maintenance and growth [111, 112].

The radioprotective function of Wnt in GSCs has been further confirmed by the observation that radioresistant GSCs expressed high levels of active β-catenin [113], whose expression levels have been previously shown to correlate with glioblastoma patients' poor prognosis [114]. The mechanisms through which Wnt/β-catenin favor GSCs radioresistance are not fully elucidated but it has been suggested that this signaling pathway may allow GSCs to tolerate extensive radiation-induced DNA damage and may induce the malignant transformation of non-tumorigenic stem cells to GSCs by promoting genomic instability [115, 116].

## PI3K/Akt/mTOR

Aberrant activation of PI3K/Akt/mTOR pathway is frequently observed in glioblastoma, and correlates with patients' poor prognosis [117, 118]. This signaling pathway has been reported to regulate migration and invasiveness of GSCs that display a preferential sensitivity to Akt inhibition as compared to non-GSCs [119].

The PI3K signaling is frequently activated in glioblastoma due to the loss of the phosphatase and tensin homologue (PTEN) tumor suppressor gene [120]. Notably, PTEN deletion promotes self-renewal and prevents differentiation of GSCs [121]. It has been demonstrated that lack of PTEN, with the subsequent activation of the PI3K/Akt pathway, confers radiation resistance in glioblastoma cell lines, while the induction of PTEN restores radiosensitivity [122, 123]. PI3K/Akt/mTOR pathway can be also activated by EGFR, whose amplified expression or mutation is frequently observed in glioblastoma and has shown to promote radioresistance of glioma cells by increasing the PI3K/Akt signaling [124, 125].

Another factor able to mediate Akt signaling activation is the Insulin-Like Growth Factor (IGF)-1/IGF type 1 receptor (IGF1R) axis. IGF1 and IGFR1 have been found overexpressed in GSCs after radiation, and have shown to protect GSCs from radiation toxicity through the activation of Akt signaling [126]. In addition, also the IGF Binding Protein 2 (IGFBP2), whose expression is often increased in glioblastoma and inversely correlates with patient outcome [127, 128], has shown to support GSCs self-renewal, growth, and radioresistance by activating the Akt pathway [5, 6, 23].

PI3K/Akt/mTOR inhibitors have shown to decrease GSCs invasiveness and tumorigenicity both in vitro and in vivo, while increasing GSCs apoptosis [124, 129, 130]. The inhibition of mTOR by the selective inhibitors rapamycin and AZD2014 showed to sensitize glioblastoma cells to radiation therapy both in vitro and in vivo studies [131–133]. These encouraging results led several mTOR inhibitors, such as everolimus, and temsirolimus, to be tested in clinical trials in association with radiochemotherapy for glioblastoma [134, 135] (http://clinicaltrials.gov, NCT00553150, NCT01062399, NCT00316849, NCT01019434). More recently, the dual inhibition of both PI3K and mTOR has been proposed as a more useful therapeutic strategy for glioblastoma, and novel molecules with dual inhibitory activity have been developed. The dual blockade of PI3K and mTOR with PI-103, which is known to reduce glioblastoma tumor volume [136], has been also proven effective in sensitizing glioblastoma cells to radiation therapy [137–139]. Furthermore, the EGFR-mediated radioresistance have been shown to be disrupted in glioma

models by EGFR tyrosine kinase inhibitors, such as ZD6474, AG1478, and ZD1839 (gefitinib) [117, 140–142] that decrease clonogenic capability and migration of glioma cells [143].

Although the promising results of preclinical studies, clinical trials testing EGFR inhibitors in patients with glioblastoma have shown mixed results [124, 144–146] (http://clinicaltrials.gov, NCT00124657, NCT00052208, NCT00187486, NCT00977431). The multitarget therapeutic approach has been suggested as a possible strategy to improve patients' outcomes. Accordingly, the EGFR inhibitor combination treatments have produced improved results as compared to monotherapy [147].

## Notch

The Notch pathway is required to support the proliferation and differentiation of normal neural stem cells [124] but its anomalous activation has been shown to promote also stemness and tumorigenicity of GSCs [148]. Notch appears to promote GSCs resistance to radiotherapy via the activation of the PI3K/Akt signaling pathway and by inducing the anti-apoptotic proteins Bcl-2 and Mcl-1 [149]. In addition, Notch signaling has been proposed to regulate GSCs resistance to radiation by driving GSCs into quiescence, similarly to normal neural stem cells [150, 151].

The γ-secretase inhibitors, Notch-targeting agents that block the release of the Notch intracellular domain, have been shown to inhibit GSCs growth and tumorigenic potential [152, 153] and to impair xenograft tumor formation in in vivo experiments [147]. Interestingly, the treatment with γ-secretase inhibitors also renders GSCs more sensitive to radiation therapy [99, 100, 154]. The novel Notch inhibitor RO4929097 is currently being evaluated, in association with radiochemotherapy, in an early clinical trial for patients with newly diagnosed malignant glioma (http://clinicaltrials.gov, NCT01119599). Moreover, a phase II trial evaluating RO4929097 as a single agent is now ongoing for patients with recurrent or progressive glioblastoma (http://clinicaltrials.gov, NCT01122901).

## Hedgehog-Gli

The Hedgehog (Hh) signaling pathway has been reported to be involved in the development of brain tumors [26], including glioma [155], where the Hh intracellular mediator Gli was firstly described [156]. In particular, the Hh-Gli signaling has been shown to regulate self-renewal, proliferation, and tumorigenic potential of GSCs through interaction with differentiated tumor cells and microenvironment [157, 158].

Moreover, the inhibition of Hh signaling increases the effect of radiation on GSCs, depletes GSCs, and significantly improves survival in a glioblastoma xenograft model [157, 159–161].

## STAT3

The STAT3 signaling pathway has been reported to be involved in mesenchymal transformation of glioblastoma and to inversely correlate with patient survival [162]. Furthermore, it has been shown that GSCs, differently from differentiated cells, exhibit the active form of STAT3, whose inhibition interrupts maintenance and growth of GSCs [163, 164]. Yang et al. [31] revealed that STAT3 activation contributes to GSCs resistance to radiation therapy. Indeed, they confirmed that radioresistant GSCs express STAT3 to a higher extent than glioma non-stem cells, and demonstrated that STAT3 inhibition reduced the percentage of GSCs, and increased their radiosensitivity. Resveratrol, a natural polyphenol found in red wine, has been shown to induce apoptosis in cancer cells, thus leading to tumor growth blockade and radiochemosensitization [165, 166], by suppressing STAT3 signaling axis [167]. Afterward, Yang et al. [31–33] observed that the inhibition of STAT3 by resveratrol suppresses stemness features and invasiveness of GSCs, and enhances their radiosensitivity.

## c-MET Tyrosine Kinase

The c-MET tyrosine kinase has been reported to promote the survival, growth, and invasion of

several cancers including glioblastoma [168]. It has been shown that this protein is overexpressed in GSCs [169], and plays a pivotal role in enhancement, maintenance, and invasiveness of GSCs [168, 170]. In addition, the observation that c-MET inhibition disrupts GSCs clonogenicity, tumorigenicity, and radioresistance demonstrate that c-MET signaling also exhibits radioprotective functions in GSCs [168]. Several molecules targeting c-MET pathway have been developed and are undergoing clinical evaluation [171–173].

## CXCL12-CXCR4/CXCR7 Axis

The signaling system formed by the chemokine CXCL12 and its receptors CXCR4/CXCR7 plays a pivotal role in growth, angiogenesis, and invasiveness of glioblastoma [118, 174]. CXCR4 and CXCL12 levels have been reported to correlate with tumor grade and poor prognosis in glioblastoma patients [174]. Moreover, the CXCL12-CXCR4/CXCR7 pathway has been described to promote survival, self-renewal, angiogenesis, metastatic potential, and resistance to radiation of GSCs [118, 174]. In vivo studies revealed that CXCR4-positive glioma cells were enriched for GSCs, and were more tumorigenic and more radioresistant than CXCR4-negative cells [22, 175, 176]. The machinery underlying CXCL12-mediated GSCs radioresistance has yet to be fully elucidated, but it has been suggested that the CXCL12 pathway acts through direct and indirect mechanisms:

1. It directly promotes GSCs survival, self-renewal, and metastatic potential [118, 174].
2. It indirectly stimulates tumor angiogenesis and vasculogenesis through the endothelial cells and tumor cells paracrine signals, and the recruitment of CXCR4-positive GSCs toward the perivascular niche [175, 177, 178].

The involvement of the CXCL12-CXCR4/CXCR7 axis in GSCs radioresistance has been strengthened by the recent observation that CXCR7 blockade after irradiation significantly reduced tumor growth and relapse, and enhanced survival in a xenograft model of glioblastoma, likely affecting GSCs [179].

Plerixafor (AMD3100), a drug that impedes the binding of CXCL12 to CXCR4, has been reported to inhibit the radiation-induced vasculogenesis in a glioblastoma xenograft model, thus preventing tumor recurrence after irradiation [96]. Interestingly, the association of AMD3100 with irradiation has shown to prevent radiation-stimulated invasion of glioma cells in irradiated normal brain [180].

A phase I/II study evaluating the plerixafor-temozolomide-radiotherapy combined treatment in patients with newly diagnosed high grade glioma is ongoing (http://clinicaltrials.gov, NCT01977677).

## TGF-β

TGF-β has been described to promote a number of cellular processes implicated in glioblastoma initiation and progression [181], and to correlate with tumor aggressiveness, degree of malignancy, and poor prognosis in glioma patients [182, 183].

TGF-β signaling has been also reported as a central actor in GSCs stemness maintenance and self-renewal promotion [10, 184, 185]. Moreover, TGF-β increases the radiation resistance in GSCs, likely through the activation of the DNA damage stress response and the inhibition of apoptosis [181, 186].

The abrogation of TGF-β signaling by the TGFβR-I kinase inhibitor LY2109761 has been reported to increase radiation response and prolongs survival in glioblastoma. LY2109761 was able to reduce GSCs self-renewal and proliferation, and potentiated the antitumor efficacy of radiation in GSCs in vitro and in GSCs-derived tumors in vivo [181]. Furthermore, the effectiveness of LY2109761 on glioblastoma was evaluated also in combination with the current clinical standard regimen, consisting in radiotherapy plus temozolomide [187]. LY2109761 showed radiosensitizing effects on glioblastoma cells, and inhibited tumor growth alone and in combination

with radiation and temozolomide both in vitro and in vivo. Currently, a phase I/II evaluating the eventual clinical benefits of the combination of the TGF-βRI kinase inhibitor LY2157299 with radiochemotherapy in patients with newly diagnosed malignant glioma is ongoing (http://clinicaltrials.gov, NCT01220271).

## SirT1

SirT1, a NAD(+)-dependent histone deacetylase, has been reported to play crucial roles in several biological processes, including stress response, DNA repair, tumorigenesis, and radiosensitivity [188, 189]. In particular, Chang et al. [190] observed that GSCs expressed SirT1 to a higher extent as compared to glioma non-stem cells. Moreover, they showed that the inhibition of SirT1 increased radiosensitivity and radiation-induced apoptosis in GSCs, thus proposing Sirt1 as a pivotal modulator of GSCs resistance to radiotherapy.

## miRNAs

MicroRNAs (miRNAs) are small non-coding RNA molecules involved in the modulation of gene expression and in the regulation of several cellular processes, such as apoptosis, proliferation, differentiation, invasiveness, stress responses, and angiogenesis [191].

miRNAs can act either as tumor suppressors or as oncogenes [191], and have been found to be implicated in glioblastoma pathogenesis [31–33] and to play a role in cancer stem cell properties, contributing to treatment resistance [192]. Indeed, an altered miRNAs expression has been observed in radioresistant glioblastoma cells [2, 3], and has been shown to predict prognosis and therapy response in glioblastoma [192–194]. Of note, it has been reported that miRNAs markedly regulated several pathways involved in glioma resistance to therapy (i.e., PI3K/Akt, ATM/Chk2 kinase, p53) [192, 195, 196].

Studies on solid tumors [197] showed that five miRNAs (miR-9, miR-21, miR-200a, miR-218, and miR-203) were associated to radioresistance. Accordingly, a miR-21 inhibitor has shown to enhance the sensitivity of glioblastoma cells to ionizing radiation-induced apoptosis and cell growth blockade, at least in part by reducing G(2)-M arrest [198]. A recent study revealed that also miR-210, a miRNA involved in cellular adaption to hypoxia and in stem cell survival and stemness maintenance, plays a role in GSCs radioresistance [199]. Other reports showed that the radiosensitivity of glioma cells was affected by a number of additional miRNAs, such as miR-7, miR-18a, miR-100, miR-101, MiR-181a, and miR-421 [152, 153, 198, 200, 201].

On the other hand, the transfection of GSCs with miR-145, a tumor-suppressive miRNA that regulates stem cells properties and inversely correlates with tumor growth and metastasis in several cancers [202, 203], has been shown to induce the differentiation of GSCs and to suppress their expression of anti-apoptotic genes, thus reducing GSCs tumorigenicity and resistance to radiation [32]. Moreover, the simultaneous administration of miR-145 and radiotherapy enhanced the survival rate of mice intra-cranially transplanted with patient-derived glioblastoma CD133+ GSCs [32].

Furthermore, miR-34-a, miR-124, miR-137, and the miR-302/367 cluster have been reported to induce GSCs differentiation and to suppress glioblastoma cells growth and invasiveness [73, 74, 204, 205]. These findings suggest that the regulation of miRNAs could become a novel therapeutic strategy to enhance the radiosensitivity of GSCs and suppress the progression of glioblastoma. However, a full knowledge of the complex biological networks controlled by miRNAs and of all the miRNAs associated to radioresistance is still lacking. Thus, further studies are needed to have a complete picture of the roles played by miRNAs in the process of radioresistance, before to introduce them in therapeutic settings.

## Conclusions and Perspectives

Growing body of data accounts for GSCs role in initiation, progression, and radioresistance of glioblastoma. Thus, GSCs are now being explored as crucial targets for novel therapeutic strategies.

Despite intensive studies, the molecular mechanisms underlying GSCs radiotherapy resistance are not yet fully understood. A better knowledge of the mechanisms of GSCs radioresistance could help to develop novel targeted therapies able to sensitize GSCs to radiation, in order to eradicate GSCs and to overcome treatment resistance, thus improving patients' outcome. Progresses in the knowledge of GSCs biology, in addition to improve the development of targeted drugs, would be useful also for the optimization of radiotherapy treatment planning. Indeed, the classical radiotherapy treatments deliver the radiation dose homogenously over the tumor, assuming that the cancer stem cells are randomly distributed [206]. More information about the total number and spatial distribution of GSCs within the tumor may allow to apply higher irradiation doses in the hypoxic/GSCs-enriched tumor regions, resulting in glioblastoma patients' improved outcome [207]. Hence, additional investigations for the identification of more direct GSCs markers to improve the biological imaging of GSCs are necessary. In addition, since GSCs can undergo a metabolic transformation as compared to the non-stem tumor cells, functional and metabolic imaging could permit a better identification and targeting of GSCs.

Nevertheless, since glioblastoma is formed by a heterogeneous cell population, targeted molecular therapies aimed to eradicate GSCs should not be sufficient alone. Thus, GSCs-targeting agents should be associated with effective chemotherapeutic drugs and/or radiotherapy in order to target both GSCs and bulk tumor cells. In addition, given the numerous evidence showing that hypoxic/perivascular niches supply nourishing and radioresistance-inducing signals to GSCs, therapeutic strategies able to target tumor microenvironment appear to be essential.

Finally, it has to be noted that since GSCs share many characteristics with normal stem cells, the targeting of GSCs could also lead to the disruption of the protective normal stem cell reservoir.

Thus, identifying the discrepancies between GSCS and normal neural stem cells is crucial for designing novel therapies able to target GSCs without affecting normal stem cells, for a safe therapy for glioblastoma.

# References

1. Schonberg DL, Lubelski D, Miller TE, Rich JN. Brain tumor stem cells: molecular characteristics and their impact on therapy. Mol Aspects Med. 2014;39:82–101.

2. Zhang B, Chen J, Ren Z, Chen Y, Li J, Miao X, Song Y, Zhao T, Li Y, Shi Y, Ren D, Liu J. A specific miRNA signature promotes radioresistance of human cervical cancer cells. Cancer Cell Int. 2013;13:118.

3. Zhang X, Zhang W, Mao XG, Zhen HN, Cao WD, Hu SJ. Targeting role of glioma stem cells for glioblastoma multiforme. Curr Med Chem. 2013;20(15):1974–84.

4. Stupp R, Mason WP, van den Bent MJ, Weller M, Fisher B, Taphoorn MJ, Belanger K, Brandes AA, Marosi C, Bogdahn U, Curschmann J, Janzer RC, Ludwin SK, Gorlia T, Allgeier A, Lacombe D, Cairncross JG, Eisenhauer E, Mirimanoff RO. European Organisation for Research and Treatment of Cancer Brain Tumor and Radiotherapy Groups; National Cancer Institute of Canada Clinical Trials Group. Radiotherapy plus concomitant and adjuvant temozolomide for glioblastoma. N Engl J Med. 2005; 352:987–96.

5. Hsieh CH, Lee CH, Liang JA, Yu CY, Shyu WC. Cycling hypoxia increases U87 glioma cell radioresistance via ROS induced higher and long-term HIF-1 signal transduction activity. Oncol Rep. 2010;24(6):1629–36.

6. Hsieh D, Hsieh A, Stea B, Ellsworth R. IGFBP2 promotes glioma tumor stem cell expansion and survival. Biochem Biophys Res Commun. 2010;397(2):367–72.

7. Eyler CE, Rich JN. Survival of the fittest: cancer stem cells in therapeutic resistance and angiogenesis. J Clin Oncol. 2008;26(17):2839–45.

8. Jamal M, Rath BH, Tsang PS, Camphausen K, Tofilon PJ. The brain microenvironment preferentially enhances the radioresistance of CD133(+) glioblastoma stem-like cells. Neoplasia. 2012; 14(2):150–8.

9. Carrasco-Garcia E, Sampron N, Aldaz P, Arrizabalaga O, Villanua J, Barrena C, Ruiz I, Arrazola M, Lawrie C, Matheu A. Therapeutic strategies targeting glioblastoma stem cells. Recent Pat Anticancer Drug Discov. 2013;8(3):216–27.

10. Bayin NS, Modrek AS, Placantonakis DG. Glioblastoma stem cells: molecular characteristics and therapeutic implications. World J Stem Cells. 2014;6(2):230–8.

11. Godlewski J, Krichevsky AM, Johnson MD, Antonio Chiocca E, Bronisz A. Belonging to a network—microRNAs, extracellular vesicles, and the glioblastoma microenvironment. Neuro Oncol. 2014;17(5): 652–62.

12. Holland EC, Gilbertson R, Glass R, Kettenmann H. The brain tumor microenvironment. Glia. 2012;60(3):502–14.

13. Charles NA, Holland EC, Gilbertson R, Glass R, Kettenmann H. The brain tumor microenvironment. Glia. 2012;60(3):502–14.

14. Jamal M, Rath BH, Williams ES, Camphausen K, Tofilon PJ. Microenvironmental regulation of glioblastoma radioresponse. Clin Cancer Res. 2010;16(24):6049–59.

15. Goel S, Duda DG, Xu L, et al. Normalization of the vasculature for treatment of cancer and other diseases. Physiol Rev. 2011;91:1071–121.

16. Jain RK. Normalizing tumor microenvironment to treat cancer: bench to bedside to biomarkers. J Clin Oncol. 2013;31(17):2205–18.

17. Jain RK. Taming vessels to treat cancer. Sci Am. 2008;298:56–63.

18. Jain RK. Normalization of tumor vasculature: an emerging concept in antiangiogenic therapy. Science. 2005;307:58–62.

19. Jain RK. Normalizing tumor vasculature with anti-angiogenic therapy: a new paradigm for combination therapy. Nat Med. 2001;7:987–9.

20. Chalmers AJ. Radioresistant glioma stem cells: therapeutic obstacle or promising target? DNA Repair (Amst). 2007;6(9):1391–4.

21. Piccirillo SG, Reynolds BA, Zanetti N, Lamore G, Binda E, Broggi G, Brem H, Olivi A, Dimeco F, Vescovi AL. Bone morphogenetic proteins inhibit the tumorigenic potential of human brain tumour-initiating cells. Nature. 2006;444:761–5.

22. Singh SK, Hawkins C, Clarke ID, Squire JA, Bayani J, Hide T, Henkelman RM, Cusimano MD, Dirks PB. Identification of human brain tumour initiating cells. Nature. 2004;432:396–401.

23. Liu Q, Nguyen DH, Dong Q, Shitaku P, Chung K, Liu OY, Tso JL, Liu JY, Konkankit V, Cloughesy TF, Mischel PS, Lane TF, Liau LM, Nelson SF, Tso CL. Molecular properties of CD133+ glioblastoma stem cells derived from treatment-refractory recurrent brain tumors. J Neurooncol. 2009;94:1–19.

24. Altaner C. Glioblastoma and stem cells. Neoplasma. 2008;55(5):369–74.

25. Bao S, Wu Q, McLendon RE, Hao Y, Shi Q, Shi Q, Hjelmeland AB, Dewhirst MW, Bigner DD, Rich JN. Glioma stem cells promote radioresistance by preferential activation of the DNA damage response. Nature. 2006;444:756–60.

26. Moncharmont C, Levy A, Gilormini M, Bertrand G, Chargari C, Alphonse G, Ardail D, Rodriguez-Lafrasse C, Magné N. Targeting a cornerstone of radiation resistance: cancer stem cell. Cancer Lett. 2012;322(2):139–47.

27. Murat A, Migliavacca E, Gorlia T, Lambiv WL, Shay T, Hamou MF, de Tribolet N, Regli L, Wick W, Kouwenhoven MC, Hainfellner JA, Heppner FL,

Dietrich PY, Zimmer Y, Cairncross JG, Janzer RC, Domany E, Delorenzi M, Stupp R, Hegi ME. Stem cell-related "self-renewal" signature and high epidermal growth factor receptor expression associated with resistance to concomitant chemoradiotherapy in glioblastoma. J Clin Oncol. 2008;26:3015–24.

28. Yamada K, Tso J, Ye F, Choe J, Liu Y, Liau LM, Tso CL. Essential gene pathways for glioblastoma stem cells: clinical implications for prevention of tumor recurrence. Cancers (Basel). 2011;3(2):1975–95.

29. Persano L, Rampazzo E, Della Puppa A, Pistollato F, Basso G. The three-layer concentric model of glioblastoma: cancer stem cells, microenvironmental regulation, and therapeutic implications. Sci World J. 2011;11:1829–41.

30. Shiao SL, Ganesan AP, Rugo HS, Coussens LM. Immune microenvironments in solid tumors: new targets for therapy. Genes Dev. 2011;25: 2559–72.

31. Yang L, Lin C, Wang L, Guo H, Wang X. Hypoxia and hypoxia-inducible factors in glioblastoma multiforme progression and therapeutic implications. Exp Cell Res. 2012;318(19):2417–26.

32. Yang YP, Chang YL, Huang PI, Chiou GY, Tseng LM, Chiou SH, Chen MH, Chen MT, Shih YH, Chang CH, Hsu CC, Ma HI, Wang CT, Tsai LL, Yu CC, Chang CJ. Resveratrol suppresses tumorigenicity and enhances radiosensitivity in primary glioblastoma tumor initiating cells by inhibiting the STAT3 axis. J Cell Physiol. 2012;227(3):976–93.

33. Yang YP, Chien Y, Chiou GY, Cherng JY, Wang ML, Lo WL, Chang YL, Huang PI, Chen YW, Shih YH, Chen MT, Chiou SH. Inhibition of cancer stem cell-like properties and reduced chemoradioresistance of glioblastoma using microRNA145 with cationic polyurethane-short branch PEI. Biomaterials. 2012;33(5):1462–76.

34. Pallini R, Ricci-Vitiani L, Banna GL, Signore M, Lombardi D, Todaro M, Stassi G, Martini M, Maira G, Larocca LM, De Maria R. Cancer stem cell analysis and clinical outcome in patients with glioblastoma multiforme. Clin Cancer Res. 2008;14(24): 8205–12.

35. Zeppernick F, Ahmadi R, Campos B, Dictus C, Helmke BM, Becker N, Lichter P, Unterberg A, Radlwimmer B, Herold-Mende CC. Stem cell marker CD133 affects clinical outcome in glioma patients. Clin Cancer Res. 2008;14(1):123–9.

36. Zhang M, Song T, Yang L, Chen R, Wu L, Yang Z, Fang J. Nestin and CD133: valuable stem cell-specific markers for determining clinical outcome of glioma patients. J Exp Clin Cancer Res. 2008; 27:85.

37. Wang J, Sakariassen PO, Tsinkalovsky O, Immervoll H, Boe SO, Svendsen A, Prestegarden L, Rosland G, Thorsen F, Stuhr L, Molven A, Bjerkvig R, Enger PØ. CD133 negative glioma cells form tumors in nude rats and give rise to CD133 positive cells. Int J Cancer. 2008;122(4):761–8.

38. Son MJ, Woolard K, Nam DH, Lee J, Fine HA. SSEA-1 is an enrichment marker for tumor-initiating cells in human glioblastoma. Cell Stem Cell. 2009;4:440–52.

39. Anido J, Sáez-Borderías A, Gonzàlez-Juncà A, Rodón L, Folch G, Carmona MA, Prieto-Sánchez RM, Barba I, Martínez-Sáez E, Prudkin L, Cuartas I, Raventós C, Martínez-Ricarte F, Poca MA, García-Dorado D, Lahn MM, Yingling JM, Rodón J, Sahuquillo J, Baselga J, Seoane J. TGF-β receptor inhibitors target the CD44(high)/Id1(high) glioma-initiating cell population in human glioblastoma. Cancer Cell. 2010;18(6):655–68.

40. He J, Liu Y, Zhu T, Zhu J, Dimeco F, Vescovi AL, Heth JA, Muraszko KM, Fan X, Lubman DM. CD90 is identified as a candidate marker for cancer stem cells in primary high-grade gliomas using tissue microarrays. Mol Cell Proteomics. 2012;11(6): M111.010744.

41. Bao S, Wu Q, Li Z, Sathornsumetee S, Wang H, McLendon RE, Hjelmeland AB, Rich JN. Targeting cancer stem cells through L1CAM suppresses glioma growth. Cancer Res. 2008;68(15):6043–8.

42. Lathia JD, Gallagher J, Heddleston JM, Wang J, Eyler CE, Macswords J, Wu Q, Vasanji A, McLendon RE, Hjelmeland AB, Rich JN. Integrin alpha 6 regulates glioblastoma stem cells. Cell Stem Cell. 2010;6(5):421–32.

43. Ogden AT, Waziri AE, Lochhead RA, Fusco D, Lopez K, Ellis JA, Kang J, Assanah M, McKhann GM, Sisti MB, McCormick PC, Canoll P, Bruce JN. Identification of A2B5+CD133- tumor-initiating cells in adult human gliomas. Neurosurgery. 2008;62(2):505–15.

44. Strojnik T, Røsland GV, Sakariassen PO, Kavalar R, Lah T. Neural stem cell markers, nestin and musashi proteins, in the progression of human glioma: correlation of nestin with prognosis of patient survival. Surg Neurol. 2007;68(2):133–44.

45. Wang J, Ma Y, Cooper MK. Cancer stem cells in glioma: challenges and opportunities. Transl Cancer Res. 2013;2(5):429–41.

46. Cheng L, Wu Q, Huang Z, Guryanova OA, Huang Q, Shou W, Rich JN, Bao S. L1CAM regulates DNA damage checkpoint response of glioblastoma stem cells through NBS1. EMBO J. 2011;30(5):800–13.

47. Harper JW, Elledge SJ. The DNA damage response: ten years after. Mol Cell. 2007;28:739–45.

48. Shiloh Y. ATM and related protein kinases: safeguarding genome integrity. Nat Rev Cancer. 2003;3:155–68.

49. Bartek J, Lukas J. DNA damage checkpoints: from initiation to recovery or adaptation. Curr Opin Cell Biol. 2007;19:238–45.

50. Reinhardt HC, Yaffe MB. Kinases that control the cell cycle in response to DNA damage: Chk1, Chk2, and MK2. Curr Opin Cell Biol. 2009;21:245–55.

51. Carruthers R, Ahmed SU, Strathdee K, Gomez-Roman N, Amoah-Buahin E, Watts C, Chalmers

AJ. Abrogation of radioresistance in glioblastoma stem-like cells by inhibition of ATM kinase. Mol Oncol. 2015;9(1):192–203.

52. Rich JN. Cancer stem cells in radiation resistance. Cancer Res. 2007;67:8980–4.

53. Venere M, Hamerlik P, Wu Q, Rasmussen RD, Song LA, Vasanji A, Tenley N, Flavahan WA, Hjelmeland AB, Bartek J, Rich JN. Therapeutic targeting of constitutive PARP activation compromises stem cell phenotype and survival of glioblastoma-initiating cells. Cell Death Differ. 2014;21(2):258–69.

54. Barazzuol L, Jena R, Burnet NG, Meira LB, Jeynes JC, Kirkby KJ, Kirkby NF. Evaluation of poly (ADP-ribose) polymerase inhibitor ABT-888 combined with radiotherapy and temozolomide in glioblastoma. Radiat Oncol. 2013;8:65.

55. Dungey FA, Löser DA, Chalmers AJ. Replication-dependent radiosensitization of human glioma cells by inhibition of poly(ADP-Ribose) polymerase: mechanisms and therapeutic potential. Int J Radiat Oncol Biol Phys. 2008;72(4):1188–97.

56. Facchino S, Abdouh M, Chatoo W, Bernier G. BMI1 confers radioresistance to normal and cancerous neural stem cells through recruitment of the DNA damage response machinery. J Neurosci. 2010; 30(30):10096–111.

57. Gieni RS, Ismail IH, Campbell S, Hendzel MJ. Polycomb group proteins in the DNA damage response: a link between radiation resistance and "stemness". Cell Cycle. 2011;10(6):883–94.

58. Hsieh A, Ellsworth R, Hsieh D. Hedgehog/GLI1 regulates IGF dependent malignant behaviors in glioma stem cells. J Cell Physiol. 2011; 226(4):1118–27.

59. Hsieh CH, Shyu WC, Chiang CY, Kuo JW, Shen WC, Liu RS. NADPH oxidase subunit 4-mediated reactive oxygen species contribute to cycling hypoxia-promoted tumor progression in glioblastoma multiforme. PLoS One. 2011;6, e23945.

60. Sheng Z, Li L, Zhu LJ, Smith TW, Demers A, Ross AH, Moser RP, Green MR. A genome-wide RNA interference screen reveals an essential CREB3L2-ATF5-MCL1 survival pathway in malignant glioma with therapeutic implications. Nat Med. 2010; 16(6):671–7.

61. Labussière M, Pinel S, Vandamme M, Plénat F, Chastagner P. Radiosensitizing properties of bortezomib depend on therapeutic schedule. Int J Radiat Oncol Biol Phys. 2011;79(3):892–900.

62. Pajonk F, Grumann T, McBride WH. The proteasome inhibitor MG-132 protects hypoxic SiHa cervical carcinoma cells after cyclic hypoxia/reoxygenation from ionizing radiation. Neoplasia. 2006;8(12):1037–41.

63. Pajonk F, Himmelsbach J, Riess K, Sommer A, McBride WH. The human immunodeficiency virus (HIV)-1 protease inhibitor saquinavir inhibits proteasome function and causes apoptosis and radiosensitization in non-HIV-associated human cancer cells. Cancer Res. 2002;62(18):5230–5.

64. Vlashi E, Mattes M, Lagadec C, Donna LD, Phillips TM, Nikolay P, McBride WH, Pajonk F. Differential effects of the proteasome inhibitor NPI-0052 against glioma cells. Transl Oncol. 2010;3(1):50–5.

65. Kubicek GJ, Werner-Wasik M, Machtay M, Mallon G, Myers T, Ramirez M, Andrews D, Curran Jr WJ, Dicker AP. Phase I trial using proteasome inhibitor bortezomib and concurrent temozolomide and radiotherapy for central nervous system malignancies. Int J Radiat Oncol Biol Phys. 2009;74(2):433–9.

66. Gozuacik D, Kimchi A. Autophagy as a cell death and tumor suppressor mechanism. Oncogene. 2004; 23:2891–906.

67. Pajonk F, Vlashi E, McBride WH. Radiation resistance of cancer stem cells: the 4 R's of radiobiology revisited. Stem Cells. 2010;28(4):639–48.

68. Guo W, Lasky JL, Chang CJ, Mosessian S, Lewis X, Xiao Y, Yeh JE, Chen JY, Iruela-Arispe ML, Varella-Garcia M, Wu H. Multi-genetic events collaboratively contribute to Pten-null leukaemia stem-cell formation. Nature. 2008;453:529–33.

69. Ye F, Zhang Y, Liu Y, Yamada K, Tso JL, Menjivar JC, Tian JY, Yong WH, Schaue D, Mischel PS, Cloughesy TF, Nelson SF, Liau LM, McBride W, Tso CL. Protective properties of radio-chemoresistant glioblastoma stem cell clones are associated with metabolic adaptation to reduced glucose dependence. PLoS One. 2013;8(11), e80397.

70. Brat DJ, Mapstone TB. Malignant glioma physiology: cellular response to hypoxia and its role in tumor progression. Ann Intern Med. 2003;138(8): 659–68.

71. Ducray F, de Reyniès A, Chinot O, Idbaih A, Figarella-Branger D, Colin C, Karayan-Tapon L, Chneiweiss H, Wager M, Vallette F, Marie Y, Rickman D, Thomas E, Delattre JY, Honnorat J, Sanson M, Berger F. An ANOCEF genomic and transcriptomic microarray study of the response to radiotherapy or to alkylating first-line chemotherapy in glioblastoma patients. Mol Cancer. 2010;9:234.

72. Jensen RL. Brain tumor hypoxia: tumorigenesis, angiogenesis, imaging, pseudoprogression, and as a therapeutic target. J Neurooncol. 2009;9:2317–35.

73. Li Y, Guessous F, Zhang Y, Dipierro C, Kefas B, Johnson E, Marcinkiewicz L, Jiang J, Yang Y, Schmittgen TD, Lopes B, Schiff D, Purow B, Abounader R. MicroRNA-34a inhibits glioblastoma growth by targeting multiple oncogenes. Cancer Res. 2009;69(19):7569–76.

74. Li Z, Bao S, Wu Q, Wang H, Eyler C, Sathornsumetee S, Shi Q, Cao Y, Lathia J, McLendon RE, Hjelmeland AB, Rich JN. Hypoxia-inducible factors regulate tumorigenic capacity of glioma stem cells. Cancer Cell. 2009;15(6):501–13.

75. McCord AM, Jamal M, Shankavaram UT, Lang FF, Camphausen K, Tofilon PJ. Physiologic oxygen con-

centration enhances the stem-like properties of CD133+ human glioblastoma cells in vitro. Mol Cancer Res. 2009;7(4):489–97.

76. Soeda A, Park M, Lee D, Mintz A, Androutsellis-Theotokis A, McKay RD, Engh J, Iwama T, Kunisada T, Kassam AB, Pollack IF, Park DM. Hypoxia promotes expansion of the CD133-positive glioma stem cells through activation of HIF-1alpha. Oncogene. 2009;28(45):3949–59.

77. Bar EE, Lin A, Mahairaki V, Matsui W, Eberhart CG. Hypoxia increases the expression of stem-cell markers and promotes clonogenicity in glioblastoma neurospheres. Am J Pathol. 2010;177(3):1491–502.

78. McGee MC, Hamner JB, Williams RF, Rosati SF, Sims TL, Ng CY, Gaber MW, Calabrese C, Wu J, Nathwani AC, Duntsch C, Merchant TE, Davidoff AM. Improved intratumoral oxygenation through vascular normalization increases glioma sensitivity to ionizing radiation. Int J Radiat Oncol Biol Phys. 2010;76(5):1537–45.

79. Chou CW, Wang CC, Wu CP, Lin YJ, Lee YC, Cheng YW, Hsieh CH. Tumor cycling hypoxia induces chemoresistance in glioblastoma multiforme by upregulating the expression and function of ABCB1. Neuro Oncol. 2012;14(10):1227–38.

80. Haensgen G, Krause U, Becker A, Stadler P, Lautenschlaeger C, Wohlrab W, Rath FW, Molls M, Dunst J. Tumor hypoxia, p53, and prognosis in cervical cancers. Int J Radiat Oncol Biol Phys. 2001;50(4):865–72.

81. Saito Y, Milross CG, Hittelman WN, Li D, Jibu T, Peters LJ, Milas L. Effect of radiation and paclitaxel on p53 expression in murine tumors sensitive or resistant to apoptosis induction. Int J Radiat Oncol Biol Phys. 1997;38(3):623–31.

82. Yamaura H, Matsuzawa T. Tumor regrowth after irradiation; an experimental approach. Int J Radiat Biol Relat Stud Phys Chem Med. 1979;35:201–19.

83. Cairns RA, Hill RP. Acute hypoxia enhances spontaneous lymph node metastasis in an orthotopic murine model of human cervical carcinoma. Cancer Res. 2004;64:2054–61.

84. Martinive P, Defresne F, Bouzin C, Saliez J, Lair F, Grégoire V, Michiels C, Dessy C, Feron O. Preconditioning of the tumor vasculature and tumor cells by intermittent hypoxia: implications for anticancer therapies. Cancer Res. 2006;66(24): 11736–44.

85. Keith B, Simon MC. Hypoxia-inducible factors, stem cells, and cancer. Cell. 2007;129:465–72.

86. Rong Y, Durden DL, Van Meir EG, Brat DJ. 'Pseudopalisading' necrosis in glioblastoma: a familiar morphologic feature that links vascular pathology, hypoxia, and angiogenesis. J Neuropathol Exp Neurol. 2006;65(6):529–39.

87. Semenza GL. HIF-1 and tumor progression: pathophysiology and therapeutics. Trends Mol Med. 2002;8:S62–7.

88. Dewhirst MW, Cao Y, Moeller B. Cycling hypoxia and free radicals regulate angiogenesis and radiotherapy response. Nat Rev Cancer. 2008;8(6): 425–37.

89. Moeller BJ, Cao Y, Li CY, Dewhirst MW. Radiation activates HIF-1 to regulate vascular radiosensitivity in tumors: role of reoxygenation, free radicals, and stress granules. Cancer Cell. 2004;5(5):429–41.

90. Holmquist-Mengelbier L, Fredlund E, Löfstedt T, Noguera R, Navarro S, Nilsson H, Pietras A, Vallon-Christersson J, Borg A, Gradin K, Poellinger L, Påhlman S. Recruitment of HIF-1alpha and HIF-2alpha to common target genes is differentially regulated in neuroblastoma: HIF-2alpha promotes an aggressive phenotype. Cancer Cell. 2006;10(5): 413–23.

91. Du R, Lu KV, Petritsch C, Liu P, Ganss R, Passegué E, Song H, Vandenberg S, Johnson RS, Werb Z, Bergers G. HIF1alpha induces the recruitment of bone marrow-derived vascular modulatory cells to regulate tumor angiogenesis and invasion. Cancer Cell. 2008;13(3):206–20.

92. Gillespie DL, Whang K, Ragel BT, Flynn JR, Kelly DA, Jensen RL. Silencing of hypoxia inducible factor-1alpha by RNA interference attenuates human glioma cell growth in vivo. Clin Cancer Res. 2007;13(8):2441–8.

93. Jensen RL. Hypoxia in the tumorigenesis of gliomas and as a potential target for therapeutic measures. Neurosurg Focus. 2006;20(4), E24.

94. Kirkpatrick J, Desjardins A, Quinn J, Rich J, Vredenburgh J, Sathornsumetee S, Gururangan S, Sidor C, Friedman H, Reardon D. Phase II open-label, safety, pharmacokinetic and efficacy study of 2-methoxyestradiol nanocrystal colloidal dispersion administered orally to patients with recurrent glioblastoma multiforme. J Clin Oncol. 2007;25:2065 [Meeting Abstracts].

95. Bao S, Wu Q, Sathornsumetee S, Hao Y, Li Z, Hjelmeland AB, Shi Q, McLendon RE, Bigner DD, Rich JN. Stem cell-like glioma cells promote tumor angiogenesis through vascular endothelial growth factor. Cancer Res. 2006;66(16):7843–8.

96. Kioi M, Vogel H, Schultz G, Hoffman RM, Harsh GR, Brown JM. Inhibition of vasculogenesis, but not angiogenesis, prevents the recurrence of glioblastoma after irradiation in mice. J Clin Invest. 2010;120(3):694–705.

97. Oka N, Soeda A, Inagaki A, Onodera M, Maruyama H, Hara A, Kunisada T, Mori H, Iwama T. VEGF promotes tumorigenesis and angiogenesis of human glioblastoma stem cells. Biochem Biophys Res Commun. 2007;360:553–9.

98. Ricci-Vitiani L, Pallini R, Biffoni M, Todaro M, Invernici G, Cenci T, Maira G, Parati EA, Stassi G, Larocca LM, De Maria R. Tumour vascularization via endothelial differentiation of glioblastoma stem-like cells. Nature. 2010;468(7325):824–8.

99. Wang J, Wakeman TP, Lathia JD, Hjelmeland AB, Wang XF, White RR, Rich JN, Sullenger BA. Notch promotes radioresistance of glioma stem cells. Stem Cells. 2010;28(1):17–28.

100. Wang R, Chadalavada K, Wilshire J, Kowalik U, Hovinga KE, Geber A, Fligelman B, Leversha M, Brennan C, Tabar V. Glioblastoma stem-like cells give rise to tumour endothelium. Nature. 2010; 468:829–33.

101. Mannino M, Chalmers AJ. Radioresistance of glioma stem cells: intrinsic characteristic or property of the 'microenvironment-stem cell unit'? Mol Oncol. 2011;5(4):374–86.

102. Cordes N, Seidler J, Durzok R, Geinitz H, Brakebusch C. beta1-integrin-mediated signaling essentially contributes to cell survival after radiation-induced genotoxic injury. Oncogene. 2006;25(9): 1378–90.

103. Monferran S, Skuli N, Delmas C, Favre G, Bonnet J, Cohen-Jonathan-Moyal E, Toulas C. Alphavbeta3 and alphavbeta5 integrins control glioma cell response to ionising radiation through ILK and RhoB. Int J Cancer. 2008;123(2):357–64.

104. Garcion E, Halilagic A, Faissner A, ffrench-Constant C. Generation of an environmental niche for neural stem cell development by the extracellular matrix molecule tenascin C. Development. 2004;131(14): 3423–32.

105. Higuchi M, Ohnishi T, Arita N, Hiraga S, Hayakawa T. Expression of tenascin in human gliomas: its relation to histological malignancy, tumor dedifferentiation and angiogenesis. Acta Neuropathol. 1993; 85(5):481–7.

106. Leins A, Riva P, Lindstedt R, Davidoff MS, Mehraein P, Weis S. Expression of tenascin-C in various human brain tumors and its relevance for survival in patients with astrocytoma. Cancer. 2003; 98(11):2430–9.

107. Charles N, Ozawa T, Squatrito M, Bleau AM, Brennan CW, Hambardzumyan D, Holland EC. Perivascular nitric oxide activates notch signaling and promotes stem-like character in PDGF-induced glioma cells. Cell Stem Cell. 2010; 6(2):141–52.

108. Diehn M, Cho RW, Lobo NA, Kalisky T, Dorie MJ, Kulp AN, Qian D, Lam JS, Ailles LE, Wong M, Joshua B, Kaplan MJ, Wapnir I, Dirbas FM, Somlo G, Garberoglio C, Paz B, Shen J, Lau SK, Quake SR, Brown JM, Weissman IL, Clarke MF. Association of reactive oxygen species levels and radioresistance in cancer stem cells. Nature. 2009;458(7239):780–3.

109. Smith J, Ladi E, Mayer-Proschel M, Noble M. Redox state is a central modulator of the balance between self-renewal and differentiation in a dividing glial precursor cell. Proc Natl Acad Sci U S A. 2000; 97(18):10032–7.

110. Venere M, Fine HA, Dirks PB, Rich JN. Cancer stem cells in gliomas: identifying and understanding the apex cell in cancer's hierarchy. Glia. 2011; 59(8):1148–54.

111. Polakis P. Wnt signaling in cancer. Cold Spring Harb Perspect Biol. 2012;4(5):a008052.

112. Reya T, Clevers H. Wnt signalling in stem cells and cancer. Nature. 2005;434(7035):843–50.

113. Kim Y, Kim KH, Lee J, Lee YA, Kim M, Lee SJ, Park K, Yang H, Jin J, Joo KM, Lee J, Nam DH. Wnt activation is implicated in glioblastoma radioresistance. Lab Invest. 2012;92(3):466–73.

114. Rossi M, Magnoni L, Miracco C, Mori E, Tosi P, Pirtoli L, Tini P, Oliveri G, Cosci E, Bakker A. β-Catenin and Gli1 are prognostic markers in glioblastoma. Cancer Biol Ther. 2011;11(8):753–61.

115. Ayyanan A, Civenni G, Ciarloni L, Morel C, Mueller N, Lefort K, Mandinova A, Raffoul W, Fiche M, Dotto GP, Brisken C. Increased Wnt signaling triggers oncogenic conversion of human breast epithelial cells by a Notch-dependent mechanism. Proc Natl Acad Sci U S A. 2006;103(10):3799–804.

116. Shiras A, Chettiar ST, Shepal V, Rajendran G, Prasad GR, Shastry P. Spontaneous transformation of human adult nontumorigenic stem cells to cancer stem cells is driven by genomic instability in a human model of glioblastoma. Stem Cells. 2007;25(6):1478–89.

117. Chakravarti A, Zhai G, Suzuki Y, Sarkesh S, Black PM, Muzikansky A, Loeffler JS. The prognostic significance of phosphatidylinositol 3-kinase pathway activation in human gliomas. J Clin Oncol. 2004;22(10):1926–33.

118. Persano L, Rampazzo E, Basso G, Viola G. Glioblastoma cancer stem cells: role of the microenvironment and therapeutic targeting. Biochem Pharmacol. 2013;85(5):612–22.

119. Eyler CE, Foo WC, LaFiura KM, McLendon RE, Hjelmeland AB, Rich JN. Brain cancer stem cells display preferential sensitivity to Akt inhibition. Stem Cells. 2008;26(12):3027–36.

120. Kao GD, Jiang Z, Fernandes AM, Gupta AK, Maity A. Inhibition of phosphatidylinositol-3-OH kinase/ Akt signaling impairs DNA repair in glioblastoma cells following ionizing radiation. J Biol Chem. 2007;282(29):21206–12.

121. Zheng H, Ying H, Yan H, Kimmelman AC, Hiller DJ, Chen AJ, Perry SR, Tonon G, Chu GC, Ding Z, Stommel JM, Dunn KL, Wiedemeyer R, You MJ, Brennan C, Wang YA, Ligon KL, Wong WH, Chin L, DePinho RA. p53 and Pten control neural and glioma stem/progenitor cell renewal and differentiation. Nature. 2008;455(7216):1129–33.

122. Jiang Z, Pore N, Cerniglia GJ, Mick R, Georgescu MM, Bernhard EJ, Hahn SM, Gupta AK, Maity A. Phosphatase and tensin homologue deficiency in glioblastoma confers resistance to radiation and temozolomide that is reversed by the protease inhibitor nelfinavir. Cancer Res. 2007;67(9):4467–73.

123. Nakamura JL, Karlsson A, Arvold ND, Gottschalk AR, Pieper RO, Stokoe D, Haas-Kogan DA. PKB/Akt mediates radiosensitization by the signaling inhibitor LY294002 in human malignant gliomas. J Neurooncol. 2005;71(3):215–22.

124. Cheng L, Bao S, Rich JN. Potential therapeutic implications of cancer stem cells in glioblastoma. Biochem Pharmacol. 2010;80(5):654–65.

125. Li B, Yuan M, Kim IA, Chang CM, Bernhard EJ, Shu HK. Mutant epidermal growth factor receptor displays increased signaling through the phosphatidylinositol-3 kinase/AKT pathway and promotes radioresistance in cells of astrocytic origin. Oncogene. 2004;23(26):4594–602.

126. Osuka S, Sampetrean O, Shimizu T, Saga I, Onishi N, Sugihara E, Okubo J, Fujita S, Takano S, Matsumura A, Saya H. IGF1 receptor signaling regulates adaptive radioprotection in glioma stem cells. Stem Cells. 2013;31(4):627–40.

127. Lin Y, Jiang T, Zhou K, Xu L, Chen B, Li G, Qiu X, Jiang T, Zhang W, Song SW. Plasma IGFBP-2 levels predict clinical outcomes of patients with high-grade gliomas. Neuro Oncol. 2009;11(5):468–76.

128. Tso CL, Freije WA, Day A, Chen Z, Merriman B, Perlina A, Lee Y, Dia EQ, Yoshimoto K, Mischel PS, Liau LM, Cloughesy TF, Nelson SF. Distinct transcription profiles of primary and secondary glioblastoma subgroups. Cancer Res. 2006;66(1):159–67.

129. Bleau AM, Hambardzumyan D, Ozawa T, Fomchenko EI, Huse JT, Brennan CW, Holland EC. PTEN/PI3K/Akt pathway regulates the side population phenotype and ABCG2 activity in glioma tumor stem-like cells. Cell Stem Cell. 2009;4(3):226–35.

130. Gallia GL, Tyler BM, Hann CL, Siu IM, Giranda VL, Vescovi AL, Brem H, Riggins GJ. Inhibition of Akt inhibits growth of glioblastoma and glioblastoma stem-like cells. Mol Cancer Ther. 2009;8(2):386–93.

131. Anandharaj A, Cinghu S, Park WY. Rapamycin-mediated mTOR inhibition attenuates survivin and sensitizes glioblastoma cells to radiation therapy. Acta Biochim Biophys Sin (Shanghai). 2011;43(4):292–300.

132. Eshleman JS, Carlson BL, Mladek AC, Kastner BD, Shide KL, Sarkaria JN. Inhibition of the mammalian target of rapamycin sensitizes U87 xenografts to fractionated radiation therapy. Cancer Res. 2002;62(24):7291–7.

133. Kahn J, Hayman TJ, Jamal M, Rath BH, Kramp T, Camphausen K, Tofilon PJ. The mTORC1/mTORC2 inhibitor AZD2014 enhances the radiosensitivity of glioblastoma stem-like cells. Neuro Oncol. 2014;16(1):29–37.

134. Hainsworth JD, Shih KC, Shepard GC, Tillinghast GW, Brinker BT, Spigel DR. Phase II study of concurrent radiation therapy, temozolomide, and bevacizumab followed by bevacizumab/everolimus as first-line treatment for patients with glioblastoma. Clin Adv Hematol Oncol. 2012;10(4):240–6.

135. Ma DJ, Galanis E, Anderson SK, Schiff D, Kaufmann TJ, Peller PJ, Giannini C, Brown PD, Uhm JH, McGraw S, Jaeckle KA, Flynn PJ, Ligon KL, Buckner JC, Sarkaria JN. A phase II trial of everolimus, temozolomide, and radiotherapy in patients with newly diagnosed glioblastoma: NCCTG N057K. Neuro Oncol. 2015;17(9):1261–9. pii: nou328.

136. Fan QW, Knight ZA, Goldenberg DD, Yu W, Mostov KE, Stokoe D, Shokat KM, Weiss WA. A dual PI3 kinase/mTOR inhibitor reveals emergent efficacy in glioma. Cancer Cell. 2006;9(5):341–9.

137. Burris 3rd HA. Overcoming acquired resistance to anticancer therapy: focus on the PI3K/AKT/mTOR pathway. Cancer Chemother Pharmacol. 2013;71(4):829–42.

138. Chen JS, Zhou LJ, Entin-Meer M, Yang X, Donker M, Knight ZA, Weiss W, Shokat KM, Haas-Kogan D, Stokoe D. Characterization of structurally distinct, isoform-selective phosphoinositide 3′-kinase inhibitors in combination with radiation in the treatment of glioblastoma. Mol Cancer Ther. 2008;7(4):841–50.

139. Prevo R, Deutsch E, Sampson O, Diplexcito J, Cengel K, Harper J, O'Neill P, McKenna WG, Patel S, Bernhard EJ. Class I PI3 kinase inhibition by the pyridinylfuranopyrimidine inhibitor PI-103 enhances tumor radiosensitivity. Cancer Res. 2008;68(14):5915–23.

140. Bianco C, Tortora G, Bianco R, Caputo R, Veneziani BM, Caputo R, Damiano V, Troiani T, Fontanini G, Raben D, Pepe S, Bianco AR, Ciardiello F. Enhancement of antitumor activity of ionizing radiation by combined treatment with the selective epidermal growth factor receptor-tyrosine kinase inhibitor ZD1839 (Iressa). Clin Cancer Res. 2002;8(10):3250–8.

141. Damiano V, Melisi D, Bianco C, Raben D, Caputo R, Fontanini G, Bianco R, Ryan A, Bianco AR, De Placido S, Ciardiello F, Tortora G. Cooperative antitumor effect of multitargeted kinase inhibitor ZD6474 and ionizing radiation in glioblastoma. Clin Cancer Res. 2005;11(15):5639–44.

142. Geoerger B, Gaspar N, Opolon P, Morizet J, Devanz P, Lecluse Y, Valent A, Lacroix L, Grill J, Vassal G. EGFR tyrosine kinase inhibition radiosensitizes and induces apoptosis in malignant glioma and childhood ependymoma xenografts. Int J Cancer. 2008;123(1):209–16.

143. Palumbo S, Tini P, Toscano M, Allavena G, Angeletti F, Manai F, Miracco C, Comincini S, Pirtoli L. Combined EGFR and autophagy modulation impairs cell migration and enhances radiosensitivity in human glioblastoma cells. J Cell Physiol. 2014;229(11):1863–73.

144. Peereboom DM, Shepard DR, Ahluwalia MS, Brewer CJ, Agarwal N, Stevens GH, Suh JH, Toms SA, Vogelbaum MA, Weil RJ, Elson P, Barnett GH. Phase II trial of erlotinib with temozolomide

and radiation in patients with newly diagnosed glioblastoma multiforme. J Neurooncol. 2010;98(1):93–9.

145. Prados MD, Chang SM, Butowski N, DeBoer R, Parvataneni R, Carliner H, Kabuubi P, Ayers-Ringler J, Rabbitt J, Page M, Fedoroff A, Sneed PK, Berger MS, McDermott MW, Parsa AT, Vandenberg S, James CD, Lamborn KR, Stokoe D, Haas-Kogan DA. Phase II study of erlotinib plus temozolomide during and after radiation therapy in patients with newly diagnosed glioblastoma multiforme or gliosarcoma. J Clin Oncol. 2009;27(4):579–84.

146. Uhm JH, Ballman KV, Wu W, Giannini C, Krauss JC, Buckner JC, James CD, Scheithauer BW, Behrens RJ, Flynn PJ, Schaefer PL, Dakhill SR, Jaeckle KA. Phase II evaluation of gefitinib in patients with newly diagnosed Grade 4 astrocytoma: Mayo/North Central Cancer Treatment Group Study N0074. Int J Radiat Oncol Biol Phys. 2011;80(2):347–53.

147. Perry J, Okamoto M, Guiou M, Shirai K, Errett A, Chakravarti A. Novel therapies in glioblastoma. Neurol Res Int. 2012;2012:428565.

148. Fan X, Khaki L, Zhu TS, Soules ME, Talsma CE, Gul N, Koh C, Zhang J, Li YM, Maciaczyk J, Nikkhah G, Dimeco F, Piccirillo S, Vescovi AL, Eberhart CG. NOTCH pathway blockade depletes CD133-positive glioblastoma cells and inhibits growth of tumor neurospheres and xenografts. Stem Cells. 2010;28(1):5–16.

149. Fassl A, Tagscherer KE, Richter J, Berriel Diaz M, Alcantara Llaguno SR, Campos B, Kopitz J, Herold-Mende C, Herzig S, Schmidt MH, Parada LF, Wiestler OD, Roth W. Notch1 signaling promotes survival of glioblastoma cells via EGFR-mediated induction of anti-apoptotic Mcl-1. Oncogene. 2012;31(44):4698–708.

150. Chapouton P, Skupien P, Hesl B, Coolen M, Moore JC, Madelaine R, Kremmer E, Faus-Kessler T, Blader P, Lawson ND, Bally-Cuif L. Notch activity levels control the balance between quiescence and recruitment of adult neural stem cells. J Neurosci. 2010;30(23):7961–74.

151. Mizutani K, Yoon K, Dang L, Tokunaga A, Gaiano N. Differential Notch signalling distinguishes neural stem cells from intermediate progenitors. Nature. 2007;449(7160):351–5.

152. Chen G, Zhu W, Shi D, Lv L, Zhang C, Liu P, Hu W. MicroRNA-181a sensitizes human malignant glioma U87MG cells to radiation by targeting Bcl-2. Oncol Rep. 2010;23:997–1003.

153. Chen J, Kesari S, Rooney C, Strack PR, Chen J, Shen H, Wu L, Griffin JD. Inhibition of notch signaling blocks growth of glioblastoma cell lines and tumor neurospheres. Genes Cancer. 2010;1(8):822–35.

154. Hovinga KE, Shimizu F, Wang R, Panagiotakos G, Van Der Heijden M, Moayedpardazi H, Correia AS, Soulet D, Major T, Menon J, Tabar V. Inhibition of

notch signaling in glioblastoma targets cancer stem cells via an endothelial cell intermediate. Stem Cells. 2010;28(6):1019–29.

155. Shahi MH, Lorente A, Castresana JS. Hedgehog signalling in medulloblastoma, glioblastoma and neuroblastoma. Oncol Rep. 2008;19:681–8.

156. Kinzler KW, Bigner SH, Bigner DD, Trent JM, Law ML, O'Brien SJ, Wong AJ, Vogelstein B. Identification of an amplified, highly expressed gene in a human glioma. Science. 1987;236:70–3.

157. Clement V, Sanchez P, de Tribolet N, Radovanovic I, Ruiz i Altaba A. HEDGEHOG-GLI1 signaling regulates human glioma growth, cancer stem cell self-renewal, and tumorigenicity. Curr Biol. 2007;17(2):165–72.

158. Takezaki T, Hide T, Takanaga H, Nakamura H, Kuratsu J, Kondo T. Essential role of the Hedgehog signaling pathway in human glioma-initiating cells. Cancer Sci. 2011;102(7):1306–12.

159. Bar EE, Chaudhry A, Lin A, Fan X, Schreck K, Matsui W, Piccirillo S, Vescovi AL, DiMeco F, Olivi A, Eberhart CG. Cyclopamine-mediated hedgehog pathway inhibition depletes stem-like cancer cells in glioblastoma. Stem Cells. 2007;25(10):2524–33.

160. Sarangi A, Valadez JG, Rush S, Abel TW, Thompson RC, Cooper MK. Targeted inhibition of the Hedgehog pathway in established malignant glioma xenografts enhances survival. Oncogene. 2009;28(39):3468–76.

161. Xu Q, Yuan X, Liu G, Black KL, Yu JS. Hedgehog signaling regulates brain tumor-initiating cell proliferation and portends shorter survival for patients with PTEN-coexpressing glioblastomas. Stem Cells. 2008;26(12):3018–26.

162. Carro MS, Lim WK, Alvarez MJ, Bollo RJ, Zhao X, Snyder EY, Sulman EP, Anne SL, Doetsch F, Colman H, Lasorella A, Aldape K, Califano A, Iavarone A. The transcriptional network for mesenchymal transformation of brain tumours. Nature. 2010;463:318–25.

163. Cao Y, Lathia JD, Eyler CE, Wu Q, Li Z, Wang H, McLendon RE, Hjelmeland AB, Rich JN. Erythropoietin receptor signaling through STAT3 is required for glioma stem cell maintenance. Genes Cancer. 2010;1:50–61.

164. Sherry MM, Reeves A, Wu JK, Cochran BH. STAT3 is required for proliferation and maintenance of multipotency in glioblastoma stem cells. Stem Cells. 2009;27:2383–92.

165. Kao CL, Huang PI, Tsai PH, Tsai ML, Lo JF, Lee YY, Chen YJ, Chen YW, Chiou SH. Resveratrol-induced apoptosis and increased radiosensitivity in CD133-positive cells derived from atypical teratoid/rhabdoid tumor. Int J Radiat Oncol Biol Phys. 2009;74:219–28.

166. Liao HF, Kuo CD, Yang YC, Lin CP, Tai HC, Chen YY, Chen YJ. Resveratrol enhances radiosensitivity of human non-small cell lung cancer NCI-H838 cells accompanied by inhibition of nuclear factor-

kappa B activation. J Radiat Res (Tokyo). 2005; 46:387–93.

167. Kotha A, SekharamM CL, Siddiquee K, Khaled A, Zervos AS, Carter B, Turkson J, Jove R. Resveratrol inhibits Src and Stat3 signaling and induces the apoptosis of malignant cells containing activated Stat3 protein. Mol Cancer Ther. 2006;5:621–9.

168. Joo KM, Jin J, Kim E, Ho Kim K, Kim Y, Gu Kang B, Kang YJ, Lathia JD, Cheong KH, Song PH, Kim H, Seol HJ, Kong DS, Lee JI, Rich JN, Lee J, Nam DH. MET signaling regulates glioblastoma stem cells. Cancer Res. 2012;72(15):3828–38.

169. Günther HS, Schmidt NO, Phillips HS, Kemming D, Kharbanda S, Soriano R, Modrusan Z, Meissner H, Westphal M, Lamszus K. Glioblastoma-derived stem cell-enriched cultures form distinct subgroups according to molecular and phenotypic criteria. Oncogene. 2008;27(20):2897–909.

170. Nicoleau C, Benzakour O, Agasse F, Thiriet N, Petit J, Prestoz L, Roger M, Jaber M, Coronas V. Endogenous hepatocyte growth factor is a niche signal for subventricular zone neural stem cell amplification and self-renewal. Stem Cells. 2009;27(2):408–19.

171. Appleman LJ. MET signaling pathway: a rational target for cancer therapy. J Clin Oncol. 2011; 29:4837–8.

172. Gherardi E, Birchmeier W, Birchmeier C, Vande WG. Targeting MET in cancer: rationale and progress. Nat Rev Cancer. 2012;12:89–103.

173. Yap TA, de Bono JS. Targeting the HGF/c-Met axis: state of play. Mol Cancer Ther. 2010;9:1077–9.

174. Würth R, Bajetto A, Harrison JK, Barbieri F, Florio T. CXCL12 modulation of CXCR4 and CXCR7 activity in human glioblastoma stem-like cells and regulation of the tumor microenvironment. Front Cell Neurosci. 2014;8:144.

175. Ehtesham M, Mapara KY, Stevenson CB, Thompson RC. CXCR4 mediates the proliferation of glioblastoma progenitor cells. Cancer Lett. 2009; 274(2):305–12.

176. Zheng X, Xie Q, Li S, Zhang W. CXCR4-positive subset of glioma is enriched for cancer stem cells. Oncol Res. 2011;19(12):555–61.

177. Folkins C, Shaked Y, Man S, Tang T, Lee CR, Zhu Z, Hoffman RM, Kerbel RS. Glioma tumor stem-like cells promote tumor angiogenesis and vasculogenesis via vascular endothelial growth factor and stromal-derived factor 1. Cancer Res. 2009; 69(18):7243–51.

178. Ping YF, Yao XH, Jiang JY, Zhao LT, Yu SC, Jiang T, Lin MC, Chen JH, Wang B, Zhang R, Cui YH, Qian C, Wang JM, Bian XW. The chemokine CXCL12 and its receptor CXCR4 promote glioma stem cell-mediated VEGF production and tumour angiogenesis via PI3K/AKT signalling. J Pathol. 2011;224(3):344–54.

179. Walters MJ, Ebsworth K, Berahovich RD, Penfold ME, Liu SC, Al Omran R, Kioi M, Chernikova SB,

Tseng D, Mulkearns-Hubert EE, Sinyuk M, Ransohoff RM, Lathia JD, Karamchandani J, Kohrt HE, Zhang P, Powers JP, Jaen JC, Schall TJ, Merchant M, Recht L, Brown JM. Inhibition of CXCR7 extends survival following irradiation of brain tumours in mice and rats. Br J Cancer. 2014;110(5):1179–88.

180. Zhou W, Xu Y, Gao G, Jiang Z, Li X. Irradiated normal brain promotes invasion of glioblastoma through vascular endothelial growth and stromal cell-derived factor 1α. Neuroreport. 2013;24(13):730–4.

181. Zhang M, Kleber S, Röhrich M, Timke C, Han N, Tuettenberg J, Martin-Villalba A, Debus J, Peschke P, Wirkner U, Lahn M, Huber PE. Blockade of TGF-β signaling by the TGFβR-I kinase inhibitor LY2109761 enhances radiation response and prolongs survival in glioblastoma. Cancer Res. 2011;71(23):7155–67.

182. Bruna A, Darken RS, Rojo F, Ocana A, Penuelas S, Arias A, Paris R, Tortosa A, Mora J, Baselga J, Seoane J. High TGFbeta-Smad activity confers poor prognosis in glioma patients and promotes cell proliferation depending on the methylation of the PDGFB gene. Cancer Cell. 2007;11:147–60.

183. Kjellman C, Olofsson SP, Hansson O, Von Schantz T, Lindvall M, Nilsson I, Salford LG, Sjögren HO, Widegren B. Expression of TGF-beta isoforms, TGF-beta receptors, and SMAD molecules at different stages of human glioma. Int J Cancer. 2000;89:251–8.

184. Ikushima H, Todo T, Ino Y, Takahashi M, Miyazawa K, Miyazono K. Autocrine TGF-beta signaling maintains tumorigenicity of glioma-initiating cells through Sry-related HMG-box factors. Cell Stem Cell. 2009;5:504–14.

185. Penuelas S, Anido J, Prieto-Sanchez RM, Folch G, Barba I, Cuartas I, García-Dorado D, Poca MA, Sahuquillo J, Baselga J, Seoane J. TGF-beta increases glioma-initiating cell self-renewal through the induction of LIF in human glioblastoma. Cancer Cell. 2009;15:315–27.

186. Hardee ME, Marciscano AE, Medina-Ramirez CM, Zagzag D, Narayana A, Lonning SM, Barcellos-Hoff MH. Resistance of glioblastoma-initiating cells to radiation mediated by the tumor microenvironment can be abolished by inhibiting transforming growth factor-β. Cancer Res. 2012;72(16):4119–29.

187. Zhang M, Herion TW, Timke C, Han N, Hauser K, Weber KJ, Peschke P, Wirkner U, Lahn M, Huber PE. Trimodal glioblastoma treatment consisting of concurrent radiotherapy, temozolomide, and the novel TGF-β receptor I kinase inhibitor LY2109761. Neoplasia. 2011;13(6):537–49.

188. Ford J, Jiang M, Milner J. Cancer-specific functions of SIRT1 enable human epithelial cancer cell growth and survival. Cancer Res. 2005;65(22):10457–63.

189. Saunders LR, Verdin E. Sirtuins: critical regulators at the crossroads between cancer and aging. Oncogene. 2007;26(37):5489–504.

190. Chang CJ, Hsu CC, Yung MC, Chen KY, Tzao C, Wu WF, Chou HY, Lee YY, Lu KH, Chiou SH, Ma HI. Enhanced radiosensitivity and radiation-induced apoptosis in glioma CD133-positive cells by knockdown of SirT1 expression. Biochem Biophys Res Commun. 2009;380(2):236–42.
191. Niemoeller OM, Niyazi M, Corradini S, Zehentmayr F, Li M, Lauber K, Belka C. MicroRNA expression profiles in human cancer cells after ionizing radiation. Radiat Oncol. 2011;6:29.
192. Mizoguchi M, Guan Y, Yoshimoto K, Hata N, Amano T, Nakamizo A, Sasaki T. Clinical implications of microRNAs in human glioblastoma. Front Oncol. 2013;3:19.
193. Pedroza-Torres A, López-Urrutia E, García-Castillo V, Jacobo-Herrera N, Herrera LA, Peralta-Zaragoza O, López-Camarillo C, De Leon DC, Fernández-Retana J, Cerna-Cortés JF, Pérez-Plasencia C. MicroRNAs in cervical cancer: evidences for a miRNA profile deregulated by HPV and its impact on radio-resistance. Molecules. 2014;19(5):6263–81.
194. Srinivasan S, Patric IR, Somasundaram K. A ten-microRNA expression signature predicts survival in glioblastoma. PLoS One. 2011;6(3), e17438.
195. Besse A, Sana J, Fadrus P, Slaby O. MicroRNAs involved in chemo- and radioresistance of high-grade gliomas. Tumour Biol. 2013;34(4):1969–78.
196. Li W, Guo F, Wang P, Hong S, Zhang C. miR-221/222 confers radioresistance in glioblastoma cells through activating Akt independent of PTEN status. Curr Mol Med. 2014;14(1):185–95.
197. Hu X, Schwarz JK, Lewis Jr JS, Huettner PC, Rader JS, Deasy JO, Grigsby PW, Wang X. A microRNA expression signature for cervical cancer prognosis. Cancer Res. 2010;70(4):1441–8.
198. Li Y, Zhao S, Zhen Y, Li Q, Teng L, Asai A, Kawamoto K. A miR-21 inhibitor enhances apoptosis and reduces G(2)-M accumulation induced by ionizing radiation in human glioblastoma U251 cells. Brain Tumor Pathol. 2011;28:209–14.
199. Yang W, Wei J, Guo T, Shen Y, Liu F. Knockdown of miR-210 decreases hypoxic glioma stem cells stemness and radioresistance. Exp Cell Res. 2014;326(1):22–35.
200. Gwak HS, Kim TH, Jo GH, Kim YJ, Kwak HJ, Kim JH, Yin J, Yoo H, Lee SH, Park JB. Silencing of MicroRNA-21 confers radio-sensitivity through inhibition of the PI3K/AKT pathway and enhancing autophagy in malignant glioma cell lines. PLoS One. 2012;7, e47449.
201. Lee KM, Choi EJ, Kim IA. microRNA-7 increases radiosensitivity of human cancer cells with activated EGFR-associated signaling. Radiother Oncol. 2011;101:171–6.
202. Michael MZ, OC SM, van Holst Pellekaan NG, Young GP, James RJ. Reduced accumulation of specific microRNAs in colorectal neoplasia. Mol Cancer Res 2003;1(12):882e91.
203. Schepeler T, Reinert JT, Ostenfeld MS, Christensen LL, Silahtaroglu AN, Dyrskjot L, Wiuf C, Sørensen FJ, Kruhøffer M, Laurberg S, Kauppinen S, Ørntoft TF, Andersen CL. Diagnostic and prognostic microRNAs in stage II colon cancer. Cancer Res. 2008;68(15):6416e24.
204. Fareh M, Turchi L, Virolle V, Debruyne D, Almairac F, de-la-Forest Divonne S, Paquis P, Preynat-Seauve O, Krause KH, Chneiweiss H, Virolle T. The miR 302-367 cluster drastically affects self-renewal and infiltration properties of glioma-initiating cells through CXCR4 repression and consequent disruption of the SHH-GLI-NANOG network. Cell Death Differ. 2012;19(2):232–44.
205. Silber J, Lim DA, Petritsch C, Persson AI, Maunakea AK, Yu M, Vandenberg SR, Ginzinger DG, James CD, Costello JF, Bergers G, Weiss WA, Alvarez-Buylla A, Hodgson JG. miR-124 and miR-137 inhibit proliferation of glioblastoma multiforme cells and induce differentiation of brain tumor stem cells. BMC Med. 2008;6:14.
206. Baumann M, Krause M, Hill R. Exploring the role of cancer stem cells in radioresistance. Nat Rev Cancer. 2008;8(7):545–54.
207. Evers P, Lee PP, DeMarco J, Agazaryan N, Sayre JW, Selch M, Pajonk F. Irradiation of the potential cancer stem cell niches in the adult brain improves progression-free survival of patients with malignant glioma. BMC Cancer. 2010;10:384.

# Cell Death Pathways, with Special Regard to Ionizing Radiation and Temozolomide

Marzia Toscano, Silvia Palumbo, Paolo Tini, Clelia Miracco, Giovanni Luca Gravina, and Sergio Comincini

## Introduction

Tumor cell death is the final goal of both radio- and chemotherapy. Radiotherapy determines various effects in cancer cells, ranging from reversible damage to death [1, 2]. Besides necrosis, one of the most known types of radiation-induced death is apoptosis, which was long thought to be the only type of programmed cell death (PCD) yielded by treatments against cancer [1–4]. In the last years, it is becoming evident that other types of PCD are triggered by both chemo- and radio-therapy [1, 2, 5]. To date, regulated necrosis (including necroptosis or PCD type III), mitotic catastrophe, apoptosis (PCD type I), and autophagy-related cell death (PCD type II) are among the known main types of cell death induced by ionizing radiation (IR) [1, 2, 6]. It is becoming even more evident that cell death pathways are not always mutually exclusive, as thought in the past. Shifts from one type towards another type of cell death pathway via complex regulatory signals can occur, which partly depend on the initiating stimuli, and vary depending on the targeted cell type [7, 8]. Furthermore, radiation triggers a series of events, which involve not only tumor cells, but also its microenvironment [4, 9].

Recently, novel approaches which aim at investigating the global tumor cell gene expression after radiation, through transcriptome analysis, and investigations on signals coming from tumor stroma, are shedding light on multiplex mechanisms induced by radiation, which are responsible for both tumor cell sensitivity and resistance to therapy [1, 9].

Temozolomide (TMZ) is a chemotherapeutic drug capable of crossing the blood–brain barrier and is today the first choice agent for human

M. Toscano (✉)
Tuscany Tumor Institute, Florence, Italy

Unit of Radiation Oncology, Department of Medicine, Surgery and Neurosciences University of Siena, Siena, Italy
e-mail: marzia.toscano@gmail.com

S. Palumbo
Unit of Radiation Oncology, Department of Medicine, Surgery and Neurosciences University of Siena, Siena, Italy

P. Tini
Tuscany Tumor Institute, Florence, Italy

Unit of Radiation Oncology, University Hospital of Siena (Azienda Ospedaliera-Universitaria Senese), Viale Bracci 11, Siena, 53100, Italy

C. Miracco
Unit of Pathological Anatomy, Department of Medicine, Surgery and Neurosciences, University of Siena, Siena, Italy

G.L. Gravina
Department of Radiological, Oncological and Anatomo-Pathological Sciences, University of Rome "La Sapienza", Rome, Italy

S. Comincini
Department of Biology and Biotechnology, University of Pavia, Pavia, Italy

© Springer International Publishing Switzerland 2016
L. Pirtoli et al. (eds.), *Radiobiology of Glioblastoma*, Current Clinical Pathology,
DOI 10.1007/978-3-319-28305-0_13

glioblastoma (GB) treatment, besides radiation [10, 11]. Data from literature indicate that TMZ effects on tumor cells include apoptosis and autophagy-related cell death, the latter being considered the most frequent type of cell death induced by this drug [5].

Given the complexity of the molecular profile of GB [12, 13], tailored, patient-oriented therapies are desirable. Advances in GB pathobiological and molecular understanding derived from large-scale omic studies are individuating an increasing number of targetable molecules for GB therapy [13]. However, to date, translation of these molecular acquisitions into clinical practice has not yet led to satisfying results, partly due to the extreme heterogeneity of GB. Molecular medicine combined with traditional radio- and chemotherapy could be a possible route to improve therapeutic efficacy. Pharmaceutical-based radiation sensitizers, as well as the combination of TMZ with other agents, that will target multiple key molecules involved in the altered molecular pathways of GB have the potential to increase the impact of both radiation and TMZ on tumor cells specifically [14–16]. In this chapter, we will address the main types of cell death induced by both IR and TMZ in cancer and possible modulation of cell death pathways to improve the efficacy of various, single or combined treatments. We will pay particular attention to apoptotic and autophagic pathways and their role in GB treatment. We will not deal with other debatable types of IR-induced cell death (i.e. senescence, which, at present, is considered either as an irreversible suppression of tumor growth or as a state of dormancy, although clonogenic survival assays seem to indicate that senescence could be also considered a type of cell death) [6, 17].

## Necrosis, Regulated Necrosis/ Necroptosis, and Mitotic Catastrophe

Necrosis is triggered in cells that enter mitosis with severely damaged DNA [6]. It is characterized by cell and mitochondrial swelling; denaturation and coagulation of proteins; disruption of cell membrane and subcellular organelles; random fragmentation of DNA and release of cytotoxins. Necrosis elicits an inflammatory response and usually follows high doses of radiation [6]. In the past, necrosis was considered a cell demise mechanism by default, to be separated from programmed types of cell death. More recently, much of the data from literature indicates that necrosis can occur in a regulated manner following specific signals, after which necrosis should be named [6]. Some investigators observed that blocking apoptosis, through chemical inhibition or molecular manipulation of caspases via receptor interaction protein kinases 1 and 3 (RIP1 and RIP3), induced a series of events resulting in cell necrosis (RIP1/RIP3-dependent regulated necrosis) [6]. Necroptosis is today considered a specific type of regulated necrosis, triggered by TNFR1 ligation, and dependent by RIP1 activation (it should be better named "RIP1-dependent regulated necrosis"). It is inducible by radiation [6] and is being explored as a possible targetable pathway in GB [18].

Mitotic catastrophe is an event that occurs during or because of aberrant mitosis, from premature or inappropriate entry of cells into mitosis, associated with various morphological and biochemical modifications [19]. It is morphologically characterized by the formation of nuclear envelopes around individual clusters of missaggregated chromosomes [6]. Various agents capable of destabilizing microtubules can induce it, and it is a major, mitotic-linked mechanism of delayed cell death following radiation of solid tumors [20]. Much of the information about this type of PCD is derived from in vitro studies on GB cell lines. Moreover, mitotic catastrophe associated with delayed apoptosis has also been observed in patient-derived p53-deficient stem-like glioma cells and differentiated cells treated with IR (5–10 Gy) [21]. Recently, transcriptome studies in vitro, through total RNA sequencing analysis, identified, after irradiation, an altered expression pattern of genes involved in the mitotic process, including G2-, spindle assembly checkpoint-, and centrosome-associated genes [1, 22].

In several experimental studies, radiosensitization of glioma cells yielded an increase in tumor cell death also through mitotic catastrophe.

To this purpose, the modulation of growth factors and kinases known to be involved in both GB growth and radioresistance is revealing to be a promising approach. In one study [23], an increase of cell death by mitotic catastrophe was observed both in vitro and in vivo in irradiated glioma cells, after modulation of the hepatocyte growth factor/MET signaling pathway. In other studies, the silencing of ILK kinase or polo-like kinase 1 enhanced radiation-induced cell death by mitotic catastrophe [24, 25].

## Apoptosis, Cancer, Ionizing Radiation, and Temozolomide (Focus on Glioblastoma)

### Apoptotic Pathway

Apoptosis (PCD I) is a common type of cell death observed in various tissues and cell types (for review see [3]). Apoptosis is an essential part of life for multicellular organisms which plays an important role in development and tissue homeostasis. In a physiological context, apoptosis is delicately regulated and balanced. Failure of this regulation results in pathological conditions such as developmental defects, autoimmune diseases, neurodegeneration, or cancer.

The earliest recognized morphological changes in apoptosis involve compaction and segregation of nuclear chromatin, condensation of the cytoplasm, and loss of adhesion to neighboring cells or to the extracellular matrix. The plasma membrane convolutes or blebs, producing fragments of cells (apoptotic bodies). These fragments are membrane-bound and contain nuclear components. The apoptotic bodies, which show changes in several cell surface molecules, are quickly taken up by nearby cells and degraded in a relatively short time, usually resulting in the elimination of dead cells without generating an inflammatory response. Biochemically, apoptosis is characterized by the double-stranded cleavage at the linker regions between nucleosomes, resulting in the formation of multiple DNA fragments, phosphatidylserine externalization, and is accompanied by the expression of a series of genes and proteins. The main actors of apoptosis are caspases.

In mammals, apoptosis may occur via two major pathways: (1) the extrinsic pathway (death receptor pathway) or (2) the intrinsic pathway (mitochondrial pathway).

Although the caspase cascade involved in extrinsic and intrinsic pathways are different, both pathways can eventually merge. Caspases can be functionally divided into two further subgroups: the apoptosis initiators including caspase-2,-8,-9,-10 and the apoptosis executors including caspase-3,-6,-7. These two pathways are regulated by several pivot proteins such as p53; Bcl-2; Nuclear Factor kappa-light-chain-enhancer of activated B cells (NFκB); and MAPKs [26, 27].

1. The extrinsic pathway, mediated by extracellular stimuli including IR and chemotherapy, is triggered by the binding death receptor (DR) family, which includes tumor necrosis factor receptor 1 (TNF-R1), Fas, DR3, TRAIL-R1/2 (DR4/5) and DR6, which contain cytoplasmic regions, namely the death domains (DD), which, when bound to their appropriate ligands, recruit the Fas-associated death domain (FADD). When death stimuli occur, Fas ligand (Fas-L) combines with Fas to form a death complex. The Fas/Fas-L composite recruits the adaptor protein FADD and pro-caspase-8, forming a death-inducing signaling complex (DISC). Auto-activation of caspase-8 at the DISC is followed by activation of effector caspases, which function as downstream effectors of the cell death program. According to the recommendations of the Nomenclature Committee on Cell Death [6], extrinsic apoptosis is defined "a caspase-dependent cell death subroutine", which "can be suppressed (at least theoretically) by pan-caspase chemical inhibitors" or "by the over-expression of viral inhibitors of caspases". The same study group [6] assessed that it can occur through three major cascades:
   (a) Death receptor signaling and activation of the caspase-8-10 and caspase-3 cascade.
   (b) Death receptor signaling and activation of the caspase-8, tBID, MOMP, caspase-9, and caspase-3.
   (c) Ligand deprivation-induced dependence receptor signaling followed by (direct or

MOMP-dependent) activation of the caspase-9 and caspase-3 cascade.

2. The intrinsic pathway is mediated by diverse apoptotic stimuli, such as extracellular stimuli (e.g., UV, IR, and cytotoxin) or intracellular signals (e.g., DNA damage, nuclear instability).

These signals lead to apoptosis via the involvement of mitochondria; apoptotic stimuli transmit death signals to the mitochondria and increase the permeability of the outer mitochondrial membrane, which leads to the release of apoptogenic proteins, such as cytochrome $c$, Smac/DIABLO, and Omi, from the mitochondria into the cytoplasm. After its release, cytochrome $c$, in the presence of ATP, associates with apoptosis protease-activating factor (Apaf-1) and pro-caspase-9 to compose the "apoptosome", which downstream triggers a caspase 9/3 signaling cascade, culminating in apoptosis. Smac/DIABLO and Omi accelerate caspase activation by inactivating the Inhibition of Apoptosis (IAPs) family members that function as endogenous caspase inhibitors. Aiming at cell homeostasis, anti-apoptotic mechanisms are also activated, which deliver signals to the mitochondrial membrane [6]. Apoptosis-associated mitochondrial membrane permeability is primarily controlled by BCL-2 family members, which include three subgroups:

(a) Anti-apoptotic proteins (Bcl-2, Bcl-xL, and Mcl-1) which, under conditions that favor cell survival, bind and inhibit pro-apoptotic BCL-2 proteins.

(b) Multi-domain pro-apoptotic proteins (Bak and Bax) which, upon death stimuli, undergo conformational change and insert into the outer mitochondrial membrane, thus increasing membrane permeability.

(c) Proteins with the BH3 domain only (Bid, Bim, Bik, Bad, Noxa, and PUMA) that bind to and inhibit the anti-apoptotic Bcl-2 family members, releasing the pro-apoptotic Bax and Bak. Bax and Bak play an essential role in the release of apoptogenic proteins. While the anti-apoptotic proteins

regulate apoptosis by blocking the mitochondrial release of cytochrome $c$, the pro-apoptotic proteins act by promoting such release. The initiation of apoptosis depends on the balance between the pro- and anti-apoptotic proteins.

According to the recommendations of the Nomenclature Committee on Cell Death (2012), the intrinsic apoptosis is a process mediated by mitochondrial outer membrane permeabilization associated with a release of inner membrane space proteins into the cytosol, a generalized and irreversible dissipation of the mitochondrial membrane potential, and the inhibition of the respiratory chain function [6]. A differentiation between caspase-dependent and caspase-independent intrinsic apoptosis is also recommended [6].

## Apoptosis and Cancer

Over 50 % of neoplasms have defects in apoptotic machinery (For review see [3]). Cancer cells often harbor mutations in pro-apoptotic proteins (e.g. Apaf-1, Bax and p53) and can also rely on the overexpression of anti-apoptotic agents (e.g. Akt, Bcl-2, Bcl-xL, and IAPs) as a means to protect them from cell death.

The increased expression of pro-survival Bcl-2 family proteins and mutations in the tumor suppressor gene TP53 are the most frequent and better characterized alteration that impact apoptosis pathways in cancer.

When there is disruption in the balance of anti-apoptotic and pro-apoptotic members of the Bcl-2 family, the result is dysregulated apoptosis in the affected cells. There are many studies that demonstrate the role of Bcl-2 family members and p53 alterations in cancer, including GB [28, 29].

Cancer cells have various modalities to block classical apoptotic pathways [3]. An efficient way for tumor cells to acquire resistance to apoptosis is through inactivation of the pro-apoptotic signaling pathways.

p53, a major mediator of the intrinsic apoptotic pathway, is a very frequently mutated gene in cancer. p53 pathways alterations may shut down both the intrinsic and extrinsic apoptotic pathways in tumors, through different mechanisms.

Dysregulation of many other genes facilitates tumorigenesis, in fact, by interfering with the downstream function of p53: p53 alterations have been found in 27.9 %, whereas the p53 pathways are dysregulated in 85.3 % of GB [13].

Dysregulation of tumor resistance-related antiapoptotic signaling includes not only antiapoptotic Bcl-2 family members and p53 pathway, but also other anti-apoptotic routes. Other relevant anti-apoptotic pathways in cancer, particularly in GB, include the phosphatidylinositol 3-kinase (PI3K)-Akt and the NFκB [13]. EGFR and its constitutively active mutated form EGFRvIII, high stimulators PI3K/Akt/ mammalian target of rapamycin (mTOR) pathway, can interact with the pro-apoptotic PUMA, resulting in its cytoplasmic sequestration and inactivation [30]. Furthermore, EGFRvIII was found to inhibit therapy-induced apoptosis via up-regulation of Bcl-xL and subsequent blockage of effector caspase activation [31]. Several IAP Family members are also dysregulated in cancer.

GB is highly heterogenous, and an array of molecular, genetic, and epigenetic alterations concurs to its progression and resistance to apoptotic and other types of cell death [13].

Overactivation of the PI3K/Akt pathway renders tumor cells resistant to apoptosis also by several other mechanisms.

It regulates NFκB and related proteins, promoting tumorigenesis through suppression of apoptosis [32].

## Apoptosis and IR

Apoptosis has long been thought to be the main form of cell death in response to cancer cell radiation.

Radiotherapy is a well-established and effective form of cancer treatment [33]. The early IR effects are usually evaluated in vitro by the MTT assay, whereas the clonogenic assay is the currently used method for assessing long-term IR effects [34]. IR can directly act on the atomic structures of nucleic acids, proteins, and lipids ([2, 35] and references therein).

An indirect damage is also caused by free radicals produced from water radiolysis ([35] and references therein).

Both the direct and indirect effects of IR initiate a series of downstream signaling events that result in the damage of macromolecules (DNA is the main target) that finally can lead to cell death. After IR, DNA undergoes single-strand breaks (SSBs) and double-strand breaks (DSBs). Unrepaired DSBs can result in cell death.

It is emerging that other mechanisms occur in determining tumor cell damage and death after IR. Cytotoxic molecules, released during treatment, may also kill neighboring cells (local bystander effects) ([35] and references therein). Furthermore, there is evidence of an IR-triggered tumor-specific immune response, which exert antineoplastic effects at the systemic level (long-range bystander, out-of field, or abscopal effects), resulting in CD8-induced apoptotic tumor cell death [36].

Among PCD types, IR-induced apoptosis has been extensively investigated for more than two decades [37]. The intrinsic pathway was found to be the main route of IR-induced apoptosis [6].

IR was also found to trigger apoptosis through the extrinsic pathway, via Fas up-regulation mediated by p53 [38].

According to some authors, IR-induced apoptosis has an effect only on the linear component of the linear-quadratic formula, which describes the initial portion of the radiation survival curve in the "low" dose range (<3–4 Gy), which grossly corresponds to doses-per-fraction used in clinical RT ([4] and references therein); it is well known that there is a direct correlation between IR sensitivity to the induction of apoptosis and loss of clonogenicity, for several tumor types. However, other authors ([4] and references therein) have instead denied correlation between IR sensitivity and sensitivity to apoptosis. Furthermore, no association between IR failure and resistance to apoptosis was found in a large series of patients affected by colorectal carcinomas ([4] and references therein). According to some authors, there is an "early" apoptosis peak occurring a few hours after IR, in several cell types (e.g. lymphoid cells), which correlates with cell loss in clonogenic assay

([4] and references therein). Instead, in other tumor types including epithelial and mesenchymal subtypes, a late apoptosis occurs ([4] and references therein), which does not correlate with cell loss in clonogenic assay and is not dose-dependent in the "low" dose range (<3–4 Gy).

In an in vivo mouse model, fractionated radiation was more efficient than single dose administration in determining apoptotic death ([4] and references therein). However, a paradox effect of IR is also observable. Tumor growth and repopulation were found via prostaglandine E2, induced by caspase-3, after tumor cell radiation ([4] and references therein).

Transcriptome analysis through total mRNA sequencing demonstrated that the expression of both pro-apoptosis and anti-apoptosis genes is altered after irradiation of the human GB cell line U-251 MG [1].

A temporal difference was found, since the majority of pro-apoptosis genes were "early continually responsive", whereas anti-apoptosis gene response occurred later [1]. Interestingly, despite the activation of an array of pro-apoptotic molecules, cell death was not induced, whereas inactivation of pro-apoptosis molecules in the nucleus, along with late activation of anti-apoptotic genes, could partly explain GB radioresistance [1].

The impact of IR in determining tumor cell death via apoptosis is today being revaluated, and some investigators claim that apoptosis actually accounts for a minor portion of cell death in solid tumors, following IR [37]. However, elucidating apoptosis-altered mechanisms could serve to identify novel targets for radiotherapy, as well as alternative pathways of cell demise inducible by IR.

## Apoptosis and TMZ

TMZ is an imidazotetrazine derivative and a novel oral cytotoxic agent that alkylates and methylates DNA [11]. One of the principal mechanisms responsible for its cytotoxicity against malignant cells is the methylation of DNA, resulting in the fragmentation of DNA and disrupted DNA replication, and thus growth suppression and apoptotic cell death. TMZ does

not require hepatic metabolism for activation and is able to penetrate the blood–brain barrier [11]. Due to this property, it is the first choice drug used against GB, besides IR [10]. It has also been adopted in advanced melanoma patients enrolled in clinical trials [39, 40]. Its therapeutic effect is also dependent on other factors. A main determinant of TMZ efficacy is known to be the methylated $O^6$-methylguanine-DNA methyltransferase (MGMT) promoter [11, 41]. Patients bearing a methylated MGMT benefit from TMZ. The possibility of increasing its chemotherapeutic efficacy is being investigated by combining TMZ with other agents [14–16].

The current standard therapy for GB patients, following surgical removal, is fractionated radiotherapy and chemotherapy with concomitant and adjuvant TMZ [10]. However, less than half of the patients bearing methylated MGMT respond to therapy and chemoresistance develops rapidly, through largely unknown routes, probably involving various factors including epigenetic regulation through miRNA [42]. Apoptosis was the main type of GB cell death observed in several studies after TMZ alone or combined with other molecules [11, 43, 44]. Roos et al. [43] found that TMZ-induced apoptosis was largely stimulated by p53 and required Fas receptor in p53 non-mutated glioma cells, whereas the mitochondrial apoptotic pathway was activated in p53-mutated glioma cells . Other investigators observed that TMZ-induced apoptosis was dependent on the pro-apoptotic protein Bak and independent of the pro-apoptotic protein Bax [45].

It is, however, also emerging that the autophagic pathway (and/or its interactions with apoptosis) is a major route determinant of GB cell death activated by TMZ.

## Autophagy, Cancer, Ionizing Radiation, and Temozolomide (Focus on Glioblastoma)

### Autophagic Pathway

Macroautophagy, hereafter referred to as autophagy, is an evolutionarily conserved, non-selective catabolic process that takes place in all eukaryotic cells, through lysosomal degradation and recycling of cytosolic components—ranging from damaged long-lived proteins, lipids, sugars, and nucleotides to whole organelles and invading pathogens ([46, 47] and references therein). Autophagy, in physiological processes, may be subdivided into "basal" autophagy, required for constitutive turnover of cytosolic components, and "induced" autophagy, which produces amino acids in response to starvation. Besides its primarily catabolic and pro-survival roles, recent investigations have ascertained that autophagy is involved in multiplex pathophysiological processes, including development, anti-aging, cell death, tumor suppression, and antigen presentation ([47] and references therein).

In general, autophagy plays a crucial pro-survival role in cell homeostasis, required during periods of starvation or following other either extra- or intracellular stresses. Its role in determining cell death is instead still controversial and likely not univocal, although it has been ascertained that autophagy is involved in death signaling ([47, 48] and references therein).

Autophagy pathways intertwine with apoptosis and other types of death routes [88]. The resulting cell type of cell demise likely depends on several other factors, including tumor type and the genetic and molecular profile of tumor cell.

It has been proposed that cells die with autophagy, and not by autophagy [49], and that apoptosis occurs concomitantly with features of autophagy [50]. Many experiments in vitro indicate that autophagic cell death occurs in cells with defective apoptosis. However, there is convincing evidence that normal neuronal cells undergo autophagic cell death following insulin starvation [51]. Furthermore, autophagic cells, when coping with excessive stress leading to autophagy over-stimulation, may commit suicide by undergoing cell death, which differs from apoptosis and other types of programmed death ("autophagy related PCD"). In order to differentiate autophagic from other types of PCD, the assessment of the autophagic flux is required [46]. Morphologically, cells that die by autophagy are characterized by an increase in the number of autophagic vacuoles in the cytoplasm, followed by cell demise.

Autophagy is a complex machinery, which is carried out in sequential steps, accompanied by the expression of specific genes. Autophagy begins with the formation of autophagosomes, double membrane-bound structures surrounding cytoplasmic macromolecules and organelles. The initiating signal for autophagosome formation is poorly understood. In yeast, 31 different autophagy-related genes (ATGs) have been identified, and many of them have mammalian orthologs. Eighteen Atg proteins (Atg1-10; Atg12-14; Atg16-18), besides Atg29 and Atg31, can be grouped according to their functions at key stages of the autophagy pathway: (1) initiation; (2) nucleation; (3) elongation and maturation; (4) transport and fusion with the lysosomes.

## Initiation

ULK1-Atg13-FIP200 complex: the macromolecular complex implicated in the initiation step of autophagosome formation is the ULK1-Atg13-FIP200 complex.

Atg13 binds ULK1 or its homolog ULK2 and mediates their interaction with FIP200.

Activities of the ULK1 kinase complex are regulated by mTOR, depending on nutrient conditions. Under normal or rich nutrient conditions, active mTORC1 interacts with the ULK1 kinase complex and phosphorylates ULK1 and mAtg13, hence blocking their activity. Under starvation conditions, Atg13 and ULK1/2 are dephosphorylated, thereby activating ULK1/2, which phosphorylates FIP200 to induce autophagosome formation.

## Nucleation

The PI3K complex: the formation of new autophagosomes requires the activity of Vps34, a PI3K class III. Phosphatidylinositol-3-phosphate (PI3P), its product, plays an essential role in the early stages of the autophagy pathway. The role of Vps34 has been established through the use of the well-known pharmacological inhibitors wortmannin and 3-methyladenine (3-MA), or the novel SAR405, who all lead to the inhibition of autophagosome formation [52].

Vps34 is part of the autophagy-regulating macromolecular complex (PI3K complex) consisting of Beclin-1/Atg6, Atg14/barkor, and p150/Vps15.

The activity of Vps34 is enhanced by its interaction with Beclin-1. The evolutionarily conserved domain of Beclin-1 is required for Vps34 binding, autophagy, and tumor suppressor function. Several Beclin-1-binding proteins have been identified, and the disruption of their interaction with Beclin-1 affects autophagosome formation. The Beclin-1-binding partners that induce autophagy include Ambra-1, UVRAG, Bif-1, and Rubicon. It interacts to regulate the lipid kinase Vps34 protein and promote formation of Beclin-1-Vps34-Vps15 core complexes. On the other hand, the binding of the anti-apoptotic proteins Bcl-2 or Bcl-xL to Beclin-1 inhibits autophagy. During starvation, the activation of c-Jun NH2-terminal kinase-1 (JNK1) results in the phosphorylation of Bcl-2 and Bcl-xL which releases their binding to Beclin-1, thus inducing autophagosome formation.

## Elongation and Autophagosome Maturation

Two ubiquitin-like reactions are involved in the elongation of the pre-autophagosomal structures:
1. In the first reaction, the ubiquitin-like protein Atg12 is covalently tagged to Atg5. Atg12 is first activated by Atg7 (E1 ubiquitin-activating enzyme-like) and then transferred to Atg10 (E2 ubiquitin-conjugating enzyme-like). Atg12 is finally covalently linked by its C-terminal glycine (Gly 186) to a lysine (Lys149) residue of Atg5 [53]. The Atg12-Atg5 then forms a conjugate with Atg16L1. This complex is essential for the elongation of the pre-autophagosomal membrane, but dissociates from fully formed autophagosomes.
2. The second ubiquitin-like reaction involves the protein microtubule-associated protein 1 light chain 3 (MAP1-LC3/LC3/Atg8). LC3 is synthesized as a precursor form and is cleaved, at its C-terminus, by the protease Atg4B, resulting in the cytosolic isoform LC3-I. LC3-I is conjugated to phosphatidylethanolamine in a reaction involving Atg7 (E1-like) and Atg3 (E2-like) to form LC3-II. Due to the relatively specific association of LC3-II with autophagosomes, LC3-II is actually the only specific autophagy marker.

## Transport to Lysosomes and Fusion

Once formed, autophagosomes first fuse with endosomes to generate amphysomes. Amphysomes are acidified by the activity of proton pumps provided by the endosomes. The amphisome than fuses with lysosomes to generate autophagolysosomes, in which lysosomal enzymes degrade the sequestered material.

The fusion steps involve proteins such as ESCRT, SNAREs, Rab7 [54]. Mutation or loss of proteins that are important for the formation of multivesicular bodies lead to an inhibition of autophagolysosome maturation [55].

Two additional processes then follow: degradation and utilization of degradation products.

Many studies have shed light on the functional role of autophagy in different cellular processes and the potential of autophagy modulation as a therapeutic strategy for different pathologic conditions, including cancer [47].

The regulation of autophagy is very complex [56]. Aminoacid starvation and the endocrine system (insulin in particular) are physiological triggers of autophagy. Numerous other factors occur in cancer. Most of them signal to the PI3K/Akt/mTOR pathway, which is a master regulator of nutrient signaling and of autophagy. mTOR, a serine/threonine kinase which belongs to the family of phosphatidylinositol kinase-related kinases, is a key component that negatively regulates the induction of autophagy. The extent of autophagy is regulated by proteins upstream of mTOR signaling, including PTEN; PDK1; Akt; and TSC1/2.

## Autophagy and Cancer

Even if resistant to apoptosis, tumor cells can still be induced to die by other mechanisms, and necrosis, senescence, and autophagy may be alternative goals for cancer therapy. The activation of autophagy represents a crucial moment in modern therapy; several lines of evidence indicate that GB cells seem to be poorly resistant to therapies that induce autophagy [57]. For example, rapamycin's disruption of the mTOR pathway induces marked autophagic processes in GB cells [58].

However, the role of autophagy in cancer is still a topic of intense debate. It is likely context-specific and presumably differs in different phases of cancer life [59]. Autophagy, in fact, may either prevent or stimulate cancer.

On the one hand, autophagy acts as a tumor suppressor, by eliminating potentially oncogenic misfolded proteins and other substrates, thus halting initial stages of cancer. Furthermore, autophagy is known to be induced by p53 and PTEN, two of the most commonly tumor suppressor genes altered in cancer [60, 61]. Conversely, autophagy is inhibited via the direct interaction of oncogenic protein Bcl-2 with Beclin-1 ([47] and references therein). These data suggest that autophagy has an anticancer role.

On the other hand, autophagy promotes tumor growth by recycling substrates that fuel cancer cells under metabolic and therapeutic stress, guaranteeing an energy source and promoting their resistance to therapy.

The view that autophagy promotes resistance to cancer treatment is largely based on its capability of conferring tumor cells with high stress tolerance and on the observation that autophagy inhibition sensitizes cancer cells to DNA damaging therapeutic agents.

However, multiple, sometimes contrasting, effects may result from autophagy activation in cancer.

Below, several tumor suppressor or cancer-promoting functions of autophagy are reported, derived from a thorough review on autophagy and cancer [48].

1. *Tumor suppressor functions of autophagy*:
   (a) Autophagy inhibits necrosis and inflammation and modulates inflammatory response.
   (b) Autophagy halts oxidative stress and genomic instability.
   (c) Autophagy leads to tumor cell death.
   (d) Autophagy positively regulates immune response, by supporting the energy demands of antigen-presenting cells and T lymphocytes within a hypoxic tumor microenvironment, and inducing a CTL epitope mimicking tumor-associated antigens.
   (e) Autophagy inhibits metastasis.
   (f) Autophagy affects the epithelial to mesenchymal transition.
   (g) Autophagy restricts expansion of dormant tumor cells.
2. *Tumor-promoting functions of autophagy*:
   (a) Autophagy induces survival of tumor cells under a variety of stresses.
   (b) Autophagy is an adaptive metabolic response to hypoxia.
   (c) Autophagy is induced by nutrient starvation.
   (d) Autophagy promotes tumor cell metastasis.
   (e) Autophagy promotes resistance to cancer therapy.
   (f) Autophagy has a negative impact on local immunity, by inducing tumor cell resistance to CTL-mediated lysis.

It is evident that autophagy may invest multiple roles and opposite functions in cancer, depending on the tumor cell context and microenvironment.

In cancer, multiple forms of exogenous stressors, including cancer chemotherapeutic drugs and radiation, almost invariably promote autophagy in tumor cells [17]. In many cases, this autophagy is cytoprotective in function, mostly by interfering with the capacity of the tumor cell to undergo apoptotic cell death [62]. However, in literature there are also multiple examples in which chemotherapeutic drugs—alone or in combination—as well as radiation in combination with chemotherapy, promote autophagic cell death [62]. It is also clear that there are cases in which the induced autophagy exhibits neither cytoprotective nor cytotoxic functions.

A direct link has been demonstrated between tumorigenesis and the disruption of autophagy. Beclin-1 is vastly the most investigated autophagic gene in cancer. It is an essential mediator of autophagy. Binding to Class III PI3K, it starts autophagosome formation, and its decreased expression is associated with a reduced autophagic vacuole formation [46, 47]. Interacting with Bcl-2, it can also induce apoptosis [46, 47]. Overexpression of Beclin-1 in MCF-7 human breast cancer cells was found to facilitate autophagy induced by serum and amino-acid deprivation, which indicates that Beclin-1 is a necessary regulator for autophagy also in cancer [63].

In mice, it was demonstrated that Beclin-1 is a haploinsufficient tumor suppressor [64, 65]. In humans, it was found monoallelically deleted in breast, ovarian, prostate cancers, and it showed a reduced expression in several types of cancers, including GB [66–68].

In recent years, the expression of Beclin-1 transcript was investigated as a prognostic factor in several cancers. Among 212 primary human brain tumors [67], medulloblastomas and most high-grade astrocytic, ependymal neoplasms and atypical meningiomas showed a significant decrease of Beclin-1 cytoplasmic protein expression when compared to the majority of low-grade tumors. Furthermore, in the same study, the expression level of Beclin-1 mRNA was significantly lower in all glial tumors when compared to all meningiomas, suggesting a possible different involvement of Beclin-1 in the different histotypes of brain neoplasms. The prognostic role of Beclin-1 expression was also investigated by immunohistochemistry in high-grade glioma patients [69], in whom high Beclin-1 protein cytoplasmic expression positively correlated with apoptosis, and negatively with cell proliferation. High Beclin-1 expression was also significantly correlated with survival, both in the univariate and multivariate analysis, with high KPS values, and with the accomplishment of an optimal postoperative therapy.

## Autophagy and IR

There are contradictory messages regarding how autophagy affects the ways through which tumor cells die when they are treated with anticancer agents. Many anticancer agents have been reported to induce autophagy, leading to the suggestion that autophagic cell death may be an important mechanism of tumor cell death by these agents [17, 70].

Many anticancer agents can induce autophagy, including IR, temozolomide, tamoxifen, rapamycin, and arsenic trioxide [70].

In different experimental investigations on various tumor cell types, IR almost uniformly has been found to promote autophagy, which is usually thought to invest a protective effect on tumor cells [17].

However, both promotion and inhibition of cancer cell radioresistance by autophagy have been documented, likely depending on experimental and tumor cell context [17].

Several investigations indicate that autophagy is cytoprotective and confers radioresistance both to spawn and to stem cancer cells [71–73]. Furthermore, silencing of Beclin-1, Atg3, and Atg4 genes sensitizes carcinoma cells to IR [74], and the number of irradiated glioma cells undergoing DNA double-strand breaks significantly increases after autophagy inhibition [75].

Other studies indicate, instead, a cytotoxic function of autophagy alone or combined with other agents in the radiosensitization of several cancer cell types, including GB [72, 76–79]. Autophagy up-regulation after apoptosis and mTOR alone or combined inhibition was identified as the main mechanism of radiosensitization in breast, lung, and glioma cancer cells [76, 77, 80].

Furthermore, an impaired therapeutic efficacy after autophagy inhibition has been observed both in experimental studies and clinical trials in a study [77].

Ionizing radiation determines the activation of multiplex pathways, which can be modulated in order to increase radiosensitization [1]. In response to radiation, the PI3K/Akt/mTOR pathway, a negative regulator of autophagy, is activated and frequently mediates resistance [81, 82]. Several studies have shown that inhibition of PI3K/Akt/mTOR signaling sensitizes tumor cells to different chemotherapeutic strategies [83]. Since GB cells appear to be dependent on this pathway for proliferation [84], targeting key molecules of this pathway could likely be a useful therapeutic strategy and has yielded promising results in several investigations. Inhibition of Akt radiosensitized U-87 MG GB cells by enhancing autophagy [76]. Rad001 (everolimus, an mTOR inhibitor) induced autophagy and radiosensitization [85]. The combined inhibition of Akt and mTOR synergized in increasing radiosensitization of U-87 MG, T98G, and U-373 MG GB cells [86].

Ionizing radiation causes genotoxic events, including DNA-double strand breaks, which activate DNA repairing usually through the DNA-dependent protein kinase, or result in cell death, usually by apoptosis. Depending on the cell type and/or IR dose, DNA-dependent protein kinase may induce autophagy, as well as inhibition of the PI3K/Akt/mTOR pathway [87].

Mitochondrial and lysosomal damage and autophagy are also being investigated in the attempt to increase tumor cell radiosensitization [72].

It is known that autophagy and apoptosis can either inhibit or stimulate each other, through key common players, including Atg5, Bcl-2, caspases, and p53 [88]. Given the complex, variously intertwined, processes of the autophagic and apoptotic pathways, a potentiation of both types of related cell death may be a common goal of novel radiosensitizing therapies. The impact of IR on PI3K/Akt/mTOR pathway activates a complex cross-talk between autophagy and apoptosis and inhibition of mTOR radiosensitized prostate cancer cells by inducing autophagy [89]. Inhibition of one of the two death pathways and concurrent potentiation of the other one, as well as the induction of both death signaling pathways, has been observed [72].

Further research is required to exploit the role of autophagy in radiosensitizing tumor cells.

## Autophagy and TMZ

TMZ is currently the most efficacious cytotoxic drug employed to combat GB. Besides the methylation status of MGMT, its effectiveness also depends on the expression level of the mTOR gene, and both TMZ and IR efficacy were improved by targeting PI3K and mTOR pathway [90]. TMZ exerts its toxicity by inducing several DNA adducts and, according to several authors, by triggering autophagic cell death [5].

In support of this conclusion, $O^6$-benzylguanine, an inhibitor of MGMT, augmented the effects of TMZ through an increase in the promotion of autophagy, with no evidence of apoptosis. Interference with autophagy via 3-methyladenine suppressed the sensitivity of malignant GB cells

to TMZ, indicating that sensitivity of GB to TMZ is mediated through autophagy.

Several studies have indicated that TMZ induces G2/M arrest and that cells subsequently die through autophagy, but not apoptosis [5, 91].

A recent study by Palumbo et al. clearly showed that response to treatment with radiation alone or combined with TMZ involved autophagy [79]. Two cell lines that differed in their sensitivity to radiation were used (T98G and U-373 MG). At low doses of radiation (~2 Gy), T98G cells showed high sensitivity to radiation compared to the U-373 MG cells, which was associated with the promotion of autophagy with minimal evidence of apoptosis. Furthermore, pretreatment of both cell lines with rapamycin, a known autophagy inducer, sensitized the resistant cells to radiation. Of critical importance, siRNA-mediated knockdown of Beclin-1 and Atg7 abrogated radiosensitivity, either alone or in combination with TMZ [79].

In other investigations, both autophagy and apoptosis were induced after TMZ at therapeutically relevant dose levels ($\leq$100 µM), in a specific time-dependent manner [92].

Senescence was induced as well, and the authors found that one of the DNA adducts produced after TMZ, the $O^6$-methylguanine (O6MeG), mispaired with thymine, inducing erroneous repair process secondary lesions, which lead to DNA double-strand breaks.

O6MeG was responsible for the temporal sequences of autophagy, senescence, and apoptosis, the latter occurring as a late response to DSBs signaling. The authors suggest that the fate of GB cells, in terms of survival or death, largely depends on the balance of players involved in the process. In this experimental set, TMZ-induced autophagy was supposed to be cytoprotective, envisaging its inhibition as pro-apoptotic in GB cells.

However, it is known that autophagy can be modulated at several points, both positively and negatively, and its inhibition at different steps likely results in its different effects [72]. For instance, Kanzawa et al. [5], in the same GB cell lines treated with TMZ, found that inhibition of early stage of autophagy by 3-methyladenine was

Novel therapeutic perspectives also derive from GB microenvironment and its modification induced by radiotherapy. GB triggers a local immune response, and tumor infiltrating lymphocytes, presenting antigen dendritic cells, and macrophages are targetable by specific antibodies. Furthermore, vaccines against heat shock protein and EGFRvIII are under study and have yielded encouraging results in some clinical trials [9, 35].

IR is known to trigger a pro-inflammatory signaling cascade and immune activation, which are further targets to be exploited for immunotherapy. Orchestrated immune and inflammatory cell modulation could improve radiation effects. This approach might open a new avenue for GB therapy; the outcome of the few ongoing trials based on a similar treatment approach will provide more information [9, 35].

In conclusion, resistance of GB to most antineoplastic agents, including IR, is a major determinant of poor cell death and is a challenge for tumor research. Due to the high heterogeneity of GB, the most promising approach is the complex one, by combining surgery, radiotherapy, chemotherapy, and targeted molecular therapy directed simultaneously towards different cellular pathogenetic mechanisms detected by suitable markers, in order to plan an even more patient-adapted treatment.

# References

1. Ma H, Rao L, Wang HL, Mao ZW, Lei RH, Yang ZY, Qing H, Deng YL. Transcriptome analysis of glioma cells for the dynamic response to γ-irradiation and dual regulation of apoptosis genes: a new insight into radiotherapy for glioblastoma. Cell Death Dis. 2013;4, e895. doi:10.1038/cddis.2013.412.
2. Mirzayans R, Andrais B, Scott A, Wang YW, Murray D. Ionizing radiation-induced responses in human cells with differing TP53 status. Int J Mol Sci. 2013;14:22409–35. doi:10.3390/ijms141122409.
3. Wong RS. Apoptosis in cancer: from pathogenesis to treatment. J Exp Clin Cancer Res. 2011;30:87. doi:10.1186/1756-9966-30-87.
4. Balcer-Kubiczek EK. Apoptosis in radiation therapy: a double-edged sword. Exp Oncol. 2012;34:277–85.
5. Kanzawa T, Germano IM, Komata T, Ito H, Kondo Y, Kondo S. Role of autophagy in temozolomide-induced cytotoxicity for malignant glioma cells. Cell Death Differ. 2004;11:448–57.
6. Galluzzi L, Vitale I, Abrams JM, Alnemri ES, Baehrecke EH, Blagosklonny MV, et al. Molecular definitions of cell death subroutines: recommendations of the Nomenclature Committee on Cell Death 2012. Cell Death Differ. 2012;19:107–20. doi:10.1038/cdd.2011.96.
7. Chaabane W, User SD, El-Gazzah M, Jaksik R, Sajjadi E, Rzeszowska-Wolny J, Los MJ. Autophagy, apoptosis, mitoptosis and necrosis: interdependence between those pathways and effects on cancer. Arch Immunol Ther Exp. 2013;61:43–58. doi:10.1007/s00005-012-0205-y.
8. Ouyang L, Shi Z, Zhao S, Wang F-T, Zhou T-T, Liu B, Bao JK. Programmed cell death pathways in cancer: a review of apoptosis, autophagy and programmed necrosis. Cell Prolif. 2012;45:487–98. doi:10.1111/j.1365-2184.2012.00845.x.
9. Patel MA, Kim JE, Ruzevick J, Li G, Lim M. The future of glioblastomatherapy: synergism of standard of care and immunotherapy. Cancers. 2014;6:1953–85. doi:10.3390/cancers6041953.
10. Stupp R, Mason WP, van den Bent MJ, et al. Radiotherapy plus concomitant and adjuvant temozolomide for glioblastoma. N Engl J Med. 2005;352:987–96.
11. Zhang J, Stevens MF, Bradshaw TD. Temozolomide: mechanisms of action, repair and resistance. Curr Mol Pharmacol. 2012;5:102–14.
12. Verhaak RG, Hoadley KA, Purdom E, Wang V, Qi Y, Wilkerson MD, et al. Integrated genomic analysis identifies clinically relevant subtypes of glioblastoma characterized by abnormalities in PDGFRA, IDH1, EGFR, and NF1. Cancer Cell. 2010;17:98–110. doi:10.1016/j.ccr.2009.12.020.
13. Brennan CW, Verhaak RG. McKenna A, et al., TCGA Research Network. The somatic genomic landscape of glioblastoma. Cell. 2013;155:462–77.
14. Shields LB, Kadner R, Vitaz TW, Spalding AC. Concurrent bevacizumab and temozolomide alter the patterns of failure in radiation treatment of glioblastoma multiforme. Radiat Oncol. 2013;8:101. doi:10.1186/1748-717X-8-101.
15. Sang D, Li R, Lan Q. Quercetin sensitizes human glioblastoma cells to temozolomide in vitro via inhibition of Hsp27. Acta Pharmacol Sin. 2014;35:832–8.
16. Noack J, Choi J, Richter K, Kopp-Schneider A, Régnier-Vigouroux A. A sphingosine kinase inhibitor combined with temozolomide induces glioblastoma cell death through accumulation of dihydrosphingosine and dihydroceramide, endoplasmic reticulum stress and autophagy. Cell Death Dis. 2014;5:e1425. doi:10.1038/cddis.2014.384.
17. Sharma K, Le N, Alotaibi M, Gewirtz DA. Cytotoxic autophagy in cancer therapy. Int J Mol Sci. 2014;15:10034–51. doi:10.3390/ijms150610034.
18. Jiang YG, Peng Y, Koussougbo KS. Necroptosis: A novel therapeutic target for glioblastoma. Med Hypotheses. 2011;76:350–2.
19. Roninson IB, Broude EV, Chang BD. If not apoptosis, then what? Treatment-induced senescence and mitotic

catastrophe in tumor cells. Drug Resist Updat. 2001;4:303–13.

20. Vakifahmetoglu H, Olsson M, Zhivotovsky B. Death through a tragedy: mitotic catastrophe. Cell Death Differ. 2008;15:1153–62.

21. Firat E, Gaedicke S, Tsurumi C, Esser N, Weyerbrock A, Niedermann G. Delayed cell death associated with mitotic catastrophe in γ-irradiated stem-like glioma cells. Radiat Oncol. 2011;6:71. doi:10.1186/1748-717X-6-71.

22. Lindgren T, Stigbrand T, Johansson L, Riklund K, Eriksson D. Alteration in gene expression during radiation-induced mitotic catasrophe in HeLa Hep2 cells. Anticancer Res. 2014;34:3875–80.

23. Buchanan IM, Scott T, Tandle AT, Burgan WE, Burgess TL, Tofilon PJ, Camphausen K. Radiosensitazion of glioma cells by modulation of Met signaling with the hepatocyte growth factor neutralizing antibody, AMG102. J Cell Mol Med. 2011;15:1999–2006.

24. Lanvin O, Monferran S, Delmas C, Couderc B, Toulas C, Cohen-Jonathan-Moyal E. Radiation-induced mitotic cell death and glioblastoma radioresistance: a new regulating pathway controlled by integrin-linked kinase, hypoxia-inducible factor 1 alpha and survivin in U87 cells. Eur J Cancer. 2013;49:2884–91. doi:10.1016/j.ejca.2013.05.003.

25. Tandle AT, Kramp T, Kil WJ, Halthore A, Gehlhaus K, Shankavaram U, Tofilon PJ, Calpen NJ, Camphausen K. Inhibition of polo-like kinase 1 in glioblastoma multiforme induces mitotic catastrophe and enhances radiosensitation. Eur J Cancer. 2013;49:3020–8. doi:10.10106/j.ejca.2013.05.013.

26. Kaltschmidt B, Kaltschmidt C, Hofmann TG, Hehner SP, Dröge W, Schmitz ML. The pro- or anti-apoptotic function of NF-kappaB is determined by the nature of the apoptotic stimulus. Eur J Biochem. 2000;267:3828–35.

27. Wada T, Penninger JM. Mitogen-activated protein kinases in apoptosis regulation. Oncogene. 2004;23:2838–49.

28. Kouri FM, Jensen SA, Stegh AH. The role of Bcl-2 family proteins in therapy responses of malignant astrocytic gliomas: Bcl2L12 and beyond. ScientificWorldJournal. 2012;2012:838916. doi:10.1100/2012/838916.

29. Milinkovic VP, Skender Gazibara MK, Manojlovic Gacic EM, Gazibara TM, Tanic NT. The impact of TP53 and RAS mutations on cerebellar glioblastomas. Exp Mol Pathol. 2014;97:202–7. doi:10.1016/j.yexmp.2014.07.009.

30. Zhu H, Cao X, Ali-Osman F, Keir S, Lo HW. EGFR and EGFRvIII interact with PUMA to inhibit mitochondrial translocalization of PUMA and PUMA-mediated apoptosis independent of EGFR kinase activity. Cancer Lett. 2010;294:101–10.

31. Nagane M, Levitzki A, Gazit A, Cavenee WK, Huang HJ. Drug resistance of human glioblastoma cells conferred by a tumor-specific mutant epidermal growth factor receptor through modulation of Bcl-XL and caspase-3-like proteases. Proc Natl Acad Sci U S A. 1998;95:5724–9.

32. Karin M. Nuclear factor-kB in cancer development and progression. Nature. 2006;441:431–6.

33. Thariat J, Hannoun-Levi JM, Sun Myint A, Vuong T, Gérard JP. Past, present, and future of radiotherapy for the benefit of patients. Nat Rev Clin Oncol. 2013;10:52-60. doi:10.1038/nrclinonc.2012.203.

34. Buch K, Peters T, Nawroth T, Sänger M, Schmidberger H, Langguth P. Determination of cell survival after irradiation via clonogenic assay versus multiple MTT assay—a comparative study. Radiat Oncol. 2012;7:1. doi:10.1186/1748-717X-7-1.

35. Vacchelli E, Vitale I, Tartour E, Eggermont A, Sautes-Fridman C, Galon J, et al. Trial Watch: anticancer radioimmunotherapy. Oncoimmunology. 2013;2, e24238. http://dx.doi.org/10.4161/onci.24238.

36. Kroemer G, Zitvogel L. Abscopal but desirable: the contribution of immune responses to the efficacy of radiotherapy. Oncoimmunology. 2012;1:407–8; PMID:22754758; doi:http://dx.doi.org/10.4161/onci.2007.

37. Verheij M, Bartelink H. Radiation-induced apoptosis. Cell Tissue Res. 2000;301:133–42.

38. Embree-Ku M, Venturini D, Boekelheide K. Fas is involved in the p53-dependent apoptotic response to ionizing radiation in mouse testis. Biol Reprod. 2002;66:1456–61.

39. Guida M, Cramarossa A, Fistola E, et al. High activity of sequential low dose chemo-modulating Temozolomide in combination with Fotemustine in metastatic melanoma. A feasibility study. J Transl Med. 2010;8:115. doi:10.1186/1479-5876-8-115. PMC 2992498.

40. Su Y, Amiri KI, Horton LW, et al. A phase I trial of bortezomib with temozolomide in patients with advanced melanoma: toxicities, antitumor effects, and modulation of therapeutic targets in Clin. Cancer Res. 2010;16:348–57. doi:10.1158/1078-0432.CCR-09-2087.

41. Hegi ME, Diserens AC, Gorlia T, et al. MGMT gene silencing and benefit from temozolomide in glioblastoma. N Engl J Med. 2005;352:997–1003.

42. Haemmig S, Baumgartner U, Gluck A, Zbinden S, Tschan MP, Kappeler A, Mariani L, Vajtai I, Vassella E. miR-125b controls apoptosis and temozolomide resistance by targeting TNFAIP3 and NKIRAS2 in glioblastomas. Cell Death Dis. 2014;5:e1279. doi:10.1038/cddis.2014.245.

43. Roos WP, Batista LF, Naumann SC, Wick W, Weller M, Menck CF, Kaina B. Apoptosis in malignant glioma cells triggered by the temozolomide-induced DNA lesion O6-methylguanine. Oncogene. 2007;26:186–97.

44. Jakubowicz-Gil J, Langner E, Bądziul D, Wertel I, Rzeski W. Apoptosis induction in human glioblastoma multiforme T98G cells upon temozolomide and quercetin treatment. Tumour Biol. 2013;34:2367–78. doi:10.1007/s13277-013-0785-0.

45. Gratas C, Séry Q, Rabé M, Oliver L, Vallette FM. Bak and Mcl-1 are essential for temozolomide induced cell death in human glioma. Oncotarget. 2014;5:2428–35.
46. Klionsky DJ, Abdalla FC, Abeliovich H, Abraham RT, Acevedo-Arozena A, Adeli K, et al. Guidelines for the use and interpretation of assays for monitoring autophagy. Autophagy. 2012;8:445–544.
47. Mizushima N. Autophagy: process and function. Genes Dev. 2015;21:2861–3.
48. Janji B, Viry E, Baginska J, Van Moer K, Berchem G. Role of autophagy in cancer and tumor progression (Chapter 9). In: Bailly Y, editor. Autophagy—a double-edged sword—cell survival or death? Croatia: InTech; 2013. p. 189–215. doi:10.5772/55388.
49. Shen S, Kepp O, Kroemer G. The end of autophagic death? Autophagy. 2012;8:1–3.
50. Kroemer G, Levine B. Autophagic cell death: the story of a misnomer. Nat Rev Mol Cell Biol. 2008;9:1004–10.
51. Yu SW, Baek SH, Brennan RT, Bradley CJ, Park SK, Lee YS, et al. Autophagic death of adult hippocampal neural stem cells following insulin withdrawal. Stem Cells. 2008;26:2602–10.
52. Ronan B, Flamand O, Vescovi L, Dureuil C, Durand L, Fassy F, et al. A highly potent and selective Vps34 inhibitor alters vesicle trafficking and autophagy. Nat Chem Biol. 2014;10:1013–9. doi:10.1038/nchembio.1681.
53. Noda NN, Fujioka Y, Hanada T, Ohsumi Y, Inagaki F. Structure of the Atg12-Atg5 conjugate reveals a platform for stimulating Atg8-PE conjugation. EMBO Rep. 2013;14:206–11. doi:10.1038/embor.2012.208.
54. Hyttinen JM, Niittykoski M, Salminen A, Kaarniranta K. Maturation of autophagosomes and endosomes: a key role for Rab7. Biochim Biophys Acta. 1833;2013:503–10. doi:10.1016/j.bbamcr.2012.11.018.
55. Manil-Segalén M, Lefebvre C, Culetto E, Legouis R. Need an ESCRT for autophagosomal maturation? Commun Integr Biol. 2012;5:566–71. doi:10.4161/cib.21522.
56. Mehrpour M, Esclatine A, Beau I, Codogno P. Overview of macroautophagy regulation in mammalian cells. Cell Res. 2010;20:748–62. doi:10.1038/cr.2010.82.
57. Lefranc F. Glioblastomas are resistant to apoptosis but less resistant to the autophagic process. Bull Mem Acad R Med Belg. 2007;162:331–8.
58. Iwamaru A, Kondo Y, Iwado E, Aoki H, Fujiwara K, Yokoyama T, Mills GB, Kondo S. Silencing mammalian target of rapamycin signaling by small interfering RNA enhances rapamycin-induced autophagy in malignant glioma cells. Oncogene. 2007;26:1840–51.
59. Martinet W, Agostinis P, Vanhoecke B, Dewaele M, De Meyer GR. Autophagy in disease: a double-edged sword with therapeutic potential. Clin Sci (Lond). 2009;116:697–712. doi:10.1042/CS20080508.
60. Arico S, Petiot A, Bauvy C, Dubbelhuis PF, Meijer AJ, Codogno P, Ogier-Denis E. The tumor suppressor PTEN positively regulates macroautophagy by inhibiting the phosphatidylinositol 3-kinase/protein kinase B pathway. J Biol Chem. 2001;276:35243–6.
61. Feng Z, Zhang H. Levine AJ, and Jin S The coordinate regulation of the p53 and mTOR pathways in cells. Proc Natl Acad Sci U S A. 2005;102:8204–9. doi:10.1073/pnas.0502857102.
62. Gewirtz DA. The four faces of autophagy: implications for cancer therapy. Cancer Res. 2014;74:647–51.
63. Liang XH, Jackson S, Seaman M, Brown K, Kempkes B, Hibshoosh H, Levine B. Induction of autophagy and inhibition of tumorigenesis by beclin 1. Nature. 1999;402:672–6.
64. Yue Z, Jin S, Yang C, Levine AJ, Heintz N. Beclin 1, an autophagy gene essential for early embryonic development, is a haploinsufficient tumor suppressor. Proc Natl Acad Sci U S A. 2003;100:15077–82.
65. Qu X, Yu J, Bhagat G, Furuya N, Hibshoosh H, Troxel A, Rosen J, Eskelinen E-L, Mizushima N, Ohsumi Y, Cattoretti G, Levine B. Promotion of tumorigenesis by heterozygous disruption of the beclin 1 autophagy gene. J Clin Invest. 2003;112:1809–20. doi:10.1172/JCI200320039.
66. Fu LL, Cheng Y, Liu B. Beclin-1: autophagic regulator and therapeutic target in cancer. Int J Biochem Cell Biol. 2013;45:921–4. doi:10.1016/j.biocel.2013.02.007.
67. Miracco C, Cosci E. OliveriG, Luzi P, Pacenti L, Monciatti I, Mannucci S, De Nisi MC, Toscano M, Malagnino V, Falzarano SM, Pirtoli L, Tosi P. Protein and mRNA expression of autophagy gene Beclin 1 in human brain tumours. Int J Oncol. 2007;30:429–36.
68. Huang X, Bai HM, Chen L, Li B, Lu YC. Reduced expression of LC3B-II and Beclin 1 in glioblastoma multiforme indicates a down-regulated autophagic capacity that relates to the progression of astrocytic tumors. J Clin Neurosci. 2010;17:1515–9. doi:10.1016/j.jocn.2010.03.051.
69. Pirtoli L, Cevenini G, Tini P, Vannini M, Oliveri G, Marsili S, et al. The prognostic role of Beclin 1 protein expression in high-grade gliomas. Autophagy. 2009;5:930–6.
70. Kondo Y, Kanzawa T, Sawaya R, Kondo S. The role of autophagy in cancer development and response to therapy. Nat Rev Cancer. 2005;5:726–34.
71. Lomonaco SL, Finniss S, Xiang C, Decarvalho A, Umansky F, Kalkanis SN, et al. The induction of autophagy by gamma-radiation contributes to the radioresistance of glioma stem cells. Int J Cancer. 2009;125:717–22.
72. Zhuang W, Qin Z, Liang Z. The role of autophagy in sensitizing malignant glioma cells to radiation therapy. Acta Biochim Biophys Sin (Shanghai). 2009;41:341–51.
73. Pajonk F, Vlashi E, McBride WH. Radiation resistance of cancer stem cells: the 4 R's of radiobiology revisited. Stem Cells. 2010;28:639–48.
74. Apel A, Herr I, Schwarz H, Rodemann HP, Mayer A. Blocked autophagy sensitizes resistant carcinoma

cells to radiation therapy. Cancer Res. 2008;68:1485–94. doi:10.1158/0008-5472.CAN-07-0562.

75. Ito H, Daido S, Kanzawa T, Kondo S, Kondo Y. Radiation-induced autophagy is associated with LC3 and its inhibition sensitizes malignant glioma cells. Int J Oncol. 2005;26:1401–10.

76. Fujiwara K, Iwado E, Mills GB, Sawaya R, Kondo S, Kondo Y. Akt inhibitor shows anticancer and radiosensitizing effects in malignant glioma cells by inducing autophagy. Int J Oncol. 2007;31:753–60.

77. Kim KW, Hwang M, Moretti L, Jaboin JJ, Cha YI, Lu B. Autophagy up-regulation by inhibitors of caspase-3 and mTOR enhances radiotherapy in a mouse model of lung cancer. Autophagy. 2008;4:659–68.

78. Bristol ML, Di X, Beckman MJ, Wilson EN, Henderson SC, Maiti A, Fan Z, Gewirtz DA. Dual functions of autophagy in the response of breast tumor cells to radiation. Cytoprotective autophagy with radiation alone and cytotoxic autophagy in radiosensitization by vitamin D3. Autophagy. 2012;8(5):739–53. doi:10.4161/auto.19313.

79. Palumbo S, Pirtoli L, Tini P, Cevenini G, Calderaro F, Toscano M, Miracco C, Comincini S. Different involvement of autophagy in human malignant glioma cell lines undergoing irradiation and temozolomide combined treatments. J Cell Biochem. 2012;113:2308–18.

80. Moretti L, Kim KW, Jung DK, Willey CD, Lu B. Radiosensitization of solid tumors by Z-VAD, a pancaspase inhibitor. Mol Cancer Ther. 2009;8:1270–9.

81. Gupta AK, Bakanauskas VJ, Cerniglia GJ, Cheng Y, Bernhard EJ, Muschel RJ, McKenna WG. The Ras radiation resistance pathway. Cancer Res. 2001;61:4278–82.

82. Wu YT, Tan HL, Huang Q, Ong CN, Shen HM. Activation of the PI3K-Akt-mTOR signaling pathway promotes necrotic cell death via suppression of autophagy. Autophagy. 2009;5:824–34.

83. Hennessy BT, Smith DL, Ram PT, Lu Y, Mills GB. Exploiting the PI3K/AKT pathway for cancer drug discovery. Nat Rev Drug Discov. 2005;4:988–1004.

84. Newton HB. Molecular neuro-oncology and development of targeted therapeutic strategies for brain tumors. Part 2: Pi3k/Akt/pten, mtor, shh/ptch and angiogenesis. Expert Rev Anticancer Ther. 2004;4:105–28.

85. Kim KW, Mutter RW, Cao C, Albert JM, Freeman M, Hallahan DE, Lu B. Autophagy for cancer therapy through inhibition of pro-apoptotic proteins and mammalian target of rapamycin signaling. J Biol Chem. 2006;281:36883–90.

86. Berger Z, Ravikumar B, Menzies FM, Oroz LG, Underwood BR, Pangalos MN, Schmitt I, Wullner U, Evert BO, O'Kane CJ, Rubinsztein DC. Rapamycin alleviates toxicity of different aggregate- prone proteins. Hum Mol Genet. 2006;15:433–42.

87. Daido S, Yamamoto A, Fujiwara K, Sawaya R, Kondo S, Kondo Y. Inhibition of the DNA-dependent protein kinase catalytic subunit radiosensitizes malignant glioma cells by inducing autophagy. Cancer Res. 2005;65(10):4368–75.

88. Eisenberg-Lerner A, Bialik S, Simon HU, Kimchi A. Life and death partners: apoptosis, autophagy and the cross-talk between them. Cell Death Differ. 2009;16:966–75. doi:10.1038/cdd.2009.33.

89. Cao C, Subhawong T, Albert JM, Kim KW, Geng L, Sekhar KR, Gi YJ, Lu B. Inhibition of mammalian target of rapamycin or apoptotic pathway induces autophagy and radiosensitizes PTEN null prostate cancer cells. Cancer Res. 2006;66:10040–7.

90. Choi EJ, Cho BJ, Lee DJ, Hwang YH, Chun SH, Kim HH, Kim IA. Enhanced cytotoxic effect of radiation and temozolomide in malignant glioma cells: targeting PI3K-AKT-mTOR signalling, HSP90 and histone deacetylases. BMC Cancer. 2014;14:17. doi:10.1186/1471-2407-14-17.

91. Kanzawa T, Bedwell J, Kondo Y, Kondo S, Germano IM. Inhibition of DNA repair for sensitizing resistant glioma cells to temozolomide. J Neurosurg. 2003; 99:1047–52.

92. Knizhnik AV, Roos WP, Nikolova T, Quiros S, Tomaszowski KH, Christmann M, Kaina B. Survival and death strategies in glioma cells: autophagy, senescence and apoptosis triggered by a single type of temozolomide-induced DNA damage. PLoS One. 2013;8, e55665. doi:10.1371/journal.pone.0055665.

93. Omuro A, DeAngelis LM. Glioblastoma and other malignant gliomas: a clinical review. JAMA. 2013;310:1842–50. doi:10.1001/jama.2013.280319.

94. Gilbert MR, Wang M, Aldape KD, Stupp R, Hegi ME, Jaeckle KA, Armstrong TS, et al. Dose-dense temozolomide for newly diagnosed glioblastoma: a randomized phase III clinical trial. J Clin Oncol. 2013;31:4085–91. doi:10.1200/JCO.2013.49.6968.

95. Zhan M, Han ZC. Phosphatidylinositide 3-kinase/AKT in radiation responses. Histol Histopathol. 2004;19:915–23.

96. Frederick L, Wang XY, Eley G, James CD. Diversity and frequency of epidermal growth factor receptor mutations in human glioblastoma. Cancer Res. 2000;60:1383–7.

97. Nakada M, Kita D, Watanabe T, Hayashi Y, Teng L, Pyko VI, Hamada J-I. Aberrant signaling pathways in glioma. Cancers. 2011;3:3242–78. doi:10.3390/cancers3033242.

Silvia Palumbo, G. Belmonte, Paolo Tini,
Marzia Toscano, Clelia Miracco,
and Sergio Comincini

## How GBM Cells Escape
## from the Effects of Radiotherapy

According to the WHO nomenclature, glioblastoma multiforme (GBM) tumors are classified based on their clinical manifestations and histological phenotypes, classified according to the World Health Organization as WHO grade IV astrocytomas [1]. Generally, brain tumors can be treated surgically based on a maximal resection and through the use of adjuvant chemoradiotherapy, which mainly leads to inhibition of the cell cycle and increased apoptosis of tumor cells [1]: nowadays, the best prognostic responses in GBM patients are those with the combined use of the alkylating agent temozolomide [2]. However, highly malignant astrocytomas (WHO grades III and IV) are more prone to anaplasia and can contain immature astrocytes or oligodendrocytes or both cell types simultaneously [3, 4]. These tumors are also characterized by high rate of cellular proliferation and invasiveness. As emphasized by the name, GBM consist of many differentiated and non-differentiated cells and these tumors are histologically extremely heterogeneous and phenotypically diverse. From a therapeutically point of view, GBM are highly chemo- and radioresistant, and this feature usually leads to tumor relapses after surgical operation [3]. As a matter of fact, the prognosis of patients with GBM is very poor with median survival of 12–15 months from diagnosis [5].

To overcome the resistant behavior of these tumor cells, several mechanisms of GBM resis-

S. Palumbo
Unit of Radiation Oncology, Department
of Medicine, Surgery and Neurosciences,
University of Siena, Siena, Italy
e-mail: silvia.palumbo@unipv.it

G. Belmonte
Tuscany Tumor Institute Unit of Radiation Oncology,
Department of Medicine, Surgery and Neurosciences,
University of Siena, Siena, Italy

P. Tini
Tuscany Tumor Institute, Florence, Italy

Unit of Radiation Oncology, University Hospital of
Siena (Azienda Ospedaliera-Universitaria Senese),
Viale Bracci 11, Siena, 53100, Italy

M. Toscano
Unit of Radiation Oncology, Department
of Medicine, Surgery and Neurosciences,
University of Siena, Siena, SI, Italy

Tuscany Tumor Institute, Florence, Italy

C. Miracco
Tuscany Tumor Institute, Florence, Italy

Unit of Pathological Anatomy, Department
of Medicine, Surgery and Neurosciences,
University of Siena, Siena, SI, Italy

S. Comincini (✉)
Department of Biology and Biotechnology,
University of Pavia, Via Ferrata 9, Pavia 27100, Italy
e-mail: sergio.comincini@unipv.it

© Springer International Publishing Switzerland 2016
L. Pirtoli et al. (eds.), *Radiobiology of Glioblastoma*, Current Clinical Pathology,
DOI 10.1007/978-3-319-28305-0_14

tance have been deeply investigated; the most important of which is the deregulation of signaling pathways such as PI3K/AKT and ATM/CHK2/p53 [6]. Importantly, locus amplification, gene overexpression, and genetic mutations of epidermal growth factor receptor (EGFR) are hallmarks of GBM that can ectopically activate downstream signaling oncogenic cascades such as PI3K/Akt/mTOR pathway. Importantly, alteration of this pathway, involved also in the regulation of autophagy process, can improve radioresistance in GBM cells, thus promoting the aggressive phenotype of this tumor [7]. However, although various pharmacological inhibitors and anti-EGFR antibodies are available, the antiglioma activity of these agents has been largely limited to preclinical models, whereas their administration to glioblastoma patients was characterized by lack of clinical benefit. Comprehensive efforts have been made within the last years to understand the underlying mechanisms that confer resistance to EGFR inhibition in glioma cells. The absence of well-known mutations that predict response to EGFR tyrosine kinase inhibitors (TKIs) in gliomas and the presence of redundant and alternative compensatory pathways are among the most important escape mechanisms that prevent potent antiglioma effects of EGFR-targeting drugs. Accordingly, an increasing number of in vitro and in vivo studies are aimed at overcoming this resistance by combinatorial approaches using anti-EGFR treatment together with one or more additional drugs [8]. In addition, the epithelial to mesenchymal transition (EMT) is a crucial biological process occurring in the early development stages of many species. However, cancer cells often obtain the ability to invade and metastasize through the EMT, which triggers the scattering of cells. The hepatocyte growth factor (HGF)/MET signaling pathway is indicative of the EMT during both embryogenesis and the invasive growth of tumors, because HGF potently induces mesenchymal transition in epithelial-driven cells. Activation of MET signaling or co-overexpression of HGF and MET frequently represents aggressive growth and poor prognosis in various cancers, including GBM. Thus, efforts to treat cancers by inhibiting MET signaling using neutralizing antibodies or

small molecule inhibitors might represent novel specific anticancer strategies [9].

Another significant component of therapeutic resistance of GBM is the presence of cancer stem cells (CSCs) and signaling pathways related to the maintenance of the stem cell-like phenotype (OCT4, SOX2, Notch, and Nanog). This resistant phenotype is further confirmed by recent findings showing that CSCs generally are highly resistant to radiotherapy in comparison to non-CSCs. Therefore, another means to overcome the GBM resistance is to regulate pathways associated with CSCs progression [10]. CSCs have a high ability for self-renewal and also for production of neurospheres [4]. CSCs express markers of undifferentiated neuronal stem cells (nestin, CD133), but do not have markers of differentiated ones (β-tubulin, glial fibrillar protein). Cultivating under certain conditions, CSCs can convert into neuronal, astroglial, or oligodendroglial cells [11]. During the differentiation, CSCs gradually stop expressing markers of stem cells and acquire markers of a specific differentiation pathway. CD133, one of the best studied markers of CSCs, is used for identification and isolation of CSCs from GBM [12]. The number of CD133-positive cells within GBM tissues varies from 0.3 to 30 % and increases with the pathological features of the tumor [13]. The population of CD133-positive CSCs isolated from the most aggressive and malignant GBM tumors displays an increased ability for self-renewal as compared with other cell populations prepared from tumors with the lower malignancy. Thus, an increased expression of CD133 is associated with bad prognosis and severe course of the disease in GBM patients [14]. The role of CD133-positive CSCs in enhancing the resistance of GBM to antitumor therapy is under active investigation. Interestingly, the percentage of CD133-positive cells in GBM after chemo- or radiotherapy treatments was higher than in untreated tumors [15]. To date, radiotherapy is thought to be the most efficient nonsurgical approach for treatment of GBM, but, as previously stated, tumor cells manifested a radio-resistant phenotype. Importantly, among the tumor-specific altered molecular pathways, it was reported that the combined expression of CD133 and MGMT was associated with an increase in the radio-resistance of

GBM [16]. Moreover, differently from CD133-negative cells, CD133-positive GBM ones can survive after irradiation due to the high efficiency of DNA repair mechanisms activated after radiation-induced damage [17, 18]. In particular, further studies on the molecular mechanisms of DNA repair in CD133-positive CSCs have shown that, as differentiated from various GBM cell lines, DNA synthesis in these cells continues after irradiation, which suggests inhibition or inactivation of cellular regulators responsible for cell cycle arrest on transition to the S-phase [19]. The data of the above-mentioned studies show an obvious contribution of CD133-positive CSCs to the increase in GBM resistance to chemo- and radio-therapy and also suggest a cardinal role of these cells in tumor progression and in metastatization. Thus, searches for approaches for suppression of the CSCs population seem promising for enhancement of efficiency of therapy of brain tumors and can be an important trend of targeted therapy [20].

## miRNA as Molecular Messengers in GBM Cells' Microenvironment

miRNA are stem-loop structures encoded by a cell's own genome. These molecules represent a population of small non-coding RNAs, with an average length of 23 nucleotides, involved in the down-regulation of expression of target genes through regions of partial complementarity, mostly in their 3′-untranslated regions (UTRs) [21]. Each miRNA can be transcribed separately from an individual transcriptional unit, or each transcriptional unit can encode a cluster of distinct miRNA. The primary miRNA transcript (often abbreviated as pri-miRNA) is typically transcribed from the genome by RNA polymerase II and is subsequently capped and polyadenylated [22]. The primary miRNA transcript folds into a stem-loop structure, which is essential for the maturation process. In animals, the primary miRNA transcript is then cleaved in the nucleus by Drosha, a RNase III endonuclease, in association with the double-stranded RNA-binding domain protein DGCR8/Pasha in a protein complex referred to as the microprocessor

complex [23]. Drosha cleaves both strands of the stem at sites near the base of the primary stem-loop [24], generating an intermediate known as the miRNA precursor (sometimes abbreviated premiRNA). The miRNA precursor is then exported out of the nucleus by Exportin-5 into the cytosol where the RNase III domain-containing nuclease, Dicer, cleaves the terminal loop to generate the nucleotide mature miRNA. Immediately after formation of the mature miRNA, the duplex is unwound and loaded onto the RNA-induced silencing complex, which ultimately carries out the silencing of target mRNA. Another important molecular player of the gene-silencing process is RISC protein trimeric complex composed by Dicer, TRBP, and a protein of the Argonaute superfamily (Ago2 in humans) [25]. It identifies target mRNA based on complementarity with the associated single-stranded miRNA and results in either mRNA cleavage or translational repression [21]. As a result, an estimated one third of all mRNAs are thought to be susceptible to post-transcriptional gene silencing by miRNA [26].

A large spectrum of aberrant expression profiles of miRNA has been detected in many types of human tumors, including gliomas [27, 28]. Recent data have shown that human tumors are characterized by globally down-regulated miRNA expression profiles due to a general defect in the miRNA production process, which strengthens the hypothesis that these molecules may mainly serve as "guardians" of biologic processes [29]. Nevertheless, miRNA have been demonstrated not only to act as tumor suppressors, but also—dependent on the function of the targeted mRNA—as oncogenes [30, 31].

The reasons for the widespread differential expression of miRNAs in malignant as compared to normal cells are not fully elucidated [32]. However, epigenetic modifications within the transcriptional regulatory sequences of miRNAs, and also genetic alterations like mutations, genomic deletions, or gene amplifications, which can affect miRNA maturation and/or interactions with mRNA targets, are thought to contribute to miRNA dysregulation [33, 34].

In GBM, high-throughput analyses have identified various miRNAs that are differentially expressed when compared to non-neoplastic brain tissues [35–37]. Functional studies have demonstrated that miRNA are important mediators of multiple biological characteristics of GBM, including cell proliferation, G1/S cell cycle progression, cell survival, cell migration, and cell invasion [38–41]. Although the exact function of all altered miRNAs in GBM and of the complex network they regulate has not been completely elucidated yet, a growing number of studies have assigned single miRNAs to distinct functions in the processes of glioma-genesis and progression. For example, miRNA that are down-regulated in GBM as compared to normal brain have been found to function as tumor suppressors by directly targeting the oncogenes c-Met, Notch [42, 43], Bmi-1 [36], the EGFR [44], receptor tyrosine kinases [45], and cell cycle components [46]. Contrarily, miRNAs with enhanced expression in GBM might be designated as oncogenes (or oncomiR); i.e., miR-21 promoting invasion by targeting regulators of matrix metalloproteinases, miR-26a targeting PTEN, and miR-10b and miR-221 targeting cell cycle inhibitors [32].

Some aggressive tumors including GBM were shown to release microvesicles (mainly exosomes) containing mRNA, DNA, enzymes, oncogenic receptors, growth factors, and miRNA, which after their uptake by surrounding non-tumors cells induce oncogenic transformation of neighbors [47–50]. The function of these circulating/secreted miRNA has not been completely explored in the context of the brain tumor microenvironment. Establishing how these regulatory molecules are involved in the modulation of oncogenic signaling networks between tumor cells and stroma is likely to add a needed additional layer of complexity to the tumor network, consisting of intercellular communication. More importantly, miRNA-exosomes signaling may provide an additional therapeutic target for this deadly disease [51]. Exosomes-miRNA interaction was also in vitro demonstrated adopting CSG cells: co-cultivating of human neural stem cell-derived astrocytes and U87-MG GBM cells resulted in the malignant-like phenotype acquired by astrocytes from tumor cells [52].

Recently, Katakowski et al. [53] observed the ability of culturing rat gliosarcoma and human GBM cell lines shares miRNA between neighboring cells through gap junctions, and these molecules exhibited functional effects in the recipient cells via inhibiting expression of target mRNAs. These findings indeed suggest that miRNA may be directly implicated in GBM malignancy as pro-oncogenes being delivered from tumor to non-tumor cells through connexin-dependent gap junction mechanism [54] or mediated by the release of cancer exosomes and their cellular internalization through endocytosis [47].

These studies highlighted that miRNA expression can manage important processes within malignant transformation of the tumor cell: on the same time, newly discovered miRNA may represent new potent anti-cancer agents for targeted therapy of GBM [55]. Hence, for selective modulation of miRNA activity, decoy antisense oligonucleotides that would interfere with oncomiRs have been developed [56]. Among those, locked nucleic acid-modified oligonucleotides (LNAs) are single-stranded bicyclic RNA analogues composed of ribonucleotides with a methylene bridge, which connects the 2-oxygen with the 4-carbon of the ribose [57, 58]. LNAs present strong advantages for application to therapy as they are resistant to exo- and endonucleases and irreversibly bind to miRNAs, leading to a constitutive inhibition of their activity [57]. As a matter of fact, the first human phase II miRNA-based therapy was developed in 2010 for hepatitis C and use LNAs synthesized as unconjugated LNA/DNA molecules (miravirsen, SPC3649, LNA antimiRTM-122, Santaris Pharma) [59]. Although the complete phosphorothioate backbone of those LNAs is assumed to improve their stability and supports delivery of naked, single-stranded, un-complexed oligonucleotides to the liver, major obstacles remain to specifically design disease-specific miRNA. Thus, many research efforts are directed to the improvement in miRNA responsive or targeted chemical design and pharmacokinetic properties [7]. In this direction, the emergence of nanotechnology and nanomedicines is offering interesting perspectives [60]. Due to their submicron size and their versatile physicochemical properties, liposomes, polymeric nanospheres, polymeric nanocapsules, lipid nanoparticles, or nano emulsions can indeed interact in unique fashion with biological systems and give new opportunities for the delivery of active molecular entities for better efficiency, specificity, and biological safety [60]. Thus, substantial benefits can be obtained concerning biological barriers crossing, kinetics of drug release, drug bioavailability in the target organs and cells, prevention of side effects, and reduction of doses [60]. As such, lipid nanocapsules (LNCs), synthesized without the use of organic solvent, can be produced to suitable therapeutic sizes (e.g., 20, 50, 100 nm) [61]. These vectors can transport conventional anticancer drug (paclitaxel, etoposide, ferrocifen derivatives, HA14-1 analogues) [62–67] or radio-pharmaceuticals [68, 69]. LNCs are also capable to perform intrinsic biological effects including having the ability to cross the plasma membrane [64], inhibition of multidrug resistance [63], and escape from the lysosomal compartment as an important pre-requisite for drugs susceptible to degradation in the endolysosomal compartment and therefore able to target specialized organelles to finally exert their action [65]. Griveau and collaborators [70] also demonstrated that surface functionalization of LNCs, especially at chains of poly (ethylene glycol) by incorporating immunoglobulins, offered the possibility of a more specific active targeting. These authors suggested as a new strategy to silence miR-21 using LNA conjugated to lipid nanocapsules (LNCs), demostrating a significant improvement of sensitivity to radiation.

## miRNA Tune the Behavior of GBM Cells to Ionizing Radiation

Radiotherapy is mainly focused on one important property of cancer cells to favorable interfere with a deregulated rate of cellular proliferation. Ionizing radiation (IR) causes water ionization within the cells giving rise to the production of reactive radicals, which subsequently interact with DNA and disrupt the phosphate DNA backbone. DNA strand breaks caused by this interaction can be either repaired or can lead to cell cycle arrest. Depending on the response to the therapy, we can observe a long-term effect of IR, which is manifested as senescence of the tumor cells, or a short term effect which is cell death via programmed cell death pathways [71, 72]. Relapse of the tumor after radiotherapy is common, and then, tumor often progresses into more aggressive forms associated with poor prognosis and resistance to further treatments [2]. It was previously described in several studies that IR triggers DNA repair mechanisms and activates several signaling pathways such as PI3K/AKT [73] or ATM/Chk2/p53 [74], which subsequently lead to higher proliferation, invasivity, and survival of GBM cells. Importantly, these innate or acquired radio-responsive molecular pathways of GBM cells are functionally crossed by the regulatory action of miRNA

The first of this pathway, PI3K/AKT/mTOR, is critical for normal brain development [75]; however, it has also been found to be hyperactivated in brain tumors [76]. Within this cascade, EGFR play an important role as an activator of this pathway since mutations in EGFR lead to tumor cell proliferation, increased survival, angiogenesis, and metastasis. One of the ways of targeting the PI3K/AKT pathway and its downstream components for intervention is offered by miRNA. Study of miRNA expression profiles after IR exposure in the U87-MG cells showed down-regulation of miR-181a. Transient overexpression of miR-181a sensitized these cells to IR and led to down-regulation of mRNA and protein level of BCL-2. BCL-2 is associated with radio-resistance, but also it plays a protective role against apoptotic cell death and is frequently overexpressed in human tumor cells [77, 78]. Another miRNA specifically involved in the AKT signaling is miR-21, which is generally classified as an oncomiR [79]. To confirm this, miR-21 was one of the first identified miRNAs to play an important role in GBM pathogenesis with an anti-apoptotic effect on tumor cells [80]. Basing on this evidence, Li and collaborators [81] reported that a specific miR-21 inhibitor can increase IR-induced growth arrest and apoptosis in U251 GBM cells by abrogating G2-M arrest. More recently, it was reported that this miR can mediate the radiation resistance of GBM cells by regulating important cell cycle genes as PDCD4 and hMSH2 [82]. In addition, Zhou et al. [83] revealed that phosphatase and tensin homolog (PTEN), a direct negative regulator of AKT, was a target gene of miR-21. In another study, PTEN was found to be regulated directly by miR-26a [84]. In particular, de-regulation of miR-26a expression can promote GBM cells growth in vitro and in vivo. Kim and collaborators have interpreted these results on the basis that cell growth can be enhanced either by decreased PTEN, RB1, or MAP3K2/MEKK2 protein expression, which subsequently leads to increased AKT activation and promotes proliferation, or by decrease of c-JUN N-terminal kinase-dependent apoptosis [37]. Additional miRNA linked to AKT regulation are miR-7 and miR-451. The involvement of miR-7 in this pathway was evaluated on U251 and U87-MG cell lines. In particular, the ectopic overexpression of miR-7 attenuated EGFR and AKT expression and radiosensitized both GBM cell lines [44], while miR-451 represses GBM in vitro and in vivo, likely through targeting calcium binding protein 39 gene (CAB39) directly and inhibiting the PI3K/AKT pathway indirectly. Moreover, AKT/cyclinD1/CDK4 survival signaling pathway is activated in radio-resistant cancer cells. Within this altered pathway, CDK4 is a member of the cyclin-dependent kinase family and its overexpression has been described in many tumor types, including oral squamous cell carcinoma [85], pancreatic endocrine tumors [86], lung cancer [87], and glioma [88]. Basing on this evidence, a combination of fractionated radiotherapy and reagents targeting the AKT/cyclin D1/CDK4 pathway, such as a CDK4 inhibitor, has been reported to abolish tumor radio-resistance [89]. Very recently, Deng and collaborators [90] identified CDK4 as a potential downstream target of miR-124 through bioinformatics analysis and by dual-firefly luciferase reporter assay. The authors reported that CDK4 knockdown can sensitize cells to radiation through the miR-124-CDK4 axis, opening new therapeutic perspectives.

In relation to the other main altered pathway, i.e., ATM/Chk2/p53, this was directly related to the radiation resistance behavior of GBM cells. In particular, in response to IR exposition, tumor cells activate the sensor kinases ATM, ATR, and DNA-PKs that in turn phosphorylate multiple downstream mediators, including the checkpoint kinases Chk1 and Chk2, which lead to bypass checkpoints and to the initiation of cell cycle [74]. As a proof of concept, a lower level of ATM was observed in the M059J radio-sensitive GBM cell line when compared to the M059K radio-resistant one, due to deficiency in DNA-PKs expression. This effect might be caused by over-expression of miR-100, which was predicted to be a direct regulator of ATM [91]. In a related study, it was reported that, after IR of both M059K and M059J cell lines, several miRNAs were up-regulated: miR-17-3p, miR-17-5p, miR-19a, miR-19b, miR-142-3p, and miR-142-5p. Moreover, miR-15a, miR-16, miR-21, miR-143, and miR-155 were found to be up-regulated only in the M059K cell line with normal DNA PK activity [92]. Furthermore, among these identified molecules, miR-143 was found to directly target fragile histidine triad (FHIT), which is often down-regulated in epithelial tumors. Cells with homozygous deletion of FHIT show higher resistance to multi-DNA damage inducers, including IR. Interestingly, the overexpression of miR-143 protects cells from DNA damage-induced killing by down-regulation of FHIT expression and leads to significant G2-phase arrest [93]. In relation to miR-155, altered expression profiles were scored in different cancer cells. In particular, it was reported that this miRNA protected the cells against IR and inhibition of this miRNA led to sensitization of cells to radiation [94]. Recently, Poltronieri and collaborators [95] have highlighted the use of miR-155 antagomirs through microvesicles as a novel GMB-targeted therapeutic strategy. The expression of miR-101 was associated with the protein levels of ATM and DNA-PK in the U87-MG cell line. It was reported that up-regulation of miR-101 by lentiviral transduction sensitized tumor cells to radiation both in vitro and in vivo [96].

It is well known that to repair nascent double-strand breaks after irradiation, chromatin remodeling protein complexes are required. To this regard, miR-99 expression was described to correlate with sensitivity to IR as it targets the SWI/SNF chromatin remodeling factor SNF2H/SMARCA5, a component of the ACF1 complex, which in turn plays an important role in double-strand break repair [75]. Moreover, it has been elucidated that reduction of BRCA1 level at the DNA damage site was the result of down-regulation of SNF2H, which was caused by induction of miR-99a and miR-100. These observations were further supported by experiments where ectopic expression of the miR-99 family in cells reduced the rate of overall efficiency of repair by both homologous recombination and non-homologous end joining [97].

Several studies demonstrated therefore that ATM kinase is activated by IR damage of DNA; it stimulates DNA repair and blocks cell cycle progression. One of the mechanisms of ATM function is by ATM-dependent phosphorylation of p53, which either arrests the cell cycle at a restriction point to allow for the DNA damage repair or leads to the apoptosis of damaged cells. The p53 is indeed a central regulator of cell response to stress and it has to be tightly regulated [98]. Bioinformatics analysis suggested that miR-125b is a negative regulator of p53-induced apoptosis [99]. Likewise, miR-34a acts as a tumor suppressor in p53-mutant U251 cells. Overexpression of miR-34a, which is transcriptionally activated through p53, led to cell growth inhibition, cell cycle arrest in G0–G1, induction of apoptosis, and significantly reduced migration and invasion capabilities. Such events could also be due to regulation of SIRT1, which is predicted to be a direct target of miR-34a [100]. This is also supported by a study, where high dosage of IR led to induction of miR-34a and reduced the p53 expression level [101].

Using a genome-wide strategy, hierarchical clustering analysis of expression 1100 miRNAs in three GBM cell lines treated with clinically relevant doses of radiation (2 Gy) revealed significant (3–4-fold) up-regulation of several

miRNA that are implicated in stimulation of survival and proliferation of tumor cells [102]. The set of up-regulated miRNAs includes miR-1285, miR-151-5p, and miR-24-1, which display beneficial effects on tumors by inhibiting the core tumor suppressor p53 (miR-1285) and supporting migration, local metastasis (miR-151-5p), and anti-apoptosis effects (miR-24-1) [103–105]. Overall, activation of these miRNAs might possibly increase tumor radio-resistance in subsequent radiotherapy sessions and stimulate motility of cancer cells, thereby at least partially explaining the evidence on enhanced migration of malignant glioma cells in response to radiotherapy [106]. It could not be excluded that stimulation of production of these miRNAs is primarily attributed to the functional activity of CSCs directed towards the generation of new populations of tumor cells, which are more radio-resistant and malignant compared to the untreated GBM cells.

The radiation treatment of GBM cell lines with normal capacity to repair radiation-induced double strand breaks (DSB) of DNA caused activation of let-7 [92, 102], a family of miRNA that suppresses proliferation of GBM cells [107]. In contrast, in the radiosensitive human GBM cell line M059J that is deficient in DNA-dependent protein kinase (DNA-PK) and has a low activity of ATM, two key members of the non-homologous end joining pathway of DNA-DSB repair, let-7 miRNA, were down-regulated [92]. Further studies showed that reduced expression of ATM in M059J cells is due to the up-regulated synthesis of miR-100, which targets the ATM mRNA [91]. Overexpression of miR-7 was shown to alter the DNA repair machinery in tested cancer cell lines including U251 and U87-MG cells [73]. This miRNA prolongs radiation-induced γH2AX foci formation and down-regulation of DNA-dependent protein kinases (DNA-PKs), thereby making cancer cells vulnerable to radiation exposure. It should be stressed that miR-7 is capable to reduce the radio-resistance of malignant invasive tumors with enhanced EGF receptor PI3K–AKT signaling, a feature that provides advantage in survival of cancer cells treated with radiation

[44]. However, how radiation induces specific miRNA and how they might regulate the DDR remain elusive. Very recently, Li and collaborators [108] found that radiation induced c-jun transcription of miR-221 and miR-222. In turn, miR-221 and miR-222 modulated DNA-PKcs expression to affect DNA damage repair by activating AKT independent of PTEN status. The authors reported that knocking down of miR-221/222 significantly increased radio-sensitivity of GBM cells. On the other side, inhibition of AKT by RNA interference (RNAi) or by LY294002 treatment may overcome miR-221/222-induced radio-resistance. Notably, these data indicated that miR-221/222 play an important role in mediating radio-induced DNA damage repair and that miR-221/222 could serve as potential therapeutic targets for increasing radio-sensitivity of GBM cells [108].

As previously reported, as specific cellular models, the human GBM cell line M059J is deficient in DNA-dependent protein kinase (DNA-PK), whereas their cognate M059K cells, isolated from the same malignant tumor, have normal DNA-PK activity. It can be reasonably argued that, within the transcriptome profile of these cell lines, miRNAs should be differentially modulated in M059J and M059K cells exposed to ionizing radiation and that the miRNA modulation might therefore contribute to the different degree of resistance to ionizing radiation. As a result, miR-15a, miR-16, miR-143, miR-155, and miR-21 were up-regulated in M059K, and the modulation of these miRNAs fluctuated in M059J cells in a time-dependent manner [92].

In another well-known GBM cell line, i.e., U87-MG, miR-181a modulation was shown to radio-sensitize tumor cells by down-regulating the anti-apoptotic protein BCL-2 [77]. This miRNA belongs to the miR-181 family, whose expression is suppressed in tumors including GBM [109]. miR-21, which is up-regulated in gliomas, enhances proliferation, malignancy, chemo- and radio-resistance by affecting a network of key tumor-suppressive pathways, targeting mitogenic kinases [45]. Treatment of U251 cells with miR-21 inhibitor led to decrease in resistance to radiation by elongating radiation-induced cell growth

arrest and increased the level of apoptosis presumably through de-repression of Cdc25A, a cell cycle regulator of the G2–M transition [81]. Because CSCs appear to be the major contributors to the radio-resistance of GBM, further identification of miRNA that substantially increase the vulnerability of brain tumors to radiation therapy may be of high clinical promise for generation of effective anti-cancer drugs that could be used supplementary to the course of radiotherapy in order to increase its efficiency in treatment of high-grade gliomas [55].

In relation to the capability of miRNA to modulate the status and the pro-death or pro-survival balance in GBM, it was recently found by our group that miR-17 modulated autophagy process in T98G GBM cell line, targeting the autophagic gene ATG7 [110]. Down-regulation of miR-17 promoted ATG7 protein expression as well as autophagy induction with a consequent decrease of cell viability and proliferation. Moreover, the combined effect of radiation or TMZ was enhanced after miR-17 down-regulation. Also, miR-21 was recently found to play a role in radio-resistance of different GBM cells [111]. The authors reported that blocking miR-21 with anti-miR-21 specific molecules resulted in radio-sensitization of U373-MG and U87-MG cells, whereas its overexpression led to a decrease in radio-sensitivity of LN18 and LN428 GBM ones. Cell cycle analysis showed a significant increase in the G2/M phase transition by anti-miR-21 administration, observed after irradiation. Interestingly, anti-miR-21 increased the expression of molecular factors associated with autophagosome formation and autophagy activity. Furthermore, augmented autophagy by anti-miR-21 resulted in an increase in the apoptotic population after irradiation [111].

Overall, these observations point to the involvement of miRNAs in the different responses of GBM cells to treatment by IR, modulating DNA repair mechanisms, sensing cell cycle arrest or progression, affecting directly or indirectly signal transduction cascades, and controlling the fate of the cell by the regulation of programmed cell death processes: all these molecular alterations are hallmarks and potential therapeutic targets within brain tumors.

Considering the development of miRNA research from its initial association to glioma to the commercial development of miRNA-based therapeutics in less than a decade, it is not beyond reasonable doubt to anticipate significant advancements in this field of study, hopefully with the ultimate conclusion of improved patient outcome.

## Conclusions

miRNA, recently defined as "small RNA molecules with an huge impact in cancer" [29], can function as potential oncogenes or oncosuppressor genes, depending on the cellular context and on the gene targets they regulate. miRNA expression profiling has indeed provided evidence of the association of these tiny molecules with tumor development and progression. They represent an emerging set of molecules that play key roles in glioma pathogenesis. Differential expression levels of specific tumor suppressive or oncogenic miRNAs can lead to signal transduction abnormalities that are associated with increased survival, growth, and proliferation. As the roles of miRNAs in glioma are better understood and novel delivery methods are developed and optimized, miRNA-based targeted therapies may emerge to possess significant therapeutic potential for tumor treatment. In particular, many intrinsic properties of glioma that contribute to its poor prognosis include difficulties in drug delivery across the blood–brain barrier (BBB). The advent of nanoparticle-mediated delivery and recent progression in RNA molecule delivery across the BBB to both CNS disease and cancer models proves encouraging to the progression of miRNA-based therapeutic efficacy in these complex diseases. miRNA can thus be reasonably considered as novel class of anticancer drugs: efforts are ongoing to develop miRNA-based drugs, either in the form of miRNA mimics, amplifying the impact of a miRNA, or miRNA inhibitors, essentially quenching the effect of the miRNA itself. Furthermore, miRNA-based drugs have the advantage that one miRNA may target and modify the expression of several genes with different roles within the same pathological pathway.

Importantly, miRNAs can also significantly modulate the effect of chemo- and radio-therapy-established protocols: many treatments require the expression of specific genes to function, and these functions can be affected by changes in the expression level of pharmacogenomic genes by means of miRNAs.

While selecting a miRNA as a potential therapeutic agent, we should take into account possible off-targets or opposing effects. For example, depending on the cellular context, miR-146a may exhibit oncogenic or antioncogenic properties. In cells with enhanced NF-κB signaling such as myeloid sarcomas and lymphomas, miR-146a shows tumor-suppressive effect through inhibiting the NF-κB activators interleukin 1 receptor-associated kinase 1 (IRAK1) and TNF receptor-associated factor 6 (TRAF6) [112]. As oncogenic miRNA, miR-146a targets BRCA1, thus preventing the pro-apoptotic effects of BRCA1 and resulting in a pro-survival response [113].

In conclusion, the miRNA-based anti-cancer therapy within glioma, and in particular, in GBM is in its infancy, but harbors a great potential for future clinical applications and interventions. This therapy could be implemented either independently or complimentary to increase the efficiency of other therapies and reduce tumor recurrence after surgical resection. Although therapeutic delivery of miRNAs is still a developing field, and there is much more work to be done before these molecules can be securely applied in clinical settings, miRNA modulation may one day have a therapeutic application in patients.

## References

1. Louis DN, Ohgaki H, Wiestler OD, Cavenee WK, Burger PC, Jouvet A, et al. The 2007 WHO classification of tumours of the central nervous system. Acta Neuropathol. 2007;114:97–109.
2. Stupp R, Mason WP, van den Bent MJ, Weller M, Fisher B, Taphoorn MJB. Radiotherapy plus concomitant and adjuvant temozolomide for glioblastoma. N Engl J Med. 2005;352:987–96.
3. Eramo A, Ricci-Vitiani L, Zeuner A, Pallini R, Lotti F, Sette G, et al. Chemotherapy resistance of glioblastoma stem cells. Cell Death Differ. 2006;13: 1238–41.

4. Singh SK, Hawkins C, Clarke ID, Squire JA, Bayani J, Hide T. Identification of a cancer stem cell in human brain tumors. Nature. 2004;432:396–401.

5. Wilson TA, Karajannis MA, Harter DH. Glioblastoma multiforme: state of the art and future therapeutics. Surg Neurol Int. 2014;5:64.

6. Nakada M, Kita D, Watanabe T, Hayashi Y, Teng L, Pyko IV, et al. Aberrant signaling pathways in glioma. Cancers. 2011;3:3242–78.

7. Palumbo S, Miracco C, Pirtoli L, Comincini S. Emerging roles of microRNA in modulating cell-death processes in malignant glioma. J Cell Physiol. 2014;229:277–86.

8. Roth P, Weller M. Challenges to targeting epidermal growth factor receptor in glioblastoma: escape mechanisms and combinatorial treatment strategies. Neuro Oncol. 2014;16:4–9.

9. Lee JK, Joo KM, Lee J, Yoon Y, Nam DH. Targeting the epithelial to mesenchymal transition in glioblastoma: the emerging role of MET signaling. Onco Targets Ther. 2014;7:1933–44.

10. Chen K, Huang YH, Chen JL. Understanding and targeting cancer stem cells: therapeutic implications and challenges. Acta Pharmacol Sin. 2013;34:732–40.

11. Galli R, Binda E, Orfanelli U, Cipelletti B, Gritti A, De Vitis S, et al. Isolation and characterization of tumorigenic, stem-like neural precursors from human glioblastoma. Cancer Res. 2004;64:7011–21.

12. Cheng JX, Liu BL, Zhang X. How powerful is CD133 as a cancer stem cell marker in brain tumours? Cancer Treat Rev. 2009;35:403–8.

13. Oka N, Soeda A, Noda S, Iwama T. Brain tumor stem cells from an adenoid glioblastoma multiforme. Neurol Med Chir. 2009;49:146–51.

14. Beier D, Wischhusen J, Dietmaier W, Hau P, Proescholdt M, Brawanski A, et al. CD133 expression and cancer stem cells predict prognosis in high-grade oligodendroglial tumors. Brain Pathol. 2008;18:370–7.

15. Liu G, Yuan X, Zeng Z, Tunici P, Ng H, Abdulkadir IR, Lu L, Irvin D, Black KL, Yu JS. Analysis of gene expression and chemoresistance of CD133+ cancer stem cells in glioblastoma. Mol Cancer. 2006;5:67–77.

16. He J, Shan Z, Li L, Liu F, Liu Z, Song M, et al. Expression of glioma stem cell marker CD133 and O6-methylguanine-DNA methyltransferase is associated with resistance to radiotherapy in gliomas. Oncol Rep. 2011;26:1305–13.

17. Bao S, Wu Q, Sathornsumetee S, Hao Y, Li Z, Hjelmeland AB. Stem cell-like glioma cells promote tumor angiogenesis through vascular endothelial growth factor. Cancer Res. 2006;66:7843–8.

18. Ropolo M, Daga A, Griffero F, Foresta M, Casartelli G, Zunino A, et al. Comparative analysis of DNA repair in stem and nonstem glioma cell cultures. Mol Cancer Res. 2009;7:383–92.

19. McCord AM, Jamal M, Williams ES, Camphausen K, Tofilon PJ. CD133+ glioblastoma stem-like cells are radiosensitive with a defective DNA damage response compared with established cell lines. Clin Cancer Res. 2009;15:5145–53.

20. Koshkin PA, Chistiakov DA, Chekhonin VP. Role of microRNAs in mechanisms of glioblastoma resistance to radio- and chemotherapy. Biochemistry. 2013;78:325–34.

21. Bartel DP. MicroRNAs: genomics, biogenesis, mechanism, and function. Cell. 2004;116:281–97.

22. Kim VN. 2005. MicroRNA biogenesis: coordinated cropping and dicing. Nat Rev Mol Cell Biol. 2005;6:376–85.

23. Denli AM, Tops BB, Plasterk RH, Ketting RF, Hannon GJ. Processing of primary microRNAs by the Microprocessor complex. Nature. 2004;432:231–5.

24. Lee Y, Ahn C, Han J, Choi H, Kim J, Yim J, et al. The nuclear RNase III Drosha initiates microRNA processing. Nature. 2003;425:415–9.

25. Gregory RI, Chendrimada TP, Cooch N, Shiekhattar R. Human RISC couples microRNA biogenesis and posttranscriptional gene silencing. Cell. 2005;123:631–40.

26. Visone R, Croce CM. 2009. MiRNAs and cancer. Am J Pathol. 2009;174:1131–8.

27. Croce CM. Causes and consequences of microRNA dysregulation in cancer. Nat Rev Genet. 2009;10:704–14.

28. Soifer HS, Rossi JJ, Saetrom P. MicroRNAs in disease and potential therapeutic applications. Mol Ther. 2007;15:2070–9.

29. Iorio MV, Croce CM. MicroRNAs in cancer: small molecules with a huge impact. J Clin Oncol. 2009;27:5848–56.

30. Lee YS, Dutta A. MicroRNAs: small but potent oncogenes or tumor suppressors. Curr Opin Investig Drugs. 2006;7:560–4.

31. Zhang B, Pan X, Cobb GP, Anderson TA. MicroRNAs as oncogenes and tumor suppressors. Dev Biol. 2007;302:1–12.

32. Kreth S, Thon N, Kreth FW. Epigenetics in human gliomas. Cancer Lett. 2014;342:185–92.

33. Calin GA, Croce CM. MicroRNAs and chromosomal abnormalities in cancer cells. Oncogene. 2006;25:6202–10.

34. Kumar MS, Lu J, Mercer KL, Golub TR, Jacks T. Impaired microRNA processing enhances cellular transformation and tumorigenesis. Nat Genet. 2007;39:673–7.

35. Gaur A, Jewell DA, Liang Y, Ridzon D, Moore JH, Chen C, Ambros VR, et al. Characterization of microRNA expression levels and their biological correlates in human cancer cell lines. Cancer Res. 2007;67:2456–68.

36. Godlewski J, Nowicki MO, Bronisz A, Williams S, Otsuki A, Nuovo G, et al. Targeting of the Bmi-1 oncogene/stem cell renewal factor by microRNA-128 inhibits glioma proliferation and self-renewal. Cancer Res. 2008;68:9125–30.

37. Kim H, Huang W, Jiang X, Pennicooke B, Park PJ, Johnson MD. Integrative genome analysis reveals an oncomir/oncogene cluster regulating glioblastoma survivorship. Proc Natl Acad Sci U S A. 2010;107:2183–8.

38. Ferretti E, De Smaele E, Po A, Di Marcotullio L, Tosi E, Espinola MS, et al. MicroRNA profiling in human medulloblastoma. Int J Cancer. 2009;124:568–77.

39. Pang JC, Kwok WK, Chen Z, Ng HK. Oncogenic role of microRNAs in brain tumors. Acta Neuropathol. 2009;117:599–611.

40. Rao SA, Santosh V, Somasundaram K. Genome-wide expression profiling identifies deregulated miRNAs in malignant astrocytoma. Mod Pathol. 2010;23:1404–17.

41. Turner JD, Williamson R, Almefty KK, Nakaji P, Porter R, Tse V, et al. The many roles of microRNAs in brain tumor biology. Neurosurg Focus. 2010;28, E3.

42. Li Y, Guessous F, Zhang Y, Dipierro C, Kefas B, Johnson E, et al. MicroRNA-34a inhibits glioblastoma growth by targeting multiple oncogenes. Cancer Res. 2009;69:7569–76.

43. Mei J, Bachoo R, Zhang CL. MicroRNA-146a inhibits glioma development by targeting Notch1. Mol Cell Biol. 2011;31:3584–92.

44. Kefas B, Godlewski J, Comeau L, Li Y, Abounader R, Hawkinson M. microRNA-7 inhibits the epidermal growth factor receptor and the Akt pathway and is down-regulated in glioblastoma. Cancer Res. 2008;68:3566–72.

45. Papagiannakopoulos T, Friedmann-Morvinski D, Neveu P, Dugas JC, Gill RM, Huillard E, et al. Pro-neural miR-128 is a glioma tumor suppressor that targets mitogenic kinases. Oncogene. 2008;31:1884–95.

46. Zhang QQ, Xu H, Huang MB, Ma LM, Huang QJ, Yao Q, et al. MicroRNA-195 plays a tumor-suppressor role in human glioblastoma cells by targeting signaling pathways involved in cellular proliferation and invasion. Neuro Oncol. 2012;14:278–87.

47. Al-Nedawi K, Meehan B, Rak J. Microvesicles: messengers and mediators of tumor progression. Cell Cycle. 2009;8:2014–8.

48. Antonyak MA, Li B, Boroughs LK, Johnson JL, Druso JE, Bryant KL, et al. Cancer cell-derived microvesicles induce transformation by transferring tissue transglutaminase and fibronectin to recipient cells. Proc Natl Acad Sci U S A. 2011;108:4852–7.

49. Graner MW, Alzate O, Dechkovskaia AM, Keene JD, Sampson JH, Mitchell DA, et al. Proteomic and immunologic analyses of brain tumor exosomes. FASEB J. 2009;23:1541–57.

50. Skog J, Würdinger T, van Rijn S, Meijer DH, Gainche L, Sena-Esteves M, et al. Glioblastoma microvesicles transport RNA and proteins that promote tumour growth and provide diagnostic biomarkers. Nat Cell Biol. 2008;10:1470–6.

51. Godlewski J, Krichevsky AM, Johnson MD, Chiocca EA, Bronisz A. Belonging to a network-microRNAs, extracellular vesicles, and the glioblastoma microenvironment. Neuro Oncol. 2015;17(5):652–62.

52. Gagliano N, Costa F, Cossetti C, Pettinari L, Bassi R, Chiriva-Internati M, et al. Glioma–astrocyte interaction modifies the astrocyte phenotype in a co-culture experimental model. Oncol Rep. 2009;22:1349–56.

53. Katakowski M, Buller B, Wang X, Rogers T, Chopp M. Functional microRNA is transferred between glioma cells. Cancer Res. 2010;70:8259–63.

54. Valiunas V, Polosina YY, Miller H, Potapova IA, Valiuniene L, Doronin S, et al. Connexin-specific cell to-cell transfer of short interfering RNA by gap junctions. J Physiol. 2005;568:459–68.

55. Chistiakov DA, Chekhonin VP. Contribution of microRNAs to radio- and chemoresistance of brain tumors and their therapeutic potential. Eur J Pharmacol. 2012;684:8–18.

56. Broderick JA, Zamore PD. MicroRNA therapeutics. Gene Ther. 2011;18:1104–10.

57. Kurreck J, Wyszko E, Gillen C, Erdmann VA. Design of antisense oligonucleotides stabilized by locked nucleic acids. Nucleic Acids Res. 2002;30:1911–8.

58. Stenvang J, Kauppinen S. MicroRNAs as targets for antisense-based therapeutics. Expert Opin Biol Ther. 2008;8:59–81.

59. Lanford RE, Hildebrandt-Eriksen ES, Petri A, Persson R, Lindow M, Munk ME, Kauppinen S, Ørum H. Therapeutic silencing of microRNA-122 in primates with chronic hepatitis C virus infection. Science. 2009;327:198–201.

60. Peer D, Karp JM, Hong S, Farokhzad OC, Margalit R, Langer R. Nanocarriers as an emerging platform for cancer therapy. Nat Nanotechnol. 2007;2:751–60.

61. Heurtault B, Saulnier P, Pech B, Proust JE, Benoit JP. A novel phase inversion-based process for the preparation of lipid nanocarriers. Pharm Res. 2002;19:875–80.

62. Allard E, Passirani C, Garcion E, Pigeon P, Vessières A, Jaouen G, et al. Lipid nanocapsules loaded with an organometallic tamoxifen derivative as a novel drug-carrier system for experimental malignant gliomas. J Control Release. 2008;130:146–53.

63. Garcion E, Lamprecht A, Heurtault B, Paillard A, Aubert-Pouessel A, Denizot B, et al. A new generation of anticancer, drug-loaded, colloidal vectors reverses multidrug resistance in glioma and reduces tumor progression in rats. Mol Cancer Ther. 2006;5:1710–22.

64. Lacoeuille F, Garcion E, Benoit JP, Lamprecht A. Lipid nanocapsules for intracellular drug delivery of anticancer drugs. J Nanosci Nanotechnol. 2007;7:4612–7.

65. Paillard A, Hindré F, Vignes-Colombeix C, Benoit JP, Garcion E. The importance of endo-lysosomal escape with lipid nanocapsules for drug subcellular bioavailability. Biomaterials. 2010;31:7542–54.

66. Roger E, Lagarce F, Garcion E, Benoit JP. Lipid nanocarriers improve paclitaxel transport throughout human intestinal epithelial cells by using vesicle-mediated transcytosis. J Control Release. 2009;140:174–81.

67. Weyland M, Manero F, Paillard A, Grée D, Viault G, Jarnet D, et al. Mitochondrial targeting by use of lipid nanocapsules loaded with SV30, an analogue of the small-molecule Bcl-2 inhibitor HA14-1. J Control Release. 2011;151:74–82.

68. Ballot S, Noiret N, Hindré F, Denizot B, Garin E, Rajerison H, et al. 99mTc/188Re-labelled lipid nanocapsules as promising radiotracers for imaging and therapy: formulation and biodistribution. Eur J Nucl Med Mol Imaging. 2006;33:602–7.

69. Vanpouille-Box C, Lacoeuille F, Roux J, Aubé C, Garcion E, Lepareur N, et al. Lipid nanocapsules loaded with rhenium-188 reduce tumor progression in a rat hepatocellular carcinoma model. PLoS One. 2011;6, e16926.

70. Griveau I, Bejaud J, Anthiya S, Avril S, Autret D, Garcion E. Silencing of miR-21 by locked nucleic acid-lipid nanocapsule complexes sensitize human glioblastoma cells to radiation-induced cell death. Int J Pharm. 2013;454:765–74.

71. Palumbo S, Comincini S. Autophagy and ionizing radiation in tumors: the "survive or not survive" dilemma. J Cell Physiol. 2013;228:1–8.

72. Yu KN, Han W. Ionizing radiation, DNA double strand break, and mutation. In: Urbano KV, editor. Advances in genetics research, vol. 4. New York: Nova Science; 2010.

73. Lee KM, Choi EJ, Kim IA. microRNA-7 increases radiosensitivity of human cancer cells with activated EGFR-associated signaling. Radiother Oncol. 2011;101:171–6.

74. Squatrito M, Brennan CW, Helmy K, Huse JT, Petrini JH, Holland EC. Loss of ATM/Chk2/p53 pathway components accelerates tumor development and contributes to radiation resistance in gliomas. Cancer Cell. 2010;18:619–29.

75. Besse A, Sana J, Fadrus P, Slaby O. MicroRNAs involved in chemo- and radioresistance of high-grade gliomas. Tumour Biol. 2013;34:1969–78.

76. Guillamo JS, de Boüard S, Valable S, Marteau L, Leuraud P, Marie Y. Molecular mechanisms underlying effects of epidermal growth factor receptor inhibition on invasion, proliferation, and angiogenesis in experimental glioma. Clin Cancer Res. 2009;15:3697–704.

77. Chen G, Zhu W, Shi D, Lv L, Zhang C, Liu P. MicroRNA-181a sensitizes human malignant glioma U87MG cells to radiation by targeting Bcl-2. Oncol Rep. 2010;23:997–1003.

78. Hara T, Omura-Minamisawa M, Kang Y, Cheng C, Inoue T. Flavopiridol potentiates the cytotoxic effects of radiation in radioresistant tumor cells in which p53 is mutated or Bcl-2 is overexpressed. Int J Radiat Oncol Biol Phys. 2008;71:1485–95.

79. Krichevsky AM, Gabriely G. miR-21: a small multi-faceted RNA. J Cell Mol Med. 2009;13:39–53.

80. Chan JA, Krichevsky AM, Kosik KS. MicroRNA-21 is an antiapoptotic factor in human glioblastoma cells. Cancer Res. 2005;65:6029–33.

81. Li Y, Zhao S, Zhen Y, Li Q, Teng L, Asai A, Kawamoto K. A miR-21 inhibitor enhances apoptosis and reduces G(2)-M accumulation induced by ionizing radiation in human glioblastoma U251 cells. Brain Tumor Pathol. 2011;28:209–14.

82. Chao TF, Xiong HH, Liu W, Chen Y, Zhang JX. MiR-21 mediates the radiation resistance of glioblastoma cells by regulating PDCD4 and hMSH2. J Huazhong Univ Sci Technolog Med Sci. 2013;33:525–9.

83. Zhou X, Ren Y, Moore L, Mei M, You Y, Mei P. Downregulation of miR-21 inhibits EGFR pathway and suppresses the growth of human glioblastoma cells independent of PTEN status. Lab Invest. 2010;90:144–55.

84. Huse JT, Brennan C, Hambardzumyan D, Wee B, Pena J, Rouhanifard SH. The PTEN-regulating microRNA miR-26a is amplified in high-grade glioma and facilitates gliomagenesis in vivo. Genes Dev. 2009;23:1327–37.

85. Poomsawat S, Buajeeb W, Khovidhunkit SO, Punyasingh J. Alteration in the expression of cdk4 and cdk6 proteins in oral cancer and premalignant lesions. J Oral Pathol Med. 2010;39:793–9.

86. Lindberg D, Hessman O, Akerstrom G, Westin G. Cyclin dependent kinase 4 (CDK4) expression in pancreatic endocrine tumors. Neuroendocrinology. 2007;86:112–8.

87. Dobashi Y, Goto A, Fukayama M, Abe A, Ooi A. Overexpression of cdk4/cyclin D1, a possible mediator of apoptosis and an indicator of prognosis in human primary lung carcinoma. Int J Cancer. 2004;110:532–41.

88. Zhang L, Yamane T, Satoh E, Amagasaki K, Kawataki T, Asahara T, et al. Establishment and partial characterization of five malignant glioma cell lines. Neuropathology. 2005;25:136–43.

89. Shimura T, Noma N, Oikawa T, Ochiai Y, Kakuda S. Activation of the AKT/cyclin D1/Cdk4 survival signaling pathway in radioresistant cancer stem cells. Oncogenesis. 2012;1:e12.

90. Deng X, Ma L, Wu M, Zhang G, Jin C, Guo Y, et al. miR-124 radiosensitizes human glioma cells by targeting CDK4. J Neurooncol. 2013;114:263–74.

91. Ng WL, Yan D, Zhang X, Mo YY, Wang Y. Overexpression of miR-100 is responsible for the low-expression of ATM in the human glioma cell line: M059J. DNA Repair. 2010;9:1170–5.

92. Chaudhry MA, Sachdeva H, Omaruddin RA. Radiation-induced micro-RNA modulation in glioblastoma cells differing in DNA-repair pathways. DNA Cell Biol. 2010;29:553–61.

93. Lin Y-X, Yu F, Gao N, Sheng J-P, Qiu J-Z, Hu B-C. microRNA-143 protects cells from DNA damage-induced killing by downregulating FHIT expression. Cancer Biother Radiopharm. 2011;26:365–72.

94. Babar IA, Czochor J, Steinmetz A, Weidhaas JB, Glazer PM, Slack FJ. Inhibition of hypoxia-induced miR-155 radiosensitizes hypoxic lung cancer cells. Cancer Biol Ther. 2011;12:908–14.

95. Poltronieri PI, D'Urso PI, Mezzolla V, D'Urso OF. Potential of anti-cancer therapy based on anti-miR-155 oligonucleotides in glioma and brain tumours. Chem Biol Drug Des. 2013;81:79–84.

96. Yan D, Ng WL, Zhang X, Wang P, Zhang Z, Mo Y-Y. Targeting DNA-PKcs and ATM with miR-101 sensitizes tumors to radiation. PLoS One. 2010;5, e11397.

97. Mueller AC, Sun D, Dutta A. The miR-99 family regulates the DNA damage response through its target SNF2H. Oncogene. 2012;32:1164–72.

98. Mirzayans R, Andrais B, Scott A, Murray D. New insights into p53 signaling and cancer cell response to DNA damage: implications for cancer therapy. J Biomed Biotechnol. 2012;2012:170325. doi:10.1155/2012/170325.

99. Le MTN, Teh C, Shyh-Chang N, Xie H, Zhou B, Korzh V. MicroRNA-125b is a novel negative regulator of p53. Genes Dev. 2009;23:862–76.

100. Luan S, Sun L, Huang F. MicroRNA-34a: a novel tumor suppressor in p53-mutant glioma cell line U251. Arch Med Res. 2010;41:67–74.

101. Sasaki A, Udaka Y, Tsunoda Y, Yamamoto G, Tsuji M, Oyamada H. Analysis of p53 and miRNA expression after irradiation of glioblastoma cell lines. Anticancer Res. 2012;32:4709–13.

102. Niemoeller OM, Niyazi M, Corradini S, Zehentmayr F, Li M, Lauber K, et al. MicroRNA expression profiles in human cancer cells after ionizing radiation. Radiat Oncol. 2011;6:29–37.

103. Ding J, Huang S, Wu S, Zhao Y, Liang L, Yan M, Ge C, et al. Gain of miR-151 on chromosome 8q24.3 facilitates tumor cell migration and spreading through downregulating RhoGDIA. Nat. Cell Biol. 2010;12:390–9.

104. Qin W, Shi Y, Zhao B, Yao C, Jin L, Ma J, et al. miR-24 regulates apoptosis by targeting the open reading frame (ORF) region of FAF1 in cancer cells. PLoS One. 2010;5:e9429.

105. Tian S, Huang S, Wu S, Guo W, Li J, He X. MicroRNA-1285 inhibits the expression of p53 by directly targeting its 3′ untranslated region. Biochem Biophys Res Commun. 2010;396:435–9.

106. Wild-Bode C, Weller M, Rimner A, Dichgans J, Wick W. Sublethal irradiation promotes migration and invasiveness of glioma cells: implications for radiotherapy of human glioblastoma. Cancer Res. 2001;61:2744–50.

107. Lee ST, Chu K, Oh HJ, Im WS, Lim JY, Kim SK, et al. Let-7 microRNA inhibits the proliferation of human glioblastoma cells. DNA Cell Biol. 2010;29:553–61.

108. Li W, Guo F, Wang P, Hong S, Zhang C. miR-221/222 confers radioresistance in glioblastoma cells through activating Akt independent of PTEN status. Curr Mol Med. 2014;14:185–95.

109. Shi L, Cheng Z, Zhang J, Li R, Zhao P, Fu Z, et al. hsa-mir-181a and hsa-mir-181b function as tumor suppressors in human glioma cells. Brain Res. 2008;1236:185–93.

110. Comincini S, Allavena G, Palumbo S, Morini M, Durando F, Angeletti F, et al. microRNA-17 regulates the expression of ATG7 and modulates the autophagy process, improving the sensitivity to temozolomide and low-dose ionizing radiation treatments in human glioblastoma cells. Cancer Biol Ther. 2013;14:574–86.

111. Gwak HS, Kim TH, Jo GH, Kim YJ, Kwak HJ, Kim JH, et al. Silencing of microRNA-21 confers radiosensitivity through inhibition of the PI3K/AKT pathway and enhancing autophagy in malignant glioma cell lines. PLoS One. 2012;7, e47449.

112. Taganov KD, Boldin MP, Chang KJ, Baltimore D. NF-kappaB-dependent induction of microRNA miR-146, an inhibitor targeted to signaling proteins of innate immune responses. Proc Natl Acad Sci U S A. 2006;103:12481–6.

113. Hsieh CH, Rau CS, Jeng SF, Lin CJ, Chen YC, Wu CJ, et al. Identification of the potential target genes of microRNA-146a induced by PMA treatment in human microvascular endothelial cells. Exp Cell Res. 2010;316:1119–26.

# NanoMaterials Technology for Research Radiobiology

## 15

### Elisa Panzarini and Luciana Dini

## Introduction

A considerable progress towards the understanding of cancer hallmarks and the consequent improvement of the detection and treatment modalities has been achieved in the past decade rendering many cancers curable [1]. A lot of diagnostic and treatment options, *i.e.*, magnetic resonance imaging (MRI), Computed Tomography (CT), biosensing, radiotherapy, chemotherapy, gene therapy, and immunotherapy, are in use for monitoring and fighting cancer. However, each of these options has limitations and side effects, thus cancer still remains leading cause of death. The recent development of nanotechnology has led to devise versatile cancer diagnostic and treatment solutions able to circumvent the limitations of the conventional therapies. A wide range of NanoMaterials (NMs)/nanodevices (NDs) has been designed, studied, and exploited in oncomedicine. These NMs/NDs include polymeric and inorganic, metallic and non-metallic NanoParticles (NPs), *i.e.*, dendrimers, liposomes, polymersomes, polymeric

micelles, nanospheres, fullerenes, quantum dots (QDs), and superparamagnetic iron oxide NPs (SPIONs) [2], and many of them are already used in medicine. Recently, nanotechnology has brought a broad array of smart multifunctional nanosized platforms that combine diagnostic/imaging and therapeutical aspects by means of advanced functionality, as for example, the internal and external stimuli-responsiveness in a highly targeted fashion to the diseased area. This emerging methodology is allowing a real-time monitoring drug delivery, release, and efficacy.

Along with surgery and chemotherapy, radiotherapy represents an important tool in cancer treatment. In fact, approximately 50 % of all cancer patients undergo radiotherapy during the course of disease, contributing to the 40 % of cancer cure [3]. Due to its importance in cancer management, both imaging and therapy, many efforts are currently done to design new radiation techniques for the improvement of survival and life quality of cancer patients.

Here we describe a comprehensive overview of the different NMs exploitable in cancer radiotherapy and imaging, shedding a light on the emerging possibilities of theranostic nanomedicines in fighting cancer. We discuss the advancements of NMs in drug delivery, imaging, diagnosis, and therapy and their future clinical application in gliomas. In fact, among different kinds of malignancies, glioblastoma multiforme (GBM) is one of the most deadly diseases affect-

E. Panzarini • L. Dini (✉)
Department of Biological and Environmental Science and Technology (Di.S.Te.B.A.), University of Salento, Prov. le Lecce-Monteroni, Lecce  73100, Italy
e-mail: elisa.panzarini@unisalento.it; luciana.dini@unisalento.it

© Springer International Publishing Switzerland 2016
L. Pirtoli et al. (eds.), *Radiobiology of Glioblastoma*, Current Clinical Pathology,
DOI 10.1007/978-3-319-28305-0_15

ing humans and represents the second cause of cancer death in adults less than 35 years old. Thus, alternative imaging/diagnostic and therapeutic approaches are urgently needed.

## NMs in Fighting Cancer

NMs consist in nanoscale (1–100 nm) constructs, synthesized from organic and inorganic materials, defined by European Commission as "A natural, incidental or manufactured material containing particles, in an unbound state or as an aggregate or as an agglomerate and where, for 50 % or more of the particles in the number size distribution, one or more external dimensions is in the size range 1–100 nm. In specific cases and where warranted by concerns for the environment, health, safety or competitiveness the number size distribution threshold of 50 % may be replaced by a threshold between 1 and 50 %" (European Commission, 18 October 2011).

Nanotechnology strongly impacts cancer medicine via development of NMs for diagnosis and therapy able to circumvent the limitations of approved clinical treatment. In fact, cancer is a major cause of death and economic constraints in human life.

A multifunctional nanosystem (payload for imaging, sensing, or therapy, and optional targeting ligands) is the essential component in nanomedicine. The design of nanosystems exploits the features of tumor cells and/or sites, such as enhanced permeability and retention (EPR) effect, pH of the tumor site environment, and proteins or glycoproteins overexpressed on cancer cell surface, to circumvent the major limitations of several therapeutic/imaging agents, *i.e.*, poor solubility, rapid deactivation, unfavorable pharmacokinetics, and limited biodistribution, improving the effectiveness of delivered molecules [2].

For the rapid and the effective clinical translation, several aspects should be controlled: (1) particle size, which dictates NMs distribution, clearance, and payload uptake; (2) biocompatibility; (3) circulating half-life, rate of aggregation, and shelf-life; (4) stealth properties, which allow immunological recognition escape and serum protein interactions; (5) functionalization to achieve differential target specificity; (6) release mechanisms of delivered molecules [4]. A wide range of NMs, whose features are reviewed in [2], has been designed to reach tumors, including polymeric NPs, liposomes, micelles, dendrimers, carbon nanotubes, gold nanoparticles, nanoshells, nanocages, and nanofibers. In Fig. 15.1, examples of the most used NMs in drug delivery are reported.

Payload may be adsorbed or attached to or encapsulated in the nanocarriers. Their targeting can be passive or active; the first exploits the characteristic biological features of target tissue, whereas in active approaches, nanocarriers are conjugated with molecules, such as proteins (mainly antibodies and their fragments), nucleic acids (aptamers), or other receptor ligands (peptides, vitamins, and carbohydrates), able to bind overexpressed antigens or receptors present on the target cell surface. In addition, active targeting can be also achieved through manipulation of physical stimuli (e.g., temperature, pH, magnetism) [5]. Although many different types of NPs have been studied for cancer diagnosis and tumor drug delivery and release, each of them can exhibit different and sometimes unique properties, allowing different applications. In Table 15.1, a list of nano-based platforms on the market whose applications span from drug delivery, imaging, and therapy and their current stage of development for cancer therapy is reported.

## Radionanomedicine: An Emerging Nanoplatform for Cancer Imaging and Therapy

Radionanomedicine is an emerging nanotechnology field exploiting NMs for cancer detection (*i.e.*, in vivo molecular and cellular imaging) and treatment. One of the most important advantages of radionanomaterials is their capability not to alter the original characteristics of the entrapped drug molecule/radionuclide. In vivo delivery of radioisotopes strictly depends on the half-life of radioisotopes, on the amount of radioisotopes ensured by carrier, on the pharmacokinetics, on the choice

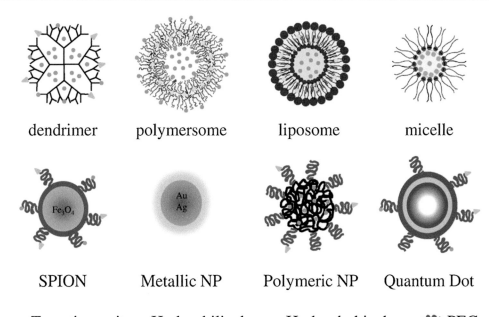

dendrimer        polymersome        liposome        micelle

SPION        Metallic NP        Polymeric NP        Quantum Dot

► Targeting unit    • Hydrophilic drug    • Hydrophobic drug    𝓃𝓌 PEG

**Fig. 15.1** Different types of NMs used in oncomedicine to deliver therapeutic molecules. Lipid-based (liposomes and micelles) and polymer-based (NPs and polymersomes) carriers, metallic and magnetic (SPIONs) NPs, dendrimers, and quantum dot are represented. Hydrophilic, attached or encapsulate, and hydrophobic encapsulated drugs, specific targeting moiety, and polymer (PEG)-stabilizing nanocarrier are represented

of tumor biomarkers to specifically drive radioisotopes into cancer cells, and on the specific tumor targeting ligands. Moreover, cancer management is taking advantage by the theranostic approach that, at the same time, ensures the delivery of therapeutic radioisotopes and provides an imaging tool to track and quantify accumulated radioisotopes. In this context, the exploitation of nanotechnology could allow an earlier detection and a better treatment of cancer [6].

## NMs in Radio-imaging

Up to date, the commonly used molecular imaging modalities include computed tomography (CT), positron emission tomography (PET), single photon emission computed tomography (SPECT), molecular magnetic resonance imaging (mMRI), contrast-enhanced ultrasound (CEU), and optical imaging, both bioluminescence and near-infrared fluorescence (NIRF). Each imaging modality has its own advantages and limitations. A great deal is deriving from the noninvasive imaging provided by NMs; thus, in recent years, a number of nanoformulations have been designed solely for diagnostic purposes. To circumvent the limitations, combinations of imaging techniques, called "multimodality imaging", are being designed [7]. Molecular imaging with multimodality and multifunction devices greatly accelerates the development of radionuclide-based multimodal molecular imaging. PET and SPECT, by measuring chemical changes that occur before the detection of macroscopic anatomical signs of a disease and by tracing in vivo biodistribution of a molecular imaging probe, are the two major radionuclide imaging modalities. Many radiolabeled NMs for multimodality tumor imaging are usually constituted by three major components: core, radionuclide, and targeting biomolecule. The last serves as carrier for specific delivery of the radionuclide conjugated to the core [8]. The NMs able to act as contrast agents for multimodality imaging have been summarized in a recent review article [8]. In

**Table 15.1** Examples of NMs in oncomedicine

| NMs (size range) | Compound (Trade name) | Applications | Target | Status | Company |
|---|---|---|---|---|---|
| Liposome (~100 nm) | Doxorubicin (Doxil/Caelyx) | Chemotherapy | Kaposi's sarcoma ovarian cancer | Approved | Ortho Biotech |
| | Daunorubicin (DaunoXome) | Chemotherapy | Breast cancer | Approved | Galen Ltd. |
| | Doxorubicin (Myocet | Chemotherapy in combination with cyclophosphamide | Metastatic breast cancer | Approved | Sopherion Therapeutics and Chepahlon, Inc. |
| | Doxorubicin (ThermoDox) | Chemotherapy | Hepatocellular carcinoma | Approved Phase III | Celsion |
| | Vincristine (Onco TCS) | Chemotherapy | Non-Hodgkin's lymphoma | Phase III | Inex Pharmaceuticals Corporation |
| | Cytarabine (DepoCyt) | Chemotherapy | Neoplastic meningitis Lymphomatous meningitis | Approved | Sigma-tau Pharmaceuticals, Inc. |
| | Cytarabine/Daunorubicin (CPX-351) | Chemotherapy | Acute myeloid leukemia | Phase III | Celator Pharmaceuticals |
| | Active metabolite of irinotecan SN38 | Chemotherapy | Metastatic colorectal cancer | Phase II | NeoPharm, Inc. |
| | Thymidylate synthase inhibitor (OSI-7904L) | Chemotherapy | Solid tumors | Phase II | OSI Pharmaceuticals |
| | Lurtotecan (OSI-211) | Chemotherapy | Topotecan-resistant ovarian cancer Metastatic or loco-regional recurrent squamous cell carcinoma of the head and neck | Phase II | OSI Pharmaceuticals |
| Polymer (50–200 nm) | Pegaspargase (Oncaspar) | Chemotherapy | Acute lymphoblastic leukemia | Approved | Sigma-tau Pharmaceuticals, Inc. |
| | Doxorubicin | Chemotherapy | Breast/Lung cancer | Phase II | Pharmacia and Upjohn |
| | Paclitaxel | Chemotherapy | Breast cancer | Phase II | Genentech, Inc. |

| Material | Agent | Application | Target | Status | Company |
|---|---|---|---|---|---|
| Iron oxide NPs (1–150 nm) | (Feridex) | MRI Imaging | Liver | Approved | Berlex Laboratories |
| | (Endorem) | MRI Imaging | Liver | Approved | Guerbet |
| | (Resovist/Supravist) | MRI Imaging | Liver | Approved | Bayer Schering Pharma AG |
| | (Lumirem), (Sinerem) | Enhanced MRI | Gastrointestinal | Approved | Guebert |
| | (Combidex) | Tumor Imaging | Prostate cancer | Phase III | Advanced Magnetics |
| | (Clariscan) | Targeted MRI contrast | Renal carcinoma | Phase III | Nycomed Amersham Imaging |
| | NanoTherm | AC Magnetic Heating | Glioblastoma | EU Approved | MagForce, Nanotechnologies AG |
| Polymeric NPs (1–150 nm) | Camptothecin (CRLX101) | Chemotherapy | Camptothecin (CRLX101) | Phase II | Cerulean Pharma, Inc. |
| | Cisplatin (NC-6004) | Chemotherapy | Breast cancer | Phase I | NanoCarrier Co. |
| | Paclitaxel (NK-105) | Chemotherapy | Ovarian, non-small cell lung, breast and stomach cancers | Phase II | Nippon Kayaku Co. Ltd. |
| | Doxorubicin (NK-911) | Chemotherapy | Solid tumors | Phase II | Nippon Kayaku Co. Ltd. |
| | Docetaxel (BIND-014) | Chemotherapy | Various cancers | Phase I | BIND Bioscience |
| Micelles (10–100 nm) | Paclitaxel (Genexol-PM) | Chemotherapy | Breast cancer | Phase IV | Samyang Biopharmaceuticals Corporation |
| | Active metabolite of irinotecan SN38 (NK-012) | Chemotherapy | Myeloma | Phase II | Nippon Kayaku Co. Ltd. |
| Dendrimers (1–10 nm) | Methotrexate | Chemotherapy | Several different cancers | In vitro/In vivo | – |
| Carbon nanotubes (1–25 nm diameter) | Paclitaxel | Chemotherapy | Breast cancer | In vivo | – |
| Quantum dots (1–10 nm) | Doxorubicin | Chemotherapy | Ovarian, breast, and prostate cancer | In vivo | – |

Table 15.2, representative radiolabeled NMs for single or multimodality tumor imaging are reported on the basis of delivery modality, *i.e.*, active or passive targeting.

## NMs in Radiotherapy

Radiotherapy (RT) utilizes high-dose ionizing radiations as X-rays, γ rays, high energy particles, *i.e.*, α- and β-particle emitters, and Auger electron emitters, to kill cancer cells preventing tumor progression and recurrence. However, one of the major limitations in the radioisotopes delivery is their rapid elimination and widespread distribution even into normal organs and tissues, thus requiring large quantity agent administration that results in undesirable toxicity. Three major approaches improve radiation therapy: enhancement of tumor radiosensitization, reversal of tumor radiation resistance, and enhancement of radioresistance of the healthy tissue. Depending on radiation modality, radiotherapy can be external, internal (named brachytherapy), or systemic. In particular, NMs offer great opportunities in internal and systemic radiotherapy.

### NMs as Radiosensitizers.

NMs play a key role in the contrast of tumor radioresistance by acting as therapeutic as well as carrier for other drugs. NMs used as radiation sensitizers are metal (Au-, Gd-, Ti-, Ag-, and Hf-based) and non-metal (silicon- and fullerene-based) NPs, QDs, and SPIONs [10].

Preclinical studies have reported that gold NPs (AuNPs) radiosensitization is a promising novel approach to enhance the effects of radiation with different photon beams mainly due to the high atomic number (Z) of gold (Z=79). The tumor dose radiation enhancement due to AuNPs is estimated by Monte Carlo simulation [11]. AuNPs are relatively easy and inexpensive to be synthetized in a wide range of sizes (2–500 nm), possess highly reactive surfaces easily modifiable to enhance targeting, and exploit EPR to accumulate in tumor cells. The first evidence of AuNPs as radiation sensitizers has been reported

by Hainfeld et al. [12], which demonstrated that 86 % mice bearing subcutaneous EMT-6 mammary carcinomas survived 1-year *vs* 20 % of mice treated with X-rays alone and 0 % with gold alone. The increase in safely tumor ablation was dependent on the amount of injected AuNPs; indeed, high metal content in tumors is necessary for significant high-Z radioenhancement, but it is not toxic for mice and largely cleared by kidney [12]. The use of an intravenous administration of AuNPs before RT was efficacious in enhancing RT outcome, as showed for the highly aggressive radiation resistant SCCCVII squamous cell carcinoma head and neck mouse tumor model [13]. AuNPs enhance RT efficacy at 42 Gy energy dose of irradiation and 68 KeV median energy into the tumor by inducing 67 % long-time survival of mice with subcutaneous SCCVII tumor. The efficacy strictly depends on radiation dose rate and energy. At the same radiation dose (about 42 Gy), AuNPs are more effective when used at 68 keV than at 157 keV; likewise, at 68 and 157 keV, radiation energy in the presence of AuNPs during irradiation is more effective at 42 Gy dose than 30 Gy and at 50.6 Gy dose than 44 Gy, respectively [13]. The possibility of utilizing AuNPs as RT adjuvant has been also demonstrated by using human U251 glioblastoma cell line [14], which expresses the relevant pathobiological features of human GBM. GBM is the most common primary malignancy of the brain representing the second cause of cancer death in adults less than 35 years old, whose average survival is approximately 15 months with only 3–5 % of patients surviving longer than 36 months [15]. AuNPs can effectively radiosensitize U251 cells to 4 Gy RT, leading to enhanced DNA damage in in vitro assay and delayed tumor growth and improved survival in in vivo experiments of xenograft-implanted mice. The synergism between RT and AuNPs results in improvement of extravasation and in-tumor deposition of AuNPs [14]. Moreover, it has been demonstrated that the use of NPs in combination with hyperthermic treatment (44 °C for 20 min) allows to reduce therapeutic radiation dose able to kill SCCVII in mice [13]. Several recent studies

**Table 15.2** Representative radiolabeled NMs for single or multimodality tumor imaging (adapted from [8, 9])

| NMs type | Radionuclides | Imaging methods | Applications |
|---|---|---|---|
| *Active targeting* | | | |
| Immunoliposome | $^{111}$In | Gamma imaging | $^{111}$In-liposome-2C5(mAb) nucleosome-specific monoclonal 2C5 targeting delivery vehicles for tumor visualization of murine Lewis lung carcinoma and human HT-29 tumor |
| Perfluorocarbon NPs | $^{111}$In | Gamma imaging | Imaging of targeted tumor angiogenesis of $\alpha_v\beta_3$-integrin in Vx-2 rabbit tumors |
| Carbon nanotubes | $^{111}$In | Gamma or SPECT imaging | Multifunctional targeted delivery and imaging with functionalized and bioconjugated $^{111}$In-DOTA-CNT-Rituximab nanoconstructs |
| QDs | $^{64}$Cu | Bifunctional PET/NIRF imaging | Dual-functional targeted delivery with amine functionalized $^{64}$Cu-DOTA-QD-RGD for tumor angiogenesis PET/NIRF imaging |
| QDs | $^{64}$Cu | Bifunctional PET/NIRF imaging | Dual-functional targeted delivery with amine functionalized $^{64}$Cu-DOTA-QD-VEGF for tumor angiogenesis PET/NIRF imaging |
| QDs | $^{18}$F | Bifunctional PET/optical imaging | $^{18}$F labeled phospholipids QD micelles for in vivo multimodal imaging |
| Iron oxide | $^{64}$Cu | Bifunctional PET/MRI imaging | $^{64}$Cu-DOTA-IO-RGD for tumor visualization of nude mice bearing U87MG tumors |
| Iron oxide | $^{18}$F | Trimodel MRI/PET-CT/optical imaging | $^{18}$F labeled iron oxide for in vivo PET-CT imaging |
| Iron oxide | $^{111}$In | SPECT/MRI | $^{111}$In-labeled antimesothelin antibody ($^{111}$In-mAbMB) with SPIONs for SPECT/MRI imaging of mesothelioma |
| Iron oxide | $^{64}$Cu | PET/MRI/Optical | $^{64}$Cu-Cy5.5-HSA-IONPs for tri-modality imaging of nude mice bearing U87MG tumors |
| Iron oxide | $^{124}$I | PET/MRI/Optical | Cross-linked, superparamagnetic iron oxide nanoparticle (TCL-SPION) labeled with $^{124}$I for PET/MRI/optical imaging of 4T1 breast tumor |

(continued)

**Table 15.2** (continued)

| NMs type | Radionuclides | Imaging methods | Applications |
|---|---|---|---|
| Lanthanide nanocrystals | $^{124}$I | PET/MRI/Optical | $^{124}$I-labeled $Er^{3+}$/$Yb^{3+}$ co-doped NaGdF4 upconversion nanophosphors (UCNPs) functionalized with RGD peptide for multimodal imaging of tumor angiogenesis |
| Micelle | $^{111}$In | SPECT/NIRF | Core cross-linked polymeric micelles conjugated with $^{111}$In-labeled annexin A5 for dual-modality SPECT/NIRF imaging of tumor apoptosis |
| Ferritin nanocages | $^{64}$Cu | PET/NIRF | Integrin $\alpha_v\beta_3$-targeted PET/NIRF imaging with Ferritin nanocages loaded with RGD peptides, $^{64}$Cu, and Cy5.5 |
| Cobalt–ferrite NPs | $^{67}$Ga | SPECT/MRI/Optical | $^{67}$Ga-labeled cobalt–ferrite NPs conjugated with the AS1411 aptamer for multimodal imaging of C6 tumor |
| Polymer | $^{99m}$Tc | Scintigraphic images of tumor targeting | Targeting tumor angiogenesis: comparison of $^{99m}$Tc-peptide and $^{99m}$Tc-polymer-peptide conjugates |
| Dendrimers | $^{76}$Br | RGD directed-dendrimers PET imaging | $^{76}$Br labeled RGD-directed-dendritic nanoprobes for PET imaging of angiogenesis |
| AuNPs | – | CT imaging | Detection of PEG-anti-Her2(mAbs) of 1.5 mm-thick mouse tumor models |
| | – | CT imaging | Detection of EGFR-AuNPs coated in mice bearing head and neck squamous tumors |
| | – | CT imaging | Accumulation of GRP-receptor-specific Au-NPs bombesin (BBN)-linked constructs in prostate-tumor-bearing immunodeficient mice |
| | – | CT imaging | AuNPs with layer-by-layer (LBL) assembly of poly(acrylic acid) (PAA) and poly(allylamine hydrochloride) (PAH) to detect human hepatocellular carcinoma cell line |
| | $^{99m}$Tc | SPECT/CT | AuNP c[RGDfk(C)] conjugates labeled with $^{99m}$Tc to detect tumor in athymic mice bearing C6 human glioma |

(continued)

**Table 15.2** (continued)

| NMs type | Radionuclides | Imaging methods | Applications |
|---|---|---|---|
| *Passive targeting* | | | |
| Liposome | $^{99m}Tc$ | Gamma imaging | Multitude diagnostics of tumor |
| | $^{111}In$ | Gamma/SPECT imaging | Clinical biodistribution, PK and imaging studies of breast, head, and neck, glioma and lung cancer patients |
| | $^{18}F$ | PET imaging | Liposomal tracking in vivo with $^{18}F$-liposome-PET imaging |
| | $^{111}In$, $^{177}Lu$ | Gamma/SPECT imaging | Gamma imaging of tumor targeting for C26 and HT29/luc animal models |
| | $^{64}Cu$ | PET imaging | Passive-targeted delivery and imaging with bioconjugated $^{64}Cu$-BAT-PEG-liposome |

(reviewed in [16]) have focused on the improved tumor radiosensitization to X-ray beams by AuNPs.

The efficacy in treating tumors of proton therapy (PT) following metal NPs administration has been recently suggested. PT is a type of external RT that uses a beam of proton to irradiate the tumor area. Due to their relatively large mass, protons have little lateral side scatter in the tissue and the beam focuses on the tumor delivering only low-dose side-effects to surrounding tissue. Furthermore, the dose delivered to tissue has its maximum of efficacy at the so-called Bragg peak. The proton-charged particles damage the DNA leading to kill cells or to block their proliferation [17]. The impact of protons on metallic NPs produces the release of secondary electrons and characteristic X-rays by the particle-induced X-ray emission (PIXE) effect that improve proton tumor dose adsorbed by the tumor cells. Kim and coworkers [18–21] demonstrated the effectiveness of therapeutic application of metallic NPs (AuNPs and FeNPs), combined with PIXE effect. 45 MeV proton beam irradiating C6 glioma cells, previously uptakening SPIONs, induces 20–28 % less cell survival compared to only irradiated sample [18]. Also, SPIONs intravenous injected before 45 meV proton beam irra-

diation induce tumor volume regression in C6 Sprague Darley rats glioma model [19]. The authors also demonstrated the efficacy of combining 45 MeV proton beam and AuNPs and FeNPs to produce PIXE effect to counteract tumor proliferation both in in vitro and in in vivo tumor model [20]. PIXE X-ray yields at 45 MeV energy and 100 Gy dose rate increases with increasing NPs concentration while the intensity depends on metal type (AuNPs<FeNPs). Cell viability decreases with increasing NPs concentration; FeNPs are more toxic than AuNPs. In in vivo model, a pre-administration of metallic NPs elicits in 20 days post-PT tumor volume regression, 90 % *vs* 75 % in AuNPs- and FeNPs-treated mice, respectively. AuNPs-treated mice showed complete tumor regression at 24 days [20]. The PIXE effect depends on ROS production [21]. Secondary electrons scattered from AuNPs upon proton beam irradiation increase ionization density within the cells, thus resulting in increased rate of death in DU145 human prostate carcinoma cells [22].

## NMs as Carriers of Radioisotopes

NPs are very promising to deliver tumor-targeted therapeutic radioisotopes for several advantages: (1) high blood retention time due to their morphology, size, coating materials, and compositions of conjugates; (2) high tumor retention time and radioisotopes concentrations; (3) improvement of delivery of radioisotopes due to the magnetization NPs property by external application of a magnetic field [23]. The insufficient delivery of radioisotopes to tumors by the currently most used targeting strategies, i.e., monoclonal antibodies (mAbs) and their fragments, limits radiotherapy outcomes. In fact, mAbs (1) can bind cell surface markers present also in healthy cells, causing systemic toxicity; (2) have few sites to conjugate radioisotopes; (3) can ignite unwanted immune responses; and (4) may be susceptible to protease degradation. These limitations can be addressed by using nanocarriers in which radioisotopes can be labeled or encapsulated via (1) encapsulation during nanocarriers synthesis; (2) labeling to nanocarriers surface after synthesis; (3) labeling of bioconjugates to nanocarriers surface after synthesis; (4) incorporation into nanocarriers lipid bilayer after synthesis; (5) after-loading of the nanocarrier's aqueous phase after synthesis, which allows the higher labeling efficiencies and the greatest in vivo stability [24, 25]. The potential benefit in systemic radiation therapy acquired by delivering of therapeutic radioisotopes by NPs is reviewed in [23].

## Radioprotection of Healthy Tissues by NMs

The main targets of radiation therapy are water and DNA, which are present in both ill and healthy cells. Thus, healthy tissues are susceptible to radiation if not properly directed. The radiotherapy efficacy strictly depends on protection from healthy tissues radiodamage. NPs have been described to exert radiation protective effects as known for amino acid cysteine [26], curcumin [27], and amifostine [28]. In particular, amifostine polymeric NPs as well as combination of amifostine and fullerenol $C_{60}$ provide significant protection from acute whole-body γ irradiation injury in mice and from oxidative stress, DNA damage, and cell death of rat lymphocytes and intestinal crypt cells [29, 30]. Citicoline when delivered as transferrin-coupled liposome has protective effects against radiation in human

ovarian adenocarcinoma OVCAR-3 cells [31], while fullerenol $C_{60}$ and cerium oxide NPs can be radioprotective per se [10].

## Reversal of Radiation Resistance by NMs

Resistance to radiation therapy based on multiple biological pathways represents the major limitation during cancer treatment. One pathway is via survivin, an inhibitor of apoptosis, known to be associated with increased tumor aggressiveness and therapy resistance. Gaca and coworkers [32] developed a human serum albumin-based nanoparticulate carrier 220 nm sized for plasmid-mediated RNA interference (miRNA) that reduces survivin expression by 50 % and increase cytotoxicity if combined with ionizing irradiation. PLGA-NPs encapsulating antisense EGFR oligonucleotides enhance radiosensitivity by inhibition of epidermal growth factor receptor (EGFR)-mediated mechanisms of radioresistance [33].

## Theranostic/Multifunctional Approaches in Radionanomedicine

The last frontier in nanomedicine is the combination of therapy with diagnosis, named theranostics. Designed to increase the efficiency and safety of treatment, the nanosystems used in theranostics have multiple functions: diagnosis, delivery of targeted therapy, and monitoring of the therapeutic response in a single setting by using combinational strategies. In this way, theranostics could allow personalized medicine and take diagnosis from the laboratory to the "point of care" [34]. To this purpose, classical drug delivery systems, such as liposomes, micelles, and NPs, can be double co-loaded with drugs and contrast agents (Fig. 15.2).

Also, Au- and iron oxide-NPs, imaging tools per se, can be conjugated with drugs.

Magnetic NPs have gained much popularity due to their unique ability to be used in magnetic resonance imaging, magnetic targeting, hyperthermia, and controlled drug release. They can be decorated with a wide variety of materials to improve their biocompatibility, carry therapeutic payloads, encapsulate/bind imaging agents, and

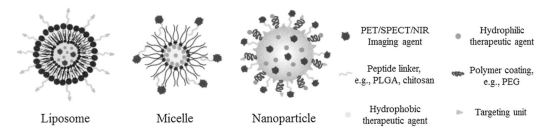

**Fig. 15.2** Representation of some nanosized constructs for multimodal imaging (PET, SPECT, NIR) and therapy (hydrophilic and hydrophobic therapeutic agents). Polymer coating, peptide linker, and targeting molecule are also represented

provide functional groups for conjugation of biomolecules that provide receptor-mediated targeting of the disease [35].

Many other types of NMs can be co-loaded with drugs and with imaging radionuclides to provide real-time feedback of drug delivery, release, and efficacy. For example, [131]I-labeled HPMA copolymers carrying DOX can be used to visualize accumulation of DOX in liver by scintigraphy and PET imaging [36]. Two liposome formulations, one encaged with vinorelbine (VNB) and [111]In-oxine [37] and the other 111In-labeled PEGylated liposomal vinorelbine [38, 39], are effective in the reduction of colorectal adenocarcinoma cells (HT-29). [111]In-chimeric L6 mAb-linked carboxylated PEG on dextran-coated iron oxide, NPs show efficient pharmacokinetics and tumor uptake, and the therapeutic effect of them upon heating induction by externally applied alternating magnetic field (AMF) has been observed [40]. A comprehensive review of the preclinical most relevant application of theranostic nanomedicines is given in [6].

## Future Perspectives: The Glioblastoma Multiforme Example

Nowadays, researchers have made great strides in developing NPs exploitable in cancer management, but many challenges still remain in screening, diagnosing, and treating some types of tumors of the central nervous system. GBM is the most common primary malignancy of the brain and despite many advances in diagnosis and treatment, the GBM prognosis, incidence, and mortality remain unpredictable. It is considered a radioresistant tumor and different radiotherapy modalities fail to control GBM, largely due to unusual responses to radiation (increased DNA damage, differential cyclo-oxygenase, HSP70 elevation, variation in cell cycle arrest, modulation of the cyclin-dependent kinase inhibitors expression, and autophagy). Moreover, although conventional treatments have found modest success in reducing the initial tumor mass, the infiltrating cancer cells that are present beyond the main mass are responsible for tumor recurrence and ultimate patient demise. Thus, it is very important in GBM fighting, the development of new strategies for the precocious diagnosis, and new treatments to combat the infiltrating cancer cells. The rising field of cancer nanotechnology holds promise in the use of multifunctional NMs for imaging and targeted therapy of GBM. NMs are strongly emerging as potential theranostic agents for the simultaneous diagnosis and therapy of GBM. Up to now, micelles, nanoshells, QDs, magnetic NPs, and nanotubes were used in the treatment of experimental GBM [41]. Recently, an innovative method that conjugates nanotechnology and the biological features of GBM for the increase in the detection and therapy of this disease has been proposed [42]. Typical feature of GBM cells is to shed microvesicles (MVs) carrying specific biomarkers (antigens and microRNAs) on their surface and/or inside the lumen into the blood [43]. Magnetic NPs could be functionalized with specific antibodies raised against the most appropriate markers of MVs. These functionalized magnetic NPs represent a highly sensitive diagnostic tool and a rapid analytical technique to profile circulating MVs directly from blood samples of GBM patients. MVs are introduced into a microfluidic chip and incubated with functionalized magnetic NPs and the eventual labeling is detected by a miniaturized NMR system. This system by integrating GBM features and nanotechnology-inspired biosensor has a high detection sensitivity and allows to monitor and predict response to GBM therapies [42].

## Conclusions

The recent years have witnessed an explosion of interest in the use of NMs in oncology research because of their potential to revolutionize the cancer diagnosis, imaging, and therapy. Significant advances have been made in synthesis methodology, such that it is now possible to prepare a variety of NMs with controlled size, shape, surface charge, and physicochemical characteristics. In addition, it is possible to use different polymers and bioactive molecules in surface tailoring and functionalization in order to improve biocompatibility, achieve active and specific targeting, increase blood circulation times, and control drug release of therapeutic payloads. Currently, there is an emerging rush to design theranostics able to permit multifactorial approaches during cancer management. Also in this field, nanotechnology plays a key role allowing the optimization of drug delivery systems, the noninvasive imaging insights on the local distribution of the drug and/or the carrier material at the target site, and the prediction of treatment responses. In the realm of cancer, the use of radioisotopes, in therapy as in diagnosis, is very important and radionanomedicine has found promising applications. In fact, the future development of multifunctional radionanomedicine should cover efficient and specific delivery of therapeutic agents, like radionuclide and anticancer drugs, bringing clinical benefits to the imaging and therapy of cancer.

## References

1. Pollack LA, Rowland JH, Crammer C, Stefanek M. Introduction: charting the landscape of cancer survivors' health-related outcomes and care. Cancer. 2009;115:4265–9. doi:10.1002/cncr.24579.
2. Nazir S, Hussain T, Ayub A, Rashid U, MacRobert AJ. Nanomaterials in fighting cancer: therapeutic applications and developments. Nanomedicine. 2014; 10:19–34. doi:10.1016/j.nano.2013.07.001.
3. Siegel R, Naishadham D, Jemal A. Cancer statistics, 2013. CA Cancer J Clin. 2013;63:11–30. doi:10.3322/caac.21166.
4. Ai J, Biazar E, Jafarpour M, Montazeri M, Majdi A, Aminifard S, et al. Nanotoxicology and nanoparticle safety in biomedical designs. Int J Nanomedicine. 2011;6:1117–27. doi:10.2147/IJN.S16603.
5. Nevozhay D, Kańska U, Budzyńska R, Boratyński J. Current status of research on conjugates and related drug delivery systems in the treatment of cancer and other diseases. Postepy Hig Med Dosw. 2007;61: 350–60.
6. Lammers T, Aime S, Hennink WE, Storm G, Kiessling F. Theranostic nanomedicine. Acc Chem Res. 2011;44:1029–38. doi:10.1021/ar200019c.
7. Patel CN, Goldstone AR, Chowdhury FU, Scarsbrook AF. FDG PET/CT in oncology: "raising the bar". Clin Radiol. 2010;65:522–35. doi:10.1016/j.crad.2010. 01.003.
8. Xing Y, Zhao J, Conti PS, Chen K. Radiolabeled nanoparticles for multimodality tumor imaging. Theranostics. 2014;4:290–306. doi:10.7150/thno.7341.
9. Ting G, Chang CH, Wang HE, Lee TW. Nanotargeted radionuclides for cancer nuclear imaging and internal radiotherapy. J Biomed Biotechnol. 2010. doi:10.1155/2010/953537.
10. Kwatra D, Venugopal A, Anant S. Nanoparticles in radiation therapy: a summary of various approaches to enhance radiosensitization in cancer. Transl Cancer Res. 2013;2:330–42. doi:10.3978/j.issn.2218-676X. 2013.08.06.
11. Lechtman E, Mashouf S, Chattopadhyay N, Keller BM, Lai P, Cai Z, et al. A Monte Carlo-based model of gold nanoparticle radiosensitization accounting for increased radiobiological effectiveness. Phys Med Biol. 2013;58:3075–87. doi: 10.1088/0031-9155/58/10/3075
12. Hainfeld JF, Slatkin DN, Smilowitz HM. The use of gold nanoparticles to enhance radiotherapy in mice. Phys Med Biol. 2004;49:N309–15. http://dx.doi.org/10.1088/0031-9155/49/18/N03
13. Hainfeld JF, Dilmanian FA, Zhong Z, Slatkin DN, Kalef-Ezra JA, Smilowitz HM. Gold nanoparticles enhance the radiation therapy of a murine squamous cell carcinoma. Phys Med Biol. 2010;55:3045–59. doi:10.1088/0031-9155/55/11/004
14. Joh DY, Sun L, Stangl M, Al Zaki A, Murty S, Santoiemma PP, Davis JJ, Baumann BC, Alonso-Basanta M, Bhang D, Kao GD, Tsourkas A, Dorsey

JF. Selective targeting of brain tumors with gold nanoparticle-induced radiosensitization. PLoS One. 2013;8(4), e62425. doi: 10.1371/journal.pone. 0062425

15. Polley MY, Lamborn KR, Chang SM, Butowski N, Clarke JL, Prados M. Conditional probability of survival in patients with newly diagnosed glioblastoma. J Clin Oncol. 2011;29:4175–80. doi:10.1200/JCO.2010.32.4343.

16. Butterworth KT, McMahon SJ, Taggart LE, Prise KM. Radiosensitization by gold nanoparticles: effective at megavoltage energies and potential role of oxidative stress. Transl Cancer Res. 2013;2:269–79. doi:10.3978/j.issn.2218-676X.2013.08.03.

17. Levin WP, Kooy H, Loeffler JS, DeLaney TF. Proton beam therapy. Br J Cancer. 2005;93:849–54. doi: 10.1038/sj.bjc.6602754

18. Kim JK, Kim HT, Kim JH, Seo SJ, Chung DS, Kim JK. Investigation of tumor cells toxicity from particle induced x-ray emission from a 45-MeV proton beam irradiated ferrite nanoparticle. Int J PIXE. 2009;19:143–55. doi:10.1142/S0129083509001837.

19. Seo SJ, Jeon JK, Jeong EJ, Chang WS, Choi GH, Kim JK. Enhancement of tumor regression by coulomb nanoradiator effect in proton treatment of iron-oxide nanoparticle-loaded orthotopic rat glioma model: implication of novel particle induced radiation therapy. J Cancer Ther. 2013;4:25–32. doi:10.4236/jct.2013.411A004.

20. Kim JK, Seo SJ, Kim KH, Kim TJ, Chung MH, Kim KR, Yang TK. Therapeutic application of metallic nanoparticles combined with particle-induced x-ray emission effect. Nanotechnology. 2010;21:425102. doi:10.1088/0957-4484/21/42/425102.

21. Kim JK, Seo SJ, Kim HT, Kim KH, Chung MH, Kim KR, Ye SJ. Enhanced proton treatment in mouse tumors through proton irradiated nanoradiator effects on metallic nanoparticles. Phys Med Biol. 2012;57:8309–23. doi:10.1088/0031-9155/57/24/8309.

22. Polf JC, Bronk LF, Driessen WH, Arap W, Pasqualini R, Gillin M. Enhanced relative biological effectiveness of proton radiotherapy in tumor cells with internalized gold nanoparticles. Appl Phys Lett. 2011;98: 193702. doi:10.1063/1.3589914

23. Zhang L, Chen H, Wang L, Liu T, Yeh J, Lu G, et al. Delivery of therapeutic radioisotopes using nanoparticle platforms: potential benefit in systemic radiation therapy. Nanotechnol Sci Appl. 2010;3:159–70. doi:10.2147/NSA.S7462.

24. Mitra A, Nan A, Line BR, Ghandehari H. Nanocarriers for nuclear imaging and radiotherapy of cancer. Curr Pharm Des. 2006;12:4729–49. doi:10.2174/138161206777902631

25. Shokeen M, Fettig NM, Rossin R. Synthesis, in vitro and in vivo evaluation of radiolabeled nanoparticles. Q J Nucl Med Mol Imaging. 2008;52:267–77.

26. Patt HM, Tyree EB, Straube RL, Smith DE. Cysteine protection against X irradiation. Science. 1949;110: 213–4. doi:10.1126/science.110.2852.213

27. Jagetia GC. Radioprotection and radiosensitization by curcumin. Adv Exp Med Biol. 2007;595:301–20. doi:10.1007/978-0-387-46401-5_13

28. Capizzi RL, Oster W. Chemoprotective and radioprotective effects of amifostine: an update of clinical trials. Int J Hematol. 2000;72:425–35.

29. Pamujula S, Kishore V, Rider B, Fermin CD, Graves RA, Agrawal KC, et al. Radioprotection in mice following oral delivery of amifostine nanoparticles. Int J Radiat Biol. 2005;81:251–7. doi:10.1080/09553000500103470

30. Theriot CA, Casey RC, Moore VC, Mitchell L, Reynolds JO, Burgoyne M, et al. Dendro[C(60)] fullerene DF-1 provides radioprotection to radiosensitive mammalian cells. Radiat Environ Biophys. 2010;49:437–45. doi:10.1007/s00411-010-0310-4.

31. Suresh Reddy J, Venkateswarlu V, Koning GA. Radioprotective effect of transferrin targeted citicoline liposomes. J Drug Target. 2006;14:13–9. doi:10.1080/10611860600613241

32. Gaca S, Reichert S, Rödel C, Rödel F, Kreuter J. Survivin-miRNA-loaded nanoparticles as auxiliary tools for radiation therapy: preparation, characterisation, drug release, cytotoxicity and therapeutic effect on colorectal cancer cells. J Microencapsul. 2012;29: 685–94. doi:10.3109/02652048.2012.680511.

33. Ping Y, Jian Z, Yi Z, Huoyu Z, Feng L, Yuqiong Y, et al. Inhibition of the EGFR with nanoparticles encapsulating antisense oligonucleotides of the EGFR enhances radiosensitivity in SCCVII cells. Med Oncol. 2010;27:715–21. doi:10.1007/s12032-009-9274-0.

34. Caldorera-Moore ME, Liechty WB, Peppas NA. Responsive theranostic systems: integration of diagnostic imaging agents and responsive controlled release drug delivery carriers. Acc Chem Res. 2011;44:1061–70. doi:10.1021/ar2001777.

35. Wadajkar AS, Menon JU, Kadapure T, Tran RT, Yang J, Nguyen KT. Design and application of magnetic-based theranostic nanoparticle systems. Recent Pat Biomed Eng. 2013;6:47–57. doi:10.2174/1874764711306010007

36. Seymour LW, Ferry DR, Anderson D, Hesslewood S, Julyan PJ, Poyner R, et al. Hepatic drug targeting: phase I evaluation of polymer-bound doxorubicin. J Clin Oncol. 2002;20:1668–76. doi:10.1200/JCO.20.6.1668

37. Lee WC, Hwang JJ, Tseng YL, Wang HE, Chang YF, Lu YC, et al. Therapeutic efficacy evaluation of 111in-VNB-liposome on human colorectal adenocarcinoma HT-29/luc mouse xenografts. Nucl Instr Methods Phys Res A. 2012;569:497–504. doi:10.1016/j.nima.2006.08.135.

38. Chow TH, Lin YY, Hwang JJ, Wang HE, Tseng YL, Pang VF, et al. Diagnostic and therapeutic evaluation of 111In-vinorelbine-liposomes in a human colorectal carcinoma HT-29/luc-bearing animal model. Nucl Med Biol. 2008;35:623–34. doi:10.1016/j.nucmedbio.2008.04.001.

39. Chow TH, Lin YY, Hwang JJ, Wang HE, Tseng YL, Pang VF, et al. Therapeutic efficacy evaluation of 111In-labeled PEGylated liposomal vinorelbine in murine colon carcinoma with multimodalities of molecular imaging. J Nucl Med. 2009;50:2073–81. doi:10.2967/jnumed.109.063503.

40. DeNardo SJ, DeNardo GL, Miers LA, Natarajan A, Foreman AR, Gruettner C, et al. Development of tumor targeting bioprobes ($^{111}$In-chimeric L6 monoclonal antibody nanoparticles) for alternating magnetic field cancer therapy. Clin Cancer Res. 2005;11:7087s–7092s. doi:10.1158/1078-0432. CCR-1004-0022

41. Hernández-Pedro NY, Rangel-López E, Magaña-Maldonado R, de la Cruz VP, del Angel AS, Pineda B, et al. Application of nanoparticles on diagnosis and therapy in gliomas. Biomed Res Int. 2013;14(1): 415–32. doi:10.1155/2013/351031.

42. Shao H, Chung J, Balaj L, Charest A, Bigner DD, Carter BS, et al. Protein typing of circulating microvesicles allows real-time monitoring of glioblastoma therapy. Nat Med. 2012;18:1835–40. doi:10.1038/nm.2994.

43. McNamara MG, Sahebjam S, Mason WP. Emerging biomarkers in glioblastoma. Cancers. 2013;5:1103–19. doi:10.3390/cancers5031103.

**Part III**

**From Bench to Bedside: Translational Perspectives**

# Preclinical Models of Glioblastoma in Radiobiology: Evolving Protocols and Research Methods

# 16

Anita Tandle, Uma Shankavaram, Cody Schlaff, Kevin Camphausen, and Andra Krauze

## Introduction

Gliomas are the most common form of primary brain tumors with glioblastoma (GBM) being the most malignant. The standard therapy for newly diagnosed malignant gliomas involves maximal surgical resection, radiotherapy, and chemotherapy. However, the invasive and diffuse nature of this malignancy together with its ill-defined borders makes a complete surgical resection nearly impossible. Following surgery, intensity modulated or image-guided radiation therapy (RT) is delivered which enhances median survival from 3 to 14 months. However, tumor recurrence occurs in 90 % of cases at the site of surgery [1]. Radiation therapy kills cells by causing DNA damage either directly or via formation of intracellular free radicals such as reactive oxygen species (ROS) [2, 3]. The ability to repair sublethal DNA damage is frequently compromised in cancer cells as compared to normal cells [3]. Thus, RT may selectively kill cancer cells compared to normal tissue. The recent technical advancement in RT delivery and dosing has increased the

precision of irradiation to the target tumor volume [2, 4]; however, this has not translated to longer survival in patients with GBM. The combination of RT with chemotherapeutic agents that sensitize tumor cells to the cytotoxic effects of RT has been studied in an attempt to enhance tumor control and minimize the radiation toxicity. Although such combination chemoradiation protocols have improved treatment outcomes in several human malignancies, they are still less than optimal, as the existing agents can cause undesirable toxicity [2]. Therefore, a continuing endeavor in experimental and translational oncology research has been to identify more effective agents to augment the radiosensitivity of tumor cells [5]. Recent efforts toward this goal have focused on molecularly targeted agents directed against certain components of intracellular signaling pathways involved in tumor growth and radioresistance [6, 7].

Keeping this background in mind the current chapter discusses the preclinical models in GBM radiobiology. The intent is to address the previous approaches to GBM research and the current research protocols in the ongoing evolution of the GBM field with special emphasis on using this information to enable rational clinical trial design for GBM patients. This chapter reviews the developments that allowed basic scientists and radiation oncologists to maximize therapeutic benefits of radiation in treating GBM. This includes progress in the field of in vitro models,

A. Tandle (✉) • U. Shankavaram • C. Schlaff
K. Camphausen • A. Krauze
Radiation Oncology Branch, National Cancer Institute, National Institutes of Health, Building 10, Room B3B100, Bethesda, MD 20892, USA
e-mail: tandlea@mail.nih.gov

© Springer International Publishing Switzerland 2016
L. Pirtoli et al. (eds.), *Radiobiology of Glioblastoma*, Current Clinical Pathology,
DOI 10.1007/978-3-319-28305-0_16

molecular profiling, and stem-cell-based assays. Preclinical models are a necessary part of radiobiology research: they provide a framework to analyze and compare data and ultimately to assist in building up theories of radiation action both in vitro and in vivo. They are necessary to relate experimental studies to clinical cancer treatment with the aim of improving therapy. The chapter discusses past, present, and future preclinical methods in optimizing treatment for GBM.

## Radiobiology of GBM Tumors

### R's of Radiobiology

In 1975, Rodney Withers published a paper entitled "The 4 R's of Radiotherapy," highlighting a short list of mechanisms that may determine the response of a biological tissues to multiple doses of radiation: Repair, Reassortment, Repopulation, and Reoxygenation [8]. Repair is the concept that the lethal damage induced by RT leads to cell death, but sublethal damage can be repaired. A complicating factor is that cells exhibit differential radiation sensitivity when they are in the different phases of the cell cycle. Cells in mitosis are most sensitive and cells in late S-phase are the most resistant to RT. As cells move from the less sensitive to the more sensitive phases of the cell cycle, termed re-assortment, an increase in cell killing occurs. However, RT damage may induce an increased rate of cell proliferation leading to tumor repopulation. Further, sensitivity to radiation increases with oxygen and the phenomenon by which hypoxic cells become oxygenated after RT is reoxygenation. Radiosensitivity is a newer member of the R's [9]. It reminds us that apart from the classic four-R's, there is an intrinsic radiosensitivity of different cell types. Radiosensitive cells include hematological cells, epithelial stem cells, gametes, and tumor cells from hematological or sex organ origin. Radioresistant cells include myocytes, neurons, stem cells, and tumor cells such as melanoma or sarcoma. In case of GBM, it has

a low alpha beta ratio (the ratio $\alpha/\beta$ gives the dose at which the linear and quadratic components of cell killing are equal)—thus is more likely to display radioresistance when treated with radiation therapy. Deacon et al. classified tumors into five categories A to E according to radioresponsiveness, with A being the most radioresponsive and E the most radioresistant [10]. GBM is part of category E tumors, which also contains other radioresistant histologies such as melanoma, osteosarcoma, and renal cell carcinoma.

Hypoxia is an important radiobiological factor as it is associated with significant radioresistance when present. This is due to the fact that oxygen, when present at the time of radiation therapy administration of within seconds thereafter, "fixes" or makes permanent the damage caused by radiation therapy and thus the damage is less likely to be repaired and will result in a greater likelihood of cell kill [11]. Previous studies have shown that the presence of hypoxia is more likely to give rise to a radioresistant stem cell population in glioma [12].

The tumor microenvironment which has bearing on hypoxia has come to the forefront of research in glioma. A number of molecular pathways have been identified that may relate both to the existence of hypoxia and radioresistance, although a direct relationship between the two in the setting of glioma has not been identified. Direct measurement of oxygen concentration in tumors including GBM has not been particularly helpful and may in fact not directly reflect the activation of hypoxia markers at the molecular levels (HIF-1$\alpha$ and HIF-2$\alpha$), although some relationship to oxygen tension has been identified [13]. Hypoxia response is mediated by the HIF family, which induces several downstream pathways related to tumor proliferation, apoptosis, and ultimately treatment resistance [14]. Hypoxia encourages the formation of stem cell populations, which in turn also foster treatment resistance [15]. Hypoxia also induces other signaling molecules such as heat shock protein 70 (HSP70/HSPA). Previous evidence has shown that HSPA is present in high levels in glioma and that this correlates with tumor grade [16].

## In Vitro Methods to Measure 5 R's

### DNA Damage Response

The DNA damage response (DDR) is a highly complex and coordinated system that determines the cellular outcome of DNA damage caused by radiation. DDR can be divided into two parts, the sensors of DNA damage and the effectors of damage repair. The sensors consist of a group of proteins that actively survey the genome for the presence of damage. These proteins then signal this damage to three main effector pathways that together determine the outcome for the cell. These effector pathways include (1) programmed cell death pathways that kill damaged cells, (2) DNA repair pathways that physically repair DNA breaks, and (3) pathways that cause temporary (or permanent) blocks in the progress of cells through the cell cycle—the damage checkpoints.

### Damage Sensors: Radiosensitivity Assessment by γH2AX and 53PB1 Foci Determination

Tumors are complex systems consisting of heterogeneous mixture of cancer and normal cells, with each having unique sensitivity to RT. The effectiveness of RT treatment could be significantly improved if tumor cells could be rendered more sensitive to ionizing radiation without altering the sensitivity of normal tissues.

### γH2AX Assay

DNA damage after RT includes nucleotide base damage, DNA single-strand breaks, and double-strand breaks (DSBs). The DNA double-strand break is the most lethal of the types of injury. DSBs can result in clastogenesis, mutagenesis, and cell death by diverse mechanisms, including mitotic catastrophe, deletions, and/or mutations [17]. An early event in DNA DSB repair is the phosphorylation of histone H2AX (γH2AX) at serine 139 by DNAPKcs, ATM, or ATR, which in less than an hour encompasses a region spanning several megabases, forming a light microscopically visible foci [18, 19]. There are four main techniques to measure γH2AX levels and kinetics: (a) immunostaining, (b) flow cytometry, (c) immunoblotting, and (d) enzyme-linked immunosorbent assay (ELISA). However, immunostaining and microscopic analysis of γH2AX foci allows the detection and quantification of damage in cell nuclei, as illustrated (Fig. 16.1). This technique is the most sensitive and specific. The number of DSBs can be directly quantified by the number of foci present in the cell shortly after DNA damage and time courses can be quantitatively determined [20]. Similar results can be obtained from xenograft samples [21]. However, the main disadvantage of using immunostaining is that the method is time-consuming and the various sizes of the foci may be difficult to count.

### 53BP1 Foci

53BP1 (also called TP53BP1) is a chromatin-associated factor that promotes immunoglobulin class switching and DNA double-strand-break (DSB) repair by non-homologous end joining. 53BP1 was first identified due to its ability to bind to the tumor suppressor protein p53 [22]. 53BP1 responds to DNA double-strand breaks in an ATM-dependent manner, quickly relocating to discrete nuclear foci after exposure to ionizing radiation. These foci co-localize with those of the Mre11-Nbs1-Rad50 complex and phosphorylated γH2AX, which are thought to facilitate the recruitment of repair factors to damaged DNA [23, 24]. It has been shown that the 53BP1-dependent repair pathway is important for survival of cells irradiated with IR during the G1 phase of the cell cycle [25].

### Radiosensitivity Assessment by Comet Assay

Another method for measuring DNA strand breaks at the level of the individual eukaryotic cells is the comet assay. It was first developed by Östling and Johansson in 1984 and later modified

**Fig. 16.1** Treatment with CUDC-101 plus radiation impairs the DNA damage repair response. U251 cells seeded in chamber slides were exposed to 2 Gy irradiation immediately followed by 0.5 μM CUDC-101 and fixed at the specified times for immunoflourescent analysis of nuclear γH2AX foci retention. Foci were evaluated in ≥50 nuclei per treatment per experiment. (**a**) Representative images obtained at 24 h from media (control), 2 Gy irradiation, 0.5 μM CUDC-101 treatment, and 0.5 μM CUDC-101 immediately following 2 Gy irradiation (drug + IR). Significant retention of γH2AX foci occurs with drug alone and combination therapy after 24 h and the combinatory effect is significantly greater than drug only. (**b**) Data represents three independent experiments. *Columns* represent the mean and error bars are the SEM. *p < 0.05 **p < 0.001, *N.S.* not significant

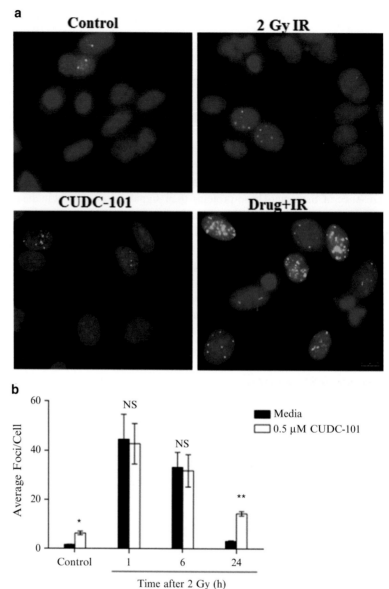

by Singh et al. in 1988 [26, 27]. Cells embedded in agarose on a microscope slide are lysed with detergent and high salt to form nucleoids containing supercoiled loops of DNA linked to the nuclear matrix. Electrophoresis at high pH results in structures resembling comets, observed by fluorescence microscopy; the intensity of the comet tail relative to the head reflects the number of DNA breaks.

The comet assay is ideally suited for use with in vitro cells. Tissues represent more of a chal-

lenge, but methods have been devised, using enzymes and/or physical maceration, to release cells or nuclei of high quality from many animal tissues and some human tissues (reviewed in [28]). Frozen cells or tissues are generally not suitable, since physical shearing of the DNA occurs as ice crystals form. Also, mitochondrial DNA is too small to be detected by comet assay as they lack typical organization of eukaryotic DNA on a nuclear matrix [29]. However, the use of the comet assay is limited due to large doses of irradiation that are typically used >10 Gy. Another practical limitation of the comet assay is the small number of samples that can be handled in one experiment, thus it cannot be used as a high throughput assay.

## DNA Repair Assessment

After DSBs are detected by DNA sensor proteins, DDR is initiated in order to repair damaged DNA. For DSBs, there are two main repair pathways, homologous recombination (HR) and nonhomologous end joining (NHEJ). These are quite different in the proteins involved, the position in the cell cycle where they primarily act and in the speed and accuracy of repair. These processes are described in more detail below.

*HR:* HR uses homologous undamaged DNA as the template to repair the damaged DNA predominantly in the S and G2 phases of cell cycle [30]. Some of the proteins involved in this process are MRN complex, RAD51, RPA and BRCA2, BLM, XRCC2, and XRCC3. Because of the use of a template, HR is the most error-free repair mechanism. There are several methods available to evaluate the HR efficiency in cultured mammalian cells, including the use of restriction fragment length polymorphisms, the measurement of functional cassettes formed through the recombination of two dysfunctional cassettes, and a newer PCR-based method.

The method using functional cassettes formed through the recombination between two dysfunctional cassettes is the more widely used assay [31]. This strategy is generally carried out by transfecting the cells with two plasmids having different defective reporter cassettes such as GFP (or other fluorescent proteins), such that only the cells containing the GFP signal are considered to contain the recombinant functional plasmid. The recombination efficiency can be expressed as the percentage of GFP-expressing cells in all the transfected cells. Other commonly used reporter genes include antibiotic-resistant genes such as the hygromycin phosphor-transferase gene, so only the cells which survive the hygromycin

selection are deemed to contain the recombinant plasmid and the recombination frequency can be calculated from the ratios between the surviving cell foci and the total transfected cells [32]. However, the sensitivity of this method is low as the cells which have the recombinant plasmid may not be able to express the transgene. In addition, it generally takes a long time for the transgene to be expressed.

A newer PCR method has been developed, by designing primers that can only anneal to the recombinant functional plasmid; the HR efficiency can be assessed using PCR/Realtime PCR. This PCR-based method is quick and sensitive to evaluate HR efficiency (Norgen Bioteck Corp.).

*NHEJ:* NHEJ joins two DNA DSB ends together without requiring homologous DNA [33]. This is a more rapid process than HR but less accurate, with small deletions or insertions frequently occurring. The NHEJ DNA repair process is functional in all phases of the cell cycle and some of the proteins involved are Ku70, Ku80, DNAPK, ATM, and XRCC4. The most commonly used in vitro assay for NHEJ uses as a substrate plasmid DNA that has been linearized with a single restriction enzyme or with two different restriction enzymes. During incubation with extract protein or partially purified fractions, circular and multimeric linear joining products are generated, which can be separated by agarose gel electrophoresis and detected by direct staining with ethidium bromide [34]. The first mammalian cell-free system for NHEJ was described by North et al. [35]. Nuclear, cytoplasmic, and whole cell extracts from various cell lines and tissues have been used to study cell-free NHEJ [34]. Antibodies have been used as more specific reagents to test the involvement of candidate proteins in cell-free NHEJ. In spite of the significant progress that has been made, NHEJ assays are still evolving and likely to become more sophisticated, automated, efficient, and sensitive in the next 20 years. HR is a pathway specific to S- and G2-phase cells; it occurs only in dividing cells. Conversely, NHEJ occurs in all phases of the cell cycle and is thus neither phase-specific nor cycle-specific.

## Effector Pathways of DDR

Three related kinases have been shown to be able to phosphorylate at sites of DSBs [36]. The phosphorylation of H2AX at sites of DSBs produced by radiation occurs primarily by the ataxia telangiectasia-mutated (ATM) protein. In cells that completely lack the ATM protein, phosphorylation of H2AX can still occur through an alternative mechanism, but with somewhat delayed kinetics. In these cells, H2AX phosphorylation is mediated by the catalytic subunit of the DNA-dependent protein kinase (DNA-PKcs). DNA-PKcs is a kinase that is structurally related to ATM and which is very important in the non-homologous end joining pathway of DNA repair. The third kinase capable of phosphorylating H2AX is ATR, which stands for AT-related kinase. Activation of ATM, DNA-PKcs, and ATR leads to the phosphorylation not only of H2AX, but also of many other cellular proteins. Recent studies have shown that as many as 700 proteins are substrates for the ATM and ATR kinases in response to DNA damage [37]. Phosphorylation of these other proteins acts as the 'signals' to activate the various different downstream effectors of the DDR (apoptosis, cell-cycle checkpoints, and DNA repair). The ATM protein plays perhaps the most important role in transmitting these signals in response to radiation-induced DSBs and is thus considered to be a master regulator of the DDR. The ATM and ATR kinases activate Chk2 and Chk1 downstream kinases to inhibit Cdc25A and Cdc25C to halt cell cycle in S- and G2-phases, respectively [38]. Measuring the phosphorylation of different kinases can help in figuring out which pathway is involved.

## Assessment of Re-assortment: Cell Cycle Analysis

The second major effector pathway of the DDR is the activation of cell cycle checkpoints. Treatment of cells with ionizing radiation causes delays in the movement of cells through the G1, S, and G2 phases of the cell cycle [39]. This occurs through the activation of DNA damage checkpoints, which are specific points in the cell cycle at which progression of the cell into the next phase can be blocked or slowed. The DDR activates four distinct checkpoints in response to irradiation that take place at different points within the cell cycle; G1 arrest, S-phase checkpoint, G2 early checkpoint, and G2 late checkpoint. The commonly used methods follow either tritiated thymidine or bromodeoxyuridine incorporation, to assess cells in S- and G2-phases of cell cycle. However, the most extensively used method to assess the relative distribution of irradiated cells in the respective phases of the cell cycle is propidium iodide (PI) staining followed by fluorescence-activated cell sorting (FACS). This method estimates phase of cell cycle based on DNA content. It has been shown that late G2 interphase cells are characterized by phosphorylation of histone H3 at serine 10. Therefore, PI staining coupled with histone H3 phosphorylation can be used to assess mitotic fraction of cell cycle after irradiation.

## Assessment of Cell Death After Irradiation

Accumulating evidences suggests that induction of cell death by apoptosis alone is insufficient to account for the therapeutic effect of radiotherapy [40]. It has become obvious in the last few years that inhibition of the proliferative capacity of malignant cells following irradiation, especially with solid tumors, can occur via alternative cell death modalities like mitotic catastrophe, senescence, and autophagy. The kind and type of cell death caused by RT is highly influenced by pathways within the DDR system [41].

*Apoptosis:* a mechanism of cell death in some normal cells can be detected by studying both the sensors and detector molecules. The apoptosis sensors are caspase 8 or caspase 9, which can activate caspase 3 as an effector molecule. The morphological changes such as chromatin condensation, nuclear fragmentation, and DNA laddering can be detected by various methods. TUNEL assay: Terminal deoxynucleotidyl transferase dUTP nick end labeling is a method for detecting DNA fragmentation by labeling the terminal end of nucleic acids. Another popular method is Annexin V staining, which detects translocation of phosphatidylserine from the inner side of the plasma membrane to the outer layer of early apoptotic cells. Other assays are caspase activity assays, detection of cells in sub-G1/Go, and changes in mitochondrial membrane potential.

*Mitotic catastrophe (MC)* is morphologically associated with the accumulation of multinucleated, giant cells containing uncondensed chromosomes and with the presence of chromosome aberrations and micronuclei [42, 43]. It is considered to be the major mechanism by which the majority of solid tumors respond to RT. The mitotic death can be detected by staining actin filaments. This involves plating of cells in a glass chamber slide. After a specific treatment, cells are fixed and stained with α-tubulin antibody to stain the cytoskeleton and DAPI to stain the nuclei. Percent cells with mitotic catastrophe can be assessed, as illustrated (Fig. 16.2). Caspase activation assays can also be used to access MC. However, these assays cannot discriminate between interphase and post-mitotic apoptosis. By combining high-resolution fluorescence videomicroscopy and automated image analysis, Rello-Varona et al. established a protocol for the simultaneous assessment of ploidy, mitosis, centrosome number, and cell death to examine MC [44]. The authors showed that this approach can be used for the high-throughput detection of mitotic catastrophe induced by three mechanistically distinct anti-mitotic agents. However, this method needs special instrumentation and technical expertise for the quantification of MC.

## Autophagy and Senescence

Autophagy, a catabolic process involving the degradation of a cell's own components through the lysosomal machinery, serves as a protective response under conditions of nutrient deprivation and is also frequently observed in tumor cells exposed to chemotherapy or radiation. The process is characterized by the formation of double-membrane cytosolic vesicles, called autophagosomes. To date, electron microscopy has been the only reliable method for monitoring autophagy. Autophagic vacuoles can be labeled with monodansylcadaverine (MDC), an autoflourescent dye which selectively labels these vacuoles [45]. Intracellular MDC can be measured by fluorescence spectrophotometer. The vacuoles could be visualized by fluorescence microscopy using an inverted microscope equipped with a filter system (excitation filter 380–420 nm, barrier filter: 450 nm). Other methods include monitoring bulk degradation of long-lived proteins and LC3, an autophagic marker localization (reviewed in [46]). There is a Cyto-ID® Autophagy Detection Kit available (Enzo Life Sciences), which measures autophagic vacuoles and monitors autophagic flux in live cells using a novel dye that selectively labels autophagosomes. The dye is a cationic amphiphilic tracer dye that allows minimal staining of lysosomes while exhibiting bright fluorescence upon incorporation into autophagolysosomes. The assay offers a rapid and quantitative approach to monitoring autophagy in live cells without the need for cell transfection.

Cellular senescence, on the other hand, is defined as a biological state in which cells have lost the ability to divide but remain metabolically active and is likewise a frequent response to radiation. Prematurely senescent cells exhibit some of the same characteristics as replicative senescent cells, including permanent cell cycle arrest, enlarged and flattened cell morphology, and increased senescence-associated β-galactosidase (SA-β-gal) activity [47]. For detection of SA-β-gal activity, cells can be washed, fixed (with 4 % formaldehyde), and stained overnight at 37 °C without $CO_2$ in freshly prepared staining buffer containing X-gal [48]. SA-ß-Gal catalyzes the hydrolysis of X-gal to produce a blue color in senescent cells which can be quantitated using a fluorescence plate reader or by flow cytometry assay. The ß-Gal staining kit is commercially available from a number of vendors.

## Assessment of Repopulation: Clonogenic Survival Assays

After exposure to RT, the majority of damaged cells die within 2–3 cell divisions and cannot clonally replicate. The first clonogenic assay was developed in 1956 by Puck and Marcus, and by

**Fig. 16.2** CUDC-101
increases mitotic catastrophe:
U251 cells were grown on
cover slips and were irradiated
(2 Gy) and exposed to
CUDC-101. At 24, 48, and 72
h after treatment, cells were
fixed for immunocytochemical
analysis of mitotic catastrophe.
Nuclear fragmentation
(defined as the presence of two
or more distinct lobes within a
single cell) was evaluated in at
least 150 cells per cohort. (**a**)
Representative fluorescent
micrographs are of cells fixed
at 72 h after treatment for
media (control), 2 Gy
irradiation, 0.5 μM CUDC-
101, and 0.5 μM CUDC-101
immediately following 2 Gy
irradiation (drug + IR). (**b**) %
mitotic catastrophe is
quantified. *=*p<0.05*;
****=*p<0.0001, N.S.* not
significant; *lower asterisk*
represents significance by
comparing the 2 Gy cohort
with the 2 Gy + 0.5 μM
CUDC-101 cohort; *upper
asterisk* represents significant
in comparing 0.5 μM
CUDC-101 cohort with the 2
Gy + 0.5 μM CUDC-101
cohort. Analysis was done
using a two-way ANOVA
with Bonferroni multiple
comparisons post-test

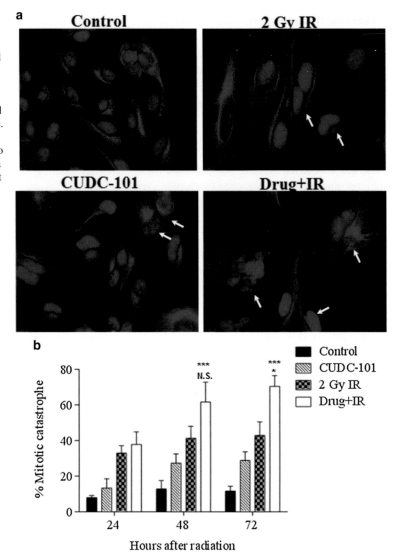

1970s, it was considered to be the "gold standard assay" in radiobiology [49, 50]. To run the assay, a single-cell suspension of tumor cells is prepared and plated. After a suitable period of incubation (3–5 doublings), the colonies are stained with crystal violet and counted. The number of colonies in the irradiated cohort is expressed as surviving fraction compared to the non-irradiated control. A cell survival curve is graphically represented by plotting the surviving fraction on a logarithmic scale on the y-axis against RT dose on a linear scale on the x-axis as illustrated (Fig. 16.3). Clonogenic survival assays have been described for tumor tissues. This requires first the production of single-cell suspensions using mechanical disaggregation followed by enzymatic digestion. However, the clonogenic assay has been shown to have negative aspects, including clump artifacts, lack of cytotoxic endpoints, and lack of normal cell–cell interactions existing in a true tissue environment. Clonogenic assays are difficult to perform in the settings of multiple drugs testing, since it is difficult to add drugs sequentially to the culture system [51]. Newer models are described utilizing cytotoxic as well as cell-proliferation end-points and maintenance of three-dimensional tissue architecture in vitro.

## Assessment of Reoxygenation

The hypothesis of reoxygenation of tumors after irradiation was proposed more than two decades ago [52]. After irradiation, which is expected to eliminate preferentially the well-oxygenated cells, it was assumed that continuous movement of previously anoxic cells into the category of well-oxygenated cells could occur. Tumor reoxygenation may result from an increase in oxygen delivery and/or a decrease in oxygen consumption by the tumor cells [53]. The increase in oxygen delivery may be due to radiation-induced acute inflammation and a decrease in interstitial fluid pressure. Early tumor reoxygenation, in addition to the cell cycle redistribution effect, significantly contributes to the radiosensitivity of tumor cells in radiotherapy protocols that use multiple daily fractions [54]. Several techniques have been developed to measure oxygenation status in tissues and tumors in living animals and humans. Three common methods are currently available to measure oxygen consumption in vitro: electron paramagnetic resonance (EPR) oximetry, the Clark oxygen electrode, and the MitoXpress fluorescent assay [55]. EPR is a powerful technology that permits continuous monitoring of oxygenation in tissues in vitro

[56]. The Clark oxygen electrode consists of an anode and a cathode in contact with an electrolyte solution and covered by a semipermeable membrane. Oxygen diffuses through the membrane to the cathode, where it is reduced. The current produced by the electrode is proportional to the oxygen tension in the solution [57]. Finally, the MitoXpress assay is based on a phosphorescent oxygen-sensitive probe available commercially. The assay is based on the ability of oxygen to quench the excited state of the MitoXpress probe. Depletion of oxygen in the surrounding solution is perceived as an increase in probe phosphorescence signal. Therefore, changes in oxygen consumption, reflecting changes in mitochondrial activity, are measured as changes in MitoXpress probe signal over time.

## In Vivo Methods to Measure 5 R's

## Preclinical Models of Glioblastoma

In the search for a more personalized approach to cancer therapy, well-defined model systems and study designs are needed to bridge the gap between promising in vitro concepts and their clinical application [58]. Animal models greatly

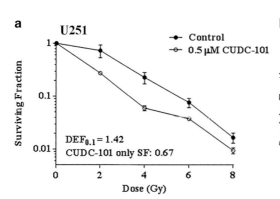
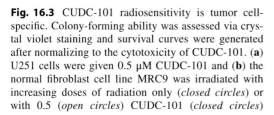
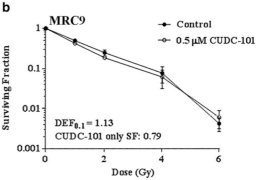

**Fig. 16.3** CUDC-101 radiosensitivity is tumor cell-specific. Colony-forming ability was assessed via crystal violet staining and survival curves were generated after normalizing to the cytotoxicity of CUDC-101. (**a**) U251 cells were given 0.5 µM CUDC-101 and (**b**) the normal fibroblast cell line MRC9 was irradiated with increasing doses of radiation only (*closed circles*) or with 0.5 (*open circles*) CUDC-101 (*closed circles*)

immediately following irradiation. Survival curves show that the radiosensitive activity of CUDC-101 is tumor cell-specific giving only a small enhancement in DEF in MRC9 cells. Dose enhancement factors (DEFs) were assessed at surviving fractions (SFs) of 0.01. Data represents three independent experiments (**a**) and two independent experiments (**b**) with points representing the mean, and error bars the SEM facilitate understanding of cancer, and importantly, serve preclinically for evaluating potential anticancer therapies. Investigations into the biology of solid tumor cells often use cell lines grown and maintained as monolayer cultures. Such experimental systems have provided a wealth of information pertaining to the critical molecules and pathways mediating tumor survival and response to therapy. The most commonly used xenograft model involves implantation of $1–10 \times 10^6$ tumor cells subcutaneously on the lateral aspect of the hind leg/flank either in SCID (severe combined immunodeficient) or Nude mouse. The endpoint is the time to reach a certain tumor volume. Tumor growth curve is plotted and the time it takes for a tumor to grow to five times the treatment volume is calculated for irradiated and control tumors. Tumor growth delay is then calculated by subtracting control tumor time from RT-treated tumor time. However, tumor cells in vitro have a different phenotype than tumor cells when grown as tumors in animal models [59]. Extensive tumor cell invasion and recurrence are the two hallmarks of GBM. Therefore, there is a compelling need for more reliable in vivo preclinical models such as orthotopic models for studying the disease and for testing new drugs and targeted therapies. An ideal model should recapitulate the key histopathological, genetic, and imaging features encountered in GBM's aggressive growth as well as being a reproducible, reliable model.

Two of the most commonly used mouse models are U251 and U87 xenograft tumors implanted into athymic nude mice. While these models enable the use of human GBM tumor cell lines, they are being tested in an immunocompromised rodent, which does not allow for adequate study of the tumor–CNS/immune microenvironment [60]. These models and other models of GBM have been available for decades; however, very few new therapies have successfully translated into the clinic during this time. Our current model systems do not have sufficient clinical predictive power and do not effectively mimic and predict human responses [61]. A systematic comparison of gene expression patterns in GBM cell lines (U87 and U251) on three different growth condi-

tions showed a high concordance between in vivo (subcutaneous and intracranial) models [59] and further evaluation with GBM patient gene expression profiles confirmed that the intracranial model simulates a subset of GBM [62]. However, the lack of complete concordance in preclinical models has led to the concept of orthotopic models and studying stem cell populations.

## New Concepts in Radiobiology

### GBM Stem Cells and Microenvironment

As mentioned earlier, drug resistance followed by a disease recurrence is the hallmark of GBM pathophysiology. An increasing number of studies suggest that GBMs are driven and maintained by a subpopulation of clonogenic cells referred to as GBM stem-like cells (GSCs). These cells have a number of in vitro properties in common with normal neural stem cells including continuous self-renewal, expression of stem cell-related genes, and the capacity to at least partially differentiate between neuronal and glial pathways [63]. Moreover, when implanted in immunodeficient mice, GSCs form a highly invasive, phenotypically heterogeneous brain tumor [64]. They also play a major role in determining radioresistance and hence are more relevant to study radioresponse of GBM [65].

Cell surface molecules such as CD133, CD15, and L1CAM are differentially expressed on GSCs and can be used for sorting or targeting GSC population. However, expression of CD133 and CD15 is not strictly related to GSCs. On the other hand, L1CAM is preferentially expressed in GSCs relative to the non-stem tumor cells and neural progenitor cells [66]. Moreover, number of studies has used CD133 as a stem cell surface marker to isolate GSCs from patient tumor samples [67]. This involves disaggregation of tumor cells, labeling with fluorescently conjugated CD133 antibody and sorting by FACS. Derived stem cells can be confirmed using neurosphere formation assay. This involves plating of single stem cells and assessing their ability to grow in suspension and form spheroids. Immunofluorescence staining can confirm spheroid expression of stem cell markers such as Sox2, Oct4, and Olig2 [68]. Other property of stem cells is to differentiate into astrocytes or oligodendrocytes by addition of serum. Some of the assays used to study radio responses of tumor cells can be employed to study radiosensitivity of stem cells; comet assay, γH2AX, and clonogenic survival assay. In vivo GSCs can be grown orthotopically in nude mice [69]. Jamal et al. have shown that the intrinsic radioresistance and effect of brain microenvironment can be studied using GSCs in nude mice [69].

## Molecular Classification of GBM: Tumor Heterogeneity

Understanding GBM heterogeneity is important to access its radioresponse. Large-scale, genomic studies of specific tumors such as The Cancer Genome Atlas (TCGA) have provided a better understanding of the alterations of pathways involved in the development of solid tumors including GBM. GBM, like other cancers, is the product of accumulated genetic and epigenetic alterations [70–72], and the application of genome-scale approaches to enumerate these genetic alterations has uncovered both molecular subclasses and common pathways mutated in this disease. Beginning with the efforts by TCGA [73, 74], and those of other groups [75, 76], GBM has been subjected to the most extensive genomic profiling of any cancer partly because it been selected as one of the first three cancers to be profiled by the National Institutes of Health's Cancer Genome Atlas (TCGA). These studies have defined a molecular landscape for GBM (Table 16.1) [77].

By leveraging TCGA data, Verhaak et al. [74] performed unsupervised hierarchical clustering of the transcriptional data from the TCGA GBM samples and integrated the results with DNA copy number and sequencing to reveal four distinct molecular subclasses that were enriched for distinct molecular alterations. These subclasses included a proneural transcriptional subclass that

is enriched for *PDGFRA* and *IDH1* mutations; classical subtype, characterized by *EGFR* amplification and *PTEN* loss; mesenchymal subtype characterized by mutation and/or loss of *NF1*, *TP53*, and *CDKN2A*. The last subtype, the neural subclass, was not clearly defined by any unique genetic signature. Furthermore, the TCGA working group recently identified DNA methylation profiles, revealing a distinct molecular subset of tumors defined by a CpG island methylator phenotype (G-CIMP) that is markedly enriched in the proneural subclass and is tightly associated with *IDH1* mutations [78]. Patients with classical subtype have better survival and patients with proneural subtype with worst prognosis [74]. The underlying changes at molecular level and hence a different subtype reflects therapeutic responses at clinical level. For example patients with IDH1 mutation are more sensitive to radiochemotherapy than IDH1 wild-type GBMs [79].

## Metabolomics in GBM

The cellular context of IDH1 mutations in GBM was first identified using metabolomics studies. Metabolomics is the global quantitative assessment of endogenous metabolites within a biological system. It allows for a global assessment of a cellular state within the context of the immediate environment, taking into account genetic regulation, altered kinetic activity of enzymes, and changes in metabolic reactions [80, 81]. Mutated IDH1 produces the oncometabolite 2-hydroxyglutarate rather than α-ketoglutarate or isocitrate. The oncometabolite is considered to be the major cause of the association between the IDH1 mutation and gliomagenesis. This association is not well-understood yet but IDH1 involvement in epigenetic silencing of *O*-6-methylguanine-DNA methyltransferase (MGMT), a DNA repair enzyme, is considered to be an important mechanism [82]. Another possible explanation is that the IDH1 mutation reduces the capacity to produce NADPH and thus reduces the capacity to scavenge ROS that are generated during irradiation and chemotherapy. IDH1 activity is responsible for two thirds of the

**Table 16.1** Compilation of established abnormalities in GBM organized by known pathways (adapted from Nicholas, Lukas et al. (2011))

| Molecular target/pathway | Abnormality | Frequency (%) | Role in primary (1°) and secondary (2°) GBM |
|---|---|---|---|
| Receptor tyrosine kinases | | | |
| EGFR | amp/mut | 30–45 | 1° > 2° |
| PDGFR | amp | 14 | 2° > 1° |
| HER2 | mut | 8 | 1° = 2° |
| c-Met | amp | 4 | 1° = 2° |
| TP53 pathway | | | |
| p53 | mut/del | 25–65 | 2° > 1° |
| MDM2 | amp | 10–25 | 1° > 2° |
| MDM4 | amp | 5–7 | 1° > 2° |
| Phosphatidyl inositol-3-kinase pathway | | | |
| PIK3CA | mut | 10–15 | 1° > 2° |
| PIK3R1 | mut | 10 | 1° > 2° |
| PTEN | mut/del | 5–40 | 1° > 2° |
| Ras pathway | | | |
| NF1 | mut/del | 10–18 | 1° > 2° |
| Cyclin-dependent kinases and retinoblastoma (RB) | | | |
| CDKN2A | mut/del | 50 | 1° = 2° |
| p16INK4A | | | 1° > 2° |
| p14ARF | | | |
| CDKN2C | | | 1° = 2° |
| p18INK4C | | | |
| CDK4 | | | 1° = 2° |
| RB | mut/del | 10–14 | 1° = 2° |
| Metabolic pathways | | | |
| IDH1, IDH2 | mut | 12–17 | 2° > 1° |

Abbreviations: *amp* amplification, *CDK4* cyclin-dependent kinase 4, *CDKN2A* cyclin-dependent kinase inhibitor 2A, *CDKN2C* cyclin-dependent kinase inhibitor 2C; *c-MET*, the MNNG HOS transforming gene, encoding a tyrosine kinase receptor that binds hepatocyte growth factor; del, deletion; *EGFR* epidermal growth factor receptor, *HER2* human epidermal growth factor Receptor 2, *IDH1* isocitrate dehydrogenase 1, *IDH2* isocitrate dehydrogenase 2, *MDM2* murine double minute 2, *MDM4* murine double minute 4, *mut* mutation, *NF1* neurofibromin 1, *p14ARF* alternate reading frame (ARF) product of the CDKN2A gene, *p16INK4A* cyclin-dependent kinase inhibitor 2A, (inhibits CDK4), *p53* tumor-suppressor protein encoded by the *TP53* gene, *PIK3CA* phosphoinositide-3-kinase catalytic alpha polypeptide, *PIK3R1* phosphoinositide-3-kinase regulatory subunit 1, *PTEN* phosphatase and tensin homolog, *Ras* a family of genes encoding small GTPases, *RB* retinoblastoma-associated protein

NADPH production capacity in normal brain, whereas the IDH1 mutation reduces this capacity by almost 40 %. Therefore, the reduced NADPH production capacity due to the IDH1 mutation renders GBM cells more vulnerable to irradiation and chemotherapy, thus prolonging survival of the patients [83]. Metabolomics can be performed on a variety of clinical samples, and as a biomarker in oncology, can be used in cancer diagnosis, assessment of response to traditional therapy and development of novel therapies.

## Computational Methods and Databases for Accessing Cancer Genomics Data

Although the data generated from the large-scale cancer genome characterization efforts have been and continue to be made publicly available, accessing and using these cancer genome data remains a major challenge. Work in this direction extended the development of computational resources and algorithms where cancer genome data can be downloaded and summarized results can be queried. Table 16.2 summarized the basic open source analytical tools or computational algorithms for manipulation and analysis of cancer genome data (Table 16.2).

## In Vivo Noninvasive Mouse Imaging

The ability to image cells, tissues, and whole animals offers an ideal solution to measure tumor burden without sacrificing the animal. Several imaging techniques have recently become available for small animals. These include 2-deoxy-2-[18F]fluoro-D-glucose positron emission tomography (FDG-PET), T2-weighted magnetic resonance imaging (T2W-MRI), and optical imaging, encompassing bioluminescence imaging (BLI) and fluorescence imaging (FLI) [84–86]. Both FDG-PET and T2W-MRI are used clinically in humans, whereas optical imaging is specifically used for research and preclinical studies. This section focuses on optical imaging in preclinical models. Most of the imaging techniques use ionizing radiation except optical imaging, which employs visible and near-infrared spectrum to visualize various cellular processes. In vivo optical imaging contributes towards the reduction in the number of animals used in basic research and drug development. For instance, the same animal can be imaged multiple times in order to monitor visually, often in real time, the progression or regression of infection or disease. In vivo optical imaging in combination with reporter gene (both fluorescent and bioluminescent reporters) technology is contributing towards a better understanding of the intricate molecular underpinnings of GBM and also is leading to the development of potential therapeutic options [86]. Several instruments are currently available to perform in vivo optical imaging and can be combined with other medical imaging modalities such as MRI and PET scans. When choosing an instrument for in vivo optical imaging, it is important to consider the method of light detection and the software used to analyze images. Due to their high sensitivity, cooled CCD cameras are most often used. When two or more reporters are used with different emission wavelengths or tissue autofluorescence is an issue, spectral unmixing can be used to tease apart the different wavelengths. Imaging of several animals simultaneously can be performed on instruments that come equipped with a multiple mouse manifold to deliver anesthetic gas, such as the IVIS series from Perkin Elmer.

Two of the most commonly used labels to locate and analyze the molecular signals are fluorescent and bioluminescent reporters. Imaging with fluorescent protein reporters has several advantages; (a) experimental setup is relatively easy, as once a reporter with certain fluorescence is chosen, it is integrated into the animal and imaged with the corresponding excitation/emission wavelengths for that fluorophore, (b) there are many fluorescent reporters available that emit light at varying wavelengths throughout the visible and near infrared spectrum. The major disadvantages are; autofluorescence of skin, and tissue, due to several cellular components that can interfere significantly with signal from fluorescent reporters if emission wavelengths overlap [87]. Additionally, chlorophyll present in standard mouse food autofluoresces, thus interfering with many common reporters [88].

Bioluminescence is most commonly used for in vivo optical imaging and refers to the light that is generated by a chemical reaction between the substrate, luciferin, and oxygen, in which luciferase acts as the enzyme to accelerate the reaction. When the electron of this reaction product returns to ground state, energy is emitted in the form of light. Unlike fluorescence imaging, there is no endogenous tissue bioluminescence; therefore, all detected light directly results from the luminescent reporter. Nevertheless, the experimental setup is slightly more challenging compared to fluorescence. You need to inject luciferin and establish the optimal dosage and the optimal time to image the animal after injection. Nevertheless, the fact that luciferin is able to cross the blood–brain barrier (BBB) is especially pertinent for GBM imaging [86, 89].

The use of in vivo optical imaging technology is emerging as an important addition to the array of tools currently available for the study

**Table 16.2** Databases for cancer genomics data (adapted and updated from Chin, Hahn et al. 2011)

| Database | Link | Data type | Type of information | Access |
|---|---|---|---|---|
| ICGC | http://dcc.icgc.org/ | Levels I–IV | Copy number, rearrangement, expression, and mutation data | Open and controlled |
| TCGA | http://cancergenome.nih.gov/dataportal | Levels I–III | Copy number, expression (mRNA and miRNA), promoter methylation, and mutation sequencing | Open and controlled |
| NCBI dbGAP | http://www.ncbi.nlm.nih.gov/gap | Levels I–II | Raw sequencing traces; second-generation sequencing BAM files by TCGA | Controlled |
| COSMIC | http://www.sanger.ac.uk/genetics/CGP/cosmic | Levels III–IV | Somatic mutations and copy number alterations by gene: amino acid position, tumor type, literature references | Open |
| Cancer Gene Census | http://www.sanger.ac.uk/genetics/CGP/Census | Level IV | Annotation of mutated or genomically altered genes | Open |
| WTSI CGP | http://www.sanger.ac.uk/genetics/CGP/Archive | Levels I–II | First-generation trace archive; SNP genotype profiles | Controlled |
| EGA | http://www.ebi.ac.uk/ega | Levels I–II | Second-generation sequencing BAM files generated by WTSI CGP | Controlled |
| Tumorscape | http://www.broadinstitute.org/tumorscape | Levels I–IV | Browsable, searchable cancer copy number viewer using SNP array data | Open |
| Oncomine | http://www.oncomine.org | Level IV | Gene expression and copy number data in readily searchable and comparable fashion | Password-protected |
| GEO | http://ncbi.nlm.nih.gov/geo | Level I | Gene expression data | Password-protected caArray |
| caArray | http://caarray.nci.nih.gov | Level I | Gene expression data | Password-protected |
| UCSC Cancer Genome Browser | https://genome-cancer.soe.ucsc.edu | Levels III–IV | Browsable viewer for cancer copy number and expression data | Open |
| The cBio Cancer Genomics Portal | http://cbioportal.org | Levels III–IV | Browsable and searchable viewer for cancer copy number and expression data | Open |
| OMIM | http://www.ncbi.nlm.nih.gov/omim | – | Inherited syndromes and causative genes for cancer and other diseases, with extensive literature review | Open |
| Mitelman | http://cgap.nci.nih.gov/Chromosomes/Mitelman | – | Copy number alterations and translocations based on cytogenetic data | Open |
| GBM-biodiscovery Portal | http://gbm-biodp.nci.nih.gov Level IV | Level IV | Browsable, searchable, and denovo prediction tool for gene expression, miRNA, and RPPA (protein) data | Open |

(Level I) Raw, (Level II) normalized/processed, (Level III) interpreted, (Level IV) summarized of GBM. The method has been successfully used to generate an optically active model of intracranial GBM that closely mimics human pathology with respect to invasion, angiogenesis, and proliferation indices [90]. Recently, Hingtgen et al. reported the development of an optical imaging and MRI approach to guide GBM resection during surgery and track tumor recurrence at multiple resolutions in mice [91]. Human or mouse glioma cells expressing luciferase can be used to monitor tumor growth, response to therapy, and to evaluate novel therapeutics using luciferase-based bioluminescence imaging (BLI) [85, 92].

## Checklist of Experiments to Develop a Sensitizer

The previous section describes various preclinical assays employed to study radiosensitization. Based on that, below we have given a checklist of experiments one could perform to develop a sensitizer:

1. Cell viability assay to examine antiproliferative effects of compound under study and to determine time and dosing kinetics.
2. Next perform the gold standard assay of radiosensitivity, i.e., clonogenic survival analysis.
3. To perform γH2AX foci, 53BP foci and comet assay in combination with radiation to analyze development of and retention of DNA damage activity.
4. If you wish to know which of the repair pathways are inhibited, then perform NHEJ and HR DNA repair assays.
5. In order to assess which are the effector pathways involved, analyze cell cycle checkpoint protein levels and cell cycle distribution.
6. Mechanism of cell death can be examined by assessment of apoptosis, mitotic catastrophe, autophagy, and senescence.
7. Finally, carry out an in vivo mouse xenograft and orthotopic models to check for radiosensitivity. The fluorescently/bioluminiscently labeled cells and tumors can be monitored using in vivo optical imaging.

## Phase II Clinical Trials Based on the Older Preclinical Models of Glioblastoma

Previous phase II studies in GBM have employed a number of agents, such as hypoxic cell radiosensitizers, cytotoxic agents, and targeted agents. The rationale for the phase I/II trials was based on (1) the understanding or assumption of the existence of tumor hypoxia and thus the need to exploit this in order to elicit therapeutic benefit, (2) previous success with the agent in question in the setting of another cancer, and (3) the understanding or perceived understanding of the signaling pathways perpetuating tumor progression and resistance to treatment. Too often have agents been selected for phase I/II trials based on the presumption that they may be effective without extensive or any preclinical research to guide dose, timing, or response. In order to increase the likelihood of an informative and practice changing phase II trial, the following two criteria can be considered necessary but not sufficient:

The drug exploits a molecular pathway known to have a significant association with tumor progression or treatment resistance and:

1. Preclinical evidence of drug effect in both in vitro and in vivo.
2. Correlation with receptor/gene, expression/tumor, and genotype/biomarkers.

Phase II trials involving GBM have evolved: new agents aimed at exploiting signaling pathways associated with glioma progression and treatment resistance, altered administration schedules for previously employed agents (e.g., dose dense TMZ), new agent combinations (erlotinib and irinotecan with TMZ), altered fractionation for RT, and new radiation modalities (e.g., carbon ions).

The introduction of new agents into phase II trials has increasingly been based on preexisting preclinical evidence. This is illustrated in phase II trials involving EGFR, mTOR, and VEGF inhibitors [93–95]. In the case of EGFR inhibitors, several have come to the forefront including EGFR tyrosine kinas inhibitors (TKI) and EGFR receptor antibodies (Cetuximab) and have led to a number of phase I and II trials. RTOG 0211 is one such trial of EGFR TKI with extensive preclinical evidence. EGFR expression and activation has been shown to be upregulated in glioma [96, 97]. Preclinical work involving the agent ZD1839 (Iressa/Gefitinib) showed that it was found to inhibit tumor proliferation in a panel of glioma cell lines, inhibit cell cycle progression through G1S and G2M, and was found to induce apoptosis [98]. Preclinical evidence thus exists for Iressa causing tumor regression both in a variety of glioma cells lines as well as tumor xenografts [96, 97, 99]. The phase II trial results found that the drug was well-tolerated, but did not improve survival beyond that seen with standard of care.

It is worthwhile noting that the standard of care changed in 2005 with the advent of the Stupp trial and the survival benefit identified with the administration of concurrent radiation and TMZ followed by adjuvant TMZ [100]. This trial also occurred before the TCGA analysis results were available and the paradigm at the time supported the conclusion that glioma signaling occurred largely through the EGFR pathway [74, 101]. No EGFR VIII stratification occurred and thus a patient subpopulation possibly responsive to gefitinib could not be identified. Other TKI's (Vandetanib) (VEGF/EGFR pathway) [94] and erlotinib [95] provided no improvement in response as single agents in the recurrent glioma setting. The mTOR inhibitors such as temsirolimus also had no single agent activity [102, 103]. Part of the reason for the failure of single agent therapy is the possibility of pathway redundancy in the heavily pretreated patient population involved in testing these agents in the recurrent glioma setting. Subsequent studies where agents were combined with standard of care concurrent chemoirradiation with TMZ (bevacizumab, erlotinib), however, also did not result in benefit [104]. As a result of the lack of clinical benefit identified in single agent phase I/II studies, horizontal (parallel pathways targeting) and vertical (downstream) rational drug combinations are being explored.

The barriers to the translation of successful preclinical results into promising new treatments in phase II trials are many and not easily overcome. They relate to the incomplete understanding of tumor heterogeneity and microenvironment [105], which leads to signaling redundancy and the impact of cancer stem cells on tumor proliferation and response [65, 106, 107]. On a more practical note, the pitfalls of phase I/II trials also relate to the often heavily pretreated patient population and selection bias inherent in the study design. Other issues are lack of molecular endpoints, and in the case of rational drug combinations, lack of preclinical data of the rational drug combination effects in vitro and vivo. Most GBM phase II trials have had some preclinical data preceding them, often a combination of tissue culture assay looking at cell survival, apoptosis, and downstream signaling as well as subcutaneous animal models. Most have not had the benefit of a molecular or genetic stratification of the patient population tested in order to determine which patients may benefit most.

## Conclusions

Despite tremendous progress in the past decade, GBM remains a challenging disease to treat. Even with the recent advances in the understanding of the molecular heterogeneity of the disease and its prognostic and predictive value, treatment options are limited. This chapter enumerates methods and protocols employed in the field of radiobiology. It highlights the more clinically relevant protocols in an attempt to find next-generation radiosensitizers. Although the current standard of care has improved overall survival to 14 months, there is no standard of care for recurrent GBM patients. After initial therapy fails, therapeutic options are limited and generally not very effective. At present, in the recurrent setting, re-irradiation is more frequently employed. Therefore, it is very important to have better understanding of GBM radiobiology, and in combination with well-designed assays, it is necessary to identify more putative radiosensitizers. The current advances in molecular studies indicate that standard of care is not always the best option for every patient. The underlying molecular aberrations could be incorporated in deciding the best treatment regimen and outcome trying to deliver a personalized medicine for individual patients. Rockne et al. have proposed a mathematical model that facilitates, based on standard clinical pre-treatment MRIs, estimation of the tumor growth in time and its response to radiotherapy [108]. The current chapter has few recommendations to improve current diagnostic and prognostic criteria as listed in the next session.

## Future Perspectives

The current WHO classification system is solely based on morphologic criteria. However, as discussed in this chapter, GBM tumors have distinct molecular signatures that could have a clinically significant impact on treatment response and survival. Molecular and genomic signatures could be incorporated into GBM classification to improvise the clinical outcomes. The routine histological classification should accompany analysis of molecular aberrations. TP53 mutations are associated with the proneural subgroup of GBM and could be used as a diagnostic biomarker by performing immunohistochemical analysis on formalin-fixed, paraffin-embedded tissue (FFPE). Moreover, drugs that potentiate p53 function and sensitize tumor cells to chemotherapy should be investigated. Currently, the EGFR status is not routinely assessed in GBM diagnosis. EGFR mutations should be routinely performed, as it can offer better therapy decisions. Also, MGMT methylation status would offer important prognostic and predictive information. The predominant tests for assessing the MGMT status include methylation-specific PCR as well as pyrosequencing. These assays can be performed on FFPE tissues [109]. Assessment of IDH-R132H protein in GBM patients who are younger than age 50 years should be done because of the relatively higher rate of IDH mutations in younger adults with GBM. This has

proven to be a reliable diagnostic, in addition to prognostic, tissue biomarker [110].

We are very hopeful that the era of personalized medicine is here, which could perhaps one day allow a therapeutic regimen that would extend patient survival well beyond current levels.

## References

1. Berens ME, Giese A. "…those left behind." Biology and oncology of invasive glioma cells. Neoplasia. 1999;1(3):208–19.
2. Connell PP, Hellman S. Advances in radiotherapy and implications for the next century: a historical perspective. Cancer Res. 2009;69(2):383–92.
3. Jeggo P, Lavin MF. Cellular radiosensitivity: how much better do we understand it? Int J Radiat Biol. 2009;85(12):1061–81.
4. Bhide SA, Nutting CM. Recent advances in radiotherapy. BMC Med. 2010;8:25.
5. Bischoff P, Altmeyer A, Dumont F. Radiosensitising agents for the radiotherapy of cancer: advances in traditional and hypoxia targeted radiosensitisers. Expert Opin Ther Pat. 2009;19(5):643–62.
6. Verheij M, Vens C, van Triest B. Novel therapeutics in combination with radiotherapy to improve cancer treatment: rationale, mechanisms of action and clinical perspective. Drug Resist Updat. 2010;13(1-2):29–43.
7. Begg AC, Stewart FA, Vens C. Strategies to improve radiotherapy with targeted drugs. Nat Rev Cancer. 2011;11(4):239–53.
8. Withers HR. The four R's of radiotherapy. In: Lett JT, Adler H, editors. Advances in radiation biology. New York: Academic Press; 1975. p. 5.
9. Steel GG, McMillan TJ, Peacock JH. The 5Rs of radiobiology. Int J Radiat Biol. 1989;56(6):1045–8.
10. Deacon J, Peckham MJ, Steel GG. The radioresponsiveness of human tumours and the initial slope of the cell survival curve. Radiother Oncol. 1984;2(4):317–23.
11. Bernier J, Hall EJ, Giaccia A. Radiation oncology: a century of achievements. Nat Rev Cancer. 2004;4(9):737–47.
12. Blazek ER, Foutch JL, Maki G. Daoy medulloblastoma cells that express CD133 are radioresistant relative to CD133- cells, and the CD133+ sector is enlarged by hypoxia. Int J Radiat Oncol Biol Phys. 2007;67(1):1–5.
13. Holmquist-Mengelbier L, et al. Recruitment of HIF-1alpha and HIF-2alpha to common target genes is differentially regulated in neuroblastoma: HIF-2alpha promotes an aggressive phenotype. Cancer Cell. 2006;10(5):413–23.

14. Bertout JA, et al. HIF2alpha inhibition promotes p53 pathway activity, tumor cell death, and radiation responses. Proc Natl Acad Sci U S A. 2009;106(34):14391–6.

15. Holmquist L, Lofstedt T, Pahlman S. Effect of hypoxia on the tumor phenotype: the neuroblastoma and breast cancer models. Adv Exp Med Biol. 2006;587:179–93.

16. Beaman GM, et al. Reliability of HSP70 (HSPA) expression as a prognostic marker in glioma. Mol Cell Biochem. 2014;393(1-2):301–7.

17. Kinner A, et al. Gamma-H2AX in recognition and signaling of DNA double-strand breaks in the context of chromatin. Nucleic Acids Res. 2008;36(17):5678–94.

18. Rogakou EP, et al. DNA double-stranded breaks induce histone H2AX phosphorylation on serine 139. J Biol Chem. 1998;273(10):5858–68.

19. Rogakou EP, et al. Megabase chromatin domains involved in DNA double-strand breaks in vivo. J Cell Biol. 1999;146(5):905–16.

20. Sedelnikova OA, et al. Quantitative detection of (125)IdU-induced DNA double-strand breaks with gamma-H2AX antibody. Radiat Res. 2002; 158(4):486–92.

21. Klokov D, et al. Phosphorylated histone H2AX in relation to cell survival in tumor cells and xenografts exposed to single and fractionated doses of X-rays. Radiother Oncol. 2006;80(2):223–9.

22. Iwabuchi K, et al. Two cellular proteins that bind to wild-type but not mutant p53. Proc Natl Acad Sci U S A. 1994;91(13):6098–102.

23. Schultz LB, et al. p53 binding protein 1 (53BP1) is an early participant in the cellular response to DNA double-strand breaks. J Cell Biol. 2000;151(7): 1381–90.

24. Anderson L, Henderson C, Adachi Y. Phosphorylation and rapid relocalization of 53BP1 to nuclear foci upon DNA damage. Mol Cell Biol. 2001;21(5):1719–29.

25. Iwabuchi K, et al. 53BP1 contributes to survival of cells irradiated with X-ray during G1 without Ku70 or Artemis. Genes Cells. 2006;11(8):935–48.

26. Ostling O, Johanson KJ. Microelectrophoretic study of radiation-induced DNA damages in individual mammalian cells. Biochem Biophys Res Commun. 1984;123(1):291–8.

27. Singh NP, et al. A simple technique for quantitation of low levels of DNA damage in individual cells. Exp Cell Res. 1988;175(1):184–91.

28. Azqueta A, Collins AR. The essential comet assay: a comprehensive guide to measuring DNA damage and repair. Arch Toxicol. 2013;87(6):949–68.

29. Shaposhnikov S, et al. Detection of Alu sequences and mtDNA in comets using padlock probes. Mutagenesis. 2006;21(4):243–7.

30. Dudas A, Chovanec M. DNA double-strand break repair by homologous recombination. Mutat Res. 2004;566(2):131–67.

31. Vasileva A, Linden RM, Jessberger R. Homologous recombination is required for AAV-mediated gene targeting. Nucleic Acids Res. 2006;34(11): 3345–60.

32. Yun S, Lie ACC, Porter AC. Discriminatory suppression of homologous recombination by p53. Nucleic Acids Res. 2004;32(22):6479–89.

33. Lieber MR. The mechanism of human nonhomologous DNA end joining. J Biol Chem. 2008;283(1): 1–5.

34. Labhart P. Nonhomologous DNA end joining in cell-free systems. Eur J Biochem. 1999;265(3):849–61.

35. North P, Ganesh A, Thacker J. The rejoining of double-strand breaks in DNA by human cell extracts. Nucleic Acids Res. 1990;18(21):6205–10.

36. Falck J, Coates J, Jackson SP. Conserved modes of recruitment of ATM, ATR and DNA-PKcs to sites of DNA damage. Nature. 2005;434(7033):605–11.

37. Matsuoka S, et al. ATM and ATR substrate analysis reveals extensive protein networks responsive to DNA damage. Science. 2007;316(5828):1160–6.

38. Yang J, et al. ATM, ATR and DNA-PK: initiators of the cellular genotoxic stress responses. Carcinogenesis. 2003;24(10):1571–80.

39. Kastan MB, Bartek J. Cell-cycle checkpoints and cancer. Nature. 2004;432(7015):316–23.

40. Brown JM, Wouters BG. Apoptosis, p53, and tumor cell sensitivity to anticancer agents. Cancer Res. 1999;59(7):1391–9.

41. Broker LE, Kruyt FA, Giaccone G. Cell death independent of caspases: a review. Clin Cancer Res. 2005;11(9):3155–62.

42. Vakifahmetoglu H, Olsson M, Zhivotovsky B. Death through a tragedy: mitotic catastrophe. Cell Death Differ. 2008;15(7):1153–62.

43. Surova O, Zhivotovsky B. Various modes of cell death induced by DNA damage. Oncogene. 2013;32(33):3789–97.

44. Rello-Varona S, et al. An automated fluorescence videomicroscopy assay for the detection of mitotic catastrophe. Cell Death Dis. 2010;1, e25.

45. Biederbick A, Kern HF, Elsasser HP. Monodansylcadaverine (MDC) is a specific in vivo marker for autophagic vacuoles. Eur J Cell Biol. 1995;66(1):3–14.

46. Mizushima N. Methods for monitoring autophagy. Int J Biochem Cell Biol. 2004;36(12):2491–502.

47. Roninson IB. Tumor cell senescence in cancer treatment. Cancer Res. 2003;63(11):2705–15.

48. Guo L, Xie B, Mao Z. Autophagy in premature senescent cells is activated via AMPK pathway. Int J Mol Sci. 2012;13(3):3563–82.

49. Puck TT, Marcus PI, Cieciura SJ. Clonal growth of mammalian cells in vitro; growth characteristics of colonies from single HeLa cells with and without a feeder layer. J Exp Med. 1956;103(2):273–83.

50. Weisenthal LM, Lippman ME. Clonogenic and non-clonogenic in vitro chemosensitivity assays. Cancer Treat Rep. 1985;69(6):615–32.

51. Hoffman RM. In vitro sensitivity assays in cancer: a review, analysis, and prognosis. J Clin Lab Anal. 1991;5(2):133–43.

52. Boucher Y, et al. Interstitial hypertension in superficial metastatic melanomas in humans. Cancer Res. 1991;51(24):6691–4.
53. Olive PL. Radiation-induced reoxygenation in the SCCVII murine tumour: evidence for a decrease in oxygen consumption and an increase in tumour perfusion. Radiother Oncol. 1994;32(1):37–46.
54. Crokart N, et al. Early reoxygenation in tumors after irradiation: determining factors and consequences for radiotherapy regimens using daily multiple fractions. Int J Radiat Oncol Biol Phys. 2005;63(3): 901–10.
55. Diepart C, et al. Comparison of methods for measuring oxygen consumption in tumor cells in vitro. Anal Biochem. 2010;396(2):250–6.
56. James PE, et al. The effects of endotoxin on oxygen consumption of various cell types in vitro: an EPR oximetry study. Free Radic Biol Med. 1995; 18(4):641–7.
57. von Heimburg D, et al. Oxygen consumption in undifferentiated versus differentiated adipogenic mesenchymal precursor cells. Respir Physiol Neurobiol. 2005;146(2-3):107–16.
58. de Jong M, Essers J, van Weerden WM. Imaging preclinical tumour models: improving translational power. Nat Rev Cancer. 2014;14(7):481–93.
59. Camphausen K, et al. Influence of in vivo growth on human glioma cell line gene expression: convergent profiles under orthotopic conditions. Proc Natl Acad Sci U S A. 2005;102(23):8287–92.
60. Jacobs VL, et al. Current review of in vivo GBM rodent models: emphasis on the CNS-1 tumour model. ASN Neuro. 2011;3(3), e00063.
61. Wilding JL, Bodmer WF. Cancer cell lines for drug discovery and development. Cancer Res. 2014;74(9):2377–84.
62. Shankavaram UT, et al. Molecular profiling indicates orthotopic xenograft of glioma cell lines simulate a subclass of human glioblastoma. J Cell Mol Med. 2012;16(3):545–54.
63. Galli R, et al. Isolation and characterization of tumorigenic, stem-like neural precursors from human glioblastoma. Cancer Res. 2004;64(19): 7011–21.
64. Singh SK, et al. Identification of a cancer stem cell in human brain tumors. Cancer Res. 2003;63(18): 5821–8.
65. Bao S, et al. Glioma stem cells promote radioresistance by preferential activation of the DNA damage response. Nature. 2006;444(7120):756–60.
66. Bao S, et al. Targeting cancer stem cells through L1CAM suppresses glioma growth. Cancer Res. 2008;68(15):6043–8.
67. Bao S, et al. Stem cell-like glioma cells promote tumor angiogenesis through vascular endothelial growth factor. Cancer Res. 2006;66(16):7843–8.
68. Huang Z, et al. Cancer stem cells in glioblastoma—molecular signaling and therapeutic targeting. Protein Cell. 2010;1(7):638–55.
69. Jamal M, et al. The brain microenvironment preferentially enhances the radioresistance of CD133(+) glioblastoma stem-like cells. Neoplasia. 2012; 14(2):150–8.
70. Stratton MR, Campbell PJ, Futreal PA. The cancer genome. Nature. 2009;458(7239):719–24.
71. Vogelstein B, Kinzler KW. Cancer genes and the pathways they control. Nat Med. 2004;10(8): 789–99.
72. Weir B, Zhao X, Meyerson M. Somatic alterations in the human cancer genome. Cancer Cell. 2004; 6(5):433–8.
73. Cancer Genome Atlas Research Network. Comprehensive genomic characterization defines human glioblastoma genes and core pathways. Nature. 2008;455(7216):1061–8.
74. Verhaak RG, et al. Integrated genomic analysis identifies clinically relevant subtypes of glioblastoma characterized by abnormalities in PDGFRA, IDH1, EGFR, and NF1. Cancer Cell. 2010;17(1):98–110.
75. Bredel M, et al. NFKBIA deletion in glioblastomas. N Engl J Med. 2011;364(7):627–37.
76. Parsons DW, et al. An integrated genomic analysis of human glioblastoma multiforme. Science. 2008;321(5897):1807–12.
77. Nicholas MK, et al. Molecular heterogeneity in glioblastoma: therapeutic opportunities and challenges. Semin Oncol. 2011;38(2):243–53.
78. Noushmehr H, et al. Identification of a CpG island methylator phenotype that defines a distinct subgroup of glioma. Cancer Cell. 2010;17(5):510–22.
79. Tran AN, et al. Increased sensitivity to radiochemotherapy in IDH1 mutant glioblastoma as demonstrated by serial quantitative MR volumetry. Neuro Oncol. 2014;16(3):414–20.
80. Griffin JL, Shockcor JP. Metabolic profiles of cancer cells. Nat Rev Cancer. 2004;4(7):551–61.
81. Spratlin JL, Serkova NJ, Eckhardt SG. Clinical applications of metabolomics in oncology: a review. Clin Cancer Res. 2009;15(2):431–40.
82. Houillier C, et al. IDH1 or IDH2 mutations predict longer survival and response to temozolomide in low-grade gliomas. Neurology. 2010;75(17): 1560–6.
83. Baldewpersad Tewarie NM, et al. NADP+-dependent IDH1 R132 mutation and its relevance for glioma patient survival. Med Hypotheses. 2013;80(6):728–31.
84. Lyons SK. Advances in imaging mouse tumour models in vivo. J Pathol. 2005;205(2):194–205.
85. Puaux AL, et al. A comparison of imaging techniques to monitor tumor growth and cancer progression in living animals. Int J Mol Imag. 2011;2011:321538.
86. Patterson AP, Booth SA, Saba R. The emerging use of in vivo optical imaging in the study of neurodegenerative diseases. Biomed Res Int. 2014; 2014:401306.

87. Monici M. Cell and tissue autofluorescence research and diagnostic applications. Biotechnol Annu Rev. 2005;11:227–56.

88. McNally JB, et al. Task-based imaging of colon cancer in the Apc(Min/+) mouse model. Appl Opt. 2006;45(13):3049–62.

89. Aswendt M, et al. Boosting bioluminescence neuroimaging: an optimized protocol for brain studies. PLoS One. 2013;8(2), e55662.

90. Jarzabek MA, et al. In vivo bioluminescence imaging validation of a human biopsy-derived orthotopic mouse model of glioblastoma multiforme. Mol Imaging. 2013;12(3):161–72.

91. Hingtgen S, et al. Real-time multi-modality imaging of glioblastoma tumor resection and recurrence. J Neurooncol. 2013;111(2):153–61.

92. Sonabend AM, et al. Murine cell line model of proneural glioma for evaluation of anti-tumor therapies. J Neurooncol. 2013;112(3):375–82.

93. Chakravarti A, et al. RTOG 0211: a phase 1/2 study of radiation therapy with concurrent gefitinib for newly diagnosed glioblastoma patients. Int J Radiat Oncol Biol Phys. 2013;85(5):1206–11.

94. Kreisl TN, et al. A phase I/II trial of vandetanib for patients with recurrent malignant glioma. Neuro Oncol. 2012;14(12):1519–26.

95. Raizer JJ, et al. A phase II trial of erlotinib in patients with recurrent malignant gliomas and nonprogressive glioblastoma multiforme postradiation therapy. Neuro Oncol. 2010;12(1):95–103.

96. Guha A, et al. Proliferation of human malignant astrocytomas is dependent on Ras activation. Oncogene. 1997;15(23):2755–65.

97. Glass TL, Liu TJ, Yung WK. Inhibition of cell growth in human glioblastoma cell lines by farnesyltransferase inhibitor SCH66336. Neuro Oncol. 2000;2(3):151–8.

98. Feldkamp MM, et al. Normoxic and hypoxic regulation of vascular endothelial growth factor (VEGF) by astrocytoma cells is mediated by Ras. Int J Cancer. 1999;81(1):118–24.

99. Kang KB, et al. Gefitinib radiosensitizes stem-like glioma cells: inhibition of epidermal growth factor receptor-Akt-DNA-PK signaling, accompanied by inhibition of DNA double-strand break repair. Int J Radiat Oncol Biol Phys. 2012;83(1):e43–52.

100. Stupp R, et al. Radiotherapy plus concomitant and adjuvant temozolomide for glioblastoma. N Engl J Med. 2005;352(10):987–96.

101. Mellinghoff IK, et al. Molecular determinants of the response of glioblastomas to EGFR kinase inhibitors. N Engl J Med. 2005;353(19):2012–24.

102. Galanis E, et al. Phase II trial of temsirolimus (CCI-779) in recurrent glioblastoma multiforme: a North Central Cancer Treatment Group Study. J Clin Oncol. 2005;23(23):5294–304.

103. Chang SM. Does temsirolimus have a role in recurrent glioblastoma multiforme? Nat Clin Pract Oncol. 2006;3(2):70–1.

104. Clarke JL, et al. A single-institution phase II trial of radiation, temozolomide, erlotinib, and bevacizumab for initial treatment of glioblastoma. Neuro Oncol. 2014;16(7):984–90.

105. Bonavia R, et al. Heterogeneity maintenance in glioblastoma: a social network. Cancer Res. 2011; 71(12):4055–60.

106. Singh S, Dirks PB. Brain tumor stem cells: identification and concepts. Neurosurg Clin N Am. 2007;18(1):31–8. viii.

107. Brescia P, et al. CD133 is essential for glioblastoma stem cell maintenance. Stem Cells. 2013;31(5):857–69.

108. Rockne R, et al. Predicting the efficacy of radiotherapy in individual glioblastoma patients in vivo: a mathematical modeling approach. Phys Med Biol. 2010;55(12):3271–85.

109. Jansen M, Yip S, Louis DN. Molecular pathology in adult gliomas: diagnostic, prognostic, and predictive markers. Lancet Neurol. 2010;9(7):717–26.

110. Horbinski C, et al. Diagnostic use of IDH1/2 mutation analysis in routine clinical testing of formalin-fixed, paraffin-embedded glioma tissues. J Neuropathol Exp Neurol. 2009;68(12):1319–25.

# From Molecular to Clinical Radiation Biology of Glioblastoma

**17**

Nadia Pasinetti, Luigi Pirtoli, Michela Buglione,
Luca Triggiani, Paolo Borghetti, Paolo Tini,
and Stefano Maria Magrini

## Premise and Background
## Mathematical Models

For a long time, the radiobiological subject of the well-known radiation resistance of glioblastoma (GB) was studied through mathematical models (MMs), not differently from other cancers. Since the early clonogenic tests on cultured

N. Pasinetti (✉) • M. Buglione • L. Triggiani
P. Borghetti
Radiation Oncology Department, University and
Spedali Civili - Brescia, Brescia 25123, Italy
e-mail: nadia_pasinetti@yhaoo.it;
michela.buglione@unibs.it; triggioluca@hotmail.it;
paolobor82@yahoo.it

L. Pirtoli
Tuscany Tumor Institute, Florence, Italy

Unit of Radiation Oncology, Department of
Medicine, Surgery and Neurosciences, University of
Siena, Siena, Italy
e-mail: luigipirtoli@gmail.com

P. Tini
Tuscany Tumor Institute, Florence, Italy

Unit of Radiation Oncology, University Hospital of
Siena (Azienda Ospedaliera Universitaria Senese),
Istituto Toscano Tumori, Viale Bracci 11, Siena, Italy
e-mail: paolo-tini@libero.it

S.M. Magrini
Radiation Oncology Department, University and
Spedali Civili - Brescia Brescia, Brescia, Italy
e-mail: stefano.magrini@unibs.it

malignant glioma cells [1] dose–response curves seem satisfactorily fitted by MMs, such as the Linear-Quadratic (LQ) model [2] and, in general, ionizing radiation (IR) sensitivity and dose-fractionation response parameters impacted on surviving fraction similarly to other tumors. More recently, some peculiarities of the IR-surviving fraction's curves in GB, diverging from LQ model at various doses, have been attributed to different cell-death pathways and/or repair mechanisms of damage to critical molecular targets, requiring more sophisticated formalisms [3]. Yet these aspects are not fully elucidated by the available MMs. Hyper-sensitivity to IR of some GB cell lines at low doses shows survival curves that have, in effect, a different behavior from that expected from the LQ MM. This behavior is not related to apoptosis, but probably to escape from the IR-induced changes that trigger increase in radiation resistance at higher doses through induction of DNA-repairing processes, or a greater access to repairing enzymes to damaged DNA [4]. We could demonstrate that in a malignant glioma cell line (T98G), the high radio-sensitivity at low and intermediate IR doses was associated with the autophagy cell-death pathway activation and can be induced by authophagy enhancement in other lines (U373MG) not spontaneously showing this behavior [5]. Thus, MMs might be inadequate to an analytic approach to some biological issues.

In the clinical scenario, presently GB patients are treated with integrated chemo-radiotherapy

© Springer International Publishing Switzerland 2016
L. Pirtoli et al. (eds.), *Radiobiology of Glioblastoma*, Current Clinical Pathology,
DOI 10.1007/978-3-319-28305-0_17

(CHT-RT) schedules, based on the alkylating agent Temozolomide (TMZ) [6]. In this domain, RT works as dichotomic parameter, with a related survival relative advantage over surgery alone, but this is not clearly dose-dependent according to a continuous dose-effect function above 60 Gy, as normally happens in solid tumors. This may be due to several factors, such as lack of data—due to the practical difficulty in safely delivering larger doses without damaging healthy brain—but generally GB recurs in the full-dose volume, thus demonstrating inherent IR resistance to high doses, in most cases. However, from a merely hypothetic point of view, the existence of a dose-response curve up to 75 Gy (that is, 34 fractions of 2.2 Gy each–Biological Effective Dose (BED)=92.1 Gy) [2] can be inferred by the LQ model (GB: $\alpha/\beta \approx 10$Gy) [7], thus indicating the possibility of a progression-free survival above 80 %. Radiobiological mathematical formalisms presently keep a role in clinical practice of RT of GB, for managing total-dose and fractionation issues on empirical grounds, but the present knowledge of genomics and signal pathways of GB warrants a mechanistic biological approach to basic, translational, and clinical research.

## Molecular Radiobiology of GB

This subject is extensively addressed in another section of this book (Chap. 9). Briefly, the DNA damage response (DDR) machinery may lead to non-homologous end joining (NHEJ) or homologous recombination (HR) repair: GB cells may exhibit enhanced DNA repair after IR through up-regulation of DNA repair genes [8], which even more effectively occurs in glioma stem-like cells (GSC). Moreover, GB cells may lose the physiological regulation of cell-cycle checkpoints, through ineffectiveness of the p53-dependent tumor-suppressing activity or inhibition of other checkpoint genes, thus resulting in a reduced yield of cell-death by IR. Some receptor tyrosine-kinase (RTK) signaling pathways, such as those downstream to the Epithelial-Growth Factor receptor (EGFR), the Platelet-Derived Growth factor receptor-alpha (PDGFRa), the

vascular endothelial growth factor receptor (VEGFR), the Tumor Necrosis factor (TNF), the human adhesion-related kinase named AXL, and the Notch cascade, may lead signals for increased aggressiveness features of GB [9], including IR-resistance. In particular, the EGFR-PI3K-Akt-mTOR pathway activation, due to amplification/overexpression of EGFR (very frequent in GB) or to its mutant form epidermal growth factor receptor variant III (EGFRvIII, lacking the extracellular domain, thus constitutively activated), is responsible for enhanced repair of DNA DSB by NHEJ after IR [10].

As for the clinical setting, the molecular classification of GB recently identified subtypes with different biological and prognostic features, but indistinguishable on morphological grounds. An aggressive postsurgical therapy, including RT, achieves a significantly reduced mortality in the classical and mesenchymal molecular subtypes, a borderline impact on survival in the neural and no effect on the proneural categories of GB [11, 12], and highlights the great heterogeneity of this disease in respect of response to current therapy. We reviewed in a chapter of this book the pathology and biological markers of prognosis in GB undergoing standard TMZ-RT at the present state-of-the-art (Chap. 7). The present therapeutic options to overcome radiation resistance of GB are the subject of another section (Chap. 2). However, no systematic formal attempt was undertaken therein to an analysis of the so-called target therapies or other ongoing research strategies against molecular determinants of aggressiveness of GB, including RT-resistance, which presently still pertains to the translational domain. This is instead the subject of the present contribution.

## Target Therapies Addressing Cell Signaling Pathways

Novel perspectives in GB treatment derive from experimental studies of targeted therapies, either alone or combined with traditional RT and CHT [13, 14]. However, clinical trials had not yet yielded significant results in terms of patient survival improvement, in spite of substantial improvements in knowledge of the biology of this disease and of technological advances and medical procedure refinements. GB is a largely heterogeneous cancer, which partly justifies failure of its treatment [13, 15]. Medical community is aware of the extreme complexity of GB since more than 30 years and attempted to individuate suitable prognostic parameters, which may help to analyze therapeutic results and to drive therapeutic management. Large scale omics analyses are unravelling GB pathobiological altered pathways, which might allow for a more comprehensive discovery of prognostic and predictive factors, as well as for novel targets for personalized therapies [15].

In particular, great expectations came from the recent assessment of the genomic landscape [16] and, in general, from the progressively improved understanding of the signal pathways of GB. The strikingly favorable impact of the tyrosine-kinase inhibitor imatinib on prognosis of chronic myeloid leukemia [17] and gastrointestinal stromal tumors (GIST) (Blanke et al., 2008), in fact, has led to a diffuse hope that unveiling biologic prognostic markers of cancers may translate into effective target therapy. Unfortunately, this is not the case of GB so far: clinical research proceeded through prospective trials testing monoclonal antibodies, tyrosine-kinase inhibitors, or other "biological" agents directed against putative determinants of aggressiveness, on the grounds of pre-clinical results indicating inherent anti-cancer properties, or radiation and/or chemotherapy enhancement, with no relevant outcome results [9, 18]. Possible hypotheses for explaining this discouraging scenario include: molecular signaling redundancy; clonal selection (or emergence) of resistant phenotypes under treatment; preclinical studies mainly addressed to tumor initiating or early-growth factors and not to late tumor progression mechanisms; difficulty in penetrating blood–brain barrier (BBB) by the drugs, etc. [18].

A shift towards new translational approaches is probably necessary. Observational studies can be implemented, grounded on large databases and heterogeneous data collection from multiple sources (i.e., clinical, imaging, laboratory, pathology, genomics, proteomics, other molecular biology data, etc.), without necessarily anticipating the possible study outcome, differently from prospective trial. More information, ontology and data standardization, "rapid-learning" machine techniques, advanced statistical methods, and external validation of the results, are necessary for this purpose. This approach could also include as a premise the yield of previous prospective trials (evidence-based medicine, EBM) or also might produce hypotheses to be confirmed by random comparisons, but in general some limits of the prospective trials, e.g., selective patients, long time, reliability of results only within a restricted domain, might be overcome.

Recent molecular and genetic studies have revealed a plethora of potential new therapeutic targets for GB. To date, however, most drugs that have made it to clinical evaluation in patients with GB have targeted the PI3K/AKT/PTEN/mTOR pathway, various RTKs (PDGFR, EGFR, VEGFR) and the p53 pathway.

In fact, the average pathway amplification rates in GB are: EGFR 35.7 %, GLI/CDK 4–13.4 %, MDM 2–9.2 %, and PIK3C2B/MDM 4–7.7 %. The CDKN2A/ CDKN2B locus was deleted in 46.4 % of the combined cases [19]. Even though other groups have found different frequency rates for these gene mutations, the pRB and p53 pathways consistently appear to be among the most frequently mutated pathways in GB. Therefore, treatment strategies targeting these signaling pathways may possess broad therapeutic potential in GB.

## PI3K/AKT/PTEN/mTOR

Despite compelling evidence that the PI3K/AKT/PTEN/mTOR pathway is a major oncogenic pathway in GB (Fig. 17.1), mTOR inhibitors have been largely unsuccessful in clinical trials to date.

Rapamycin, temsirolimus, and everolimus, first-generation mTOR inhibitors, have been studied in phase 2 trials both as monotherapy [20–22] and in combination with other targeted therapies [23–25]. Responses were generally transient; significant improvements in progression-free survival and overall survival have not been seen despite radiographic responses suggestive of biological activity [20, 23–25].

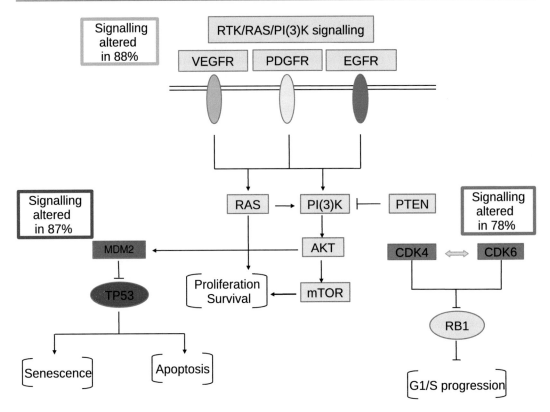

**Fig. 17.1** Three core signaling pathways altered in malignant gliomas: RTK/RAS/PI3K, RB, and p53 (see more details Paragraph 2)

Several explanations for the lack of clinical activity have been elucidated or suggested. Between them, activation of mTORC2 and AKT stimulated by mTORC1 inhibition is one of the reasons that could promote rapamycin resistance [26].

Currently, rapamycin analogs, dual-targeted mTOR complex 1 and 2 agents as well as dual mTOR and PI3K-targeted inhibitors are being investigated experimentally and in clinical trials [27].

## RTKs: VEGFR/PDGFR/EGFR

Abnormal angiogenesis is one of the hallmarks of malignant gliomas as evidenced by gadolinium-enhancement on magnetic resonance imaging and endothelial proliferation on pathology. Specifically, tumor growth depends on angiogenesis induced by VEGF expression.

Bevacizumab, a monoclonal antibody that targets the VEGF-A ligand, is the most successful targeted agent approved for recurrent glioblastoma due to high response rates. Based on two phase II trials, bevacizumab received accelerated FDA approval in 2009 for recurrent adult glioblastoma [23, 25, 28].

Recently, association of bevacizumab to initial chemoradiation showed a significantly improved progression-free survival in comparison with standard chemoradiation alone, without overall survival changing [29, 30].

Small-molecule tyrosine kinase inhibitors such as imatinib mesylate (which targets PDGFR-a, PDGFR-b, c-kit, and c-abl) and sunitinib (which targets VEGFR1-3, PDGFR-a, PDGFR-b, Kit, Fms-like tyrosine kinase 3 (Flt-3), and colony stimulating factor 1 receptor (CSF-1R)) have been tested with only limited success in GB therapy [30–32].

Other VEGFR/PDGFR inhibitors (e.g., sorafenib, pazopanib, and vatalanib) [33] and EGFR/ErB2 inhibitors (e.g., lapatinib, erlotinib, and gefitinib) have shown no significant clinical and survival benefits for GB patients [34–37]. *EGFR* is altered in about half of GB, resulting from gene mutation, amplification, and gene fusion [38, 39]. First-generation EGFR inhibitors, including erlotinib, gefitinib, and cetuximab, a chimeric EGFR monoclonal antibody, have demonstrated limited activity in GB [35–37, 40]. In the study by Mellinghoff et al. [40], primary glioblastoma cell lines from patients were treated with gefitinib or erlotinib. They found that responsiveness to EGFR kinase inhibitors was strongly associated with coexpression by the tumor of EGFRvIII and PTEN. EGFRvIII, a constitutively active mutant variant of EGFR, preferentially activates PI3K–Akt signaling and can sensitize glioblastoma cells to EGFR kinase inhibitors. Loss of PTEN, a tumor-suppressor protein that inhibits the PI3K signalling pathway (Fig. 17.1), may promote resistance to EGFR kinase inhibitors. However, they found this in a small cohort and their results were not reproduced in several subsequent studies [41, 42]: resistance mechanisms to these agents are probably more complicated. A second generation of EGFR-targeted agents includes: irreversible inhibitors; pan-Her inhibitors; and multitargeted tyrosine kinase inhibitors targeting EGFR and other tyrosine kinases, currently under evaluation. Potential explanations for the general failure of EGFR, PDGFR, and VEGFR inhibitors may be the poor ability of some inhibitors to penetrate the BBB [43]. Another potential obstacle to better clinical outcomes may be the concomitant activation of multiple RTKs, which undermine the efficacy of single-agent RTK inhibition [44–46]. Clonal subpopulations of cells that mutually express different RTKs (EGFR, MET, and PDGFR) can coexist within single tumors and the stable coexistence of different clones within the same tumor will have important clinical implications for tumor resistance to targeted therapies. The application of combined regimens is probably a better approach to targeting the heterogeneity in RTK signalling.

## p53/RB/CDKN2A

p53 mutations play a particularly significant role in the development of secondary GBs and are often the earliest detectable genetic alteration in primary brain tumors, as they are present in 65 % of precursor low-grade diffuse astrocytomas (Fig. 17.1). Mutations in the p53 pathway are also detected in primary gliomas, although less frequently [43]. There are currently only a few clinical studies targeting p53 in GB. In a phase I trial, Lang and colleagues [47] showed that intratumoral injection of a p53-containing adenovirus vector resulted in the transfer of the p53 gene and expression of functional exogenous p53 in all patients. Moreover, transfected cells were only found within a short distance from the injection site, suggesting the additional benefit of no systemic viral dissemination. Unfortunately, no clear-cut clinical benefit has been shown.

Two additional phase I trials evaluating the transduction efficiency and effectiveness of wild-type Ad5CMV-p53 gene therapy (NCT00004041) or recombinant adenovirus-p53 SCH-58500 (NCT00004080) in combination with surgery have also been completed, but reports have not been published to date [48, 49].

Since the pRB pathway, leading to mithosis and downregulated by wild-type p53, is inhibited by the kinase activity of the CDK4/CDK6/Cyclin D complex (Fig. 17.1), inhibition of CDK4/6 may be a novel treatment strategy in GB patients with aberrantly expressed pRB. A phase II study to determine the efficacy of PD 0332991 (Palbociclib), a novel small molecule inhibitor of CDK4 and CDK6, in patients with recurrent Rb-positive glioblastoma [50] has also been completed, but reports have not been published to date.

## Current Immunotherapies

The term "cancer immunosurveillance" no longer suffices to accurately describe the complex interactions that occur between a developing tumor and the immune system of the host.

Both the innate and adaptive compartments participate in the immune process and functions not only to protect the host from tumor development, but also to "edit" the immunogenicity of tumors that may eventually arise in the body.

Dunn and colleagues [51] have appropriately proposed the broader term "cancer immunoediting", to emphasize the dual roles of immunity not only to prevent but also for the shaping of neoplastic disease. Therefore, the immune system itself may be part of the problem and the mechanisms of tumor escape from immunologic control are much more complex than previously thought.

Cancer immunoediting process includes three phases, the "Three E's of immunoediting": *Elimination, Equilibrium, and Escape* [51].

*Elimination* involves the immunosurveillance of the tumor, as the immune system destroys the tumor cells it recognizes. If this phase successfully eradicates the developing tumor, it represents the complete immunoediting process without progression to the subsequent phases.

In the *equilibrium phase,* the host immune system and any tumor cell variant that has survived the previous phase enter into a dynamic equilibrium, wherein lymphocytes exert potent and relentless selection pressure on the tumor cells that is enough to contain, but not fully extinguish, a tumor bed containing many genetically unstable and mutating tumor cells.

In the *escape phase*, tumor cell variants selected in the equilibrium phase can grow in an immunologically intact environment. This breach of the host's immune defenses most likely occurs when genetic and epigenetic changes in the tumor cell confer resistance to immune detection and/or elimination, allowing the tumors to expand, become clinically detectable, and often outpace even the destructive effects of chemotherapy and radiation.

Targeted immunotherapies provide promise for inhibiting tumor growth through immune activation of tumor-infiltrating lymphocytes (TILs) and decreasing immune tolerance within the tumor microenvironment [52]. There are three basic strategies underlying immunotherapy: immune-modulating cytokine therapy, passive therapy, and active immune therapy including cancer vaccines.

The latest immunotherapy approaches have improved patient survival, provided a greater understanding of antitumor immune mechanisms, and resulted in FDA-approved agents for an expanding number of malignancies. Recent immunotherapy trials have highlighted the importance of heterogeneity in the immune microenvironment, including wide variability in the degree of intrinsic immunogenicity exhibited by different tumors.

Considerable energy and resources have been devoted to developing effective immunotherapies for GB. Modern progress in both systemic cancers and GB suggests that these efforts may be promising. Tumor-associated factors involved with suppression of cellular immune responses, in patients with GB, are partially known [53]. The brain parenchyma, in fact, is known to be immunosuppressive and GB (which originates from brain matter itself) has been shown to usurp these mechanisms [54]. Furthermore, the immunosuppressive effects of GB are not limited to its microenvironment. GB is able to induce systemic immunosuppression, limiting the innate defense to tumor growth and the efficacy of adaptive immunotherapy [55, 56].

## Passive Immunotherapy

Today, the best established type of tumor immunotherapy is passive treatment with monoclonal antibodies (mAbs). Antibody molecules are too large to passively cross the normal BBB. Even so, the same mAbs that are effective outside the brain may also benefit brain tumor patients [57]. Several factors may contribute. The BBB is dynamic, affected by both tumor growth and conventional therapies. Generally, complexes formed by a mAb and its target antigen can act as strong immunogens, to stimulate an active immune response [54].

Outside the brain, immune system components may act to modulate an active response: mAbs against non-tumor antigens are another form of indirect activity. Once an active response is stimulated, the BBB's relevance changes [54]. Activated lymphocytes are motile and their normal traffic pattern is to survey the brain; these metabolically active cells are not blocked by the BBB. Both T cells and antibody-forming cells can be found in the central nervous system and, in turn, can modify the BBB.

**Passive Cells (Adoptive Transfer)**

Passive immunotherapy can utilize activated lymphocytes, usually T cells, directly. However, for brain and other tumors, adoptive transfer of activated T cells does not yet give consistent, predictable, long-term tumor control [58, 59].

It is increasingly necessary to focus on specific roadblocks. One goal is to improve the efficacy and survival of the injected cells [58, 59]. Their survival can be increased by preliminary depletion of the patient's own lymphocytes. The fact that lymphodepletion can be a byproduct of radiation [59] or chemotherapy [60] provides one rationale for combining conventional treatments and immunotherapy for brain tumors. Advantages of passive immunotherapy include immediacy, fine control, and independence from normal immune regulation. The short expected survival for many brain tumor patients makes immediacy important.

**Active Immunization**

**Vaccines**

Active immunotherapy aims to stimulate or amplify the patient's own immune response [54]. A common strategy is to provide antigen presenting cells (APCs), usually dendritic cells (DCs), that have been made to express the target antigen (DC vaccine). A technically simpler alternative is to combine the antigen with a non-cellular adjuvant (peptide or protein vaccine), and developing new adjuvants is an ongoing goal [61]. As with

adoptive transfer, active immunization has shown promise against brain tumors and others, but is still under development. DCVax-L® by Northwest Biotherapeutics is currently under scrutiny in a phase III trial for newly diagnosed GB cases. The phase I/II clinical trials showed that median life expectancy for DCVax-L®-treated patients increased to nearly 3 years. DCVax-L® uses patient-derived tumor and healthy dendritic cell tissues to "educate" the innate immune response to recognize GB tissue for elimination and has been shown to be safe [62, 63].

A recent press release from Agenus on their Prophage G100 vaccine details the positive outcomes of a phase II trial (www.agenusbio.com). Prophage Series vaccines are individualized cancer vaccines being tested in clinical trials. Each Prophage Series vaccine is designed to contain the precise signals (antigenic fingerprint) of the patient's particular cancer and allow the body's immune system to target only cells bearing this specific fingerprint. Vaccine candidates in the Prophage Series contain the heat shock protein, gp96. This vaccine is used in conjunction with the standard treatment of care. The released results of the phase II study indicate that the median survival rate had increased to 23.3 months from the 14.6 months with standard treatment alone (Bloch et al., 2013 Abstract). The positive outcome of the multi-institutional phase II study has clear promise as a combination therapy. Prophage G100 has not as yet entered a randomized phase III trial.

Along this research avenue, Sampson et al. [64] presented the results of their phase II multicenter trial using the rindopepimut vaccine in patients with newly diagnosed EGFRvIII-expressing GB. The EGFRvIII is an immunogenic, tumor-specific mutant protein expressed on the cell surface of about one third of GB. EGFRvIII functions as a constitutively active tyrosine kinase that enhances tumorigenicity and tumor cell migration while conferring radiation and chemotherapeutic resistance. Expression of EGFRvIII is also an independent negative prognostic indicator for long-term survival for patients with GB. Thus, EGFRvIII makes an ideal potential immunotherapy target.

Preclinical studies have demonstrated that an EGFRvIII-targeted peptide vaccine is immunogenic and efficacious against established intracerebral tumors [65].

Vaccination eliminated cells expressing the EGFRvIII antigen and was associated with significantly longer PFS and OS than expected. Rindopepimut and standard adjuvant TMZ chemotherapy were administered to 65 patients with newly diagnosed EGFRvIII-expressing (EGFRvIII+) GB after gross total resection and chemoradiation. The toxicity profile was favorable. Grade 3 or 4 events were minimal, and the most common adverse event was injection site reactions. PFS at 5.5 months was 66 %, median PFS was 9.2 months, and median OS was 21.8 months. As a control, the authors looked at the EGFRvIII+ patients from the RTOG 0525 trial who matched the eligibility criteria for the ACT III trial. They reported that the median OS of the ACT III patients (21.8 months) was superior to the median OS of the matched RTOG 0525 patients (16.0 months) [66].

There are several phase II trials and one phase III trial underway for evaluation of tumor lysate vaccines. The phase II trial from the same group that conducted the phase I study has been recruiting patients since 2010 and compares the efficacy of tumor lysate-pulsed DCs with two adjuvants—resiquimod, a topical agent to boost cytotoxic T cell response, and polyinosinic-polycytidylic acid stabilized by lysine and carboxymethylcellulose (poly-ICLC), an agent shown to promote T cell infiltration of gliomas [67].

## Anti-PD-1

Another attractive approach that is also beginning to receive some clinical validation is targeting immunosuppression in the tumor bed. Even if a vaccine or T-cell modulation therapy is successful, the ability of tumors to counteract immune effectors may act to limit clinical benefit. Of current clinical interest is the PD-1/PD-L1(-L2) axis. PD-1 is expressed by T cells, particularly activated T cells, and binds to its ligands PD-L1/L2 that can be expressed by potential target cells, thereby rendering the T cell unresponsive or "exhausted" [68]. This axis is well-characterized as limiting T cell responses in chronic virus infection, but increasingly it is thought to play a role in limiting immune responses in cancer as well.

A variety of tumors, including glioblastoma, have been found to express PD-L1 (and occasionally PD-L2). A phase I/II trial of anti-PD-1 therapy in relapsed GB is currently underway (NCT01952769) (Table 17.1) [71].

## Cytokine Therapy

Cytokine therapy utilizes mediators of immune activation and proliferation to broadly induce an anti-tumor immune response. Importantly, while cytokine therapy is effective at immune activation, the immune effects are non-specific and often lead to extensive systemic toxicities, limiting their use [72]. Cytokines that have been studied include gamma-chain cytokines, such as the interleukins (IL)-2, IL-7, IL-15, and IL-21 [72]. Cytokines that signal through the common-gamma chain are potent growth factors for T cells and natural killer cells. IL-2, the $\gamma c$ prototype, can mediate antitumor effects as a single agent or in the context of multimodality regimens, but is limited by side effects and a propensity for expansion of regulatory T cells. IL-7, IL-15, and IL-21 each possesses properties that can be exploited in the context of immunotherapy for cancer. Each has been demonstrated to mediate potent vaccine adjuvant effects in tumor models, and each can enhance the effectiveness of adoptive immunotherapies. Although the overlap among the agents is significant, IL-7 is uniquely immunorestorative and preferentially augments reactivity of naive populations; IL-15 potently augments reactivity of CD8.

Produced by APCs, IL-12 is responsible for inducing Th1 immune responses and augmenting proliferation of NK and CD8+ T-cells, as well as engendering the production of IFN-$\gamma$, a marker of T-cell activation. IL-12 therapy has resulted in increased tumor rejection and local inflammatory responses in mouse models of glioma [73]. A phase I trial [74]), currently recruiting participants, involves two investigational drugs: an

**Table 17.1** Current immunotherapies (Paragraph 3)

| Target | Trial names | Phases | Protocol | Status | References |
|---|---|---|---|---|---|
| EGFRvIII + | VICTORI | I | Autologous Dcs + Rindopepimut | Completed | [69] |
| | ACTIVATE | II | Rindopepimut + GM-CSF | Completed | [64] |
| | ACT II | II | Rindopepimut + GM-CSF ± TMZ | Completed | [64] |
| | ACT III | II | Rindopepimut + GM-CSF + TMZ | Completed | [70] |
| | ReACT | II | Rindopepimut + GM-CSF ± Bevacizumab | Ongoing | https://clinicaltrials.gov/ct2/show/NCT01498328 |
| | ACT IV | III | Rindopepimut + GM-CSF + TMZ vs. standard care TMZ | Ongoing | https://clinicaltrials.gov/ct2/show/NCT01480479 |
| PD-1/PD-L1 | NCT01952769 | I-II | Pidilizumab (CT-011) | Ongoing | https://clinicaltrials.gov/ct2/show/NCT01952769 |
| Cytokines | NCT02026271 | I | Veledimex + INXN-2001 | Ongoing | https://clinicaltrials.gov/ct2/show/NCT02026271 |

activator ligand (veledimex—INXN-1001) in combination with an Adenovirus Vector Engineered to Express hIL-12 (INXN-2001) (Table 17.1).

While cytokine therapy showed some potential in preclinical studies, initial clinical results in tumor regression have been disappointing. This may be due to the multiplicity of mechanisms of tumor immune evasion in the tumor microenvironment, such as immune checkpoint interactions, that continues to suppress immune activity despite the effects of cytokine therapy. Alternatively, local delivery of cytokine may be necessary to deliver an intratumoral dose high enough to be effective [75].

## Oncolytic Viruses

Also oncolytic viruses have potential use as a treatment for GB [76]. These viruses are replication-incompetent except in specific cell populations such as tumors. Once the selected viruses find their host cell through surface marker identification, the viruses undergo lytic expansion, thus destroying the cell population, and remain replicative incompetent once the cell population is eradicated. Selectivity of these viruses depends on the cell surface expression of targeted receptors. EGFRvIII, PDGFR, and IL-13R have all been used as selectivity receptors for GB in oncolytic virus production. Oncolytic viruses, including Herpes Simplex 1, are under investigation for use in GB. HSV-1M032 is being explored as it lacks the γ134.5 neurovirulence loci, which prevents virus latency and has appropriate biodistribution after intracerebral injection in nonhuman primates with no adverse clinical signs [77]. HSV-1M032 is in a phase I trial, which has not been opened for recruitment to date [78].

GB Adenovirus trials have also begun using DNX-2401. Formerly known as Delta-24, this adenovirus is selective for GB due to the deregulation of retinoblastoma protein. Delta-24 replication is dependent on functionally inactive retinoblastoma protein. The addition of an RGD-4C peptide increases oncolytic activity against GB compared to non-RGD-containing

analogs [79]. In mouse xenograft models, single-dose injections of Delta-24-RGD-4C decreased tumor size and increased mouse survival. In a phase I trial, 52 % of the 24 patients who received a single intratumoral injection of the DNX-2401 as first-line therapy showed stabilization or partial or complete regression of their disease [80].

## Synergism with Chemo- and Radiation-therapy

## Vaccines and Chemotherapy

Chemotherapy and immunotherapy have often been regarded as independent or antagonistic treatment modalities. This assumption is based on two considerations. First, cytotoxic chemotherapy is associated with severe lymphopenia, due to non-specific cell death of proliferating cells [81]. Second, chemotherapy-induced cell death was presumed to occur through a non-inflammatory apoptotic process or by induction of immune tolerance [81]. In the first case, lymphopenia could theoretically curtail immunotherapy's effectiveness by depleting the peripheral pool of immune cells available for mounting an antitumor response. In the second case, chemotherapy effects would be either a passive lack of immune activation and proliferation or an active suppression of antigen presentation by tumor-infiltrating T cells. However, chemo- and immunotherapy are no longer considered to be a priori antagonistic [82] and the concept of combined chemo-immuno therapy is receiving more attention [83].

Antigens suspected to play a role in synergy between drug and vaccines therapies included EGFRvIII (Table 17.1). As previously described, a phase II trial (ACT II) compared the use of standard TMZ doses of 200 mg/m$^2$ for 5 days out of 4 weeks in conjunction with the EGFRvIII vaccine and GM-CSF versus TMZ doses of 100 mg/m$^2$ for 21 days out of 4 weeks in conjunction with the EGFRvIII vaccine and GM-CSF [64].

A multicenter, single-arm phase II clinical trial (ACT III) was performed to confirm these results [70].

The EGFRvIII peptide vaccine (rindopepimut) has now moved on to a phase III trial (ACT-IV). This 2-arm, randomized, phase III study will investigate the efficacy and safety of the addition of rindopepimut to the current standard of care (TMZ) in patients with recently diagnosed glioblastoma [84]. This study is ongoing but not recruiting participants, and the results are not complete.

The phase II trial with relapsed EGFRvIII-positive glioblastoma, ReACT, is also ongoing for administration of EGFRvIII peptide vaccine and GM-CSF in combination with bevacizumab [85]. Another phase III trial is designed to evaluate the impact on disease progression and survival time, as well as safety, in patients following treatment with DCVax-L®. Patients will receive the standard of care, including radiation and TMZ therapy, and two out of three will additionally receive DCVax-L®, with the remaining one third receiving a placebo.

Patients randomized to the placebo arm will have the option to receive DCVax-L® in a crossover arm upon documented disease progression [86].

These studies serve to emphasize the delicate immune balance that can ultimately determine the success of a treatment protocol. In practice, clinicians may either administer vaccines concurrently with chemoradiation (Table 17.2) or use an interdigitated alternating regimen as a strategy to minimize cytotoxic T lymphocytes (CTL) depletion and maximize Treg inhibition. In addition to harnessing chemotherapy immune-activating effects, immunotherapy may also be used as a chemo-sensitizing agent that renders drug-resistant tumors more amenable to standard therapeutic options.

A significant advance in our understanding of the plethoric immunomodulatory properties of many conventional chemotherapeutic drugs and targeted therapeutic agents has been a driving force behind the design and development of chemoimmunotherapeutic strategies. Selected antineoplastic agents, by inducing rapid tumor shrinkage, reversing cancer-induced immunosuppression, and promoting antitumor cytotoxic immune effectors, may create a favorable environment, allowing immune-based therapies [87].

## Vaccines and Radiation Therapy

Ionizing radiation exhibits immunomodulatory properties. Historically, RT is considered to be an immunosuppressive agent [88]; T lymphocytes, in particular, have been shown to be extremely sensitive to ionizing radiation [88]. Thus, it has been easy to assume that radiotherapy is counterproductive to immunotherapy.

However, multiple preclinical and clinical observations in recent years have indicated that certain patients with cancer obtain greater clinical benefit from immunotherapy regimens if they have been previously treated with RT [89].

The immunogenic effects of RT can be exploited to promote synergistic clinical benefits for patients receiving combination regimens with therapeutic cancer vaccines.

RT evokes a spectrum of molecular alterations in the biology of surviving tumor cells, defined as immunogenic modulation, that renders tumor cells more sensitive to attack by antigen-specific $CD8^+$ cytotoxic T lymphocytes. The molecular mechanisms associated with immunogenic modulation include (1) changes in tumor cell surface phenotype, (2) modulation of anti-apoptotic or survival genes, or immune-responsive genes or both, (3) modulation of antigen-processing machinery components, and (4) translocation of calreticulin to the tumor cell surface [90].

Immune activation secondary to apoptotic cell death suggests a synergistic role for radiation therapy and immunotherapy. Furthermore, recent findings strongly show a proinflammatory effect of radiotherapy that may synergize with therapeutic immune modulators.

The synergistic effects of radiation and immunotherapy have also been reported. The phase I study [91] evaluated a Gene-Mediated Cytotoxic Immunotherapy approach for malignant gliomas. The purpose of this study was to assess the safety and feasibility of delivering an experimental approach called GliAtak, which uses AdV-tk, an adenoviral vector containing the Herpes Simplex thymidine kinase gene, plus an oral anti-herpetic prodrug, valacyclovir, in combination with standard of care radiation.

**Table 17.2** Synergism with chemo- and radiation-therapy (Paragraph 5)

| Trial names | Phases | Protocol | Status | References |
|---|---|---|---|---|
| ReACT | II | Rindopepimut + GM-CSF ± Bevacizumab | Ongoing | https://clinicaltrials.gov/ct2/show/NCT01498328 |
| ACT IV | III | Rindopepimut + GM-CSF + TMZ vs. standard care TMZ | Ongoing | https://clinicaltrials.gov/ct2/show/NCT01480479 |
| NCT00045968 | III | TMZ + RT + DCVax®-L vs. TMZ (+RT) + placebo | Ongoing | https://clinicaltrials.gov/ct2/show/NCT00045968 |
| NCT00751270 | Ib | AdV-tk + Valacyclovir + RT | Completed — no results published | https://clinicaltrials.gov/ct2/show/NCT00751270 |

Another important implication for the potential use of immunotherapies against GB was downregulation of MHC class I and II genes in migrating and invading glioma cells [92]. RT increases expression of MHC molecules, thereby counteracting a principal strategy for immune evasion by GB. Newcomb et al. showed in a mouse model that RT increases the expression of MHC class I on GL261 glioma cells in vitro and increases the expression of β2-microglobulin in vivo. When RT is combined with peripheral vaccination, it achieves significant long-term survival rates in animals bearing established, measurable intracranial tumors with an invasive phenotype [93]. The fact that modest doses of radiation were required to recover MHC class I expression supports the safety of combining radiotherapy in trials of immunotherapy for patients with recurrent high-grade gliomas who are likely to have already received first-line radiotherapy.

Several additional preclinical and clinical experiences have been reported for DCs immunotherapy of malignant gliomas and specifically of glioblastoma multiforme. Pellegatta et al. demonstrated the prolonged survival of mice with GL261 malignant gliomas treated by intratumoral (IT)-pulsed-(p)DC only or in combination with subcutaneous-pDC [94].

Yamanaka et al. have found that patients with both IT and intradermal (ID) administration of DC ($n=7$) had a longer survival time than the patients with intradermal administration only ($n=11$; $P=.043$) [95].

Results support the idea that IT delivery of DC may increase anti-tumor efficacy by creating an IT environment more favorable to the development of T-cell-mediated immune responses.

Numerous studies showed the synergistic effects of EGFR vaccines and RT (Table 17.2). As published by Heimberger et al. [69], EGFRvIII overexpression is a poor prognostic indicator in patients surviving $\geq 1$ year and the expression of EGFRvIII is a negative prognosticator for long-term survival. Radiation exposure has been shown to result in robust stimulation of the EGFRvIII mutant receptor, leading to increased tumor survival and expansion. PEPvIII

(an EGFRvIII-targeted peptide vaccine) was administered after the completion of radiation in many different trials. In the first clinical trial (VICTORI) conducted at Duke University Medical Center, PEPvIII was loaded onto autologous DCs, which were matured and used for immunization. In a phase 2 study clinical trial (A Complimentary Trial of an Immunotherapy Vaccine Against Tumor Specific EGFRvIII (ACTIVATE)), the OS of vaccinated patients was greater than that observed in a control group matched for eligibility criteria, prognostic factors, and TMZ treatment. [96].

The preclinical studies and early clinical trials described here demonstrate that RT can enhance the efficacy of therapeutic cancer vaccines. Although these outcomes provide the rationale for current clinical trials employing both modalities, further investigation is required to achieve synergy and realize the full potential of the combination. Radiation induces a spectrum of immunogenic alterations in tumor biology, ranging from immunogenic modulation to immunogenic cell death (ICD). These may be harnessed to achieve optimal synergy with therapeutic cancer vaccines, mAb, and other immunotherapy regimens to maximize clinical benefit, even for patients in whom RT failed or those who have limited treatment options [97].

## Heavy Ion Radiotherapy

In GB, a multiplicity of approaches has been investigated in the efforts to enhance traditional treatments (RT and CHT). In particular, signaling cascades involved in cell proliferation, apoptosis, and angiogenesis achieved major importance as targets for GB therapy. Combining molecular-targeted therapies and RT or/and CHT may allow for reducing toxicities and improving treatment outcomes. Also other modalities applying charged particles can be improved in parallel to traditional photon therapy. The emergence of heavy ion radiotherapy using carbon ions constitutes an innovative development in the field of high-precision radiotherapy. Carbon ions are less dependent on the oxygen enhancement ratio

(OER) and carbon irradiation-induced apoptosis, autophagy, and cellular senescence [98]. A synergistic role for RT and immunotherapy through immune activation secondary to apoptotic cell death is recognized. Moreover, via decreased expression of integrins, it was shown to inhibit glioma migration. Japanese data indicate beneficial effects of chemo-radiation in combination with carbon irradiation in treatment of GB. In a preliminary phase I/II clinical trial, the survival of patients with glioblastoma treated with carbon radiotherapy increased in a dose-dependent manner [99]. A retrospective analysis published by Combs et al. [100] showed that, for GB, an increase in OS by addition of a carbon ion boost may be expected in combination with TMZ. Based on the preclinical experience, an additive effect of carbon ions may be expected to potentially increase outcome. This question is currently being evaluated in the CLEOPATRA trial. In the Phase II-CLEOPATRA study, a carbon ion boost was compared to a proton boost applied to the macroscopic tumor after surgery at primary diagnosis in patients with GB in combination with after standard RT-CHT with TMZ [101]. No study results are actually posted.

## Conclusions and Future Perspectives

The power of molecular-targeted therapy has been limited by multiple factors, from complexity of molecular biology underlying gliomagenesis to challenges of patient selection to specific therapies, drug delivery, and evaluation of treatment response.

The project that catalogs genomic abnormalities involved in the development of cancer, named The Cancer Genome Atlas (TCGA) [102, 103], published the results of its first study in a large GB cohort consisting of 206 patient samples. Recently, Verhaak et al. subclassified GB into proneural, neural, classical, and mesenchymal subtypes by integrating multidimensional data on gene expression, somatic mutations, and DNA copy number [11, 12]. This classification might lead to establishment of personalized therapies for groups of patients with GB.

In malignant glioma, other several factors such as drug delivery, pharmacological effects, and so on limited success of molecular targeted therapies in clinical trials.

Redundancy and complexity of signaling pathways often lead to failure of clinical studies with single molecular-targeted agents. While research and development of more promising molecular-targeted agents are needed in the laboratory, known molecular-targeted agents are likely to have synergistic antitumor effects in combination. Therefore, adding other therapeutic modalities to molecular targeted therapy might create new avenues for success.

Failure of molecular-targeted therapies may be also caused by the discrepancy between PFS and OS as endpoints; also the question when and how to integrate new therapies into the backbone of standard therapy still remains.

Similarly, these aspects concern immunotherapy, where major obstacles to broad clinical applicability become progressively more evident. Most strategies define only a short-lasting tumor rejection, with many patients responding poorly to treatment. The precise processes behind this high variability of therapeutic efficacy remain to be clarified, but most likely involve high heterogeneity of different tumor types as well as poor immunogenicity and evolving capability to escape immune recognition [104].

Another area of interest is drug development that penetrates or bypasses BBB (like liposomal carriers and nanoscale particles). The BBB becomes the obstacle for entrance of large or water-soluble molecules and limits the ability of drugs to reach sufficient concentration in glioma tissue. Focus the attention on new drugs generation is always more relevant.

Some questions also concern RT techniques and doses remain open. It's necessary to maximize RT effects combining new molecular target agents with different radiation schedule, leading to management of toxicities without losing the possibility of a good tumor response.

In summary, global gene expression analysis incorporated into patient glioma analysis and treatment management might identify predictive and therapeutic biomarkers, stratify patients based on molecular characteristics, and provide individualized therapies. Additionally, development in the investigation of novel molecular-targeted agents, multiple combined treatments, and integration with standard therapies might allow the "molecularly tailored" therapeutic strategies to cure GB in the future.

# References

1. Gerweck LE, Komblith PL, Burlett P, et al. Radiation sensitivity of cultured glioblastoma cells. Radiology. 1977;125:231–4.
2. Fowler JF. A review: the linear quadratic formula and progress in fractionated radiotherapy. Br J Radiol. 1989;62:679–94.
3. Williams JR, Gridley DS, Slater JB. Radiobiology of resistant glioblastoma cells. www.intechopen 2011; 3–22.
4. Joiner MC, Marples B, Lamblin P. Low-dose hypersensitivity: current status and possible mechanism. Int J Radiat Oncol Biol Phys. 2001;49:379–89.
5. Palumbo S, Pirtoli L, Tini P, et al. Different involvement of autophagy in human malignant glioma cell lines undergoing irradiation and temozolomide combined treatment. J Cell Biochem. 2012;113: 2308–18.
6. Stupp R, Mason WP, van den Bent MJ, et al. Radiotherapy plus concomitant and adjuvant temozolomide for glioblastoma. N Engl J Med. 2005; 352:987–96.
7. Pedicini P, Fiorentino A, Simeon V, et al. Clinical radiobiology of glioblastoma multiforme. Estimation of tumor control probability from various radiotherapy fractionation schemes. Strahlenther Onkol. 2014;190:925–32.
8. Otomo T, Hishii M, Arai H, et al. Microarray analysis of temporal gene responses to ionizing radiation in two glioblastoma cell lines: up-regulation of DNA repair genes. J Radiat Res. 2004;45:53–60.
9. Veliz I, Loo Y, Castillo O, et al. Advances and challenges in the molecular biology and treatment of glioblastoma—is there any hope for the future? Ann Transl Med. 2015;3(1):7.
10. Hatampaa KJ, Burma S, Zhao D, Habib AA. Epidermal growth factor receptor in glioma: signal transduction, neuropathology, imaging, and radioresistance. Neoplasia. 2010;12:675–84.
11. Verhaak RGW, Hoadley KA, Purdom E, et al. An integrated genomic analysis identifies clinically relevant subtypes of glioblastoma characterized by abnormalities in PDGFRA, IDH1, EGFR and NF1. Cancer Cell. 2010;17(1):98–110. doi:10.1016/J. ccr2009.12.020.
12. Verhaak RGW, Hoadley KA, Purdom E, et al. Integrated genomic analysis identifies clinically relevant subtypes of glioblastoma characterized by abnormalities in PDGFRA, IDH1, EGFR, and NF1. Cancer Cell. 2010;17(1):98–110.
13. Ohka F, Natsume A, Wakabayashi T. Current trends in targeted therapies for glioblastoma multiforme. Neurol Res Int. 2012;2012:878425.
14. Mrugala MM. Advances and challenges in the treatment of glioblastoma: a clinician's perspective. Discov Med. 2013;15(83):221–30.
15. Cloughesy TF, Cavenee WK, Mischel PS. Glioblastoma: from molecular pathology to targeted treatment. Annu Rev Pathol. 2014;9:1–25.
16. Brennan CW, Verhaak RG, McKenna A, et al. The somatic genomic landscape of glioblastoma. Cell. 2013;155(2):462–77.
17. Druker BJ, Guilhot F, O'Brien SG, et al. Five-year follow-up of patients receiving imatinib for chronic myeloid leukemia. N Engl J Med. 2006;355(23): 2408–17.
18. Bastien JI, McNeill KA, Fine HA. Molecular characterizations of glioblastoma, targeted therapy, and clinical results to date. Cancer. 2015;121(4): 502–16.
19. Rao SK, Edwards J, Joshi AD, Siu IM, Riggins GJ. A survey of glioblastoma genomic amplifications and deletions. J Neurooncol. 2010;96: 169–79.
20. Galanis E, Buckner JC, Maurer MJ, et al. Phase II trial of temsirolimus (CCI-779) in recurrent glioblastoma multiforme: a North Central Cancer Treatment Group study. J Clin Oncol. 2005;23:5294–304.
21. Chang SM, Wen P, Cloughesy T, et al. Phase II study of CCI-779 in patients with recurrent glioblastoma multiforme. Invest New Drugs. 2005;23:357–61.
22. Cloughesy T, Raizer J, Drappatz J, et al. A phase II trial of everolimus in patients with recurrent glioblastoma multiforme. Neuro Oncol. 2011;13 suppl 3:42–3.
23. Kreisl TN, Lassman AB, Mischel PS, et al. A pilot study of everolimus and gefitinib in the treatment of recurrent glioblastoma (GBM). J Neurooncol. 2009;92:99–105.
24. Lee EQ, Kuhn J, Lamborn KR, et al. Phase I/II study of sorafenibin combination with temsirolimus for recurrent glioblastoma or gliosarcoma: North American Brain Tumor Consortium study 05-02. Neuro Oncol. 2012;14:1511–8.
25. Kreisl TN, Kim L, Moore K, et al. Phase II trial of single agent bevacizumab followed by bevacizumab plus irinotecan at tumor progression in recurrent glioblastoma. J Clin Oncol. 2009;27(5):740–5.
26. Tanaka K, Babic I, Nathanson D, et al. Oncogenic EGFR signaling activates an mTORC2-NF-jB pathway that promotes chemotherapy resistance. Cancer Discov. 2011;1:524–38.
27. Sami A, Karsy M. Targeting the PI3K/AKT/mTOR signaling pathway in glioblastoma: novel therapeutic agents and advances in understanding. Tumour Biol. 2013;34:1991–2002.

28. Vredenburgh JJ, Desjardins A, Herndon JE, et al. Bevacizumab plus irinotecan in recurrent glioblastoma multiforme. J Clin Oncol. 2007;25(30):4722–9.

29. Chinot OL, Wick W, Mason W, et al. Bevacizumab plus radiotherapy-temozolomide for newly diagnosed glioblastoma. N Engl J Med. 2014;370:709–22.

30. Gilbert MR, Dignam JJ, Armstrong TS, et al. A randomized trial of bevacizumab for newly diagnosed glioblastoma. N Engl J Med. 2014;370:699–708.

31. Fine HA. Bevacizumab in glioblastoma—still much to learn. N Engl J Med. 2014;370:764–5.

32. Kreisl TN, Smith P, Sul J, Salgado C, Iwamoto FM, Shih JH, Fine HA. Continuous daily sunitinib for recurrent glioblastoma. J Neurooncol. 2013;111(1):41–8.

33. Reardon DA, Vredenburgh JJ, Desjardins A, et al. Effect of CYP3A-inducing anti-epileptics on sorafenib exposure: results of a phase II study of sorafenib plus daily temozolomide in adults with recurrent glioblastoma. J Neurooncol. 2011;101:57–66.

34. Thiessen B, Stewart C, Tsao M, et al. A phase I/II trial of GW572016 (lapatinib) in recurrent glioblastoma multiforme: clinical outcomes, pharmacokinetics and molecular correlation. Cancer Chemother Pharmacol. 2010;65:353–61.

35. Raizer JJ, Abrey LE, Lassman AB, et al. A phase I trial of erlotinib in patients with nonprogressive glioblastoma multiforme postradiation therapy, and recurrent malignant gliomas and meningiomas. Neuro Oncol. 2010;12:87–94.

36. Uhm JH, Ballman KV, Wu W, et al. Phase II evaluation of gefitinib in patients with newly diagnosed grade 4 astrocytoma: Mayo/North Central Cancer Treatment Group Study N0074. Int J Radiat Oncol Biol Phys. 2011;80:347–53.

37. Raizer JJ, Abrey LE, Lassman AB, et al. A phase II trial of erlotinib in patients with recurrent malignant gliomas and nonprogressive glioblastoma multiforme postradiation therapy. Neuro Oncol. 2010;12:95–103.

38. Fuller GN, Bigner SH. Amplified cellular oncogenes in neoplasms of the human central nervous system. Mutat Res. 1992;276:299–306.

39. Frattini V, Trifonov V, Chan JM, et al. The integrated landscape of driver genomic alterations in glioblastoma. Nat Genet. 2013;4510:1141–9.

40. Mellinghoff IK, Wang MY, Vivanco I, et al. Molecular determinants of the response of glioblastomas to EGFR kinase inhibitors. N Engl J Med. 2005;353:2012–24.

41. Van den Bent MJ, Brandes AA, Rampling R, et al. Randomized phase II trial of erlotinib versus temozolomide or carmustine in recurrent glioblastoma: EORTC Brain Tumor Group Study 26034. J Clin Oncol. 2009;27:1268–74.

42. Yung WK, Vredenburgh JJ, Cloughesy TF, et al. Safety and efficacy of erlotinib in first-relapse glioblastoma: a phase II open-label study. Neuro Oncol. 2010;12:1061–70.

43. Mao H, Lebrun DG, Yang J, Zhu VF, Li M. Deregulated signaling pathways in glioblastoma multiforme: molecular mechanisms and therapeutic targets. Cancer Invest. 2012;30:48–56.

44. Snuderl M, Fazlollahi L, Le LP, et al. Mosaic amplification of multiple receptor tyrosine kinase genes in glioblastoma. Cancer Cell. 2011;20:810–7.

45. Szerlip NJ, Pedraza A, Chakravarty D, et al. Intratumoral heterogeneity of receptor tyrosine kinases EGFR and PDGFRA amplification in glioblastoma defines subpopulations with distinct growth factor response. Proc Natl Acad Sci U S A. 2012;109:3041–6.

46. Inda MM, Bonavia R, Mukasa A, et al. Tumor heterogeneity is an active process maintained by a mutant EGFR-induced cytokine circuit in glioblastoma. Genes Dev. 2010;24:1731–45.

47. Lang FF, Bruner JM, Fuller GN, Aldape K, Prados MD, Chang S, Berger MS, McDermott MW, Kunwar SM, Junck LR, Chandler W, Zwiebel JA, Kaplan RS, Yung WK. Phase I trial of adenovirus-mediated p53 gene therapy for recurrent glioma: biological and clinical results. J Clin Oncol. 2003;21:2508–18.

48. ClinicalTrials.gov. Gene therapy in treating patients with recurrent malignant gliomas. http://clinicaltrials.gov/ct2/show/NCT00004041. Accessed June 2014.

49. ClinicalTrials.gov. Gene therapy in treating patients with recurrent or progressive brain tumors. http://clinicaltrials.gov/ct2/show/NCT00004080. Accessed June 2014.

50. ClinicalTrials.gov. A study of PD 0332991 in patients with recurrent Rb positive glioblastoma. http://clinicaltrials.gov/ct2/show/NCT01227434.

51. Dunn GP, Old LJ, Schreiber RD. The three Es of cancer immunoediting. Annu Rev Immunol. 2004;22:329–60.

52. Topalian SL, Weiner GJ, Pardoll DM. Cancer immunotherapy comes of age. J Clin Oncol. 2011;29:4828–36.

53. Waziri A. Glioblastoma-derived mechanisms of systemic immunosuppression. Neurosurg Clin N Am. 2010;21(1):31–42.

54. Lampson LA. Brain tumor immunotherapy: seeing the brain in the body. Drug Discov Today. 2013;18(7–8):399–406.

55. Bloch O, Crane CA, Kaur R, et al. Gliomas promote immunosuppression through induction of B7-H1 expression in tumor-associated macrophages. Clin Cancer Res. 2013;19(12):3165–75.

56. Bloch O, Kaur T, Aghi M, et al. Progression-free survival in a trial of immunotherapy for glioblastoma (abstract). In: Proceedings of the 81st Annual Meetings of the American Association of Neurological Surgeons; 2013 April 28–May 1, New Orleans, LA: J Neurosurgery 2013;119. p. A565. Abstract no. 801.

57. Lampson LA. Monoclonal antibodies in neuro-oncology: getting past the blood–brain barrier. MAbs. 2011;3:153–60.

58. Wölfl M, et al. Primed tumor-reactive multifunctional CD62L1 human CD81 T cells for immunotherapy. Cancer Immunol Immunother. 2011;60:173–86.

59. Tatum AM, et al. CD81 T cells targeting a single immunodominant epitope are sufficient for elimination of established SV40T antigen-induced brain tumors. J Immunol. 2008;181:4406–17.

60. Dietrich PY, et al. T-cell immunotherapy for malignant glioma: toward a combined approach. Curr Opin Oncol. 2010;22:604–10.

61. Mellman I, et al. Cancer immunotherapy comes of age. Nature. 2011;480:480–9.

62. Yu JS, Liu G, Ying H, Yong WH, Black KL, Wheeler CJ. Vaccination with tumor lysate-pulsed dendritic cells elicits antigen-specific, cytotoxic T-cells in patients with malignant glioma. Cancer Res. 2004;64:4973–9.

63. Prins RM, Soto H, Konkankit V, Odesa SK, Eskin A, Yong WH, Nelson SF, Liau LM. Gene expression profile correlates with T-cell infiltration and relative survival in glioblastoma patients vaccinated with dendritic cell immunotherapy. Clin Cancer Res. 2011;17:1603–15.

64. Sampson JH, Aldape KD, Archer GE, Coan A, et al. Greater chemotherapy-induced lymphopenia enhances tumor-specific immune responses that eliminate EGFRvIII-expressing tumor cells in patients with glioblastoma. Neuro Oncol. 2011;13(3):324–33.

65. Jackson CM, Lim M, Drake CG. Immunotherapy for brain cancer: recent progress and future promise. Clin Cancer Res. 2014;20(14):3651–9.

66. Lim M. Immunotherapy for glioblastoma: are we finally getting closer? Neuro Oncol. 2015;17(6):771–2.

67. ClinicalTrials.gov. Dendritic cell vaccine for patients with brain tumors. https://clinicaltrials.gov/ct2/show/NCT01204684.

68. Keir ME, Butte MJ, Freeman GJ, et al. PD-1 and its ligands in tolerance and immunity. Annu Rev Immunol. 2008;26:677–704.

69. Heimberger AB, Sampson JH. PEP-3-KLH (CDX-110) vaccine in glioblastoma multiforme patients. Expert Opin Biol Ther. 2009;9(8):1087–98.

70. Schuster J, Lai RK, Recht LD, et al. A phase II, multicenter trial of rindopepimut (CDX-110) in newly diagnosed glioblastoma: the ACT III study. Neuro Oncol. 2015;17(6):854–61.

71. ClinicalTrials.gov. Anti PD1 antibody in diffuse intrinsic pontine glioma and relapsed glioblastoma multiforme. https://clinicaltrials.gov/show/NCT01952769.

72. Fewkes NM, Mackall CL. Novel gamma-chain cytokines as candidate immune modulators in immune therapies for cancer. Cancer J. 2010;16:392–8.

73. DiMeco F, Rhines LD, Hanes J, Tyler BM, Brat D, Torchiana E, Guarnieri M, Colombo MP, Pardoll DM, Finocchiaro G, et al. Paracrine delivery of IL-12 against intracranial 9L gliosarcoma in rats. J Neurosurg. 2000;92:419–27.

74. ClinicalTrials.gov. A study of Ad-RTS-hIL-12 WITH Veledimex in subjects with glioblastoma or malignant glioma. http://clinicaltrials.gov/ct2/show/NCT02026271.

75. Patel MA, Kim JE, Ruzevick J, Li G, Lim M. The future of glioblastoma therapy: synergism of standard of care and immunotherapy. Cancers (Basel). 2014;6(4):1953–85.

76. Carlsson SK, Brothers SP, Wahlestedt C. Emerging treatment strategies for glioblastoma multiforme. EMBO Mol Med. 2014;6(11):1359–70.

77. Roth JC, Cassady KA, Cody JJ, Parker JN, Price KH, Coleman JM, Peggins JO, Noker PE, Powers NW, Grimes SD, et al. Evaluation of the safety and biodistribution of M032, an attenuated herpes simplex virus type 1 expressing hIL-12, after intracerebral administration to aotus nonhuman primates. Hum Gene Ther Clin Dev. 2014;25:16–27.

78. ClinicalTrials.gov. Genetically engineered HSV-1 Phase 1 Study (M032-HSV-1) http://clinicaltrials.gov/ct2/show/NCT02062827.

79. Fueyo J, Alemany R, Gomez-Manzano C, Fuller GN, Khan A, Conrad CA, Liu TJ, Jiang H, Lemoine MG, Suzuki K, et al. Preclinical characterization of the antiglioma activity of a tropism-enhanced adenovirus targeted to the retinoblastoma pathway. J Natl Cancer Inst. 2003;95:652–60.

80. Pol JG, Marguerie M, Arulanandam R, Bell JC, Lichty BD. Panorama from the oncolytic virotherapy summit. Mol Ther. 2013;21:1814–8.

81. Prins RM, Odesa SK, Liau LM. Immunotherapeutic targeting of shared melanoma-associated antigens in a murine glioma model. Cancer Res. 2003;63:8487–91.

82. Lake RA, Robinson BWS. Immunotherapy and chemotherapy—a practical partnership. Nat Rev Cancer. 2005;5:397–405.

83. Haynes NM, Van der Most RG, Lake RA, Smyth MJ. Immunogenic anti-cancer chemotherapy as an emerging concept. 2008. Curr Opin Immunol.

84. ClinicalTrials.gov. Phase III STUDY of Rindopepimut/GM-CSF in patients with newly diagnosed glioblastoma (ACT IV). https://clinicaltrials.gov/ct2/show/NCT01480479.

85. ClinicalTrials.gov. A study of Rindopepimut/GM-CSF in patients with relapsed EGFRvIII-positive glioblastoma (ReACT). https://clinicaltrials.gov/ct2/show/NCT01498328.

86. ClinicalTrials.gov. Study of a Drug [DCVax®-L] to treat newly diagnosed gbm brain cancer (ReACT). https://clinicaltrials.gov/ct2/show/NCT00045968.

87. Alizadeh D, Larmonier N. Chemotherapeutic targeting of cancer-induced immunosuppressive cells. Cancer Res. 2014;74(10):2663–8.

88. Gough MJ, Crittenden MR. Combination approaches to immunotherapy: the radiotherapy example. Immunotherapy. 2009;1:1025–37.

89. Formenti SC, Demaria S. Combining radiotherapy and cancer immunotherapy: a paradigm shift. J Natl Cancer Inst. 2013;105(4):256–65.

90. Garnett-Benson C, Hodge JW, Gameiro SR. Combination regimens of radiation therapy and therapeutic cancer vaccines: mechanisms and opportunities. Semin Radiat Oncol. 2015;25(1):46–53.

91. ClinicalTrials.gov. Phase 1b Study of AdV-tk + Valacyclovir combined with radiation therapy for malignant gliomas (BrTK01). https://clinicaltrials.gov/ct2/show/NCT00751270.

92. Zagzag D, Salnikow K, Chiriboga L, Yee H, Lan L, Ali MA, Garcia R, Demaria S, Newcomb EW. Downregulation of major histocompatibility complex antigens in invading glioma cells: stealth invasion of the brain. Lab Invest. 2005;85(3):328–41.

93. Newcomb EW, Demaria S, Lukyanov Y, Shao Y, Schnee T, Kawashima N, Lan L, Dewyngaert JK, Zagzag D, McBride WH, Formenti SC. The combination of ionizing radiation and peripheral vaccination produces long-term survival of mice bearing established invasive GL261 gliomas. Clin Cancer Res. 2006;12(15):4730–7.

94. Pellegatta S, Poliani PL, Stucchi E, et al. Intratumoral dendritic cells increase efficacy of peripheral vaccination by modulation of glioma microenvironment. Neuro Oncol. 2010;12(4):377–88.

95. Yamanaka R, Homma J, Yajima N, et al. Clinical evaluation of dendritic cell vaccination for patients with recurrent glioma: results of a clinical phase I/II trial. Clin Cancer Res. 2005;11(11):4160–7.

96. Sampson JH, Heimberger AB, Archer GE, et al. Immunologic escape after prolonged progression-free survival with epidermal growth factor receptor variant III peptide vaccination in patients with newly diagnosed glioblastoma. J Clin Oncol. 2010;28(31):4722–9.

97. Soukup K, Wang X. Radiation meets immunotherapy—a perfect match in the era of combination therapy? Int J Radiat Biol. 2015;91(4):299–305.

98. Debus J, Abdollahi A. For the next trick: new discoveries in radiobiology applied to glioblastoma. Am Soc Clin Oncol Educ Book. 2014:e95-9. doi:10.14694/EdBook_AM.2014.34.e95, Review.

99. Mizoe JE, Tsujii H, Hasegawa A, et al. Phase I/II clinical trial of carbon ion radiotherapy for malignant gliomas: combined X-ray radiotherapy, chemotherapy, and carbon ion radiotherapy. Int J Radiat Oncol Biol Phys. 2007;69(2):390–6.

100. Combs SE, Bruckner T, Mizoe JE, Kamada T, Tsujii H, Kieser M, Debus J. Comparison of carbon ion radiotherapy to photon radiation alone or in combination with temozolomide in patients with high-grade gliomas: explorative hypothesis-generating retrospective analysis. Radiother Oncol. 2013;108(1):132–5.

101. Combs SE, Kieser M, Rieken S, et al. Randomized phase II study evaluating a carbon ion boost applied after combined radiochemotherapy with temozolomide versus a proton boost after radiochemotherapy with temozolomide in patients with primary glioblastoma: the CLEOPATRA trial. BMC Cancer. 2010;10:478.

102. McLendon R, Friedman A, Bigner D, et al. Comprehensive genomic characterization defines human glioblastoma genes and core pathways. Nature. 2008;455(7216):1061–8.

103. Parsons DW, Jones S, Zhang X, et al. An integrated genomic analysis of human glioblastoma multiforme. Science. 2008;321(5897):1807–12.

104. Kalbasi A, June CH, Haas N, Vapiwala N. Radiation and immunotherapy: a synergistic combination. J Clin Invest. 2013;123:2756–63.

# Perspective of the Large Databases and Ontologic Models of Creation of Preclinical and Clinical Results

**18**

Elisa Meldolesi, Mario Balducci, Silvia Chiesa, Andrea Damiani, Nicola Dinapoli, Roberto Gatta, and Vincenzo Valentini

## General Introduction

Over the past decade, remarkable advances in the medical field, and in particular, in cancer care have occurred, leading to a tremendous transformation in the internal medical concept [1]. Starting from an inflexible "one size fits all similar groups" approach, where the same treatment is used for the same kind of tumor, clinical practice is moving towards a personalized medicine concept with an essential role of decision support systems (DSS).

Glioblastoma multiforme (GM) is the most common primary brain tumor with only few available therapies providing significant improvement in survival. Therefore, the development of new diagnostic and treatment technologies beside the concomitant research progress in pathology, biologic biomarkers (e.g., MGMT promoter, DNA metilation, IDH, EGFR, etc. [2]), genomics, and proteomics justifies the growing trend towards "individualized medicine".

The use and role of medical imaging technologies in clinical oncology has also greatly expanded during the last decade from a primarily diagnostic and qualitative tool to award a central role in the context of individualized medicine with a quantitative value. Several studies have been developed to analyze and quantify different imaging features (e.g., descriptors of intensity distribution, spatial relationships between the various intensity levels, texture heterogeneity patterns, descriptors of shape, etc.) and the relations of the tumor with the surrounding tissues to identify their possible relationship with treatment outcomes or gene expressions [3, 4].

Furthermore, multidisciplinary management of cancer patients has been proven essential to reach a highly individualized treatment. The integration between different specialists leads to a mortality reduction not only cancer-related, but also related to concomitant diseases [5, 6].

In this context of progressive technologies and treatment innovation, the development of predictive models can answer to the increasing necessity of individualized medicine. Based on individual patient features, in fact, predictive models, complementing existing consensus or guidelines, allow physicians deliver tailored treatment. Patient care is transforming from an evidence-based treatment into a personalized medicine concept (build on an evidence base) going from prescription by consensus to prescription by numbers.

E. Meldolesi (✉) • M. Balducci • S. Chiesa
• N. Dinapoli • R. Gatta • V. Valentini
Radiation Oncology Department, Gemelli-ART,
Università Cattolica S. Cuore, Largo A. Gemelli 8,
Rome 00168, Italy
e-mail: elimlds@gmail.com;
mario.balducci.1955@gmail.com;
silvia.chiesa.md@gmail.com;
nicola.dinapoli.74@gmail.com;
roberto.gatta.bs@alice.it; vvalentini@rm.unicatt.it

© Springer International Publishing Switzerland 2016
L. Pirtoli et al. (eds.), *Radiobiology of Glioblastoma*, Current Clinical Pathology,
DOI 10.1007/978-3-319-28305-0_18

## Personalized Medicine

Personalized medicine is defined by the National Cancer Institute as "a form of medicine that uses information about a person's genes, proteins, and environment to prevent, diagnose, and treat disease. In cancer, personalized medicine uses specific information about a person's tumor to help diagnose, plan treatment, find out how well treatment is working, or make a prognosis" [7].

To date, in the medical field and inherently also in oncology, clinical practice is based on evidence-based guidelines and protocols as results of the outcome of randomized clinical trials (RCTs). Although in the past decades they have had a key role in the definition of the treatment strategies in cancer care, RTCs's population is often constituted by a selective group of patients, very different from the population seen in routine clinical practice. Some patients groups are under-represented, including elderly, those with comorbidities [8, 9], and patients from under-represented ethnic and socioeconomic backgrounds [10–12]. Furthermore, the long time that it is usually requested to reach the pre-established outcome is an intrinsic limitation of this kind of research. As a result, the presented evidence is often valid for only a subgroup of patients and trial results are quickly outdated.

Beside RCTs, a complementary form of research is progressively emerging that has, in the population-based observational studies, its major expression. The role of this new research is mostly to ensure that the result of clinical trials translates into tangible benefits in the general population [13]. Given the differences between patients recruited to trials and those seen in routine practice, in fact, small benefit observed in highly selected trial patients is likely to disappear when the same treatments are applied in routine practice. Observational studies are essential to identify whether practice has changed appropriately, to document harms of therapy in a wider population, in patients of different age and with different comorbidities, and to determine whether patients in routine practice are reaching the expected outcomes with the expected toxicity [14, 15].

In this new era of individualized medicine, it is more and more important to develop supporting decision tool, based on models able to predict different outcomes starting from large heterogeneous datasets. Essential, for the development of this kind of DSS, is the creation of large databases, archives of heterogeneous data coming from multiple sources. Numerous information that are routinely collected in clinical practice as diagnostic and clinical imaging, laboratory data, treatment outcome data, biologic environment, genomics, and proteomics are included into large databases. Using innovative "rapid-learning" research techniques, these data are simultaneously analyzed in order to obtain, from the extraction of knowledge of the masses, a benefit of the individual [16]. From a technical point of view, this large amount of data required to create a predictive model is necessary not only to provide sufficient statistical power to act as an efficient and reliable predictive tool, but also to validate the obtained model. Therefore, a secondary dataset is needed for validation of the model, preferably by external (from a different institution) datasets [17]. Only after external validation, a prediction model can be implemented as an acceptable decision support tool.

In this context, the idea of research is totally changed. Heterogeneity of data is now assuming a key role against the ab initio definition of the collecting variables (as in the RCTs). Large databases approach requires gathering data without knowing beforehand what would be the outcomes of the research, which is quite different from the fixed design of a prospective randomized controlled trial. Therefore, a flexible strategy for data collection, data mining, and outcome reporting is needed with the possibility to add new variables to the large databases in an ad-hoc manner.

Considering that large database can be created combining data coming from various departments of a single hospital or from multiple institutes different on a regional, national, and international level, integration of information is a big challenge for data-sharing initiatives.

## Ontology and Data Standardization

The standardization process, essential to universally define data and procedures that will constitute a large database, is obtained through the creation of an ontology.

"Ontology" is a compound word, composed of onto-, from the Greek ὄντος (òntos) which is the present participle of the verb εἰμί (eimi), i.e., "to be, I am", and λόγία (lògia), i.e., "science, study, theory". Ontology formally represents knowledge as a set of concepts within a domain and the relationships between those concepts. In practice, an ontology is a terminological system where all the information, related in this case to medical disciplines and treatment, are specified and organized in a well-defined data collection model. An ontology collects uniform and unambiguous definition for each variable and the relationship between different variables into the space and the time concept. Eventually, better and unambiguous understanding leads to an approach where the research data could be made available without differences in interpretation; for now and the future. From the perspective of computer science, different kind of data can be represented in any ontology starting from a generic "registry" layer with purely epidemiologic information, to a "procedural" level, where treatment information and related toxicities are reported, up to a higher "research" level where dimensional data, such as images, genomics, proteomics, etc., are collected [18]. Therefore, in the development of an ontology, the information can grow both in terms of variety and granularity, until the idea of clinical large database [18].

Furthermore, the formalization of any ontology can grow from a simple dictionary, where the meaning of the terms is described in natural language, toward a more and more formal expression resulting also from the sharing of the definitions between different institutions on a local, national, or international level. At the cost of increasing complexity and formalism that enriches the language with more and more complex constructs representing relationships between variables, different techniques can be used for representing richer knowledge contents. In this context, the most frequently used model to represent data distribution is the Semantic Web, developed by Tim Berners-Lee [19]. For the Semantic Web technology, data is represented by triplets (subject, predicate, object) using the Resource Description Framework (RDF) language [20].

The interaction between elements of multiple triplets is defined inside an ontology through a different language (RDFS or OWL) allowing informatics system to automatically generate inference from any exploitable data source. Software agents can easily parse and make inference on big data repositories applying formal-ontologies on explicitly declared facts to infer the entire set of facts logically inferable.

The power of the semantic web is the extremely simple, however flexible RDF representation (one table with three columns) (Table 18.1), as well as the federated nature of the web where both data and knowledge can reside at multiple locations on the internet and can be queried using SPARQL, the query language of the Semantic Web [21].

Furthermore, a distributed learning approach is able to learn from the collected data creating a

**Table 18.1** Examples of "semantic" triple representation [18]

| Subject | Predicate | Object example (URL) | Reference |
|---|---|---|---|
| Patient | hasBeenDiagnosedWith | Malignant neoplasm of rectum, http://purl.bioontology.org/ontology/ICD10/C19 | ICD-10 |
| Patient | hasBiologicalSex | Male, http://ncicb.nci.nih.gov/xml/owl/EVS/Thesaurus.owl#C20197 | NCI Thesaurus |
| | | Female, http://ncicb.nci.nih.gov/xml/owl/EVS/Thesaurus.owl#C16576 | |
| Disease | hasStageFinding | T1 Stage finding, http://ncicb.nci.nih.gov/xml/owl/EVS/Thesaurus.owl#C48720 | NCI Thesaurus |

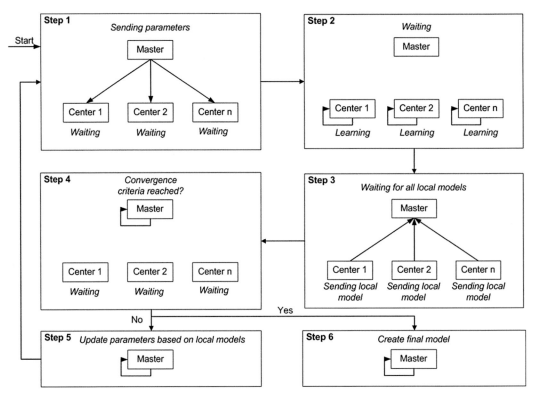

**Fig 18.1** Distributed machine learning flow [23]

model without the need for data to leave the individual hospital. A distributed machine learning algorithm is able, through a local learning application which is installed at each hospital, to create a local model that is sent to the central server. Starting from the integration of all the single models, a consensus model is generated and sent back to each hospital for refinement. After pre-established convergence criteria are met, it is possible to create a final consensus model (Fig. 18.1). This method works for a variety of models as described in literature [22].

## Radiomics and Imaging Analysis

In medical field and inherently also in oncology, the imaging technologies have always had a key role in the identification and staging of a cancer disease being fundamental for the definition of the treatment procedure. During the last decade, we have witnessed an important change of the medical imaging concept coming from a diagnostic, qualitative position to award a central role in the context of individualized medicine with the identification of numerous measurable features.

The term "Radiomics" is a relatively new term that was used in several studies to indicate the extraction of large amounts of features from radiographic images with the intent of creating mineable databases [3]. The goal of Radiomics is to convert images into mineable data, with high fidelity and high throughput [4].

Until last decade, texture heterogeneity, characteristics of shape, volume, and intensity distribution of the tumor, were only analyzable, on the acquired images, in a qualitative way. In this new Radiomics era, images are fractionated in order to identify specific patterns and/or descriptor that could be quantified and easily reproduced in a consistent manner in different institutions.

Considering the different gray scales inside the tumor image, it was possible to identify and quantify not only some descriptors (e.g., descriptors of shape, texture, and optical porosity), but also the relationship between the tumor and the surrounding tissues in a bidimensional and tridimensional way [3, 4].

Despite all this technological progress, it is still a long way to identify the numerous heterogeneity's patterns characteristics of different tumors. However, it is clear how these patterns could highly contribute to choose the better treatment strategy for each single patient.

## Prediction Models

Over the past decade, medical doctor had to face numerous and remarkable challenges in oncology that have progressively moved toward a personalization of the treatments. In this context of growing technologies and treatment's innovation, predictive models achieve a relevant role, beside the existing consensus and/or guidelines, in helping clinicians in daily clinical practice.

The methodological process to develop a DSS is depicted in Fig. 18.2 [1].

A large heterogeneous database is required to store all the information without knowing beforehand what would be the research's topic. From the hypothesis, it is determined which features should be included in the learning effort. Bayesian network is usually considered the best approach [24] to impute for the missing data and to detect and correct bias into the initial dataset, to improve data quality. After this pre-processing step, it is possible, through a machine learning procedure, to analyze the different features listed in the large database and obtain a model representing the distribution of the same features and their relationship inside the dataset.

Beside common medical statistics approaches (Cox proportional hazard model [25], logistic regression [26] etc), the usage of different machine learning algorithms (Bayesian network [27, 28], decision trees [29], support vector machines [30], neural networks [31], genetic algorithm [32], etc.) leads to the possibility of creating predictors characterized by different performance and usage related to the final outcome. To obtain a reliable and consistent DSS and able to work properly

also in a different environment from where it was created, it is necessary to validate the new model (training set) preferably by external dataset (validation set) [1, 17].

Considering the performance, the Receiving Operating Characteristic (ROC) and its equivalent Area Under the Curve (AUC) are the most used measurement units (Fig. 18.3). However, it is important to know that the ROC is not always applicable to all the predictor: in such cases different indicators could be used (accuracy, sensitivity, specificity, F-score, etc.).

To date, European Organization for Research and Treatment Cancer (EORTC) has developed several interactive DSS related to either primary or recurrent glioblastoma (Table 18.2). These survival's prediction models are currently used in clinical practice beside the existing consensus and/or guidelines, helping clinicians in choosing the better treatment strategy for each single patient.

Medical doctors and/or patients can use predictive models in a variety of ways. Graphical calculating devices as nomograms [25, 33] are one of the most common forms of predictive device, beside the even more appealing interactive website (Table 18.2). Furthermore, in this era of technological progress, the possibility to create specific applications for devices of new generation is also very interesting (e.g., cell-phones, tablet, etc.).

## Perspectives in Glioblastoma

GM is the most common primary brain tumor, but, even now, only few available therapies providing significant improvement in survival are known. In the past decade, the possibility to use more and more sophisticated technologies allowed to deal with numerous challenges obtaining a tremendous influx of data describing molecular and genomic alterations in the pathogenesis of GM [34]. Notwithstanding this explosion of knowledge, the early clinical data from the usage of selective therapies developed on these identified aberrations are largely disappointing. The wide heterogeneous nature of this disease and the possibility for the tumor to change mutations during its progression, beside the well-known difficulty of neuro-oncology

**Fig 18.2**

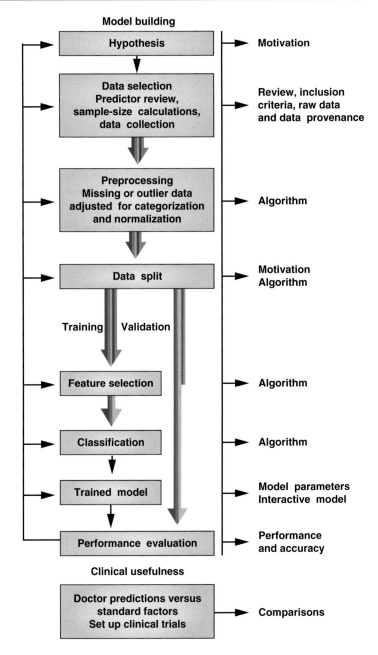

Figure 1| Schematic overview of methodological
processes in clinical decision-support system
devolopment, describing model development, assessment
of clinical usefulness and what ideally to publish. The
coloured, parallel lines represent heterogeneous. The
which have been split early for independent validation
(but without internal cross-validation).

**Table 18.2** Examples of interactive decisional support systems (DSS) related to glioblastoma, currently used in clinical practice

| Institution | Prediction model | Web link (URL) |
|---|---|---|
| European Organisation for Research and Treatment of Cancer (EORTC) | Prediction of survival in general GMB population | https://www.eortc.be/tools/gbmcalculator/model1.aspx |
| European Organisation for Research and Treatment of Cancer (EORTC) | Prediction of survival in patients treated by RT/TMZ (MGMT methylation status unavailable) | https://www.eortc.be/tools/gbmcalculator/model2.aspx |
| European Organisation for Research and Treatment of Cancer (EORTC) | Prediction of survival in patients treated by RT/TMZ (MGMT methylation status available) | https://www.eortc.be/tools/gbmcalculator/model3.aspx |
| European Organisation for Research and Treatment of Cancer (EORTC) | Prediction of survival in patients with recurrent glioblastoma | http://www.eortc.be/tools/recgbmcalculator/calculator.aspx |

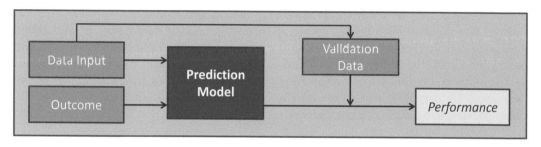

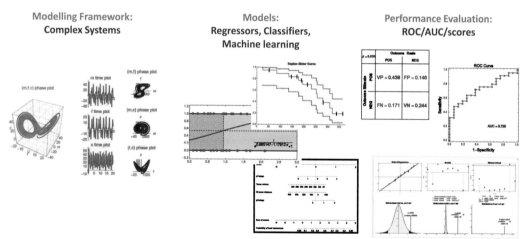

**Fig 18.3** Predictive models

drugs to penetrate the blood–brain barrier, can partially justify the large ineffectiveness of the most current molecular-targeted therapies. Despite these discouraging initial results, it is still very reasonable to believe that in the era of "individualized medicine" genomically and molecularly driven research in combination with multiple patients-specific data (clinical, pathological, biological, proteomics, imaging, etc.) will ultimately be successful.

Recent studies have demonstrated how the interaction between an imaging's quantitative analysis and specific gene and microRNA tumor expression can be useful as a robust initial prognostic tool in order to personalize therapy for GBM patients [35, 36]. Therefore, only through the understanding of the gene regulatory network and the study of the interaction between molecular alteration and different GM's characteristic features, it will be possible to develop better preclinical models that will help physicians to choose the best drug or the best combination of drugs for each patient in the most efficient possible way.

## Conclusions

The interaction between the implementation of new technologies and the usage of automated computer bots has allowed, in the last decade, a broad range of researches to be expanded, due to the very generalizable and flexible technology utilized. In oncology, the availability of reliable and consistent prediction tools makes possible to stratify population in specific risk groups for different selected outcomes, identifying patients who better than other can benefit from a specific treatment procedure. Furthermore, it will also stimulate research focused on specific risk groups, trying to find new treatment options or other combinations of treatment options for these subgroups. Therefore, personalized medicine can be expected not only to save patients from unnecessary toxicity and inconvenience, but also to facilitate the choice of the most appropriate treatment.

Clinicians are now facing two new challenges. The first one is represented by the trend towards "individualized medicine" trying to consider several potential options for each patient in place of inflexible "one size fits all similar groups" approach. Secondly, the new concept of "prescription by numbers" support the moving towards a "shared decision making" approach, where doctors and patients, evaluating pros and cons of different treatment strategy, can actively discuss and decide on therapeutic interventions.

The development and validation of predictive models is a fundamental step to create new software able to give the knowledge a different dimension. Guidelines and protocols currently used in a daily clinical practice will be optimized by the usage of predictive models, considering that medical doctor will have a more accurate idea of the treatment's possibilities for each patient in terms of both survival and side effects.

The behavior of specific tumor is very difficult to predict due to their huge intrinsic heterogeneity. However, treatment can only become more personalized if accurate, science-based decision aids are developed, which can offer assistance in clinical decision-making in daily practice.

Therefore, the poor human cognitive capacity, able to discriminate and use not more than 5 features in a daily clinical practice [37], can find in DSS a valuable help able to compensate for this human intrinsic limitation.

Finally, considering the important role that predictive models could play in the clinical practice, clinicians must be aware that although they can be very useful with great performances and sometimes with a great $p$-value, they remain only DSS, not decision-makers.

## References

1. Lambin P, van Stiphout RGPM, Starmans MHW, Rios-Velazquez E, Nalbantov G, Aerts HJWL, et al. Predicting outcomes in radiation oncology—multifactorial decision support systems. Nat Rev Clin Oncol. 2013;10(1):27–40. http://www.ncbi.nlm.nih.gov/pubmed/23165123.
2. McNamara MG, Sahebjam S, Mason WP. Emerging biomarkers in glioblastoma. Cancers (Basel). 2013;5(3):1103–19. http://www.pubmedcentral.nih.gov/articlerender.fcgi?artid=3795381&tool=pmcentrez&rendertype=abstract.
3. Lambin P, Rios-Velazquez E, Leijenaar R, Carvalho S, van Stiphout RGPM, Granton P, et al. Radiomics: extracting more information from medical images using advanced feature analysis. Eur J Cancer. 2012;48(4):441–6. http://www.ncbi.nlm.nih.gov/pubmed/22257792.
4. Kumar V, Gu Y, Basu S, Berglund A, Eschrich SA, Schabath MB, et al. Radiomics: the process and the challenges. Magn Reson Imaging. 2012;30(9):1234–48.
5. Mason WP, Del Maestro R, Eisenstat D, Forsyth P, Fulton D, Laperrière N, et al. Canadian recommendations for the treatment of glioblastoma multiforme. Curr Oncol. 2007;14(3):110–7. http://www.ncbi.nlm.nih.gov/pubmed/17593983.
6. Friedland PL, Bozic B, Dewar J, Kuan R, Meyer C, Phillips M. Impact of multidisciplinary team management in head and neck cancer patients. Br J Cancer.

2011;104(8):1246–8. http://www.pubmedcentral.nih.gov/articlerender.fcgi?artid=3078600&tool=pmcentrez&rendertype=abstract.

7. NCI. NCI Dictionary of terms: personalized medicine. http://www.cancer.gov/dictionary?cdrid=561717. http://www.cancer.gov/dictionary?cdrid=561717

8. Tyldesley S, Zhang-Salomons J, Groome PA, Zhou S, Schulze K, Paszat LF, et al. Association between age and the utilization of radiotherapy in Ontario. Int J Radiat Oncol Biol Phys. 2000;47(2):469–80. http://www.ncbi.nlm.nih.gov/pubmed/10802375.

9. Faivre J, Lemmens VEPP, Quipourt V. Bouvier a M. Management and survival of colorectal cancer in the elderly in population-based studies. Eur J Cancer. 2007;43(15):2279–84. http://www.ncbi.nlm.nih.gov/pubmed/17904353.

10. Bach PB, Cramer LD, Warren JLBC. Racial differences in the treatment of early-stage lung cancer. N Engl J Med. 1999;341(16):1198. http://www.nejm.org/doi/full/10.1056/NEJM199910143411606.

11. Boyd C, Zhang-Salomons JY, Groome PA, Mackillop WJ. Associations between community income and cancer survival in Ontario, Canada, and the United States. J Clin Oncol. 1999;17(7):2244–55. http://www.ncbi.nlm.nih.gov/pubmed/10561282.

12. Hershman D, McBride R, Jacobson JS, Lamerato L, Roberts K, Grann VR, et al. Racial disparities in treatment and survival among women with early-stage breast cancer. J Clin Oncol. 2005;23(27):6639–46. http://www.ncbi.nlm.nih.gov/pubmed/16170171.

13. Booth CM, Tannock IF. Randomised controlled trials and population-based observational research: partners in the evolution of medical evidence. Br J Cancer Nature Publishing Group. 2014;110(3):551–5. http://www.pubmedcentral.nih.gov/articlerender.fcgi?artid=3915111&tool=pmcentrez&rendertype=abstract.

14. Booth CM. Evaluating patient-centered outcomes in the randomized controlled trial and beyond: informing the future with lessons from the past. Clin Cancer Res. 2010;16(24):5963–71. http://www.ncbi.nlm.nih.gov/pubmed/21169249.

15. Fuentes-Raspall R, Puig-Vives M, Guerra-Prio S, Perez-Bueno F, Marcos-Gragera R. Population-based survival analyses of central nervous system tumors from 1994 to 2008. An up-dated study in the temozolomide-era. Cancer Epidemiol. 2014;38(3):244–7. http://www.ncbi.nlm.nih.gov/pubmed/24794586.

16. Lambin P, Roelofs E, Reymen B, Velazquez ER, Buijsen J, Zegers CML, et al. 'Rapid Learning health care in oncology'—an approach towards decision support systems enabling customised radiotherapy. Radiother Oncol. 2013;109(1):159–64. http://www.ncbi.nlm.nih.gov/pubmed/23993399.

17. Vickers AJ. Prediction models: revolutionary in principle, but do they do more good than harm? J Clin Oncol. 2011;29(22):2951–2. from: http://www.ncbi.nlm.nih.gov/pubmed/21690474.

18. Meldolesi E, van Soest J, Dinapoli N, Dekker A, Damiani A, Gambacorta MA, et al. An umbrella protocol for standardized data collection (SDC) in rectal cancer: a prospective uniform naming and procedure convention to support personalized medicine. Radiother Oncol. 2014;112(1):59–62. http://www.ncbi.nlm.nih.gov/pubmed/24853366.

19. Tim B-L, Hendler James LO. "The Semantic Web" A new form of Web content that is meaningful to computers will unleash a revolution of new possibilities. Sci Am Mag. 2001;284:35–43. http://www.cs.umd.edu/~golbeck/LBSC690/SemanticWeb.html.

20. Graham Klyne JJC. Resource Description Framework (RDF): concepts and abstract syntax. 2004. http://www.w3.org/TR/2004/REC-rdf-concepts-20040210/.

21. Assélé Kama A, Choquet R, Mels G, Daniel C, Charlet J, Jaulent M-C. An ontological approach for the exploitation of clinical data. Stud Health Technol Inform. 2013;192:142–6. http://www.ncbi.nlm.nih.gov/pubmed/23920532.

22. Boyd S. Distributed Optimization and Statistical Learning via the alternating direction method of multipliers. Found Trends® Mach Learn. 2010;3(1):1–122. http://www.nowpublishers.com/product.aspx?product=MAL&doi=2200000016

23. Meldolesi E, van Soest J, Alitto AR, Autorino R, Dinapoli N, Dekker A, et al. VATE: VAlidation of high TEchnology based on large database analysis by learning machine. Color Cancer. 2014;3(5):435–50. http://www.futuremedicine.com/doi/abs/10.2217/crc.14.34.

24. Luta G, Ford MB, Bondy M, Shields PG, Stamey JD. Bayesian sensitivity analysis methods to evaluate bias due to misclassification and missing data using informative priors and external validation data. Cancer Epidemiol. 2013;37(2):121–6. http://www.pubmedcentral.nih.gov/articlerender.fcgi?artid=3834354&tool=pmcentrez&rendertype=abstract.

25. Valentini V, van Stiphout RGPM, Lammering G, Gambacorta MA, Barba MC, Bebenek M, et al. Nomograms for predicting local recurrence, distant metastases, and overall survival for patients with locally advanced rectal cancer on the basis of European randomized clinical trials. J Clin Oncol. 2011;29(23):3163–72. http://www.ncbi.nlm.nih.gov/pubmed/21747092.

26. Bagley SC, White H, Golomb BA. Logistic regression in the medical literature. J Clin Epidemiol. 2001;54(10):979–85. http://linkinghub.elsevier.com/retrieve/pii/S0895435601003729.

27. Jayasurya K, Fung G, Yu S, Dehing-Oberije C, De Ruysscher D, Hope A, et al. Comparison of Bayesian network and support vector machine models for two-year survival prediction in lung cancer patients treated with radiotherapy. Med Phys. 2010;37(4):1401–7. http://www.ncbi.nlm.nih.gov/pubmed/20443461.

28. Oh JH, Craft J, Al Lozi R, Vaidya M, Meng Y, Deasy JO, et al. A Bayesian network approach for modeling local failure in lung cancer. Phys Med Biol. 2011;56(6):1635–51. http://www.ncbi.nlm.nih.gov/pubmed/21335651.

29. Hu R. Medical Data Mining Based on Decision Tree Algorithm. Comput Inf Sci. 2011;4(5):14–9. http://www.ccsenet.org/journal/index.php/cis/article/view/11950.

30. Van Stiphout RGPM, Lammering G, Buijsen J, Janssen MHM, Gambacorta MA, Slagmolen P, et al. Development and external validation of a predictive model for pathological complete response of rectal cancer patients including sequential PET-CT imaging. Radiother Oncol. 2011;98(1):126–33. http://www.ncbi.nlm.nih.gov/pubmed/21176986.

31. Patel JL, Goyal RK. Applications of artificial neural networks in medical science. Curr Clin Pharmacol. 2007;2(3):217–26. http://www.eurekaselect.com/openurl/content.php?genre=article&issn=1574-8847&volume=2&issue=3&spage=217.

32. Wiggins M, Saad A, Litt B, Vachtsevanos G. Genetic Algorithm-Evolved Bayesian Network Classifier for Medical Applications.

33. Gorlia T, van den Bent MJ, Hegi ME, Mirimanoff RO, Weller M, Cairncross JG, et al. Nomograms for predicting survival of patients with newly diagnosed glioblastoma: prognostic factor analysis of EORTC and NCIC trial 26981-22981/CE.3. Lancet Oncol. 2008;9(1):29–38. http://www.ncbi.nlm.nih.gov/pubmed/18082451.

34. Bastien JIL, McNeill KA, Fine HA. Molecular characterizations of glioblastoma, targeted therapy, and clinical results to date. Cancer. 2015;121(4):502–16.

35. Zinn PO, Mahajan B, Majadan B, Sathyan P, Singh SK, Majumder S, et al. Radiogenomic mapping of edema/cellular invasion MRI-phenotypes in glioblastoma multiforme. PLoS One. 2011;6(10), e25451. http://www.pubmedcentral.nih.gov/articlerender.fcgi?artid=3187774&tool=pmcentrez&rendertype=abstract.

36. Zinn PO, Sathyan P, Mahajan B, Bruyere J, Hegi M, Majumder S, et al. A novel volume-age-KPS (VAK) glioblastoma classification identifies a prognostic cognate microRNA-gene signature. PLoS One. 2012;7(8), e41522. http://www.pubmedcentral.nih.gov/articlerender.fcgi?artid=3411674&tool=pmcentrez&rendertype=abstract.

37. Abernethy AP, Etheredge LM, Ganz PA, Wallace P, German RR, Neti C, et al. Rapid-learning system for cancer care. J Clin Oncol. 2010;28(27):4268–74. http://www.pubmedcentral.nih.gov/articlerender.fcgi?artid=2953977&tool=pmcentrez&rendertype=abstract.

# Concluding Remarks and Perspectives for Future Research

## 19

Antonio Giordano, Giovanni Luca Gravina, and Luigi Pirtoli

After early reports of the usefulness of postoperative radiotherapy (RT) in improving survival outcomes of Glioblastoma (GB) after surgery [1, 2], the almost unanimous opinion in the oncology community at present is that the most significant, recent improvement in the prognosis of GB patients is due to Temozolomide (TMZ) chemotherapy (CHT). The results of the well-known EORTC/NCIC phase III trial have shown, in fact, better outcomes with TMZ CHT concurrently and sequentially delivered, as compared to postoperative RT only; that is, there is a higher median (14.6 vs. 12.1 months) and 2-year survival (26.5 % vs. 10.4 %), with a 37 % decrease of risk-of-death [3]. However, the above results should be critically considered, in light of the subsequent reports of large database collections (Patterns-of-Care Studies) also showing a highly significant role and deep impact of modern conformal radiation therapy (3D-CRT) on prognosis, a result that cannot be demonstrated as the yield of random studies, for obvious ethical reasons. In a comparison between two large series of GB patients collected over subsequent periods (633 cases, 1997–2001; 1059 cases, 2002–2007) by the Italian Patterns of Care Study Group on Gliomas, improved survival results were significantly related to the adoption of 3D-CRT vs. outdated techniques ($p < .001$). This corresponds to the same significance level of the introduction of TMZ chemotherapy [4]. However, the overall survival results remained poor (median survival: 9.5 months; 1-, 2-, and 5-year survival, respectively: 62.3, 24.8, and 3.9 %) in this report as well as in previous and subsequent similar studies [5, 6]. In the context of considering that the present state-of-the-art treatments affect GB patients' prognosis only to a limited extent, in fact, the possibility of further improving the efficiency of RT in disease control by safely increasing radiation effectiveness is relevant.

From a radiobiological point of view, radiation dose escalation has not achieved valuable results, due both to the radiation vulnerability of the brain and to the well-known resistance of GB to radiation. These observations emerge from the clinical setting, as widely reported in several contributions in the first section of this book, to

A. Giordano
Sbarro Institute for Cancer Research and Molecular Medicine and Center for Biotechnology, Temple University, Philadelphia, PA, USA

Department of Medicine, Surgery & Neurosciences, University of Siena, Siena, Italy

G.L. Gravina
Department of Radiological, Oncological, and Anatomo-Pathological Sciences, University of Rome "La Sapienza", Rome, Italy

L. Pirtoli (✉)
Tuscany Tumor Institute, Florence, Italy

Unit of Radiation Oncology, Department of Medicine, Surgery and Neurosciences, University of Siena, Siena, Italy
e-mail: luigipirtoli@gmail.com

© Springer International Publishing Switzerland 2016
L. Pirtoli et al. (eds.), *Radiobiology of Glioblastoma*, Current Clinical Pathology,
DOI 10.1007/978-3-319-28305-0_19

be major limitations of the therapeutic outcomes. So far, in clinical series, a radiation dose-response curve is not demonstrated beyond the dose of 60 Gy, even if it may be hypothesized on theoretical grounds [7]. The difficulty of increasing tumor doses without severe healthy brain damage, even with the most advanced RT techniques (with the possible exception of particle radiation), may partly account for this observation, but the GB's radio-resistance is likely an inherent feature of the tumor, linked to an "active" adaptation to the radiation threat, probably more efficient than in other neoplasms.

This intriguing aspect is presently the subject of intensive radiobiology (RB) preclinical research, aimed at circumventing the obstacle instead of, or besides, escalating radiation dose. We dedicated the second part of the book to this subject, and the collected papers exhaustively address possible radiation enhancement strategies by manipulations active on genetic and epigenetic determinants, cell-death pathways, microenvironment and hypoxia, glioma stem cells, immune system, nanoparticle technology, etc., showing many promising results in this regard. Nevertheless, revolutionary disclosures do not seem to be around the corner and much more research is needed. It is our opinion that RB research should be aimed at taking into account primarily those cues stemming from clinical studies, in a closer cooperation between basic and clinical investigators than in the past, in order to achieve optimal results. Ultimately, clinical and preclinical RB of GB cannot satisfactorily progress without researchers taking into account the continuously evolving, related pathobiology, as indicated in the title of this book.

Translational aspects are, in fact, the subject of the third, and last, section of this book. An impressive number of rationales for multimodal therapies combining RT with agents hypothetically effective in modifying radiation sensitivity in the above-indicated domains have been the subject of recent clinical phase I to III trials and continue to emerge as plausible working hypotheses. The general lack of significantly improved results by these studies over those achieved by the present standard-of-care demands a reflection

on translational issues. Targeting putative key factors of radiation resistance in clinical trials requires previous proofs-of-principle, soundly grounded by preclinical in vitro and in vivo experiments. This accomplishment is difficult to achieve in an extremely complex disease, such as GB is, due to a limited knowledge of the biological–clinical correlations [8] and the unfulfilling reliability of many markers. These subjects should be addressed by further research, even if important goals have already been reached through the analysis of large datasets, e.g.: those regarding the "somatic genomic landscape" of GB [9]. Another limitation for the successful translation of preclinical into clinical research concerns the usefulness of the yield of clinical prospective trials. Some limitations are, in fact, relatively small series, selective patients, long time periods, and reliability of results only within a restricted domain, which make it difficult to translate the results into generally improved clinical outcomes.

In conclusion, both evolved preclinical protocols and research methods are warranted, as well as data mining techniques and ontology platforms, based on suitably constructed large databases including both pathobiology and clinical parameters. This process may produce very reliable working hypotheses for random comparisons of radiation-based competitive treatment schedules for GB.

A final remark might be that the field of radiation sciences, including RB, is different, as compared to pharmacological research, in that in the former there usually is not any pressure from the industry to obtain a commercial product as soon as possible. This is an advantage and a disadvantage at the same time. The advantage is represented by an independent and not cursory preclinical phase, which could be carried out as a rule over a suitable time and thoroughly in academic institutions; the disadvantage by severe funding limitations. Funding constraints might have contributed to the limited number of significant disclosures on radio-sensitizing agents against tumors, in particular GB, of relevant clinical value after reliable trials. Public funding and the interest of health authorities in encouraging cooperation between independent researchers and industry are of the utmost importance and should by all means be solicited by the investigators involved in RB research.

## References

1. Salazar OM, Rubin P, Donald JF, Feldstein ML. High-dose radiation therapy in the treatment of glioblastoma multiforme. Int J Radiat Oncol Biol Phys. 1976;1:717–27.
2. Walker MD, Strike TA, Sheline GE. Analysis of dose-effect relationship in the radiotherapy of malignant gliomas. Int J Radiat Oncol Biol Phys. 1979;5:1715–31.
3. Stupp R, Mason WP, van den Bent MJ, et al. Radiotherapy plus concomitant and adjuvant temozolomide for glioblastoma. N Engl J Med. 2005;352:987–96.
4. Scoccianti S, Magrini SM, Ricardi U, et al. Patterns of care and survival in a retrospective analysis of 1059 patients with glioblastoma multiforme treated between 2002 and 2007: a multicenter study by the Central Nervous System Study Group of Airo (Italian Association of Radiation Oncology). Neurosurgery. 2010;67:446–58.
5. Chang SM, Parney IF, Huang W, et al. Patterns of care for adults with newly diagnosed malignant glioma. JAMA. 2005;293:557–64.
6. Brandes AA, Franceschi E, Ermani M, et al. Pattern of care and effectiveness of treatment for glioblastoma patients in the real world: Results from a prospective population-based registry. Could survival differ in a high-volume center? Neurooncol Pract. 2014;1:166–71.
7. Pedicini P, Fiorentino A, Simeon V, et al. Clinical radiobiology of glioblastoma multiforme: estimation of tumor control probability from various radiotherapy fractionation schemes. Strahlenther Onkol. 2014;190:925–32.
8. Cohen-Jonathan Moyal E. Du laboratoire vers la clinique: expérience du glioblastoma pur moduler la radiosensibilité tumorale. Cancer/Radiothérapie. 2012;16:25–8.
9. Brennan C, Verhaak RGW, McKenna A, et al. The somatic genomic landscape of glioblastoma. Cell. 2013;155:462–77.

Printed in the United States
By Bookmasters

cytoprotective, whereas autophagy inhibition at a late stage through bafilomycin induced apoptosis. Furthermore, the GB cell type and the therapeutic dose are also determinants for the pro-survival or pro-death role of autophagy.

All these data further support the hypothesis that autophagy modulation could increase the sensitivity of GB cells to therapy, and that caution is required on the desired effect based on tumor context.

## Glioblastoma Therapy: Status-of-the-Art and New Perspectives

Gliobastoma (GB) is the most common and aggressive primary brain tumor, with a median survival of only about 4 months in patients without therapy. A significant, although limited (16–19 months), improvement of the median survival is obtained with current multimodal approach, which includes maximal surgical resection, with adjuvant radiotherapy and TMZ, with approximately 25–30 % of the patients alive at 2 years after diagnosis, and a <10 % 5-year survival rate [10, 93, 94].

Recurrences are, in fact, the rule, given the high invasiveness of GB cells between normal brain cells, which makes them elusive targets for effective surgical management, and GB cell resistant to both IR and TMZ [11, 90].

The high proliferative capability of GB and massive angiogenesis also contribute to GB's poor prognosis. Moreover, GB is highly heterogenous, which impairs treatment effects, and thus requires novel therapeutic approaches and/or novel agents to be combined with the current standard of care. Therapeutic strategies are based on cellular and molecular mechanisms leading to: activation of apoptosis and/or other types of PCD, inhibition of growth factors and receptors, and blocking of angiogenesis. In the last decade, intensified research efforts have been invested into studying the molecular pathways altered in GB, in order to identify novel therapy targets. Recently, the GB project Study Group of The Genome Cancer Atlas (TGCA) [13] identified several molecular subtypes of GB, which could

differently affect current therapy efficacy, shedding light on novel potential molecular drug targets. However, several genetic and epigenetic alterations are common to most GBs. Clinical and experimental data have demonstrated that the natural resistance of GB to apoptosis, and thus to IR and conventional chemotherapy, is largely based on the constitutive activation of several intracellular signaling pathways, of which the most relevant identified to date is the PTEN/PI3K/Akt/mTOR/NFκB pathway and its regulators. The PI3K/Akt/mTOR signaling pathway is a main determinant of several processes related to cancer growth, invasiveness, and radioresistance [95]. In GB, it is often over-activated through a loss-of-function of the phosphatase and tensin homolog (PTEN) tumor suppressor gene, and/or a hyper-activation of EGFR. The EGFRvIII variant activates persistent downstream PI3K/Akt/mTOR and RAS/RAF/MAPK signaling, inducing GB cell proliferation and survival [96]. Loss of PTEN tumor suppressor gene function, as well as overexpression of EGFR, occurring in 30–40 % and 57.4 % of GB, respectively, are the most common alterations that promote GB growth and therapy resistance [13]. Alterations of the platelet-derived growth factor receptor (PDGFR), found in about 13.1 % of GB [13], may also induce PI3K/Akt/mTOR pathway over-activation [97].

Besides targeting growth factors and angiogenesis, combining IR/TMZ with the modulation of key determinants of GB metabolism may be a more effective treatment option. Autophagy sustains metabolic pathways required for tumor growth and is altered in GB, therefore its modulation could be envisaged as a possible support tool to IR and TMZ treatment. Furthermore, autophagy is the main pathway activated by both IR and TMZ.

In GB, it has been ascertained that radio- and chemoresistance largely depend on cancer stem cells, which have been found to express higher basal levels of Atg5, Atg12, and LC3 autophagic proteins than any other cancer cells [71], and which are more capable of repairing damaged DNA. Targeting stem cells by IR and combined therapy is a novel treatment paradigm for GB patients.